ABC of
Pleural Diseases

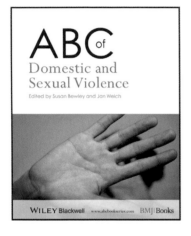
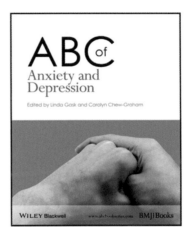
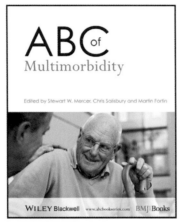
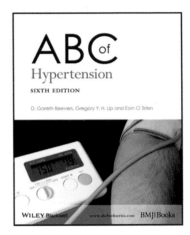
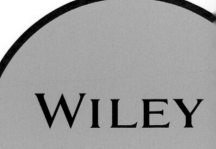

ABC of

Pleural Diseases

EDITED BY

Najib M. Rahman
University of Oxford, Oxford, UK

Ian Hunt
St. George's Hospital, London, UK

Fergus V. Gleeson
Churchill Hospital, Oxford, UK

Nick A. Maskell
Academic Respiratory Unit, University of Bristol, UK

WILEY Blackwell   **BMJ** | Books

Registered Office(s)
John Wiley & Sons, Inc., 111 River Street, Hoboken, NJ 07030, USA
John Wiley & Sons Ltd, The Atrium, Southern Gate, Chichester, West Sussex, PO19 8SQ, UK

Editorial Office
9600 Garsington Road, Oxford, OX4 2DQ, UK

For details of our global editorial offices, customer services, and more information about Wiley products visit us at www.wiley.com.

Wiley also publishes its books in a variety of electronic formats and by print-on-demand. Some content that appears in standard print versions of this book may not be available in other formats.

Library of Congress Cataloging-in-Publication Data
Names: Rahman, Najib M., editor. | Hunt, Ian, M.D., editor. | Gleeson,
    Fergus V., editor. | Maskell, Nick A., editor.
Title: ABC of pleural diseases / edited By Najib M. Rahman, Ian Hunt,
    Fergus V. Gleeson and Nick A. Maskell.
Description: Hoboken, NJ : Wiley, 2017. | Series: ABC series | Includes
    bibliographical references and index. |
Identifiers: LCCN 2017043481 (print) | LCCN 2017045215 (ebook) | ISBN
    9781118527115 (pdf) | ISBN 9781118527108 (epub) | ISBN 9780470654743 (pbk.)
Subjects: | MESH: Pleural Diseases
Classification: LCC RC751 (ebook) | LCC RC751 (print) | NLM WF 140 | DDC
    616.2/5–dc23
LC record available at https://lccn.loc.gov/2017043481

Cover Design: Wiley
Cover Image: © stockdevil/Gettyimages

Set in 9.25/12pt Minion by SPi Global, Pondicherry, India
Printed and bound in Singapore by Markono Print Media Pte Ltd

10   9   8   7   6   5   4   3   2   1

Contents

Contributors

Rahul Bhatnagar
Academic Respiratory Unit, University of Bristol, UK

Anna C. Bibby
Academic Respiratory Unit, University of Bristol, UK

John P. Corcoran
Oxford Centre for Respiratory Medicine, Churchill Hospital, Oxford, UK

Matthew Evison
Wythenshaw Hospital, Manchester, UK

Stephanie Fraser
Thoracic Surgery, Guy's Hospital, London, UK

David Feller-Kopman
Johns Hopkins Medical School, Baltimore, MD, USA

Fergus V. Gleeson
Churchill Hospital, Oxford, UK

Rob J. Hallifax
Oxford Centre for Respiratory Medicine, Churchill Hospital, Oxford, UK

John Harvey
North Bristol NHS Trust, Bristol, UK

Clare E. Hooper
Worcestershire NHS Trust, UK

Ian Hunt
St. George's Hospital, London, UK

Y.C. Gary Lee
University of Western Australia, Perth, Australia

Nick A. Maskell
Academic Respiratory Unit, University of Bristol, UK

Andrew McDuff
New Cross Hospital, Wolverhampton, UK

Mohammed Munavvar
Royal Preston Hospital, Preston, UK

Najib M. Rahman
Oxford Centre for Respiratory Medicine, Churchill Hospital, Oxford, UK

Carol Tan
St George's Hospital, London, UK

Ambika Talwar
Churchill Hospital, Oxford, UK

Brendan Tinwell
St George's Hospital, London, UK

Ahmed Yousuf
Glenfield Hospital, Leicester, UK

CHAPTER 1

Anatomy and Physiology of the Pleura

John P. Corcoran and Najib M. Rahman

Oxford Centre for Respiratory Medicine, Churchill Hospital, Oxford, UK

OVERVIEW

- The pleural space is a real rather than potential space, containing a small amount (<20 mL) of pleural fluid.
- Mesothelial cells line the visceral and parietal pleura, with size and shape varying according to position. They are metabolically active and can perform a variety of functions.
- The parietal pleura is innervated whereas the visceral pleura has no nerve supply (and hence does not produce pain in pathological conditions).
- The pleural space is normally under negative pressure.
- Pleural fluid is secreted from the systemic vessels of the parietal pleura, and is drained through lymphatic channels in the parietal pleura. The normal drainage capacity is very large compared to the secretion capacity.

The pleural cavity is a real rather than potential space, containing a thin layer of fluid and lined with a double-layered membrane covering the thoracic cavity (*parietal* pleura) and outer lung surface (*visceral* pleura) whose precise purpose and structure are incompletely understood. The gaps in our knowledge are best illustrated by the unexplained anatomical variations among different mammals. In humans, the left and right pleural cavities are separated by the mediastinum, but in species as diverse as the mouse and bison there is a single pleural cavity, allowing free communication of fluid and air between right and left. The elephant has evolved to have no cavity at all – instead having loose connective tissue between the two pleural membranes. In time, it may be that describing how and why these differences have evolved will help us to understand the role the pleural cavity has in humans. This chapter focuses on the key features of human pleural anatomy and physiology.

Embryology

The human body contains three mesothelium-lined cavities – two large (pleural, peritoneal) and one small (pericardial) – derived from a continuous mesodermal structure called the intra-embryonic coelom as it is partitioned at 4–7 weeks' gestation. Arising from a medially placed foregut structure that will ultimately form

the mediastinum, primordial lung buds grow out into the laterally placed pericardio-peritoneal canals, taking a layer of lining mesothelium that will become the visceral pleura in the process. As the lungs rapidly enlarge, they enclose the heart and widen the pericardio-peritoneal canals to form the pleural cavities. These are separated from the pericardial space by the pleuro-pericardial membranes, whilst the septum transversum (an early partial diaphragm) joins the pleuro-peritoneal membranes to partition each pleural cavity from the peritoneal space. The mesothelium lining the pericardio-peritoneal canals as they become the pleural cavities goes on to form the parietal pleura.

Macroscopic anatomy

The pleura is a double-layered serous membrane overlying the inner surface of the thoracic cage (diaphragm, mediastinum and rib cage) and outer surface of the lung, with an estimated total area of 2000 cm^2 in the average adult male. Between lies the pleural cavity, a sealed space maintained 10–20 micrometres across and filled with a thin layer of fluid to maintain apposition and provide lubrication during respiratory movement. The left and right pleural cavities are completely separated by the mediastinum.

The visceral pleura is tightly adherent to the entire lung surface, not only where it is in contact with chest wall, mediastinum and diaphragm, but also into the interlobar fissures. The parietal pleura is subdivided into four sections according to the associated intrathoracic structures: costal (overlying ribs, intercostal muscles, costal cartilage and sternum); cervical (extending above the first rib over the medial end of the clavicle); mediastinal; and diaphragmatic. Inferiorly, the parietal pleura mirrors the lower border of the thoracic cage but may extend beyond the costal margin, notably at the right lower sternal edge and posterior costovertebral junctions.

The visceral and parietal pleura meet at the lung hilae, through which the major airways and pulmonary vessels pass. Posteriorly, where a double layer of parietal pleura has been pulled into the thoracic cavity during lung development, lie the pulmonary ligaments extending from hilum to diaphragm bilaterally. These are thought to prevent torsion of the lower lobes, and are important intra-operatively as they may contain vessels, lymphatics or tumour.

ABC of Pleural Diseases, First Edition. Edited by Najib M. Rahman, Ian Hunt, Fergus V. Gleeson and Nick A. Maskell.
© 2018 John Wiley & Sons Ltd. Published 2018 by John Wiley & Sons Ltd.

Microscopic anatomy

The pleura is composed of a monolayer of mesothelial cells overlying layers of connective tissue; its precise structure varies between visceral and parietal pleura and according to anatomical position. Up to five layers can be identified histologically, consisting of the mesothelial cellular surface and four subcellular layers (basal lamina and thin connective tissue; thin superficial elastic tissue; loose connective tissue containing nerves, vessels and lymphatics; and a deep fibroelastic layer, often fused to the underlying tissue). These subcellular layers tend to be better defined when overlying looser substructures such as the mediastinum, than rigid tissue such as ribs or intercostal muscle. The parietal pleura is approximately 30 micrometres thick and overlies the deeper endothoracic fascia. The visceral pleura is between 30 and 80 micrometres thick with denser connective tissue layers that both contribute to elastic recoil of the lungs during expiration, and protect the lungs during inspiration by limiting their volume and expansion.

Mesothelial cells

The mesothelial cells lining the visceral and parietal pleura are the predominant cell type within the pleural cavity, forming an active multipotent layer capable of sensing and responding to external stimuli. Mesothelial cells dislodged from the pleural surface to float freely within the fluid-filled space can transform into macrophages with immunological roles; whilst various studies have also proven them capable of producing growth factors, extracellular matrix proteins and a range of cytokines. They are metabolically active and have both secretory and absorptive roles, with electron microscopy demonstrating abundant pinocytic vesicles, polyribosomes and mitochondria amongst their intracellular structures. Injury or disruption of the monolayer is repaired through mitosis and migration of adjoining cells or incorporation of free-floating mesothelial cells from pleural fluid.

Their size, shape and surface structure vary subtly according to location within the pleural space, although no major cytological differences have been found between mesothelial cells of pleural, pericardial or peritoneal origin. Each cell has a carpet of microvilli at the pleural surface whose precise role is still unknown; however, the density of microvilli is greatest in the inferior parts of the thorax, and greater in visceral than parietal pleura at corresponding levels. Parietal mesothelial cells in the apices are flatter with fewer microvilli; whilst basally the cells are cuboidal, more numerous per unit area and have a higher density of microvilli. These adaptations may relate to variable lung and chest wall movement at different thoracic levels.

Innervation, blood supply and lymphatics

Innervation

The visceral pleura is innervated by the vagal and sympathetic trunks which do not have pain fibres. Only the parietal pleura contains pain fibres, with pleuritic pain consequently implying involvement of this surface. It is innervated by intercostal nerves and refers pain to the corresponding area of the chest wall; with the exception of the diaphragm which being supplied by the phrenic nerve refers pain to the ipsilateral shoulder.

Blood supply

The parietal pleura is supplied by systemic capillaries according to anatomical location. (Figure 1.1) These originate from the intercostal and internal mammary arteries for the costal pleura; pericardiophrenic artery for the mediastinal pleura; subclavian arteries for the cervical pleura; and superior phrenic and musculophrenic arteries for the diaphragmatic pleura. Venous drainage follows arterial supply into either the superior or inferior vena cava depending on location.

The arterial supply of the visceral pleura is somewhat controversial. It is generally agreed that the bronchial arteries supply the majority of the visceral pleura, although supply of the lung apex and its convex surface is debated and may involve the pulmonary circulation. Venous drainage occurs via the pulmonary veins.

Lymphatics

The visceral pleural lymphatics constitute a superficial network of interconnecting vessels over the surface of and through the lung along the interlobular septae. Lymph flows via the bronchovascular bundles towards the lung hilae, with a greater density of lymphatics in dependent areas of lung with higher intravascular pressures.

Lymphatic plexuses are found in the parietal pleura overlying intercostal spaces, mediastinum and the diaphragm, but are essentially absent over the ribs. The costal pleura drains anteriorly into internal mammary nodes and posteriorly into intercostal nodes at the rib heads. The mediastinal lymphatics drain to tracheobronchial and mediastinal nodes; whilst those in the diaphragm pass to parasternal, middle phrenic and mediastinal nodes.

Whilst the visceral pleura is separate from the pleural space, the parietal pleura is unique in containing stomata that allow direct communication with the underlying lymphatic network and removal of large particles from the pleural space. These stomata are 2–6 micrometres in diameter at rest and found in greatest density in the mediastinum and lower thorax. Beneath the stomata lie dilated spaces called lacunae which drain into the lymphatic network via valves to maintain unidirectional flow. Associated with the stomata in some areas are modified mesothelial cells and immune aggregates

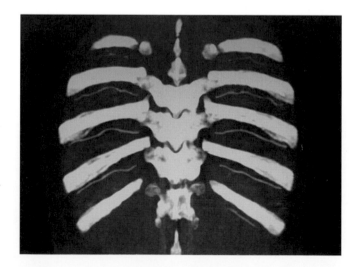

Figure 1.1 CT angiogram demonstrating the course and variability of the intercostal arteries posteriorly.

(lymphocytes, plasma cells and monocytes) surrounding a central lymphatic vessel. These are Kampmeier's foci, thought to have a similar role to Peyer's patches in the gut in local host defence mechanisms.

Physiology of the pleural space

Pleural pressure

The pressure in the pleural space is normally sub-atmospheric, with the tendency of lungs to collapse being countered by the chest wall trying to expand. This negative pressure is not uniform, with a gradient from apex (most negative) to base (least) of more than 8 cm H_2O in an upright position caused by gravity, weight of intrathoracic structures and differences in lung and chest wall shape. This pressure gradient causes different distension pressures in individual lung regions, explaining variation in alveolar size (larger apically) and ventilation (better basally).

Pleural fluid formation and constituents

The volume of pleural fluid in health is small, with mammalian studies placing it between 0.1 and 0.2 mL/kg, whilst a single human study reported a mean volume of 8.4 mL per hemithorax (0.26 mL/kg). This fluid forms a thin continuous film of relatively even thickness (10–20 micrometres) between visceral and parietal pleura.

Pleural fluid is derived from systemic vessels of the pleural membranes, with the vast majority produced by the parietal pleura in the upper thorax. This source fits with anatomical and physiological features of the parietal pleura, with its microvessels being closer to the surface and subject to higher filtration pressures than those of the visceral pleura. Fluid filters from these microvessels through the extrapleural interstitium and into the pleural space down a small gradient. The high-pressure nature of the filtration means pleural fluid has a low protein concentration relative to plasma (approximately 15% of plasma protein levels), with smaller liquid molecules more easily crossing into the pleural space than larger proteins.

However, the electrolyte composition of pleural fluid implies an additional active process in its formation though this has not been identified. Pleural fluid has a greater bicarbonate concentration relative to plasma, and lower concentrations of sodium and chloride. Consequently, pleural fluid is alkaline relative to plasma, with a normal pH of 7.6.

The same human study reported above also informs our knowledge of the cellular content of pleural fluid. This showed a mean of 700 red cells per mm³ and 1700 white blood cells per mm³, with the majority of these being macrophages (75%) or lymphocytes (23%).

Mesothelial cells, neutrophils and eosinophils make up the remainder. These data are again largely consistent with mammalian studies.

Pleural fluid absorption

Various routes by which fluid exits the pleural space have been proposed, including via capillaries in the visceral pleura or reabsorption by mesothelial cells. It is now accepted that drainage occurs predominantly via lymphatic stomata in the parietal pleura, whose main location in the lower thorax contrasts with the source of pleural fluid production. Support for bulk flow drainage through the stomata rather than membrane diffusion or active transport comes from various factors, including the constant rate of fluid absorption despite variation in protein concentration and ability of comparatively large erythrocytes to leave the pleural space intact. Distal lymphatic flow is influenced by intrinsic vessel contractility and respiratory movements, the latter of which also encourage fluid circulation within the pleural space.

Pleural fluid production and absorption are normally in equilibrium, with their baseline rate estimated to be 0.01–0.02 mL/kg/hour. Should production increase (e.g. during exercise) the rate of drainage responds via a negative feedback mechanism. Studies in patients with heart failure have shown the lymphatic stomata can increase their rate of absorption almost 20-fold, equivalent to over 500 mL/day in the average adult male. This system is extremely effective at regulating pleural fluid volume close to steady-state conditions; it is only once the rate of filtration and production exceeds maximum absorption that pleural effusions occur.

Role of the pleural space

The main function of pleural fluid is to ensure close apposition of visceral and parietal pleura, and allow frictionless movement of these surfaces during breathing. However, there is no evidence for the pleural space itself having an essential role. Human studies on pleurodesis – the intentional obliteration of the pleural space to treat recurrent effusions or pneumothoraces – show no significant impairment of lung function or gaseous exchange post-procedure. Just as we cannot explain variations in pleural anatomy among species, we are unable to answer why the space should exist or have been preserved during evolution.

Further reading

Rahman NM and Wang NS. (2008) Anatomy of the pleura, in *Textbook of Pleural Diseases*, 2nd edn (eds Light RW, Lee YCG), pp.13–36, Taylor & Francis, Boca Raton.

CHAPTER 2

Radiology of Pleural Disease

Rob J. Hallifax, John P. Corcoran and Najib M. Rahman

Oxford Centre for Respiratory Medicine, Churchill Hospital, Oxford, UK

OVERVIEW

- The majority of the pleura is not visible in health on chest radiographs.
- Small pleural effusions (<200 mL) may not be visible on chest X-ray.
- Thoracic ultrasound is a highly sensitive test for the detection of pleural fluid and is mandatory for interventions in the pleural space when fluid is present.
- Computed tomography (CT) is the investigation of choice for patients with undiagnosed pleural effusions. It can detect pleural thickening, pleural plaques and malignant pleural disease including mesothelioma, and may demonstrate evidence of disease elsewhere in the thorax.
- CT has a high sensitivity and specificity for the detection of malignant pleural disease.
- Magnetic resonance imaging and positron emission tomography with CT scanning are used in specific circumstances in the investigation and management of pleural disease.

The standard postero-anterior (PA) chest radiograph (CXR) has been augmented by the use of thoracic ultrasound and multi-slice computed tomography (CT) scans in imaging the pleural space. Ultrasound is now routinely used in the assessment of suspected pleural effusions and guidelines strongly recommend its usage in all pleural procedures (pleural aspiration, biopsy and chest drain insertion). Ultrasound can easily distinguish between pleural fluid and collapsed or consolidated lung, which on CXR can both appear as similar areas of opacification. The safety of pleural procedures has been enhanced by routine use of ultrasound. Pleural thickening and pleural plaques are often best visualised on CT. CT provides cross-sectional images which can also distinguish pleural and chest wall diseases from diseases of the lung parenchyma. The combination of positron emission tomography (PET) with CT scanning allows identification of metabolically active cells which can differentiate malignant from non-malignant tissue. This chapter describes each imaging modality, highlighting advantages and disadvantages of each technique with respect to pleural disease.

Plain radiography

In health, the pleura is usually only visible on plain PA CXR in the fissures. In the horizontal and oblique fissures there are double layers of visceral pleura; visible when tangential to the X-ray beam. The visceral pleura is also visualised in patients with a pneumothorax. Identifying the edge of the pleura as a thin white line on CXR, with no normal lung markings distally, is key to making the diagnosis (Figure 2.1). The parietal pleura are never normally visualised in health. However, pleural plaques and pleural thickening may be seen on CXR. Pleural plaques, which can be idiopathic or related to asbestos exposure, are often calcified which increases radiological visibility (Figure 2.2). The sensitivity of a CXR in the detection of plaques is in the range of 30–80% and the specificity is in the range of 60–80%, depending on the number of plaques, their distribution and the quality of the CXR. Diffuse non-calcified pleural thickening is more difficult to identify on CXR. CT scanning is the definitive imaging technique for pleural thickening.

Pleural effusions are often first identified on plain CXR. Increased opacification at the lung base or visible fluid level (meniscus) may be seen on CXR. However, CXR is not a sensitive test as tumour, enlarged/dilated left ventricle (on left) or pleural thickening provide a similar CXR appearance. Conversely, a small effusion may not be evident on CXR. Ultrasound is the imaging investigation of choice for pleural effusions.

Ultrasound

Ultrasound is a low-cost, portable, radiation-free imaging option. It is an ideal next step investigation after CXR for investigation of pleural disease. There is a trade-off between the optimal spatial resolution (often provided by higher frequency probes) and depth penetration to allow visualisation of large effusions. Therefore, variable transducers (3–5 MHz) are often used. Probes with smaller footprints are easiest for intercostal access, to avoid rib 'shadows'. Ultrasound relies on reflection of high frequency sound waves from tissues. Any interface with air, including normal aerated lung, will produce large reflections and therefore appear white, whereas soft tissue and fluid interfaces do not reflect and so pleural effusions appear dark (black).

ABC of Pleural Diseases, First Edition. Edited by Najib M. Rahman, Ian Hunt, Fergus V. Gleeson and Nick A. Maskell.
© 2018 John Wiley & Sons Ltd. Published 2018 by John Wiley & Sons Ltd.

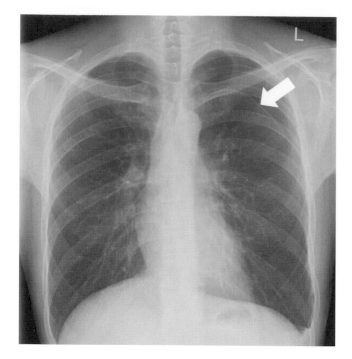

Figure 2.1 Postero-anterior (PA) chest radiograph (CXR) showing pneumothorax. The white arrow indicates the edge of the visceral pleural.

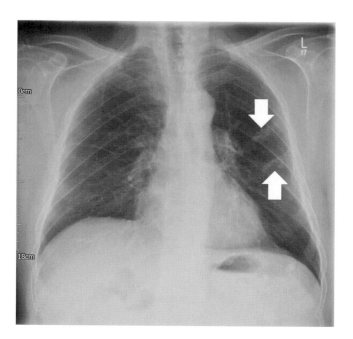

Figure 2.2 PA-CXR showing pleural plaques in left midzone (white arrows).

Ultrasound of the normal lung and pleura reveals a characteristic echogenic 'stripe' of the two opposing pleural layers (Figure 2.3). During respiration, the lung and hence the pleura move, producing a shimmering movement known as the 'lung sliding' sign. Distal to the pleural 'stripe', reverberation artefacts known as 'comet tails' are usually seen extending from the pleural surface deeper into the image in the plane of the scanning probe. These 'comet tails' can be produced by different structures at the pleural surface (e.g. foci of calcification or small foreign bodies) or from the lung parenchyma.

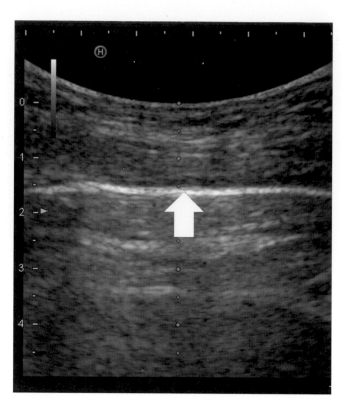

Figure 2.3 Ultrasound appearance of the normal lung and pleura. Echogenic 'stripe' of the two opposing pleural layers (white arrow).

Although usually seen in health, many conditions, such as pulmonary oedema or even pulmonary fibrosis, can increase the number of 'comet tails', although their true significance in disease has not been formally evaluated. The absence of 'comet tail' and 'lung sliding' signs is useful to confirm the diagnosis of pneumothorax (as the two pleural layers are no longer opposed). Ultrasound was shown to be more sensitive than CXR for detection of pneumothorax in post lung biopsy patients. However, ultrasound may give false positive results in patients with impaired lung function, particularly those with chronic obstructive pulmonary disease.

Once a pleural effusion has been identified using CXR, ultrasound is the best next line of investigation to visualise and characterise the fluid. Fluid is seen as dark on ultrasound, ranging from entirely anechoic (black) to hypoechoic or echogenic (grey) (Figure 2.4). The area is often delineated by the diaphragm basally and the echogenic line of the visceral pleural and/or lung. Transudates always appear anechoic whereas exudates can be either anechoic or echoic.

Heterogeneous echogenic effusions can provide a 'swirling' pattern on ultrasound. Malignant effusions are more likely to be echogenic, but these signs alone are not sufficient to be diagnostic. Homogenous echogenic effusions are often caused by a haemorrhagic effusion or intrapleural infection (empyema). Exudative effusions, particularly if long-standing and related to empyema or malignancy, can form septations – fine fibrinous strands – which divide the fluid into separate pockets (Figure 2.5), and can eventually become thickened and vascularised. The presence of fluid allows ultrasound visualisation of underlying structures such as the diaphragm and pericardium. Detection of a diaphragmatic nodule

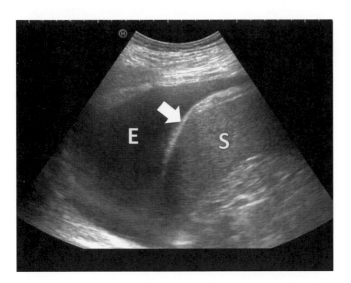

Figure 2.4 Ultrasound appearance of a pleural effusion (E) with diaphragm (white arrow) and spleen (S) visible.

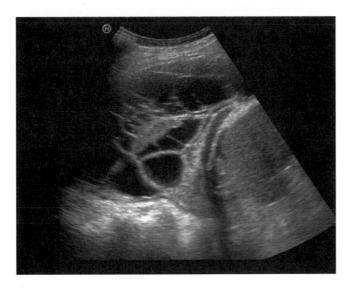

Figure 2.5 Ultrasound image showing heavily septated pleural effusion.

is strongly suggestive of malignancy. Identification of an inverted or flattened hemidiaphragm, which either does not move or paradoxically moves upwards on inspiration, is suggestive of raised intrapleural pressure. Performing a therapeutic aspiration in these cases is likely to result in symptomatic benefit to the patient.

Ultrasound is now an essential tool for pleural procedures in assessing the site for diagnostic and therapeutic aspirations, insertion of chest drains and for real-time ultrasound-guided procedures strongly recommended by current UK guidelines.

CT scan

Modern multi-slice CT scanners have the ability to acquire images of the entire thorax in one breath hold (<10 seconds) which reduces movement artefact. These images are often reconstructed in the coronal and sagittal planes to aid diagnostic evaluation. The administration of intravenous contrast allows differentiation between

pleural surface and any associated pathology, as well as characterising the tissue itself (e.g. areas of necrosis).

CT has become the imaging modality of choice (over ultrasound and CXR) for the assessment of pleural thickening and nodules, particularly if malignancy is suspected. Pleural plaques appear on CT as well-defined areas of pleural thickening, with a 'rolled edge' (i.e. thicker at the edges than centrally). They are distinct from underlying rib and extrapleural fat, separated by a thin layer of fatty tissue. Lipomas (benign tumours originating from fatty tissue) are often an incidental finding whose CT appearance is of a uniform pleural mass with the density of fat.

Around 10% of patients exposed to asbestos will develop asbestos-related diffuse pleural thickening. CT is a valuable tool in the assessment of these patients with possible diffuse pleural thickening seen on a CXR, allowing differentiation from malignant disease and extrapleural fat. CT criteria for diffuse pleural thickening is a continuous sheet of pleural thickening ($\geq$3 mm thick) extending at least 5 cm laterally and 8–10 cm craniocaudally.

Pleural metastases are the most common cause of pleural thickening, most likely primaries including lung, breast, lymphoproliferative, ovarian and gastrointestinal. The CT features associated with a high probability of malignant pleural disease are nodular pleural thickening, mediastinal pleural thickening, parietal pleural thickening >1 cm and circumferential pleural thickening (with specificities of 94%, 94%, 88% and 100%, respectively, but sensitivities of 51%, 36%, 56% and 41%) (Figure 2.6).

Although diffuse malignant mesothelioma may be identified on CXR as irregular nodular opacities peripherally, CT is the investigation of choice for suspected mesothelioma. Nodular pleural thickening is seen in 94% of cases, usually in the lower zones. An associated effusion is present in 60% of patients, usually unilateral, with only 5% of patients having bilateral disease. The disease may be limited to focal masses or involve the entire pleural surface resulting in thoracic volume loss with rib crowding. Exposure to asbestos can cause benign asbestos-related plaque disease, and differentiation from malignant mesothelioma can be difficult. However, malignant pleural disease tends to involve the entire pleural surface whereas benign disease does not involve the mediastinal pleura.

In patients presenting with a pleural effusion and suspected malignancy, CT scanning with late venous phase contrast can more readily distinguish pleural nodularity if some pleural fluid remains. Therefore, in these patients, complete drainage of the fluid prior to CT scanning is not beneficial to the diagnostic process.

PET CT

Positron emission tomography (PET) combined with CT scanning can provide additional information in the investigation of pleural malignancy. Malignant cells are more metabolically active than non-malignant cells. Injection of a radioactive isotope, 18-fluorodeoxy-glucose (18FDG) can highlight these cells because 18FDG is more avidly concentrated in malignant tissue rather than normal tissue. PET may be relatively specific for pleural malignancy, as one study of 98 patients showed 18FDG activity in 61 of 63 patients with pleural malignancy compared to an absence of activity in 31 of 35 patients

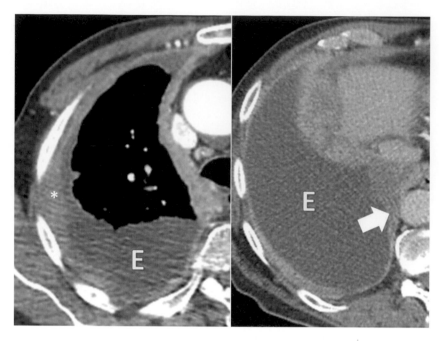

Figure 2.6 Two cross-sectional computed tomography (CT) images showing nodular thickening (asterisk) and mediastinal involvement (arrow) in the presence of pleural effusion (E).

with benign disease. However, any cause of significantly metabolically active disease may result in increased 18FDG activity; for example, in the increased activity seen in patients post talc pleurodesis. Additionally, tumours that are relatively inactive metabolically may not be detected, and it is unlikely that small volume pleural disease would be successfully detected, resulting in reduced sensitivity.

MRI

Given the high specificity of CT, magnetic resonance imaging (MRI) is not routinely used in the diagnosis of malignant pleural thickening. MRI delineates the extent of soft tissue involvement and inflammation of the chest wall without requiring intravenous contrast. Therefore, MRI can be employed if intravenous contrast is contraindicated or if detailed soft tissue images are required, such as suspected chest wall or diaphragm invasion, peripheral nerve tumours or vascular tumours.

Further reading

Duysinx B, Nguyen D, Louis R, Cataldo D, Belhocine T, Bartsch P *et al.* (2004) Evaluation of pleural disease with 18-fluorodeoxyglucose positron emission tomography imaging. *Chest*, **125**, 489–493.

Epler GR, McLoud TC, Munn CS and Colby TV. (1986) Pleural lipoma: diagnosis by computed tomography. *Chest*, **90**, 265–268.

Goodman TR, Traill ZC, Phillips AJ, Berger J and Gleeson FV. (1999) Ultrasound detection of pneumothorax. *Clinical Radiology*, **54**, 736–739.

Hooper C, Lee G and Maskell N. (2010) British Thoracic Society Pleural Disease Guideline 2010. *Thorax*, **65**, Suppl 2.

International Labour Office. (1980) Guidelines for the use of the ILO classification of radiographs of pnuemoconiosis: revised edition. *Occupational Health and Safety Series, no.22 (rev.80)*, International Labour Office, Geneva.

Kawashima A and Libshitz HI. (1990) Malignant pleural mesothelioma: CT manifestations in 50 cases. *American Journal of Roentgenology*, **155**, 965–969.

Leung AN, Muller NL and Miller RR. (1990) CT in differential diagnosis of diffuse pleural disease. *American Journal of Roentgenology*, **154**, 487–492.

Lynch DA, Gamsu G, Ray CS and Aberle DR. (1988) Asbestos-related focal lung masses: manifestations on conventional and high-resolution CT scans. *Radiology*, **169**, 603–607.

Peacock C, Copley SJ and Hansell DM. (2000) Asbestos-related benign pleural disease. *Clinical Radiology*, **55**, 422–432.

Sistrom CL, Reiheld CT, Gay SB and Wallace KK. (1996) Detection and estimation of the volume of pneumothorax using real-time sonography: efficacy determined by receiver operating characteristic analysis. *American Journal of Roentgenology*, **166**, 317–321.

Yang PC, Luh KT, Chang DB, Wu HD, Yu CJ and Kuo SH. (1992) Value of sonography in determining the nature of pleural effusion: analysis of 320 cases. *American Journal of Roentgenology*, **159**, 29–33.

CHAPTER 3

Pneumothorax

John Harvey[1], Andrew McDuff[2] and Ian Hunt[3]

[1] North Bristol NHS Trust, Bristol, UK
[2] New Cross Hospital, Wolverhampton, UK
[3] St. George's Hospital, London, UK

> **OVERVIEW**
>
> - Pneumothorax is common and associated with cigarette smoking.
> - It is not usually life-threatening but it can be a medical emergency.
> - Recommended management differs between patients with and without previous lung disease.
> - Pneumothorax can be a recurrent problem and early liaison with thoracic surgeons improves management in selected patients.

Definition, epidemiology, risk factors and aetiology

Pneumothorax describes the presence of air in the pleural space. Classification of pneumothorax depends on whether there is underlying lung disease or the presence of identifiable trauma (Box 3.1).

Hospital admission rates for spontaneous pneumothorax in the UK have been reported as 16.7/100 000 for men and 5.8/100 000 for women, with corresponding mortality rates of 1.26/million and 0.62/million per annum between 1991 and 1995. The incidence of iatrogenic pneumothorax is not precisely known; however, the most common causes are subclavian vein cannulation, thoracentesis and positive pressure ventilation.

Anatomical abnormalities have been demonstrated, even in patients without clinically apparent underlying lung disease. Sub-pleural blebs and bullae (termed emphysema-like changes) are found at the lung apices at thoracoscopy and on computed tomography (CT) scanning in up to 90% of cases of primary pneumothorax and are thought to be involved in the development of pneumothorax.

Small airway obstruction, mediated by an influx of inflammatory cells, often characterises pneumothorax. Smoking has been implicated in this aetiological pathway. Smoking is associated with a 12% lifetime risk of developing pneumothorax in men who smoke heavily, compared to 0.1% in those who have never smoked. Patients with primary spontaneous pneumothorax tend to be taller than control patients. The gradient of negative pleural pressure increases from the lung base to the apex, so that alveoli at the lung apex in tall individuals are subject to significantly greater distending forces than those at the base of the lung, and this may in theory predispose to the development of apical sub-pleural blebs.

Unfortunately, despite the clear relationship between smoking and pneumothorax, over 80% of patients continue to smoke after a primary pneumothorax. The risk of recurrence is as high as 54% within the first 4 years. Risk factors for recurrence are smoking, height and age over 60 years, pulmonary fibrosis and emphysema. Determined efforts should be directed at smoking cessation after the development of a pneumothorax.

Presentation

Classically, patients present with an episode of pleuritic chest pain and dyspnoea. Clinical examination reveals the reduced movement of the chest wall, hyper-resonance on percussion and absence of breath sounds on the affected side.

However, the symptoms are often minor, particularly in primary pneumothorax, and in busy emergency and admission units the signs may be difficult to detect. A high clinical index of suspicion must therefore be maintained, especially in thin, young smokers.

Symptoms and signs are often more obvious in secondary pneumothorax because of underlying lung disease.

Tension pneumothorax is a medical emergency which requires immediate treatment prior to any further examination or imaging (Box 3.2).

Investigations

The standard imaging for diagnosis is the postero-anterior chest X-ray (PA-CXR) (Figure 3.1). Expiratory films are no longer recommended as they have not been shown to improve detection. Management is guided by the X-ray findings as the plain PA-CXR has been used to quantify the pneumothorax size. However, it should be remembered that it tends to underestimate the size because a radiograph is a two-dimensional image whilst the pleural cavity is a three-dimensional structure. A 2 cm rim of air between chest wall and lung edge measured at the level of the hilum

---

ABC of Pleural Diseases, First Edition. Edited by Najib M. Rahman, Ian Hunt, Fergus V. Gleeson and Nick A. Maskell.
© 2018 John Wiley & Sons Ltd. Published 2018 by John Wiley & Sons Ltd.

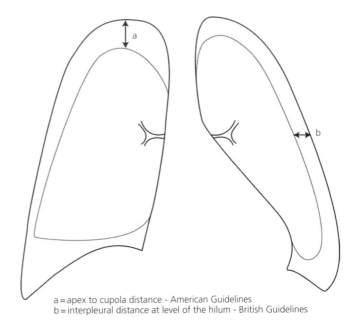

a = apex to cupola distance - American Guidelines
b = interpleural distance at level of the hilum - British Guidelines

Figure 3.2 Standard methodology for measurement of pneumothorax size.

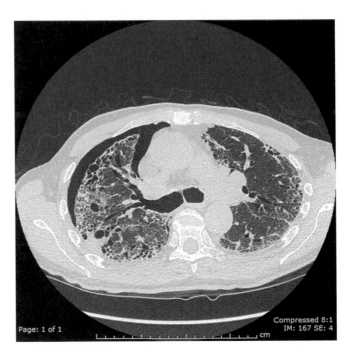

Figure 3.3 Secondary pneumothorax with evidence of interstitial lung disease.

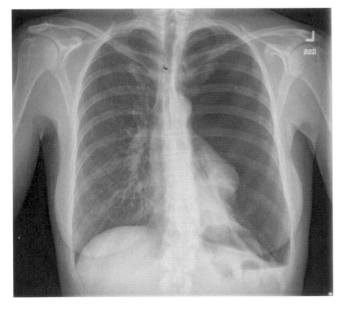

Figure 3.1 Tension pneumothorax with evidence of early tracheal shift.

represents a 50% pneumothorax (Figure 3.2, line b). There are alternative strategies for estimating the size (e.g. Figure 3.2, line a), but these tend to overestimate size and are not recommended. A 2 cm (i.e. 50%) pneumothorax is classified as large and expert opinion typically favours active intervention in these patients.

In cases of uncertainty where underlying lung disease (e.g. bullous emphysema) or where previous thoracic surgery makes interpreting the CXR difficult, then CT scanning is the 'gold' standard (Figure 3.3) and should be undertaken prior to intervention.

There is increasing interest in the role of ultrasound scanning in the diagnosis of pneumothorax especially in critical care environ-ments where traditional imaging techniques may be more challenging. However, there are few data on the value of this modality and it requires specialist sonographic skills and its place in routine management pathways is unclear.

Management

The aim of managing patients with pneumothorax is to relieve symptoms using the minimal intervention necessary in order to allow a prompt return to their usual activities of daily living.

The current British Thoracic Society guidelines for management are summarised in Figure 3.4.

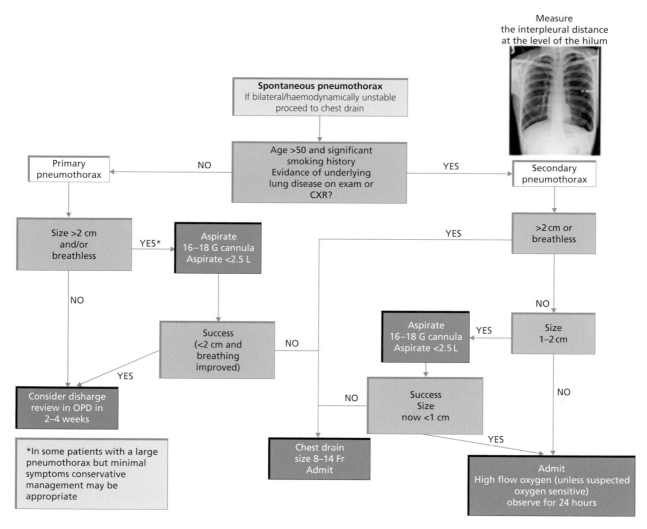

Figure 3.4 British Thoracic Society 2010 guideline algorithm for the management of pneumothorax.

Tension (i.e. haemodynamically unstable) pneumothoraces

This is a medical emergency and intervention should not be delayed for any reason (including CXR). The affected side should undergo immediate needle decompression with an 18 G (i.e. green), or larger, cannula. A chest drain will be inserted afterwards.

Haemodynamically stable

It is important to make the distinction between primary (i.e. no underlying lung disease) and secondary pneumothoraces as this is the key step in determining management of haemodynamically stable patients.

The intervention options are needle aspiration or insertion of a chest drain.

Conservative management

Some patients with pneumothorax have mild symptoms. Some patients, particularly those with primary pneumothorax and a small pneumothorax, do not require specific treatment. A pneumothorax will slowly resolve over time as the air is reabsorbed and some haemodynamically stable patients may be safely managed without an immediate procedure to remove the air.

Needle aspiration

It is known that aspiration (Box 3.3) of primary spontaneous pneumothorax is safe, effective and allows early discharge from hospital. Needle aspiration works as the air leak causing the pneumothorax heals rapidly and there is frequently no ongoing air leak when the patient is seen. Needle aspiration is also less painful than chest drain insertion and requires less operator skill. This is therefore the recommended first intervention in primary pneumothoraces. It has a success rate of 50–70% in clinical trials. No more than 2.5 L of air should be aspirated as this is likely to signify the presence of a persistent air leak and suggests that further re-expansion of the lung is unlikely at this point.

Chest drains

Chest drain insertion is usually required for secondary pneumothoraces as the abnormal lung is less likely to heal quickly and there is a tendency for a persistent air leak. Chest drains are also required in primary pneumothoraces that fail to improve with needle aspiration.

Guidelines now recommend that small bore (i.e. 14 Fr or less) drains are used for the management of pneumothorax. They are known to be as effective in draining the pleural space as large bore drains and are more comfortable. These are frequently inserted using the Seldinger technique.

Box 3.3 **Summarised needle aspiration technique**

- Confirm the affected side by looking at the CXR yourself (do not take someone else's word for it!)
- Identify the 2nd or 3rd intercostal space mid-clavicular line
- Clean the area with chlorhexidine
- Inject 1% lidocaine to the skin and infiltrate down to pleura
- Confirm aspiration of air with green needle
- Advance 18 G cannula until air aspirated
- Remove stylet
- Using 50 mL syringe and three-way tap, aspirate until resistance is felt or 2.5 L (50 × 50 mL syringe) is aspirated
- Repeat CXR
- Success is defined by a smaller pneumothorax (<2 cm at the level of the hilum with improved symptoms
- In case of failure, proceed to chest drain insertion

Heimlich valves

Heimlich valves are an ambulatory treatment option that provide an alternative to chest drain insertion. Heimlich valves function with enclosed valves allowing air to escape from the chest and not re-enter. They allow selected patients to be discharged home following insertion of the device.

Digital thoracic drainage

An alternative to the conventional arrangement of a chest drain connected to an underwater seal is a digital thoracic drainage system. These devices are frequently used following thoracic surgery and allow a digitally recorded measure of air leak and regulated portable suction which offers advantages over 'wall' suction in both preserving patient mobility and providing a more consistent pressure. The accurate measurement of air leak potentially allows an earlier distinction to be made between patients likely to have an ongoing air leak from those whose air leak will resolve over time.

Referral of patients

All patients with pneumothorax should be referred to a respiratory physician either as an inpatient (within 24 hours ideally) or as an outpatient if needle aspiration is successful (within 2 weeks). Respiratory physicians have the specialist knowledge and skills required to manage these patients and have a close working relationship with their thoracic surgery colleagues whose skills may be required in the presence of an ongoing air leak.

Patients with an ongoing air leak should be discussed with a thoracic surgeon 48 hours after the insertion of the chest drain. Following this there will need to be a decision on whether to proceed to early surgical intervention or to continue with non-operative management.

Surgical interventions for persistent air leak include: video-assisted thoracic surgery (VATS) or open thoracotomy with pleurectomy, chemical pleurodesis or pleural abrasion. The aim of these approaches is to obliterate the pleural space by causing a fibrinous reaction between the lung surface and chest wall.

Recurrent pneumothorax

Patients with primary spontaneous pneumothorax have a recurrence risk of 30–50% and should be warned of this on discharge and told to seek medical advice if symptoms recur.

Patients with a second pneumothorax either on the same or the opposite side should be referred to a thoracic surgeon. Patients with a second pneumothorax are at an extremely high risk (>80%) of a further episode and should be considered for definitive treatment to obliterate the pleural space.

Patients in whom a recurrence could have disastrous consequences (e.g. pilots, divers) should be referred to a thoracic surgeon after their first episode.

Further reading

Baumann MH, Strange C, Heffner JE, Light R, Kirby TJ, Klein J *et al*; AACP Pneumothorax Consensus Group. (2001) Management of spontaneous pneumothorax: an American College of Chest Physicians Delphi consensus statement. *Chest* **119** (2), 590–602.

Havelock T, Teoh R, Laws D, Gleeson F on behalf of the BTS Pleural Disease Guideline Group. (2010) Pleural procedures and thoracic ultrasound: British Thoracic Society pleural disease guideline 2010. *Thorax* **65**, i61–i76. doi:10.1136/thx.2010.137026

MacDuff A, Arnold A, Harvey J on behalf of the BTS Pleural Disease Guideline Group. (2010) Management of spontaneous pneumothorax: British Thoracic Society pleural disease guideline 2010. *Thorax* **65**, ii18–ii31. doi:10.1136/thx.2010.136986

CHAPTER 4

Investigation of Pleural Effusions

Clare E. Hooper

Worcestershire NHS Trust, UK

OVERVIEW

- Selection of optimum pleural procedures, with both diagnostic and therapeutic intent, streamlines investigation and reduces patient risk and discomfort.
- Thoracic ultrasound is an essential tool for diagnosis and safe pleural procedure guidance.
- The division of exudates and transudates by Light's criteria helps to focus investigation and management but dual diagnoses giving a mixed picture are common.
- Pleural biopsy is essential to exclude or confirm malignancy or tuberculosis in patients with persistent undiagnosed effusions.
- Benign asbestos effusion and idiopathic pleuritis are diagnoses of exclusion and should be followed up for a minimum of 12 months because of the small risk of underlying malignancy.

Pleural effusions are a common presentation with a large number of possible causes. They may result from systemic disease or processes local to the pleura and lung. The guiding principle of investigation should be to minimise the number of invasive tests performed by selecting procedures with the best diagnostic yield and both diagnostic and therapeutic benefits. As malignancy accounts for a substantial proportion of symptomatic unilateral pleural effusions, it is important that it is robustly excluded. Figure 4.1 details a suggested algorithm for investigating pleural effusions in countries of low tuberculosis (TB) prevalence (such as the UK).

Bilateral pleural effusions in patients with a clear history or clinical features suggesting a transudate (i.e. congestive cardiac failure, renal failure, hypoproteinaemia) do not require specific investigation with aspiration or cross-sectional imaging unless they fail to respond to appropriate medical management. Although the division of pleural effusions by their unilateral or bilateral appearance on chest X-ray and their protein content (exudates or transudates) is helpful in focusing initial tests, some effusions are of multi-factorial origin and present with a mixed picture, requiring a particularly flexible approach to investigation.

Clinical presentation

Pleural effusions are associated with dyspnoea, pleuritic chest pain and cough (caused by extrinsic bronchial compression by a large effusion) but patients may also present with an asymptomatic chest X-ray finding. Whether an effusion is associated with dyspnoea is determined by its size, the degree of associated pleural thickening and the presence of coexistent parenchymal lung disease or the respiratory reserve of the patient.

History taking

The following aspects of the history are particularly important:

- Duration of symptoms.
- Severity of dyspnoea (is a therapeutic pleural aspiration indicated urgently for symptomatic relief?)
- Preceding lower respiratory tract infection.
- Systemic symptoms of sepsis or malignancy (fevers, sweats, weight loss).
- History of cardiac or respiratory disease.
- Past history of malignant disease.
- Risk factors for TB: ethnic origin, contacts, immunocompromise.
- Drug history, including new drugs with a possible association with the onset of symptoms, change to diuretic dosage and any anticoagulants/antiplatelet agents (which require consideration before invasive procedures).
- Symptoms or history of connective tissue disease.
- Occupational history with an emphasis on asbestos exposure.
- Smoking.
- Performance status (to determine appropriateness of more invasive and physically stressful diagnostic and management strategies).

Examination

A thorough multi-system examination is important. This should include the following:

- Confirmation of clinical signs of a pleural effusion.
- Assessment of dyspnoea at rest and on minor exertion.

ABC of Pleural Diseases, First Edition. Edited by Najib M. Rahman, Ian Hunt, Fergus V. Gleeson and Nick A. Maskell.
© 2018 John Wiley & Sons Ltd. Published 2018 by John Wiley & Sons Ltd.

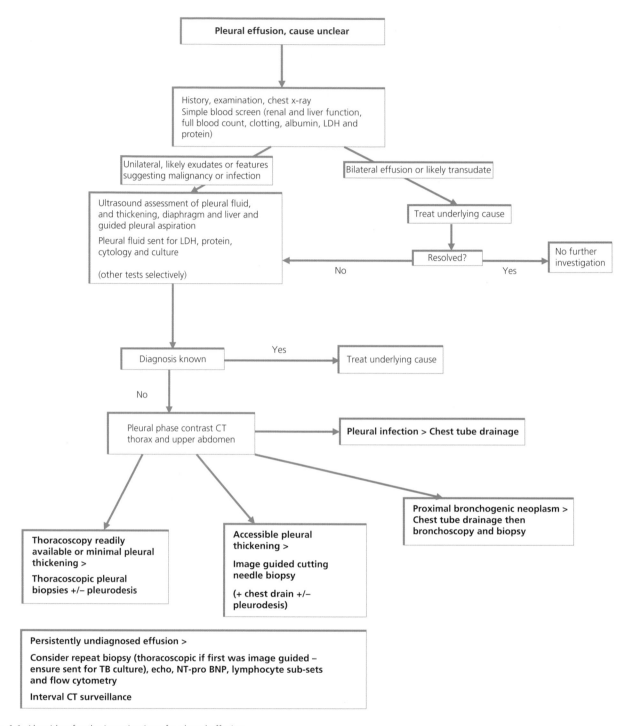

Figure 4.1 Algorithm for the investigation of a pleural effusion.

- Examination for signs of disseminated malignancy (lymph nodes, abdominal organomegaly, breast examination).
- Joints and skin.
- Signs of cardiac failure.

Initial imaging

Chest X-ray

Costophrenic angle blunting or loss of diaphragmatic contour is seen on erect postero-anterior (PA) chest X-ray in the presence of 200 mL or more of pleural fluid. In the erect position, simple pleural effusions have a surface meniscus as shown in Figure 4.2(a). Loculated effusions can appear as discrete smooth sub-pleural opacities and loculated pleural infection or empyema is often seen as a classic D-shaped opacity (Figure 4.2b).

A useful convention for classifying the size of effusion on PA chest X-ray is the proportion of the hemithorax that is occupied by fluid: small <1/3; moderate 1/3 to 1/2; large >1/2. Massive pleural effusions, occupying the entire hemithorax and causing mediastinal shift to the contralateral side, are most often seen with pleural malignancy.

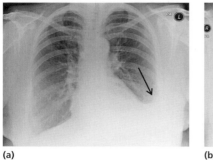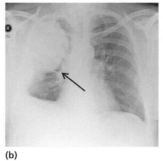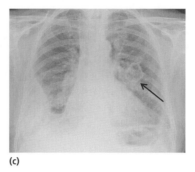

(a)　　　　　　　　　　　(b)　　　　　　　　　　　(c)

Figure 4.2 Chest X-rays: (a) meniscus of left pleural effusion; (b) D-shaped appearance of loculated pleural empyema; (c) asbestos-related pleural plaques.

In a supine patient, particularly on antero-posterior (AP) chest X-ray (e.g. in the critical care setting), pleural effusions distribute posteriorly and appear as a general haze over the hemithorax with preservation of vascular markings.

Other important observations that may provide clues to the cause of effusion include the presence of parenchymal consolidation or masses, bulky hila and abnormal mediastinal contours, cardiomegaly and evidence of previous cardiac surgery, diffuse pleural thickening and pleural plaques (associated with asbestos exposure; Figure 4.2c).

Thoracic ultrasound

Ultrasound is the next essential step after chest X-ray for patients who require further investigation. It should be performed by the physician who will plan and perform any subsequent invasive investigations.

Ultrasound is more sensitive than chest X-ray in detecting small effusions, allows accurate characterisation of the nature and distribution of pleural fluid, guidance of safe pleural aspiration and often the detection of signs of malignancy or underlying lung consolidation.

Pleural fluid may appear anechoic (simple), echogenic/complex or septated on ultrasound (Figure 4.3). The presence of echogenicity or septation positively confirms that the effusion is an exudate, while anechoic appearances can occur with either transudates or exudates.

The observation of significant pleural or diaphragmatic thickening or nodularity on thoracic ultrasound has a high specificity (95–100%) for identifying a malignant cause for the pleural effusion (Figure 4.4).

Real-time ultrasound guidance of diagnostic pleural aspiration has been shown to improve success rates and reduce the risk of organ puncture and iatrogenic pneumothorax.

A visual assessment of pleural fluid volume on ultrasound along with an impression of patient dyspnoea is helpful in determining what volume of fluid to remove at initial aspiration while awaiting more definitive procedures.

Pleural fluid tests

All unilateral pleural effusions of unknown cause should be sampled and sent for assessment of protein and lactate dehydrogenase (LDH), cytological examination and microscopy and culture.

Additional tests are useful in specific circumstances. The aspiration procedure is described elsewhere in this book.

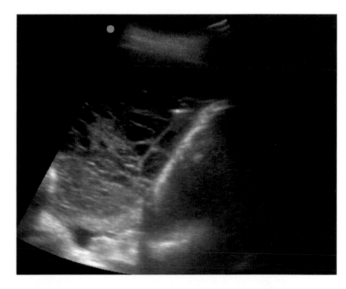

Figure 4.3 Thoracic ultrasound image of a complex septated pleural effusion.

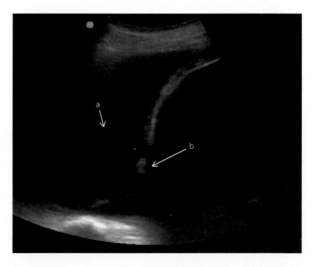

Figure 4.4 Thoracic ultrasound demonstrating large anechoic pleural effusion (a) and nodularity and thickening of the diaphragmatic pleura (b).

Fluid appearance

Pleural fluid appearance can provide some information regarding the likely cause of effusion but is often non-specific. Straw coloured fluid may indicate a transudate or a paucicellular exudate. Blood-tinged fluid is non-specific but frankly bloody pleural effusions suggest malignancy, benign asbestos effusion, post cardiac injury syndrome, pulmonary infarction or haemothorax. Brown fluid is usually a marker of a long-standing bloody effusion. Milky fluid suggests a lipid effusion (chylous or pseudochylous) but can be difficult to distinguish from the turbid or purulent fluid of empyema.

Distinguishing exudates and transudates

The dichotomous division of pleural effusions into exudates and transudates is a standard approach that is useful in focusing investigations towards a smaller number of diagnostic possibilities. Table 4.1 lists causes of pleural exudates and transudates.

Pleural fluid protein alone gives a rough guide: >30 g/L suggests an exudate and <30 g/L a transudate. This division is not accurate when fluid protein approaches the cut-off or in the presence of abnormal serum protein.

Light's criteria have been shown to be the most accurate method of dividing exudates and transudates. The system requires the concurrent measurement of paired serum and pleural fluid protein and LDH (Box 4.1).

Light's criteria sacrifice specificity for high sensitivity in the identification of pleural exudates, misclassifying approximately 20% of transudates as exudates, often in patients with cardiac failure who have been treated with diuretics.

It is also important to note that effusions of mixed aetiology are not uncommon, such that about 5% of malignant pleural effusions are transudative. This probably reflects coexistent cardiac failure, renal failure or hypo-albuminaemia.

Table 4.1 Causes of pleural exudates and transudates.

Exudates	Transudates
Common	*Common*
Simple parapneumonic effusion	Left ventricular failure
Pleural infection	Hepatic failure (hepatic hydrothorax)
Malignant pleural effusion	Renal failure
	Hypo-albuminaemia
Less common	*Less common*
Post CABG effusion	Peritoneal dialysis
Benign asbestos effusion	Hypothyroidism
Tuberculous pleuritis	Nephrotic syndrome
Rheumatoid arthritis	
Post myocardial infarction	
Haemothorax	
Pulmonary embolism with infarction	
Pancreatitis	
Rare	*Rare*
Drug reaction	Constrictive pericarditis
Sarcoidosis	Urinothorax
Other connective tissue disease (SLE, Sjögren syndrome)	Meigs syndrome

CABG, coronary artery bypass graft; SLE, systemic lupus erythematosus.

Pleural fluid cytology and differential cell counts

Approximately 60% of malignant pleural effusions can be diagnosed by cytological examination of the pleural fluid. Most are diagnosed at the first aspiration and diagnostic yield is not significantly improved by sending more than two samples. Higher volume samples do have a better yield; 50–60 mL is optimum.

In health, pleural fluid contains mesothelial cells and a small number of inflammatory cells. The presence of cells of another line (e.g. squamous cell, adenocarcinoma, sarcoma) implies malignancy. When malignant cells have been confirmed, immuno-cytochemical staining is used to help define their precise type.

When 'atypical' cells are reported, the differential lies between an inflammatory process and malignancy; in this circumstance, examining further fluid samples may help to identify malignant cells.

Adenocarcinoma that has metastasised to the pleura gives positive malignant cytology in a large proportion of cases because of ready shedding of malignant cells into fluid but diagnostic yield for other malignancies is often poor. Sensitivity of pleural fluid cytology in pleural mesothelioma for example is just 5–20%, necessitating a pleural biopsy in most cases.

In the absence of malignant cells, a cellular differential is helpful in narrowing the diagnostic possibilities. The percentage of nucleated cells taken up by each inflammatory cell type is reported.

Lymphocytic effusions contain ≥50% lymphocytes and occur with chronic pleural effusions of any cause. In the UK, they are most commonly seen with effusions caused by left ventricular failure and malignancy but worldwide tuberculous pleuritis is the leading cause. Intensely lymphocytic effusions (≥80% lymphocytes) occur with lymphoma, TB, chronic rheumatoid pleurisy, late post coronary artery bypass effusion and sarcoidosis.

Neutrophil predominant effusions (≥50% neutrophils) occur in acute inflammatory processes such as parapneumonic effusions, pleural infection, acute TB and the early stages of benign asbestos effusions.

Eosinophilic effusions have ≥10% eosinophils. Blood or air in the pleural space, drug reactions, Churg–Strauss syndrome and parasitic infections are often associated with pleural eosinophilia but overall it is a non-specific finding and is also commonly observed in patients with pleural malignancy.

Microscopy and culture

If sent in both plain and blood culture bottles, the yield for pleural fluid culture in pleural infection is up to 60%. This sample collection approach also maximises the growth of multiple organisms.

The sensitivity of pleural fluid culture in TB pleuritis is just 5%. Fluid should still be sent when TB is suspected but pleural biopsy culture and histology is required to exclude the diagnosis.

Pleural fluid pH (and glucose)

Limited available human data (and more extensive animal studies) tell us that the pH of pleural fluid in the healthy state is alkaline (>7.6). Transudative pleural effusion fluid has a pH of 7.45–7.55, while most exudates are in the range of 7.30–7.45. Pleural fluid acidosis (pH <7.30) occurs when there is a particularly high level of metabolic activity in the pleural space with accumulation of lactic acid and carbon dioxide, creating hydrogen ions which do not leave the pleural space at a normal rate because of diseased and thickened pleura. Pleural fluid acidosis is a non-specific finding (common causes are listed in Box 4.2) and is therefore not useful diagnostically.

In routine clinical practice, pleural fluid pH measurement only has utility as the most accurate means of discriminating between a simple parapneumonic effusion that will resolve with antibiotics and/or conservative management and complicated parapneumonic effusions or pleural infection that require chest tube drainage. The pH cut-off value with optimum diagnostic characteristics has been shown in a large meta-analysis to be ≤7.2.

When the clinical diagnosis is infection, pleural fluid should be drawn up into an arterial blood gas syringe and processed using a blood gas analyser to provide the pH result. There is no clinical need to analyse frankly purulent fluid (empyema) and this should be avoided because of the risk of damage to the machine. Exposure of fluid to air and lidocaine should be minimised as these significantly increase and reduce the measured pH, respectively.

Although measured routinely in the past, pleural fluid glucose has not been shown to add anything to the standard diagnostic process when pH can be measured accurately as described earlier. When the pleural membranes are functioning normally, glucose passes freely and reflects blood glucose (which has relevance in diabetes and other systemic states of abnormal blood glucose control). Low pleural fluid glucose (<3.4 mmol/L) occurs in parallel with pleural fluid acidosis via a similar mechanism.

Lipids

Milky pleural fluid may be brought about by chylothorax, pseudochylothorax or empyema. Bench centrifugation will cause the cellular and serous component of empyema fluid to separate, while lipid effusions retain their homogenous appearance.

It is important to distinguish between chylous and pseudochylous effusions in order to identify the underlying cause. This is achieved by measuring a lipid profile demonstrating high triglyceride levels (usually >1.24 mmol/L) and the presence of chylomicrons in chylothorax and high cholesterol levels (usually >5.18 mmol/L) with or without cholesterol crystals in pseudochylothorax.

Box 4.2 **Common causes of low pH (<7.3) pleural effusions**

- Pleural infection or complicated parapneumonic effusion
- Malignancy
- Tuberculosis
- Rheumatoid effusion
- Oesophageal rupture

Chylothorax results from disruption of the thoracic duct or its tributaries so that chyle leaks into the pleural space. Causes include thoracic surgery, trauma, lymphoma, TB and lymphatic malformations.

Pseudochyothorax arises in the context of chronic inflammatory pleural effusions with extensive pleural thickening, such that the products of cell death are retained within an encapsulated pleural space, resulting in cholesterol-rich fluid and cholesterol deposition over the pleura in a self-perpetuating process. Chronic rheumatoid arthritis associated effusion is the most common cause in the UK, but worldwide chronic tuberculous pleuritis represents the primary aetiology.

Biomarkers and auto-antibodies

Pleural effusions often represent a significant diagnostic challenge, not least because presenting clinical features are frequently non-specific. It is common for pleural infection and pleural malignancy to be confused in the early stages of investigation, with concomitant mismanagement and delayed diagnosis. Biomarkers that would resolve the key diagnostic dilemmas, perhaps without recourse to pleural biopsy, are an attractive possibility, but most examined to date have demonstrated inadequate diagnostic characteristics to have clinical utility.

Table 4.2 summarises biomarkers that have shown promise in limited patient sub-groups and/or are the subject of ongoing study.

When there is a suspicion of connective tissue disease (CTD) associated pleural effusion, sending a serum auto-immune profile including rheumatoid factor is essential. Rheumatoid arthritis (RA) and systemic lupus erythematosus (SLE) account for the vast majority of CTD associated pleural effusions. Measurement of pleural fluid antibodies simply reflects levels in the circulation and is of no additional value. An absence of joint symptoms or pre-existing diagnosis of CTD does not exclude RA or SLE as an underlying cause of effusion (in 25% of rheumatoid effusions, the effusion precedes or occurs simultaneously with the first onset of joint symptoms).

Cross-sectional imaging

A CT scan is an important next step in investigating an exudative pleural effusion when the diagnosis is not clear following initial fluid tests and clinical assessment.

CT scanning in this setting should be performed with pleural phase contrast (images taken 25–45 seconds post contrast) and before complete drainage of the effusion to optimise pleural visualisation. Scans performed in this way have excellent specificity for detecting pleural thickening with malignant characteristics (nodular, circumferential, >1 cm thick, extending over the mediastinal surface; Figure 4.5).

The distribution and nature of pleural thickening on CT helps to guide decisions regarding the optimum mode of pleural biopsy.

The presence of a proximal mass lesion may warrant bronchoscopy and biopsy if pleural fluid cytology is negative for malignant cells and parenchymal, mediastinal and upper abdominal appearances may provide information regarding the origin and extent of a malignant process involving the pleura.

Table 4.2 Biomarkers in the investigation of pleural effusions.

Biomarker	Diagnostic problem considered	Diagnostic characteristics	Potential clinical utility
Adenosine deaminase			
Enzyme produced by activated macrophages, neutrophils and lymphocytes as a non-specific marker of inflammation	Diagnosis of tuberculous pleuritis	Pleural fluid test Sensitivity 56–100% Specificity 55–100% Accuracy highly variable between clinical settings	In common use in USA for good NPV in low TB prevalence populations Discriminates TB from pleural malignancy with specificity of 95% in this setting
γ-Interferon release assays			
Detect IFN-γ secreted by pre-sensitised lymphocytes following in vitro stimulation by *Mycobacterium tuberculosis* specific antigens	Diagnosis of tuberculous pleuritis	Validated with blood. Use of pleural fluid is subject of studies Commercially available assays have slightly different performance characteristics Sensitivity using blood 60–100%, with pleural fluid 40–100% Specificity with blood 70–100%, with pleural fluid 60–98%	Limited by cost and inability to discriminate latent from active TB NPV good in low prevalence settings in the absence of immunosuppression but ADA is of superior/equivalent utility
Mesothelin			
Glycoprotein product of mesothelial cells that is over-expressed in malignancy	Diagnosis of malignant pleural mesothelioma	Validated with blood. Use of pleural fluid is subject of studies and probably gives superior diagnostic accuracy Summary estimates for blood: Sensitivity 64%, specificity 89% Pleural fluid sensitivity 60–70%, specificity 80–98%	May have value in clarifying suspicious cytology, particularly in frail patients unable to tolerate thoracoscopy Limitations include frequent false positive results in non-mesothelioma malignancy (particularly gynaecological, gastrointestinal and primary lung cancers) More studies needed before clinical adoption. May have a larger role in disease monitoring than diagnosis
NT-pro BNP			
Vasoactive peptide produced by cardiac ventricles in response to pressure or volume overload	Discrimination of effusions of cardiac origin	Validated with blood. Use of pleural fluid is subject of studies – appears equivalent due to free passage from circulation into pleural fluid Diagnostic accuracy highly variable by cut-off level selected and between heterogeneous patient groups studied	May have value in detecting comorbid cardiac failure in patients with effusions of a non-primary cardiac cause – moderate cut-off level (1500 pg/mL) likely to be optimum Good NPV may be used to rapidly exclude the need for cardiac investigations Poor specificity limits diagnostic utility of a positive result
Procalcitonin			
Hormokine produced systemically as a highly specific response to bacterial infection. Validated for monitoring of sepsis	Discrimination of effusions of infective origin Discrimination between pleural infection and simple parapneumonic effusion	Few data. Studies ongoing Area under the receiver operating characteristics curve for discriminating pleural infection from other causes of effusion appears to be >0.8	May have superior specificity to established markers of infection (e.g. CRP) in discriminating pleural infection from pleural malignancy May have a role in disease monitoring in pleural infection

ADA, adenosine deaminase; CRP, C-reactive protein; IGRA, γ-interferon release assay; NPV, negative predictive value; NT-pro BNP, N-terminal prohormone of brain natriuretic peptide.

Cross-sectional imaging is particularly important in the assessment of chylous effusions when pleural biopsy is usually unhelpful diagnostically.

Magnetic resonance imaging (MRI) is more expensive and less freely available than CT in the UK but does allow an accurate assessment of the pleura and should be considered for selected patients if radiation exposure or contrast allergy are particular clinical concerns.

Metabolic and dynamic imaging

Integrated positron emission tomography with computed tomography (PET-CT) combines the excellent spacial resolution of CT with a measure of metabolic activity via assessment of radio-labelled glucose uptake in the pleura. This modality in particular has the potential to focus image-guided pleural biopsies more accurately with trials awaited to confirm clinical utility (Figure 4.6).

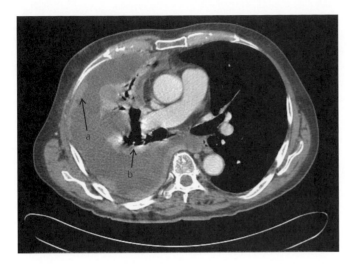

Figure 4.5 Pleural phase contrast CT scan demonstrating the thick, nodular pleural thickening of pleural malignancy (a). Note extension over the mediastinal surface (b).

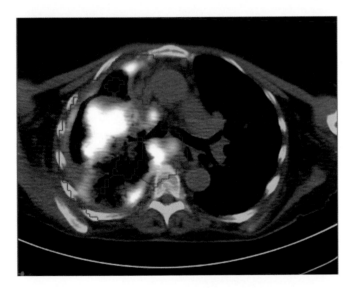

Figure 4.6 Integrated positron emission tomography with computed tomography (PET-CT) scan of right malignant pleural mesothelioma demonstrating intense areas of pleural FDG avidity. Courtesy of Professor Iain Lyburn. Cobalt Imaging Centre, Cheltenham, UK.

Dynamic MRI provides a measure of blood flow and angiogenesis within tissues and diffusion-weighted MRI measures water diffusion between cells. Early observational evidence is emerging that both modalities may have value diagnostically and prognostically in the evaluation of pleural disease.

Pleural biopsy

Biopsy of the pleura with histological examination, including immunohistochemistry and TB culture, should be performed for all patients with a persistent effusion, who are fit for the procedure, when a diagnosis has not been achieved by examination of pleural fluid and cross-sectional imaging.

The two key means of obtaining pleural tissue are via image-guided cutting needle biopsy (CT or ultrasound) or by a thoracoscopic approach. The choice between the two depends on the percutaneous accessibility of pleural thickening as assessed by CT, the need to drain pleural fluid and the relative local availability of each technique.

CT-guided cutting needle biopsy has a sensitivity of 80–90% for the diagnosis of malignant pleural disease and thoracoscopy 90–95%. Both techniques have been shown in randomised controlled trials to have superior sensitivity for malignancy and pleural TB over blind closed needle biopsy and have superseded this technique in modern practice.

Thoracoscopy can be performed under conscious sedation (local anaesthetic thoracoscopy) or general anaesthetic (video-assisted thoracoscopy). It has the advantage of allowing a visual examination of the pleural surface, and facilitating fluid drainage and pleurodesis within a single procedure. Thoracoscopy and thoracic surgery are covered in detail elsewhere in this book.

Diagnostic challenges

Despite adoption of a systematic approach as described, a proportion of patients with persistent pleural effusions remain undiagnosed. In these cases it is important to revisit the possibility of the following:

- Underlying cardiac cause (consider and echocardiogram with reporting for both systolic and diastolic failure. Send N-terminal prohormone of brain natriuretic peptide (NT-pro BNP)).
- Lymphoma (consider sending lymphocytic fluid for flow cytometry and lymphocyte sub-sets).
- Pleural TB (avoid empirical treatment but consider thoracoscopic biopsies and adenosine deaminase (ADA) or γ-interferon release assay (IGRA) for their negative predictive value).

Biopsy diagnoses of benign asbestos effusion and idiopathic pleuritis warrant clinical and radiographical follow-up for at least 12 months. Around 9% of patients with a thoracoscopic diagnosis of idiopathic pleuritis are ultimately diagnosed with malignancy. Closer surveillance is required when tissue has been obtained by percutaneous biopsy alone.

Further reading

Hooper CE, Lee YC, Maskell N; BTS Pleural Guideline Group. (2010) British Thoracic Society guidelines for the investigation of a unilateral pleural effusion in adults. *Thorax* **64**, ii4–ii17.

Light W and Lee YCG (eds). (2008) *Textbook of Pleural Diseases*, 2nd edition. Hodder Arnold.

Maskell NA, Gleeson FV and Davies RJ. (2003) Standard pleural biopsy versus CT-guided cutting-needle for the diagnosis of malignant disease in pleural effusions: a randomised controlled trial. *Lancet* **361**, 1326–1331.

Qureshi NR, Rahman NM and Gleeson FV. (2009) Thoracic ultrasound in the diagnosis of malignant pleural effusion. *Thorax* **64**, 139–143.

Venekamp LN, Velkeniers B and Noppen M. (2005) Does idiopathic pleuritis exist? Natural history of non-specific pleuritis patients diagnosed after thoracoscopy. *Respiration* **72**, 74–78.

CHAPTER 5

Pleural Pathology

Brendan Tinwell and Ian Hunt

St George's Hospital, London, UK

OVERVIEW

- The visceral and parietal pleura cover the lungs and chest wall respectively, forming a potential space which usually contains <1 mL of fluid.
- Patients with pleural disease commonly present with chest pain or shortness of breath, and can be related to pleural effusion, diffuse thickening or large mass lesions.
- Primary pleural disease (neoplastic or non-neoplastic) is much less common than secondary involvement of the pleura by disease located elsewhere.
- A range of benign and malignant neoplasms and tumour-like conditions involve the pleura, and accurate diagnosis often depends on histological examination of an adequate surgical biopsy specimen interpreted in conjunction with detailed clinical and radiological findings.

Normal anatomy and histology of the pleura

The lungs are invested by a thin serous membrane, the visceral pleura, which is reflected on to the chest wall at the hilum of each lung to form the parietal pleura, which is also reflected on to the mediastinum and diaphragm. The parietal pleura extends superiorly into the root of the neck (approximately 3 cm above the midpoint of the clavicle) and inferiorly into the costodiaphragmatic recesses at the level of the 12th rib (overlying the kidney). The visceral pleura further extends into the lung as major fissures, dividing the lungs into lobes, and can be regarded as consisting of three layers:

1 A single continuous layer of flattened mesothelial cells resting on a layer of loose collagen and elastic fibres;
2 An external elastic lamina; and
3 A vascular (interstitial) layer containing small blood vessels and lymphatics, which is continuous with interlobular septa of the lung and itself rests on an internal elastic lamina surrounding the entire lung.

Pathological processes involving the pleura

The pathological processes involving the pleura may be conveniently classified into **neoplastic** and **non-neoplastic**, the latter including inflammatory and tumour-like conditions. Primary diseases of the pleura of any type are rare (e.g. solitary fibrous tumour or malignant mesothelioma), and the pleura is usually involved secondarily by disease processes located elsewhere (e.g. bacterial pneumonia leading to empyema, or lung carcinoma with metastases to the pleura).

Pleural effusion (accumulation of fluid in the pleural space) is a common manifestation of many of these primary and secondary pleural disorders and most are related to infections, malignancy, heart failure or pulmonary emboli. Normally, there is less than 1 mL of fluid within the pleural cavity, this being maintained by a balance between hydrostatic and oncotic pressure within parietal and visceral pleural vessels, and by an extensive network of lymphatic channels which drain fluid away. Inflammatory disorders result in increased vascular permeability and therefore leakage of protein-rich serous or haemorrhagic exudate into the pleural cavity causing an **exudative pleural effusion**. Similarly, malignancies cause vascular alterations and obstruction of lymphatics resulting in an exudate forming within the pleural space.

A non-inflammatory or **transudative pleural effusion**, also referred to as hydrothorax, is typically bilateral, low in protein and usually results from increased capillary hydrostatic pressure (such as in heart failure) or reduced colloid osmotic pressure (such as in hypo-albuminaemia caused by cirrhosis or nephrotic syndrome).

Measurement of pH, glucose, protein and lactate dehydrogenase (LDH) concentrations in pleural fluid and blood may aid the distinction between exudates and transudates, but more specialised pleural fluid assays (e.g. natriuretic peptides in heart failure or chylomicrons in chylothorax) may be employed in certain cases.

Chylothorax (or chylous pleural effusion) is a special type of effusion (usually exudative) referring to accumulation of lymphocytes,

---

ABC of Pleural Diseases, First Edition. Edited by Najib M. Rahman, Ian Hunt, Fergus V. Gleeson and Nick A. Maskell.
© 2018 John Wiley & Sons Ltd. Published 2018 by John Wiley & Sons Ltd.

immunoglobulin and lipid-rich milky fluid in the pleural cavity. Chylothorax may be secondary to traumatic rupture of major lymphatic ducts or obstruction thereof by tumour, most of which are malignant lymphomas. The chylous fluid forms a creamy or fatty supernatant when left to stand and contains a high concentration of chylomicrons and triglyceride (although the latter may be low). Pseudochylothorax is caused by cholesterol crystal accumulation in any chronic pleural effusion (especially those related to tuberculosis, rheumatoid disease or chronic haemothorax) and is usually neutrophil-rich and lacking chylomicrons. Urinothorax is a rare cause of pleural effusion which may be considered in patients with undiagnosed pleural effusion associated with obstructive uropathy, urological trauma (including surgical injury) or kidney biopsy.

Of **neoplasms** involving the pleura, metastatic cancers are much more common than primary pleural tumours, greatly outnumbering the most common and most important of these, diffuse malignant mesothelioma. In the USA, for example, there are approximately 130 cases of metastatic tumour to the pleura for each case of diffuse malignant mesothelioma of the pleura. It is worth noting here that lung cancer is one of the most common tumours to metastasise to the pleura, and that there has recently been a reclassification of the American Joint Committee on Cancer (AJCC) TNM staging of lung cancer (7th edition) to reflect the fact that lung cancer patients with pleural metastases – either pleural nodules or malignant effusion, demonstrate similar survival as patients with contralateral lung nodules (both M1a) and that patients with distant visceral metastases (M1b) have significantly worse survival. Benign and malignant tumours of the pleura are listed in Table 5.1.

Table 5.1 Classification of benign and malignant neoplasms of the pleura, including tumour-like conditions.

Benign neoplasms	Primary malignant neoplasms (other than mesothelioma)
Solitary fibrous tumour	Malignant solitary fibrous tumour
Adenomatoid tumour	Pleuropulmonary blastoma
Calcifying fibrous pseudotumour	Synovial sarcoma
	Angiosarcoma
Lipoma	Epithelioid haemangioendothelioma
Lipoblastoma	Primary effusion lymphoma
Schwannoma	Pyothorax-associated lymphoma
Neurofibroma	Ewing sarcoma/PNET (Askin tumour)
	Desmoplastic small round cell tumour
	Pleural liposarcoma
	Pleural thymoma (low malignant potential)
	Pleural desmoid tumour (low malignant potential)
	Pleural Rosai–Dorfman disease

Tumour-like conditions	Secondary malignant neoplasms
Reactive eosinophilic pleuritis	Metastatic carcinoma (especially lung, breast, gastrointestinal tract, ovary and kidney)
Nodular pleural plaque	Malignant lymphoma
Amyloid deposition	Metastatic malignant melanoma
Pleuropulmonary endometriosis	Metastatic sarcoma

PNET, primitive neuroectodermal tumour.

Neoplasia (other than diffuse malignant mesothelioma) – primary pleural neoplasms and tumour-like proliferations

Benign
Solitary fibrous tumour

Solitary fibrous tumour (SFT) is the second most common primary pleural neoplasm (and the most common benign primary pleural tumour) but is far outnumbered by diffuse malignant mesothelioma of the pleura, such that SFT accounts for <5% of all primary pleural tumours. This tumour is more frequently encountered in extrapleural sites including the head and neck region, retroperitoneum, soft tissues, liver, breast, and so on and pleural tumours were previously erroneously referred to as 'localised fibrous mesothelioma'.

SFT of the pleura is thought to arise from fibroblast-like, submesothelial mesenchymal cells and affects individuals of both sexes over a wide age range (usually sixth decade), where up to 25% present with an incidental, pleural-based mass on a chest radiograph performed for other reasons. It is benign, slow-growing and not associated with asbestos exposure. Patients with malignant SFT (one-third of cases) are more likely to present with cough, chest pain, dyspnoea or pleural effusion.

Two unusual clinical syndromes are encountered with SFT:

• Pierre Marie–Bamberg syndrome (10–20%) in which patients with SFT present with digital clubbing and hypertrophic pulmonary osteoarthropathy; and
• Doege–Potter syndrome (<5%) where elaboration of insulin-like growth factor by the tumour results in episodes of refractory hypoglycaemia which resolve after surgical resection.

SFTs are typically solitary, well-circumscribed and attached to the visceral pleura by a narrow pedicle, and range in size from a few centimetres to over 25 cm. Approximately half demonstrate a sessile growth pattern and may displace the underlying lung. The cut surface of SFT is usually light grey and fibrous but may have a whorled or focally cystic appearance. Large tumours with areas of haemorrhage, necrosis or lung invasion are more likely to be malignant. The histological appearance is varied, but is often a solid, variably cellular proliferation of uniform spindle-shaped cells separated by 'ropey' collagen fibres, arranged in a short-storiform or 'patternless' pattern and associated with branching, 'staghorn' vessels (haemangiopericytoma-like pattern) (Figures 5.1 and 5.2).

A diffuse sclerosing pattern is also common, while other tumours are more cellular, consisting of sheets and fascicles of spindle cells (may mimic synovial sarcoma or fibrosarcoma). Some of these tumours have neural features and need to be differentiated from nerve sheath tumours (schwannoma) or neurofibroma. The variable histological patterns are more readily appreciated on resection specimens, and therefore care must be taken on smaller biopsy specimens as the differential diagnosis is wide.

Immunohistochemistry is important in diagnosis (especially biopsy material) and a panel incorporating epithelial markers (cytokeratin, epithelial membrane antigen), vascular markers (CD31, CD34), neural markers (S100), smooth muscle markers (smooth muscle actin and desmin) and mesothelial markers (calretinin, WT1,

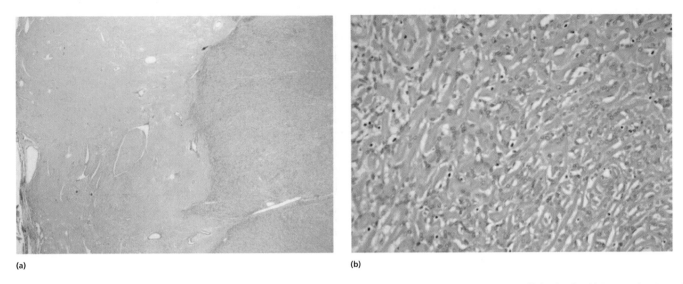

(a)   (b)

Figure 5.1 Solitary fibrous tumour (SFT): variable cellularity and branching vasculature (a) with 'patternless' arrangement of bland cells with intervening 'ropey' collagen (b).

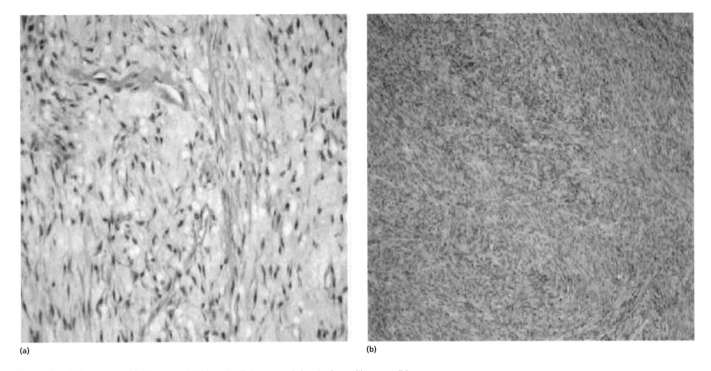

(a)   (b)

Figure 5.2 SFT: tumour exhibiting myxoid (a) and cellular, vaguely herringbone-like areas (b).

thrombomodulin) and less specific immunostains vimentin, bcl-2, CD99 and CD117 may be necessary. SFT is consistently positive for vimentin, CD34, CD99 and bcl-2, and negative for epithelial markers, S100, CD31 and smooth muscle markers (note that the positively expressed immunostains are not specific for SFT, and therefore the final diagnosis depends on consideration of the clinical, radiological, histological and panel of immunohistochemical findings).

The treatment of choice is complete surgical resection and prediction of behaviour depends on the resectability of the tumour as well as the histological appearances.

Adenomatoid tumour

Adenomatoid tumours are rare benign mesothelial neoplasms more often seen in the male or female genital tract, but are very seldom reported in the pleura, where they usually represent an incidental finding of a pleural nodule (or nodules) up to 3 cm in size.

Histologically, these tumours comprise nodular, non-invasive, expansile proliferations of tubular structures lined by flattened, vacuolated epithelioid cells expressing cytokeratin and calretinin (vascular markers are negative, and the vacuoles do not contain mucin). These tumours are distinguished from diffuse malignant mesothelioma by the lack of diffuse or invasive growth and from localised malignant mesothelioma by the characteristic adenomatoid pattern.

Calcifying fibrous pseudotumour

This is a distinctive, rare soft tissue lesion usually described in the extremities, trunk, groin or axilla, but infrequently seen in the pleura, primarily affecting young adults of either sex. It is not clear whether they represent a specific neoplasm or a reactive process.

Imaging (usually for other reasons) reveals lobular, pleural-based mass or masses, sometimes measuring up to 12 cm in size and containing areas of calcification. The nodules are well-circumscribed and demonstrate a gritty cut surface, consisting of hyalinised fibrous tissue containing bland spindle-shaped cells and scattered psammomatous microcalcifications. A sparse, perivascular chronic inflammatory cell infiltrate is usually identified. The spindle cells do not express cytokeratin or CD34 (distinguishing them from sarcomatoid malignant mesothelioma and solitary fibrous tumour, respectively).

These lesions behave in a benign fashion and local excision is usually adequate therapy, but rare recurrences have been reported.

Lipoma and lipoblastoma

These represent rare, incidental adipocytic tumours that are more commonly seen in children, and need to be distinguished from chest wall lipomas protruding into the pleural cavity. Patients may very rarely present with pain resulting from torsion and infarction.

Schwannoma and neurofibroma

These are very rare primary pleural tumours of neural origin, with only isolated cases reported. Tumours arising within the chest wall should be excluded, and it is also important to recognise that neurofibroma may also coexpress S100 and CD34, the latter marker usually associated with SFT.

Tumour-like conditions

Reactive eosinophilic pleuritis

This refers to a reactive, nodular or diffuse proliferation of inflammatory cells, including eosinophils, histiocytes, giant cells and other inflammatory cells, which is seen in the visceral pleura as a consequence of spontaneous pneumothorax. It may need to be distinguished from pleural involvement by Langerhans histiocytosis (characteristic radiographical features of this are absent and the histiocytic cells lack immunoreactivity for S100 and CD1a).

Nodular pleural plaque

This may resemble a solitary pleural nodule on chest radiography when seen 'en face', but is readily distinguished from a discrete lesion on cross-sectional computed tomography (CT) (Figure 5.3).

Amyloid deposition

Amyloid deposition in the pleura may mimic malignant mesothelioma by virtue of causing chest pain, dyspnoea and pleural effusion with diffuse nodular pleural thickening. Histological examination reveals amorphous eosinophilic material which may be associated with a foreign body giant cell reaction, and which produces a characteristic 'apple-green' birefringence when stained with Congo red and viewed under polarised light.

Pleuropulmonary endometriosis

This usually affects women of reproductive age in whom it presents with dyspnoea (related to spontaneous pneumothorax), cough (sometimes with haemoptysis) and pleuritic chest pain. A distinct pleural nodule may be seen, causing clinical and radiological confusion with a neoplasm, and histologically the presence of proliferative endometrial glands and stroma may be misdiagnosed as adenocarcinoma, biphasic mesothelioma or even pleuropulmonary blastoma.

The differential diagnoses may be readily excluded if attention is paid to the clinical context (pleuropulmonary blastoma, for instance, is practically only seen in children under 6 years of age)

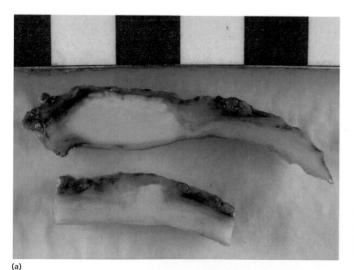

(a)

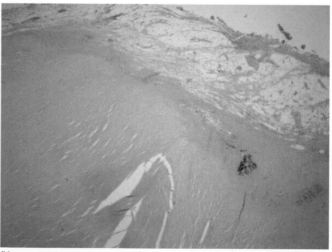

(b)

Figure 5.3 Nodular pleural plaque: macroscopic appearance of solid, 10 × 20 mm yellowish nodule (a) mimicking an expansile tumour nodule, but histology (b) reveals dense, hyalinised, 'basket-weave' collagen only.

and lack of significant glandular or stromal atypia (immunohisto-chemistry may be helpful in small biopsies).

Malignant pleural neoplasms (other than malignant mesothelioma)

Malignant solitary fibrous tumour

Malignant SFTs make up approximately one-third of cases of SFT, and are generally symptomatic. They are characterised by frequent local recurrence, and may metastasise, but do not involve the pleural surface in a diffuse manner like malignant mesothelioma. There are no unifying histological criteria for malignancy, and resectability is perhaps the most important indicator of malignant behaviour.

Reported histological findings associated with malignancy include increased mitotic activity (>4 mitotic figures/10 high power fields), high cellularity with nuclear crowding and overlapping and the presence of coagulative tumour cell necrosis and significant nuclear pleomorphism. The presence of these histological features in the context of a sessile tumour are predictive of recurrence.

Pleuropulmonary blastoma

This is a rare paediatric neoplasm characterised by a biphasic histo-logical appearance which includes benign epithelial elements and primitive, embryonic-like mesenchymal stroma. It is not to be con-fused with pulmonary blastoma which affects adults (mean age at diagnosis of 35 years). These tumours have a variable cystic and solid appearance and may present with hydropneumothorax. Radical surgery followed by chemoradiotherapy may be associated with long-term survival.

Synovial sarcoma

Synovial sarcoma (SS) is typically a biphasic spindle cell tumour with a cytokeratin expressing epithelioid component (except for monophasic spindle cell variants) that is usually seen around joints in the extremities of young adults. Rare primary pleural SS are described, exhibiting a wide age range (9–69 years) and usually pre-senting with chest pain, dyspnoea, cough or effusion related to pre-dominantly solid, pleural-based masses. Detection of the t(X:18) translocation within surgical biopsy specimens is a very useful adjunctive test to confirm the diagnosis.

Epithelioid haemangioendothelioma

This tumour, derived from vascular endothelium, usually develops in the lungs as multiple nodules, but occasionally mimics malig-nant mesothelioma clinically and radiologically. Patients are usu-ally over 45 years of age and may have a history of asbestos exposure. The tumour cells may appear epithelioid or spindled, and the pres-ence of intracytoplasmic lumina may impart a signet ring like appearance, causing confusion with metastatic adenocarcinoma. Focal positivity for cytokeratin immunostains may cause further confusion with mesothelioma, but positive staining for vascular markers, CD31 and CD34, confirms the diagnosis.

Pleural thymoma

Pleural involvement by thymoma is usually in the context of an anterior mediastinal mass that spreads to the pleura, but rare cases involve the pleura in a diffuse fashion without evidence of a primary mediastinal mass. Primary pleural thymomas typically present in adults (6th decade) as nodular or diffuse thickening of the pleura, and may be indistinguishable clinically or radiologically from malignant mesothelioma. Patients infrequently present with myasthaenia gravis or haematological abnormalities. Recognition of a lobular architecture and dense lymphocytic infiltrate (predom-inantly T cells with immature TdT positive phenotype) with an arborising network of cytokeratin-positive cells aids correct diag-nosis of typical cases but confusion may occur with lymphocyte-poor tumours or cases with spindle cell morphology. The histological differential diagnosis includes pleural invasion from mediastinal thymoma, lymphoma, metastatic carcinoma, meta-static seminoma, mesothelioma and pleural sarcoma. The progno-sis of these tumours depends on the extent of disease and thus resectability thereof (Figure 5.4).

Inflammation

Inflammation of the pleura histologically (pleuritis) is usually either fibrinous (acute), fibrous (chronic) or a combination of both (organising acute process). Inflammatory diseases of the lung, for example bacterial pneumonia, pulmonary infarction or bronchiectasis, are common causes of acute fibrinous pleuritis, but rarely the pleura may become primarily infected as a result of haematogenous seeding during the course of transient bacteraemia.

Pleural empyema refers to the presence of frank pus within the pleural cavity (representing the most severe form of acute fibrinous pleuritis), which may be a complication of pneumonia, ruptured lung abscess, penetrating chest trauma (including surgical proce-dures or thoracentesis), oesophageal perforation or extension from paravertebral, subdiaphragmatic or hepatic abscesses (Figure 5.5). An empyema may become loculated or undergo organisation, forming a pleural peel or dense fibrous adhesions between the chest wall and the lung (restriction of lung function is rare, but may occur with so-called fibrothorax; Figure 5.6).

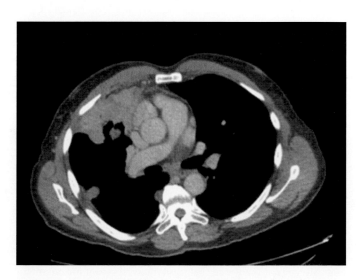

Figure 5.4 Chest CT demonstarting pleural thymoma.

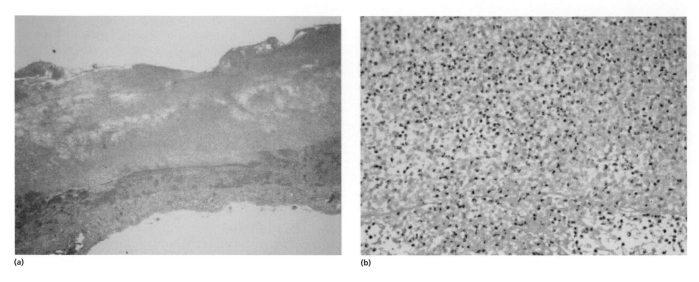

(a) (b)

Figure 5.5 Histology of acute pleural empyema showing a thick layer of fibrinopurulent exudate overlying congested parietal pleura (a) and containing numerous neutrophils and necrotic inflammatory cells (b).

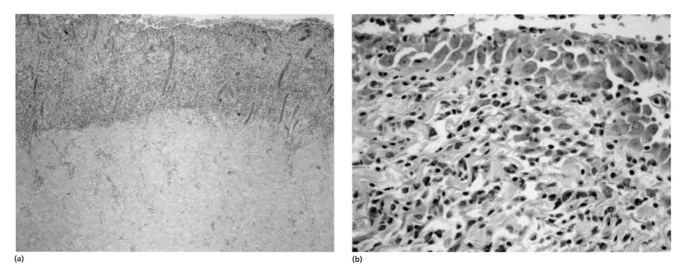

(a) (b)

Figure 5.6 Organising fibrinous pleuritis demonstrating fibrosis, dense chronic inflammation and vertically oriented vessels (a) and an example of eosinophilic pleuritis associated with mesothelial hyperplasia (b).

Chronic fibrous pleuritis is a relatively non-specific pattern of inflammation which may be secondary to a wide variety of conditions. Discrimination of reactive fibrous pleuritis from desmoplastic sarcomatoid mesothelioma may be problematic in small biopsies.

Eosinophilic pleuritis is typically associated with spontaneous pneumothorax in young adults, but may be so exuberant as to mimic tumours of the pleura. Eosinophilic inflammation may also be associated with Langerhans cell histiocytosis, parasitic infestation, drug reactions, lymphangioleiomyomatosis and Hodgkin lymphoma.

Granulomatous pleuritis is a specific form of chronic pleuritis characterised by the presence of aggregates of epithelioid histiocytes (granulomas) often with multinucleated giant cells, which may be associated with areas of necrosis also referred to as 'caseation' (Figure 5.7). Granulomatous pleuritis is often infective in nature (e.g. tuberculosis or fungal infection) and, if this is considered clinically, it is advised that fresh material is sent for microbiological investigation at the time of surgical biopsy as special histological stains may be negative for organisms despite the

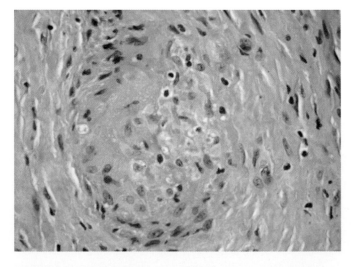

Figure 5.7 Granulomatous pleuritis: a discrete aggregate of epithelioid histiocytes forming a granuloma.

presence of infection. Non-infective causes of granulomatous inflammation in the pleura include sarcoidosis and rheumatoid nodules.

Further reading

Cagle PT and Allen TC. (2011) Pathology of the pleura: what the pulmonologists need to know. *Respirology* **16**, 430–438.

Granville L, Laga AC, Allen TC, Dishop M, Roggli, VL, Churg A *et al.* (2005) Review and update of uncommon primary pleural tumours: a practical approach to diagnosis. *Archives of Pathology and Laboratory Medicine* **129**, 1428–1443.

Guinee DG and Allen TC. (2008) Primary pleural neoplasia: entities other than diffuse malignant mesothelioma. *Archives of Pathology and Laboratory Medicine* **132**, 1149–1170.

Kumar V, Abbas AK and Fausto N. (eds) (2014) *Robbins and Cotran Pathologic Basis of Disease*, 9th edn. Elsevier.

Moran CA and Suster S. (2010) *Tumours and Tumour-like Conditions of the Lung and Pleura*, Saunders Elsevier.

Ryu JH, Tomassetti S and Maldonado F. (2011) Update on uncommon pleural effusions. *Respirology* **16**, 238–243.

CHAPTER 6

Unusual Causes of Pleural Disease

David Feller-Kopman

Johns Hopkins Medical School, Baltimore, MD, USA

OVERVIEW

- Become familiar with the more uncommon aetiologies of pleural effusions.
- Learn the proper clinical context in which one should suspect a more uncommon aetiology for pleural effusion.
- Identify proper evaluation of the more uncommon causes (i.e. additional pleural fluid testing, additional imaging) of pleural effusions.
- Become familiar with management strategies, including proper follow-up, for uncommon pleural effusions.

Urinothorax

Urinothorax is defined by the presence of urine within the pleural space and is most often associated with an obstructive uropathy. The mechanism behind the accumulation of urinothorax has not been consistently demonstrated in animals models, but many believe direct cephalad extension through the diaphragm and/or lymphatic transport are responsible.

The true incidence of urinothorax is difficult to obtain as a recent review noted only 58 cases reported in the human literature. Some authors believe the true incidence is under-reported, though it appears that the highest risk patients are those undergoing renal and/or ureteral manipulation, those with obstructive calculi, blunt abdominal trauma or those with genitourinary malignancy or infection.

Aspiration of a urinothorax should reveal a straw-coloured fluid, possibly even smelling like urine. The fluid is transudative and may present with a low pH, as urinary pH is often in the 5.0–7.0 range. Pleural glucose and protein levels are traditionally low; however, lactate dehydrogenase (LDH) levels may be high and run the risk of misclassifying the effusion as an exudate. A biochemical diagnosis has been classically obtained from a pleural fluid creatinine to serum creatinine ratio of greater than one. If further diagnostic studies are needed, the use of radionuclide scintigraphy (99mTc ethylene dicysteine) has been reported to be helpful.

Treatment involves addressing the underlying genitourinary disease, as resolution of the effusion follows correction of the obstructive uropathy. If the effusion does not resolve within a few weeks, an alternative diagnosis should be sought.

Yellow nail syndrome

Yellow nail syndrome is a rare entity initially described in the 1960s associated with yellow or abnormal nails, lymphoedema, and respiratory symptoms including cough, dyspnoea and recurrent pleural effusions (Figures 6.1–6.3). The underlying mechanism has still not been elucidated but most believe functional and anatomical lymphatic problems are to blame.

Approximately 150 cases of yellow nail syndrome have been reported in the literature. Most patients present in the 4th–6th decade with bilateral pleural effusions. Yellow nail syndrome is a clinical diagnosis and though there are no pathognomonic features in pleural fluid analysis, they are typically exudative in nature. Thirty percent of patients present with a chylothorax. Effusions in yellow nail syndrome tend to be recurrent and difficult to control, but in those with chylothorax, thoracic duct ligation may be an option as are ventriculo-peritoneal shunts (Figure 6.4).

Ovarian hyperstimulation syndrome

Ovarian hyperstimulation syndrome (OHS) is a well-described adverse reaction to human chorionic gonadotrophin presenting with symptoms related to a diffuse capillary leakage syndrome. OHS can occur in up to 5% of patients receiving human chorionic gonadotrophin stimulation for fertility treatments. Varying degrees of abdominal pain, dyspnoea, anasarca, ascites, pleural or pericardial effusion, renal insufficiency and haemoconcentration can be present. The syndrome appears to be closely related to the lifespan of the corpus luteum and most commonly presents 5–7 days after receiving human chorionic gonadotropin. The presence of significantly enlarged ovaries in the setting of recent human chorionic gonadotrophin administration or pregnancy should suggest the diagnosis.

In those with severe disease requiring hospital admission, thoracic radiographs can be abnormal in up to 80%, with bilateral pleural effusion being present in approximately one-third. Pleural fluid has been reported as a characteristic protein-rich exudate with normal LDH levels. However, a number of other reports have simply described a hydrothorax.

ABC of Pleural Diseases, First Edition. Edited by Najib M. Rahman, Ian Hunt, Fergus V. Gleeson and Nick A. Maskell.

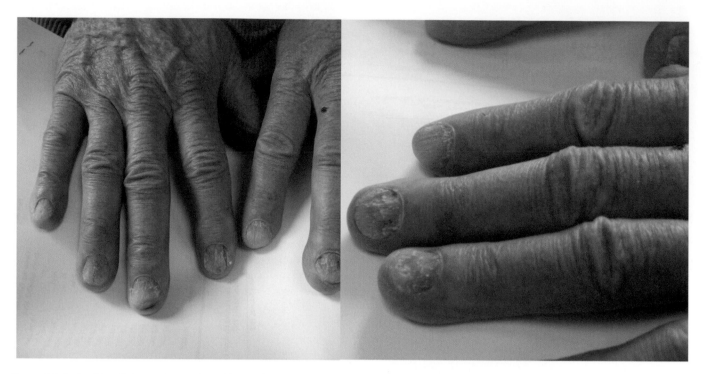

Figure 6.1 Dystrophic nail changes in a patient with typical yellow nail syndrome.

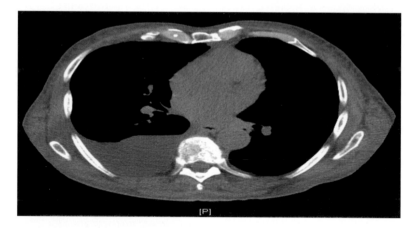

Figure 6.2 CT of the thorax demonstrating a bland-looking effusion in a patient with nail changes.

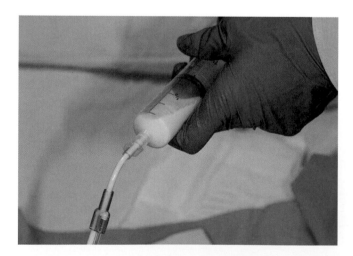

Figure 6.3 Thoracentesis of fluid, demonstrating milky pleural fluid.

Treatment remains supportive, with pleural drainage for symptomatic relief or to rule out infection. The effusion typically resolves over the following 1–2 weeks without further intervention.

Meigs syndrome

Meigs syndrome, initially described in 1937, is defined as the presence of ascites and pleural effusions with complete resolution after removal of benign ovarian tumours. The pathophysiology of Meigs syndrome has not been clearly defined but theories such as excessive tumour surface fluid transudation, lymphatic obstruction or increased vasculature permeability secondary to vasoactive growth factors have all been advocated.

Patients presenting with a pleural effusion and a gynaecological mass should undergo pleural fluid sampling as part of a malignancy diagnostic work-up, with Meigs syndrome remaining a diagnosis of

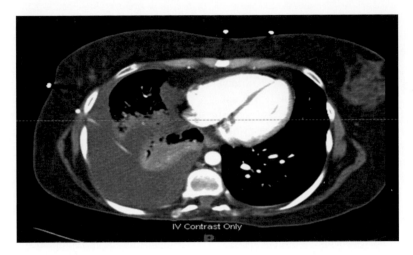

Figure 6.4 CT scan demonstrating a ventriculo-peritoneal shunt.

exclusion. The pleural fluid in Meigs syndrome is typically a transudate, and though suggestive of a benign aetiology, work-up of the pelvic mass should continue. Pleural effusions are commonly right-sided but a large series found 10% can be left-sided and 22% were bilateral.

Treatment options are purely supportive as pleural effusions should resolve after removal of the ovarian tumour. If this does not occur, another diagnosis should be entertained. Repeat thoracentesis may be required for symptomatic relief until surgical removal of the ovarian tumour can be completed.

Dural-pleural fistula

Dural-pleural fistulae are defined by an abnormal connection between the subarachnoid space and pleural space. They have been reported after spinal trauma and vertebral neoplasms but have also been seen after thoracotomy.

Patients present with varying neurological symptoms ranging from headaches to recurrent meningitis along with pulmonary symptoms related to recurrent pleural effusions. The pleural fluid is transudative and more representative of cerebrospinal fluid with normal glucose, protein and chloride levels. Beta-2-transferrin is found only in cerebrospinal fluid and inner ear perilymph, making its presence in pleural fluid diagnostic of dural-pleural fistula. The clear identification of cerebrospinal fluid or beta-2-transferrin may be difficult as there is often mixing of pleural and cerebrospinal fluid within the pleural space. Some authors have even reported cases of exudative effusions related to dural-pleural fistulas, but believe this phenomenon was related to a concomitant haemothorax. The presence of beta-2-transferrin in pleural fluid is diagnostic of a dural-pleural fistula, but its absence does not rule one out.

Multiple imaging techniques are available for diagnosis including radioisotope cisternography, myelogram and computed tomography myelogram, with the latter offering the best anatomical definition to plan surgical interventions preoperatively.

Treatment varies, and because of the paucity of literature it has been recommended a single therapeutic approach should not be utilised. In general, if a leak is properly identified, the prognosis is good. Multi-disciplinary evaluation is suggested as treatment regimens have included observation with spontaneous resolution, chest drainage with tube thoracostomy, lumbar drainage, local exploration and closure of defect, or more advanced procedures including thoracoplasty and muscle flap placements.

Central venous catheter migration

Identifying the presence of intravenous infusate within the pleural space defines an effusion resulting from extravascular migration of a central venous catheter. One is typically able to identify an abnormal radiograph with malpositioning of the catheter, but attention to detail in examining the radiograph is crucial.

The presence of a rapidly expanding pleural effusion in the setting of a recently placed central venous catheter should raise the suspicion of extravascular placement or migration. The pleural fluid may be either transudative or exudative, depending on the nature of the infusate the patient is receiving. Pleural fluid may appear milky if the patient is receiving a lipid infusion through the extravasated line, and have a high pleural fluid : serum glucose ratio in patients receiving parental glucose infusions. One may suspect that most catheter-related pleural effusions would be unilateral and ipsilateral; however, reports of contralateral and bilateral effusions have been reported.

Management relies on prompt recognition and removal of the migrated catheter. Some have advocated observation of small, asymptomatic pleural effusions, with plans for intervention in those effusions causing respiratory embarrassment or haemothorax.

Chylothorax

Chyle in the pleural space, or chylothorax, is highly suggestive of a disruption of the thoracic duct. Chyle is a lymphocyte-rich fluid combined with immunoglobulins and lipids, being described as milky white in appearance. The aetiology of chylothorax can be broadly separated into traumatic and non-traumatic causes, with trauma being the underlying aetiology in 40% of cases.

Chylothorax is often not suspected until after milky-white pleural fluid is visualised, but should be included in the differential in certain situations. Non-traumatic chylothorax is most commonly seen in malignancies such as lymphoma, and should also be suspected in cases of pleural effusions with concomitant significant mediastinal lymphadenopathy. Traumatic chylothorax is commonly seen after oesophageal surgery, but can be seen after almost any other cardiac, thoracic, neurosurgical or neck surgery where thoracic duct injury is possible. Chylothorax has also been reported after penetrating injuries, motor vehicles accidents or even severe coughing.

Traditional teaching has been that pleural fluid triglyceride levels greater than 110 mg/dL were diagnostic for chylothorax, less than 50 mg/dL essentially ruled out chylothorax and the range of 50–110 mg/dL required further analysis with lipoprotein analysis. More recent study has called this teaching into question, based on the fact that up to 15% of patients with chylothorax had triglyceride levels of less than 110 mg/dL, including some with levels less than 50 mg/dL. Chylothorax is ultimately diagnosed with a pleural fluid lipoprotein analysis that is positive for chylomicrons. Imaging studies including lymphangiography and lymphoscintigraphy have been utilised by some to identify the site of leak, but the impact on patient management remains undefined.

Treatment remains highly dependent on the underlying aetiology and therefore consensus guidelines have not been identified. Therapeutic aspiration of pleural fluid is clearly indicated for symptomatic relief, with some patients requiring tube thoracostomy for continued drainage. Non-surgical management has been generally advocated in traumatic chylothorax, as resolution occurs in up to 80%. Dietary modifications including the use of medium chain triglycerides, low-fat diet and total parental nutrition have all been advocated attempting to minimise the production of chyle. Medications such as somatostatin and octreotide have also been utilised with some success.

In patients with poorly responsive malignancies who are poor surgical candidates, the use of tunnelled pleural catheters may provide palliative relief. Another non-surgical intervention is thoracic duct embolisation, with a recent report claiming a success rate of greater than 80%.

Surgical intervention is suggested in those with continued pleural output of more than 1.5 L/day, no decrease in pleural output over 2 weeks or signs of worsening malnutrition or immunosuppression resultant from the continued loss of chyle. Surgical management options include pleurodesis, thoracic duct repair/ligation, lympho-venous anastamosis and pleurectomy.

Pseudochylothorax

A pseudochylothorax, also known as a cholesterol effusion, may develop as an asymptomatic pleural effusion in patients with lung entrapment. It is often related to a chronic underlying pleural space 'problem'; such as tuberculous pleurisy, rheumatoid pleuritis, chronic pneumothorax or empyema. The exact mechanism for increased cholesterol levels in the pleural space has not been identified, but some believe the abnormal parietal pleura prevents cholesterol efflux, and therefore cholesterol accumulates within the pleural space.

Patients may be asymptomatic one-third of the time. The gross appearance of fluid may appear similar to a classic chylothorax; however, unlike a chylothorax presenting with elevated triglyceride levels, the hallmark of a pseudochylothorax is the presence of an elevated pleural fluid cholesterol level with relatively low triglyceride levels. The diagnosis is established by a pleural fluid cholesterol level of more than 200 mg/dL (>5.18 mmol/L) or the presence of cholesterol crystals and absence of chylomicrons. Pleural fluid protein levels are often higher than 50 mg/dL along with a pleural fluid cholesterol to triglyceride ratio greater than one.

Management of pseudochylothorax is directed at the underlying pleural space disease process along with symptomatic relief directly related to the pleural effusion. Therapeutic thoracentesis, decortication and pleurodesis have been used with some success, but often the effusion will resolve if the underlying disease is treated effectively.

Further reading

Garcia-Pachon E and Romero S. (2006) Urinothorax: a new approach. *Current Opinion in Pulmonary Medicine* **12** (4), 259–263.

Lloyd C and Sahn SA. (2002) Subarachnoid pleural fistula due to penetrating trauma: case report and review of the literature. *Chest* **122** (6), 2252–2256.

Maldonado F and Ryu J. (2009) Yellow nail syndrome. *Current Opinion in Pulmonary Medicine* **15**, 371–375.

Man A, Schwarz Y and Greif J. (1997) Pleural effusion as a presenting symptom of ovarian hyperstimulation syndrome. *European Respiratory Journal* **10**, 2425–2426.

Sahn SA. (2008) The value of pleural fluid analysis. *American Journal of Medical Sciences* **335** (1), 7–15.

CHAPTER 7

Pleural Infection

Ian Hunt[1] and Najib M. Rahman[2]

[1] St. George's Hospital, London, UK
[2] Oxford Centre for Respiratory Medicine, Churchill Hospital, Oxford, UK

OVERVIEW

- Pleural infection in the presence of bacteria within the pleural space is usually a complication of underlying pneumonia.

- Overall, around 8% of patients with pneumonia will develop pleural infection.

- Symptoms may be those of sepsis or a longer term indolent illness.

- Diagnosis is made based on radiological findings and then pleural aspirate under ultrasound guidance.

- The presence of frank pus (empyema), low pleural pH (complicated parapneumonic effusion) or positive pleural fluid microbiology are diagnostic of pleural infection. All of these conditions require prompt intercostal drainage (under image guidance).

- Treatment includes broad-spectrum antibiotics (for a total of 4–6 weeks with 1 week of intravenous therapy) and chest drainage.

- Around 70% of patients will respond to antibiotics and chest drainage – those not responding clinically should be referred promptly for thoracic surgical intervention.

- Surgical treatment of pleural infection aims to debride the pleural cavity and re-expand the underlying lung to avoid the long-term complications of persistent pleural infection and trapped lung.

Pleural infection is the presence of infected fluid or material in the pleural space, and includes both empyema (the presence of frank pus) and complicated parapneumonic effusion (the presence of bacteria or evidence of bacterial infection). Pleural infection is a life-threatening condition, even in young people. In the UK, the mortality is 20%, the risk of death being higher in the elderly. Early medical intervention is associated with better outcomes. A significant proportion (20%) will require a thoracic surgical procedure to treat the acute illness or prevent long-term complications.

Pleural infection typically develops from a parapneumonic effusion although an iatrogenic pleural infection may complicate thoracic or oesophageal surgery or chest drain insertion (Box 7.1). The origins of cardiothoracic surgery can probably be traced back to the management of empyema in Ancient Greece. Hippocrates described how those afflicted, often from battlefield chest wounds,

were typically sweaty and feverish with sunken eyes, curled fingernails and warm fingers. Those that survived the initial illness developed spontaneous discharge of pus through the chest wall (empyema necessitans). This was sometimes assisted by cautery or incision. There was a recognition even then that assisted open drainage performed too early resulted in death, although it would take another two thousand years to relearn these lessons.

The management of empyema changed little for two millennia. However, the advent of the underwater seal prevented death from pneumothorax (or sucking chest wound) seen with open drainage performed too early in the disease process. During the First World War, the US Army Empyema Commission investigated the high mortality associated with empyema treatment. Their subsequent recommendations on nutrition, obliteration of the pleural space, closed tube drainage and timing of intervention reduced death rates significantly. The discovery of antibiotics and advances in anaesthetic techniques in the first half of the twentieth century enabled the development of the medical and surgical treatment of empyema that forms the basis of present day care. In particular, modern keyhole video-assisted thoracic surgery (VATS) techniques allow effective treatment of even the most severe forms of pleural infection.

Pathology

It is estimated that over 50% of patients with pneumonia will develop a parapneumonic effusion. The majority of these are 'simple' effusions (i.e. will resolve with antibiotic treatment alone). However, in a proportion, bacteria translocate to the pleural fluid and establish infection, at which point antibiotics alone will not resolve the infection. Overall, around 8% of patients with pneumonia develop an infected pleural collection.

There are three stages in the development of a pleural infection:

1 *Exudative/simple.* A simple effusion forms adjacent to the infected lung, resulting from increased vascular permeability and the production of inflammatory mediators.
2 *Fibrinopurulent/complicated.* The effusion becomes complicated by infection as a result of translocation of bacteria across the

---

ABC of Pleural Diseases, First Edition. Edited by Najib M. Rahman, Ian Hunt, Fergus V. Gleeson and Nick A. Maskell.
© 2018 John Wiley & Sons Ltd. Published 2018 by John Wiley & Sons Ltd.

visceral pleura. Pleural fluid pH and glucose fall while lactate dehydrogenase (LDH) rises (complicated parapnuemonic effusion). A macroscopically purulent effusion then develops with fibrin deposition (empyema). Fibrin strands may cause the effusion to become septated (formation of several pockets of fluid rather than one larger collection) and loculated (distinct areas of pleural fluid in separate parts of the pleural space).

3 *Organising/chronic.* Both the visceral and parietal pleura become thickened and the lung is encased by a fibrous peel or cortex.

Bacteriology

Around 60% of patients with pleural infection have positive pleural fluid cultures while only 12% have positive blood cultures. Therefore, throughout treatment, in around 40% of cases there will be no identifiable causative organism.

Streptococcus species and *Staphylococcus aureus* are most often seen in community-acquired parapneumonic empyemas. Gram-negative bacteria (e.g. *Escherichia coli, Haemophilus influenzae* and enterococci) and anaerobes (e.g. *Bacteroides* species) are also commonly isolated. Hospital-acquired empyemas (both iatrogenic and parapneumonic) are often caused by methicillin-resistant *Staphylococcus aureus* (MRSA), *Staphylococcus aureus*, enterococci and *Pseudomonas aeruginosa.*

Natural history

Untreated, pleural infection may resolve spontaneously but this is highly unlikely. The patient is at risk of a complication of the empyema:

- Septicaemia
- Invasion into the bronchial tree (bronchopleural fistula)
- Invasion through the chest wall with spontaneous external drainage (empyema necessitans)
- Chronic lung fibrosis with hemithorax contraction
- Osteomyelitis
- Death.

Symptoms and signs

The patient's condition may range from asymptomatic to severely septic. There is not always a history of a predisposing pneumonia. The patient's signs and symptoms will depend on their age, comorbidities, severity of the underlying pneumonia, and the size and stage of the pleural infection. Symptoms include shortness of breath, chest pain, cough and fever.

Unlike other infections, pleural infection can develop as an indolent illness over weeks to months with weight loss, cachexia and general malaise. In association with the chest X-ray findings, this is often referred as a potential cancer.

Hypoxia and fever are common findings. Cardiovascular signs (hypotension and tachycardia) are present in toxic patients, while examination of the chest may reveal a dull percussion note with reduced vocal resonance and air entry consistent with a pleural effusion. In longer term pleural infections, digital clubbing and contraction of the hemithorax may occur.

Diagnosis

The diagnosis of pleural infection should be suspected if a patient fails to respond clinically to adequate treatment of pneumonia within 48–72 hours. Inflammatory markers (white cell count (WCC) and C-reactive protein (CRP)) remain raised and an effusion may be present on chest X-ray. Blood cultures should be performed as they may reveal the underlying organism. A thoracic ultrasound and pleural fluid aspiration should be performed.

Thoracic ultrasound scan

Thoracic ultrasound will confirm the presence of an effusion. Ultrasound is now mandatory for guiding aspiration or drainage of pleural fluid, and it may demonstrate additional diagnostic information – ultrasound is highly sensitive (more than CT) for the detection of septations (Figure 7.1).

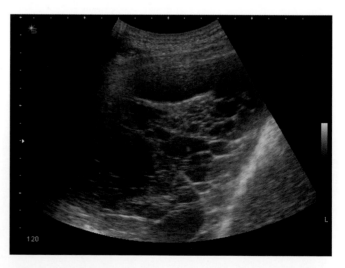

Figure 7.1 Thoracic ultrasound showing heavily septated complicated parapneumonic effusion.

Pleural fluid aspiration

Diagnostic aspiration and analysis of pleural fluid is the most important test in guiding management. Aspiration of frank pus or turbid fluid is diagnostic of an empyema. Non-purulent fluid should be checked for pH (using a blood gas analyser); an acidic pleural aspirate (pH <7.2) is diagnostic of complicated parapneumonic infection. This is usually associated with a low pleural glucose (<3.4 mmol/L) and high LDH (>1000 IU/L). The fluid should also be sent for Gram stain and culture, and recent evidence suggests sending pleural fluid in 'blood culture bottle' media can increase microbiological yield. Additionally, it should be sent for cytological analysis if an underlying malignancy is suspected.

Further imaging

CT scanning can be helpful if doubt remains around the diagnosis of empyema or if an underlying cause such as malignancy is suspected. CT in pleural infection will typically demonstrate the presence of enhancing visceral and parietal pleural surfaces (known as the 'split pleura' sign) and may demonstrate underlying lung consolidation and other abnormalities such as parenchymal lung abscess. Pleural thickening is almost always seen. There is often an associated reactive mediastinal lymphadenopathy. A CT scan is essential in those patients being considered for surgery as it helps the surgeon decide the best approach and type of operation and may guide the position of the surgical ports. Magnetic resonance imaging (MRI) does not generally provide any additional information, but may be useful in selected younger patients to reduce radiation dose.

Medical management

The goals are to treat the underlying cause of the pleural infection, drain the infected pleural fluid and eliminate the pleural space while simultaneously addressing nutrition, mobility and the prevention of thromboembolic disease. Antibiotics and chest drainage are the cornerstones of initial medical management.

Initial care

While some patients with empyema can be relatively asymptomatic, others may be profoundly septic and moribund. There may be respiratory compromise secondary to the original pneumonia. In addition, the mass effect of the fluid or pus may compress the underlying lung causing further respiratory embarrassment. Signs of sepsis and haemodynamic compromise may also be present. It is essential therefore that resuscitation and restoration of normal physiological parameters are performed first. This may involve the administration of oxygen, respiratory support, fluid boluses or the use of vasopressors.

Antibiotics

Antibiotic therapy should be started immediately and cover all likely bacteria as dictated by the probable underlying cause. The microbiology of community-acquired and hospital-acquired pleural infection are distinct, and different from pneumonia. Antibiotics may later be rationalised in the light of positive pleural or blood cultures. Initial treatment should cover Gram positives and anaerobes in community-acquired infection, and cover MRSA and resistant Gram negatives in hospital-acquired infection until culture results are known. The optimal duration of treatment is unknown but a total treatment course of around 4–6 weeks is typical, with at least 1 week of intravenous treatment. Penicillins and cephalosporins have good pleural penetration but aminoglycosides are not effective in the pleural space and should be avoided.

Chest tube drainage

Box 7.2 details the indications for drainage of the effusion. An intercostal chest drain should only be inserted under ultrasound guidance, and ideally should be placed in a dependent position. Although it has been a widely held view that a large bore drain (>20 Fr) should be used, there is no conclusive evidence for this, and smaller bore drains appear to be equally effective. Smaller bore drains should receive regular sterile saline flushes to maintain patency.

Fibrinolytics

Fibrinolytics (e.g. streptokinase, t-PA) have been assessed for their efficacy in breaking down fibrin strands and encouraging complete pleural drainage in pleural infection. Randomised evidence and meta-analysis of methodologically sound trials suggest fibrinolytics alone do not alter clinically important outcomes and should not be used. However, a recent randomised trial demonstrates that the combination of intrapleural tPA and DNase significantly improves drainage and may prevent the need for surgery. Further trials are required before routine use.

There is early evidence that intrapleural lavage using saline may help to improve the radiographic appearance and reduce surgical referral in pleural infection, but further trials are required to assess this potentially highly accessible treatment further.

If pleural infection is treated appropriately at an early stage, non-surgical management is curative in around 70% of cases. Drains should remain in place until there is radiological and clinical improvement and the amount of fluid drainage each day is minimal.

Surgery

Surgery should be considered when sepsis and a pleural effusion or empyema remain despite appropriate non-surgical treatment. A surgical opinion should be sought early after starting treatment in the absence of clear clinical improvement. Other indications for surgery include the presence of a multi-loculated pleural collection or the presence of a thick cortex 'trapping' the lung in the context of a continuingly septic patient.

Box 7.2 **Indications for drainage of an empyema**

- Frank pus
- Organisms in the pleural fluid
- Pleural fluid pH <7.2
- Loculated effusion
- Symptomatic large effusion

The earlier the patient is referred in the disease process, the more likely the pleural infection can be dealt with through a minimally invasive VATS technique with the advantage of quicker recovery and lower risks of complications from the surgery.

VATS debridement and decortication

A VATS approach, usually performed through two or three port incisions, aims to break down any loculations, drain the pleural collection, remove fibrin debris and, if necessary, remove the thickened visceral fibrous cortex for lung re-expansion and obliteration of the pleural space (Figure 7.2). Drains are placed under direct vision and with early mobilisation and physiotherapy termination of the pleural infection and early discharge can be achieved. With early referral the majority of pleural infections requiring surgical intervention are now managed in this way.

Rib resection and drainage

Through a technique described during the Napoleonic Wars, resection of a small (5 cm) portion of rib in a dependent position allows access to the pleural space and enables the breakdown of loculations with the evacuation of fluid, pus or debris. It is often combined with placing a large-bore 'empyema' drain which is gradually shortened over time as the infection abates. It is a quick, uncomplicated, safe and effective method of draining empyemas. Furthermore, it can be performed under local anaesthetic in patients who are too frail to tolerate general anaesthesia.

Thoracotomy decortication

On occasion, thoracotomy and decortication (peeling of the fibrous cortex off the lung surface) with drainage of the empyema and re-expansion of the 'trapped' lung is needed. However, with better medical management and early referral for surgical intervention in those who are failing to respond to antibiotics and drainage, the need to perform such potentially extensive procedures has reduced significantly over the last decade. It tends to be offered now to patients who have gone on to develop long-term complications of their original empyema with significant lung entrapment and contraction of the hemithorax.

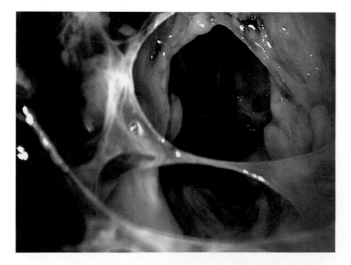

Figure 7.2 Empyema at the time of video-assisted thoracic surgery (VATS).

Open window thoracostomy

Rarely, a chest wall stoma, or fenestration, can be fashioned in those patients with trapped lung who are too frail to withstand major surgery. Originally a technique for managing pneumonectomy (lung removed) space pleural infection, two or more ribs are resected in a dependent position. The pleural cavity is marsupialised by suturing the skin to the parietal pleura, thus creating a stoma. This allows free drainage of pleural pus into a stoma bag or dressing. The stoma may need to be kept patent with an empyema tube.

Thoracoplasty

Thoracoplasty, or collapse of the chest wall by resecting or dividing ribs, was originally used to control upper lobe disease or pleural space issues in the context of tuberculosis. However, it is still very occasionally used today to manage a persistent pleural space in the setting of empyema (often fungal) and a diseased lung that fails to fill the chest cavity. It would normally only be considered once other options (e.g. decortication) had failed. The advantage over a thoracostomy is that there is no long-term open drainage. Surgery should draw a line under matters, although it can be disfiguring.

Trapped lung

The phenomenon of trapped lung describes the situation in which the lung fails to re-expand after drainage of a pleural effusion. The cause is a thickened cortex of fibrotic tissue overlying or incorporating the visceral pleura, encasing the lung.

Prognosis and long-term outcomes

Empyema can be a fatal disease if not treated promptly and appropriately. Several factors are thought to be associated with poor outcomes (Box 7.3), but these have not been shown to be consistently predictive of poor outcome in studies. Currently, 20% of all patients in the UK die as a result of their empyema.

The mortality associated with surgical intervention is 2–6% but depends very much on age, frailty of the patient and type of surgical approach.

While there are few data available detailing quality of life after surgery or non-surgical treatment, most patients would appear to regain their pre-morbid functional status. Occasionally, however, a patient may be left with a chronic contracted fibrothorax causing respiratory compromise and incapacitation. A surgical decortication and pleurectomy may help restore respiratory function.

Box 7.3 **Factors associated with poor outcomes**

- Increasing age
- Poor nutritional status
- Hypo-albuminaemia
- Delay to pleural drainage
- Chest malignancy

Conclusions

A pleural effusion will develop in a significant proportion of patients with pneumonia. Pleural infection is therefore relatively common and prompt and appropriate treatment can prevent complications or the need for surgical intervention. A respiratory physician should be involved early in the disease process. Similarly, a thoracic surgeon should be consulted promptly if more conservative measures fail to produce a quick improvement in the patient's condition.

Further reading

Davies HE, Davies RJO and Davies CWH. (2010) Management of pleural infection in adults: British Thoracic Society pleural disease guideline 2010. *Thorax* **65** (Suppl 2), ii41–ii53.

Hooper CE, Edey AJ, Wallis A, Clive AO, Morley A, White P *et al.* (2015) Pleural irrigation trial (PIT): a randomised controlled trial of pleural irrigation with normal saline versus standard care in patients with pleural infection. *European Respiratory Journal* **46** (2), 456–463.

[No authors listed]. (2006) Managing empyema in adults. *Drug and Therapeutics Bulletin* **44**, 17–21.

Rahman NM, Maskell NA, West A, Teoh R, Arnold A, Mackinley C *et al.* (2011) Intrapleural use of tissue plasminogen activator and DNase in pleural infection. *New England Journal of Medicine* **365**, 518–526.

Zahid I, Nagendran M, Routledge T and Scarci M. (2011) Comparison of video-assisted thoracoscopic surgery and open surgery in the management of primary empyema. *Current Opinion in Pulmonary Medicine* **17** (4), 255–259.

CHAPTER 8

Management of Malignant Pleural Effusions

Anna C. Bibby, Nick A. Maskell and Rahul Bhatnagar

Academic Respiratory Unit, University of Bristol, UK

OVERVIEW

- Malignant pleural effusions are common and are associated with poor prognosis.

- Symptoms are not always related to size of effusion, as rapidity of fluid accumulation and comorbidities may contribute.

- A definitive procedure to remove fluid and prevent its return should be undertaken as soon as diagnosis is confirmed.

- Choice of intervention should be driven by need to relieve symptoms.

- Patient preference must be accounted for when deciding on management.

Malignant pleural effusions account for up to 70% of exudative effusions. They can be the result of primary tumours in the lung or pleura, or metastatic spread from distant malignancy. Lung and breast cancers are the most common underlying causes in men and women, respectively – together these two diseases account for over 50% of all malignant effusions. Lymphoma, ovarian and prostate cancer are also common pathologies (Figure 8.1).

Unfortunately, malignant pleural effusions are associated with a poor prognosis as their presence usually signifies advanced or metastatic disease. Median survival from diagnosis currently ranges from 3 to 12 months, depending on the underlying tumour type, with effusions related to lung cancer associated with the shortest survival times. Recently, a prognostic scoring system (the LENT score) has been developed and validated to help determine the predicted life expectancy of patients who present with malignant pleural effusions.

Pathophysiology

Malignant effusions occur as a result of direct invasion of the pleural space by tumour; however, indirect tumour effects, such as blockage of pleural lymphatics or increased permeability of adjacent blood vessels, also contribute to fluid accumulation. The time taken for an effusion to develop varies between individuals and influences the degree and severity of their symptoms.

Symptoms

Patients with malignant pleural effusions are usually symptomatic. Breathlessness is the most common feature, and is the result of reduced lung volumes caused by compression by fluid (Figure 8.2). The dynamics of the chest wall and diaphragm may be altered by pressure from the fluid, and this will contribute to the sensation of breathlessness. Pre-existing respiratory conditions (e.g. chronic obstructive pulmonary disease (COPD)) or malignancy within the lungs will exacerbate the severity of this symptom.

Additional symptoms include a dry cough caused by pleural irritation, and chest wall or neuropathic pain resulting from tumour invasion. Systemic symptoms such as malaise, lethargy and anorexia are also common. In addition to symptoms from their effusion, patients may also have symptoms relating to their primary malignancy (e.g. haemoptysis), a breast lump or 'B' symptoms of lymphoma.

The severity of symptoms does not always relate to the size of the effusion. For instance, a patient may have a large effusion that does not cause them significant symptoms. Alternatively, their functional status may be limited by comorbidities to such a degree that they do not exert themselves to a point where breathlessness occurs. Factors that contribute to symptom severity include the time the fluid has taken to accumulate and the patient's underlying physiological reserve, including respiratory comorbidities.

Management – general considerations

The most common options for managing malignant pleural effusions are shown in Box 8.1. Choice of intervention should be driven by two guiding principles: the need for diagnosis and the aim to improve symptoms. The wishes of the patient should be considered throughout the decision-making process.

Until the underlying malignant diagnosis is established, it is important that the chosen pleural intervention does not limit future investigations or treatment options. Simple pleural aspiration is an appropriate initial investigation, as it can transiently improve symptoms. Additionally, simple aspiration may yield a cytological

---

ABC of Pleural Diseases, First Edition. Edited by Najib M. Rahman, Ian Hunt, Fergus V. Gleeson and Nick A. Maskell.

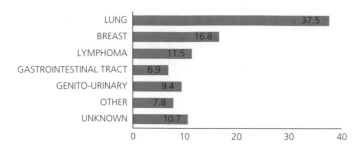

Figure 8.1 Site of primary tumour (%) of 2040 patients with malignant pleural effusions. (Adapted from BTS Guidelines for managing malignant pleural effusions, 2010.)

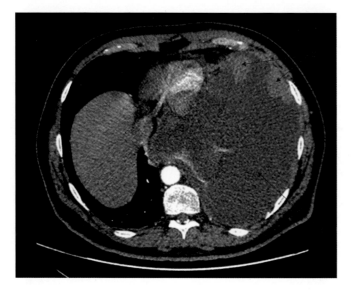

Figure 8.2 CT scan showing a large left-sided pleural effusion (arrow A), causing complete compression of the left lung. Two pleurally based soft tissue masses are seen on the left (arrow B) with associated pleural thickening.

Box 8.1 **Potential interventions for malignant pleural effusions**

- Observation/conservative management
- Simple aspiration
- Insertion of chest drain with talc pleurodesis
- Thoracoscopy and talc poudrage
- Insertion of an indwelling pleural catheter (IPC)
- Video-assisted thoracoscopic surgery

---

diagnosis in a proportion of cases, although sensitivity is less than 60%. If pleural aspiration does not lead to a conclusive diagnosis, then a targeted biopsy will usually be necessary. This can be obtained surgically; using a radiologically guided technique; or by local anaesthetic thoracoscopy.

Once the histo-cytological diagnosis is confirmed, a definitive procedure to remove the fluid and prevent re-accumulation can be undertaken. The appropriate definitive procedure should be adapted to each individual, with consideration given to the patient's wishes, symptoms, physical fitness and prognosis.

The goal of definitive pleural procedures is to control symptoms. Consequently, if a patient is asymptomatic, and the underlying disease is known, conservative management and watchful waiting may be entirely appropriate. Most patients will become symptomatic in time and at that stage further intervention can be decided on.

For symptomatic patients, a decision on which definitive intervention to undertake should be made as soon as possible after obtaining the causal diagnosis. The different management options are described next, with consideration given to the benefits and disadvantages of each procedure.

Simple pleural aspiration

An approximate maximum of 1.5 L pleural fluid can be withdrawn via simple aspiration under local anaesthetic. It is a straightforward, rapid and effective way to relieve breathlessness. Patients can undergo a therapeutic procedure in clinic, and return home immediately. Additionally, simple aspiration can yield diagnostic information without compromising future investigations or treatment. Most patients will undergo simple aspiration at some point during their diagnostic and therapeutic pathway.

As malignant pleural effusions usually recur, simple aspiration is an effective temporising measure but is not ideal as a definitive intervention. Occasionally, it may be appropriate to undertake repeated aspirations if a patient is very frail, has a limited life expectancy or if an effusion is slow to re-accumulate. However, for most patients a procedure that will remove the fluid and reduce the need for further interventions is to be preferred.

Intercostal chest drainage and pleurodesis

Chest tube drainage is an effective way of draining effusions to 'dryness' (Figure 8.3). Chest drains come in a range of sizes, and can be inserted either via Seldinger technique or blunt dissection. The TIME 1 (First Therapeutic Intervention in Malignant Effusion) trial found no clinically significant difference in patient-reported pain scores between people who had large and small bore chest drains for malignant pleural effusions. The insertion of Seldinger chest drains is described in another chapter of this book.

Once the pleural space is 'dry', pleurodesis can be undertaken. The aim of this is to obliterate the pleural space by instilling an irritant agent to generate inflammation and subsequent adhesion. Several pleurodesis agents have been used in the past, including antibiotics and chemotherapy agents; however, sterile talc powder has been shown to be the most efficacious agent, and is now the sole agent used in the UK.

Success of pleurodesis relies on even distribution of the irritant across the pleural space by respiratory motion, and sustained pleural apposition which can sometimes be achieved with thoracic suction. Success rates of up to 80% are reported for talc pleurodesis in the literature, although in clinical practice this figure is probably lower. The results of a recent multi-centre study suggests that pleurodesis via wide-bore chest tube may be more likely to succeed than if a small-bore tube is used.

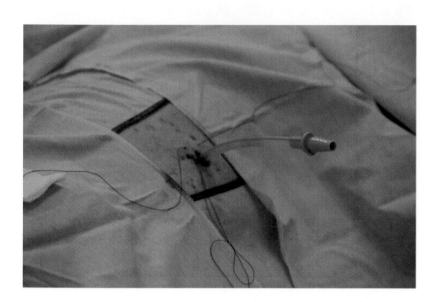
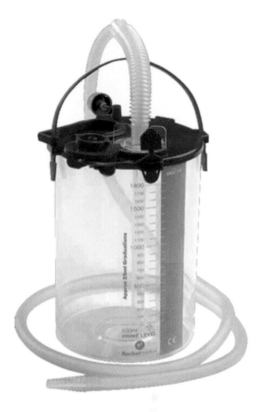

Figure 8.3 A wide-bore chest drain and drainage bottle.

Potential complications of talc pleurodesis via a chest drain include pain, failure of the procedure because of drain blockage or dislodgement and unsuccessful pleurodesis. The inconvenience of a 5–7 day inpatient stay, some of which may be spent confined to the bedside on thoracic suction, is a significant disadvantage.

Thoracoscopy and talc poudrage

Thoracoscopy with talc poudrage is an effective means of achieving fluid control in patients who are fit enough to undergo the procedure. Patients who can tolerate general anaesthesia can undergo video-assisted thoracoscopic surgery (VATS), whilst frailer patients, or those disinclined towards surgery may be offered local anaesthetic thoracoscopy (LAT) under conscious sedation (Figure 8.4). A small proportion of patients will be too frail for either procedure, and will need to have alternative management strategies considered.

One of the major benefits of thoracoscopy is that biopsies can be taken, fluid drained and pleurodesis performed in the same procedure. For many people, a single procedure with both diagnostic and therapeutic benefits is an attractive prospect, although some may be deterred by its invasive nature.

The sensitivity of pleural biopsies taken at thoracoscopy for the detection of malignancy is reported as up to 93% in some articles. Once biopsies have been taken, talc poudrage can be undertaken. Poudrage involves spraying a fine film of talc across both pleural surfaces via the thoracoscopy port (Figure 8.5). Thoracoscopic poudrage appears to be marginally more effective at preventing recurrence of pleural effusions than talc slurry via a chest drain, but more will be known when results become available from the TAPPS trial (Thoracoscopy And talc Poudrage versus Pleurodesis using talc Slurry), a multi-centre, randomised controlled trial which directly compares the two methods.

LAT carries a shorter inpatient stay of 2–3 days on average. Some centres offer a day-case thoracoscopy service (without poudrage), and this practice is likely to become more commonplace in the future.

Thoracoscopy has some disadvantages, however. Patients must be fit enough to undergo the procedure, which in the context of advanced malignancy is not always the case. Additionally, some patients prefer to undergo the least invasive procedure possible, particularly in the context of limited life expectancy. It also requires the insertion of a large chest drain at the end of the procedure, which may be painful.

A specific complication associated with thoracoscopy is the potential spread of tumours along the thoracoscopy tract. Mesothelioma is particularly prone to local seeding in this fashion, to the extent that in some centres prophylactic radiotherapy to the thoracoscopy site is offered when mesothelioma is diagnosed. However, a recently published multi-centre randomised trial (SMART – Surgical and large bore pleural procedures in malignant pleural Mesothelioma and Radiotherapy Trial) found no benefit of giving prophylactic radiotherapy to this group of patients.

Access to services is also an issue. Surgical VATS is undertaken by thoracic surgeons in tertiary centres, which means a long journey to an unfamiliar city for many patients. Similarly, LAT, although more prevalent in secondary care, is not universally available and travel may again be necessary. Fortunately, as the field of pleural

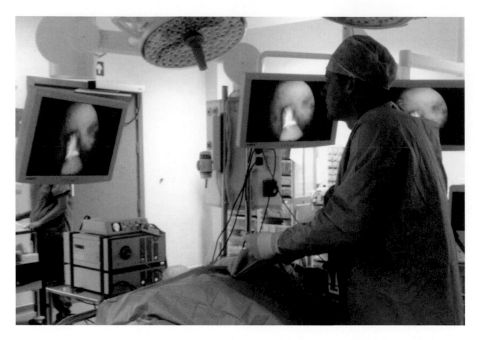

Figure 8.4 A patient undergoing local anaesthetic thoracoscopy. The monitor screens show pleural biopsies being taken.

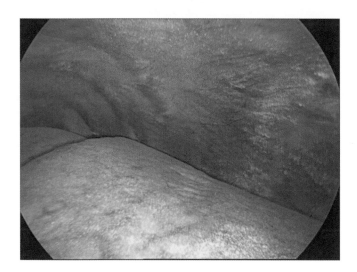

Figure 8.5 Talc poudrage seen via a thoracoscope. A fine film of talc is seen covering the parietal pleura in the top of the picture, with deflated lung visible inferiorly.

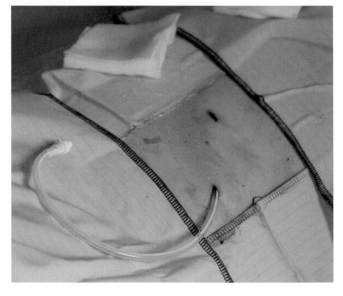

Figure 8.6 An indwelling pleural catheter immediately after insertion.

medicine has expanded over the past decade, LAT provision has increased and is likely to continue to do so as more hospitals establish independent LAT services.

Indwelling pleural catheters

Indwelling pleural catheters are tunnelled chest drains that can remain in place for many months or even years (Figure 8.6). They are typically inserted as a day-case procedure, under local anaesthetic, and provide immediate relief of symptoms. Thereafter they can be drained at home, as required, either by a district nurse or the patient's family. They offer the patient an unobtrusive method of long-term fluid control that minimises hospital admission, empowers the patient and enhances quality of life.

There are some patients whose lungs do not re-expand even after fluid has been removed. If extensive tumour is present across the pleural surface, it can form a thick rind that encases the underlying lung. This is known as a trapped lung (Figure 8.7). The lung may also fail to re-inflate if there is a central lung tumour obstructing a proximal bronchus and preventing air from entering the lung. Nonetheless, these patients may experience symptomatic benefit from removal of fluid, because of relief of local pressure effects, and restoration of normal chest wall and diaphragm dynamics. In these patients, an indwelling pleural catheter (IPC) is an effective option for fluid management and symptom relief.

IPCs are also effective in patients without trapped lungs. The TIME 2 trial demonstrated that patients with IPCs had a similar reduction in breathlessness and chest pain as patients who underwent chest tube drainage and talc pleurodesis. As a result, IPCs can now be offered to patients with symptomatic malignant pleural effusions instead of talc pleurodesis, with patient preference being the main determining factor.

With regular drainage, the presence of an IPC can lead to spontaneous pleurodesis in up to 60% of patients. If this occurs, the IPC can be removed. A multi-centre trial (IPC-PLUS) is currently

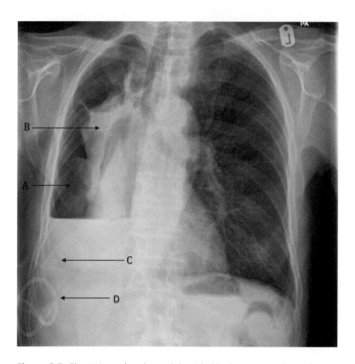

Figure 8.7 Chest X-ray showing a right-sided hydro-pneumothorax (arrow A) secondary to trapped lung (arrow B), with an indwelling pleura catheter (IPC) in situ. Arrow C illustrates the IPC entering the pleural space and arrow D shows it coiled up externally against the skin.

underway examining the effectiveness of using talc slurry via indwelling catheters to encourage pleurodesis.

The most common complication of IPCs is infection, the risk of which increases the longer the catheter stays in place. Case series and review articles report infection rates of 2–5%, with many episodes able to be managed with oral antibiotics and the need for drain removal rare. The use of chemotherapy has not been shown to increase the rate of pleural infection once an IPC is in place, although careful consideration should be given to the timing of insertion. Interestingly, there is some evidence that the inflammatory effects of pleural infection may increase the chance of pleurodesis, and therefore it may not always be an entirely negative occurrence.

Another potential disadvantage of IPCs is the availability of local services. As well as requiring a specialist hospital team to insert the catheter, community services are sometimes required if the patient or their family are unable to undertake regular drainage independently. Fortunately, experience of these catheters is increasing rapidly as more pleural teams are inserting them and more patients are choosing to have them inserted.

Which procedure is best?

Each intervention has advantages and disadvantages and will suit different patients at different stages in their pathway. It is important to evaluate the risks and benefits of each procedure on an individual patient basis. In addition, it is essential to determine the patient's wishes in order to maximise their quality of life and satisfaction with the service provided. Table 8.1 shows a summary of the advantages and disadvantages of each procedure, whilst Figure 8.8 shows a flowchart that may assist this complex decision-making process.

The future

The management of malignant pleural effusion is an exciting and rapidly developing area with many well-designed clinical trials currently underway. These trials promise to enhance our

Table 8.1 Advantages and disadvantages of pleural procedures.

Procedure	Advantages	Disadvantages
Simple aspiration	Simple, swift procedure Patient able to return home immediately Can yield diagnostic material Can be repeated Does not jeopardise future interventions	Temporary measure
Chest drain and talc pleurodesis	Definitive procedure Up to 80% successful pleurodesis rates Patient discharged with no visible reminder of disease	Pain 5–7 day inpatient stay Failure rate (drain and pleurodesis)
Thoracoscopy and talc poudrage	Single procedure allowing diagnosis, drainage and pleurodesis 1–2 day inpatient stay Excellent biopsy sensitivity Poudrage may be more effective than talc slurry Accessibility improving	Limited to patients with acceptable performance status Not universally accessible Some patients may not wish to undergo invasive procedure Potential risk of tumour seeding
Indwelling pleural catheter	Day-case procedure with home drainage Effective for patients with trapped lung Empowers patients and improves quality of life Spontaneous pleurodesis in ~60%	Some patients may not want permanent reminder of disease in situ Risk of infection Risk of tumour seeding Need to coordinate insertion with timing of chemotherapy

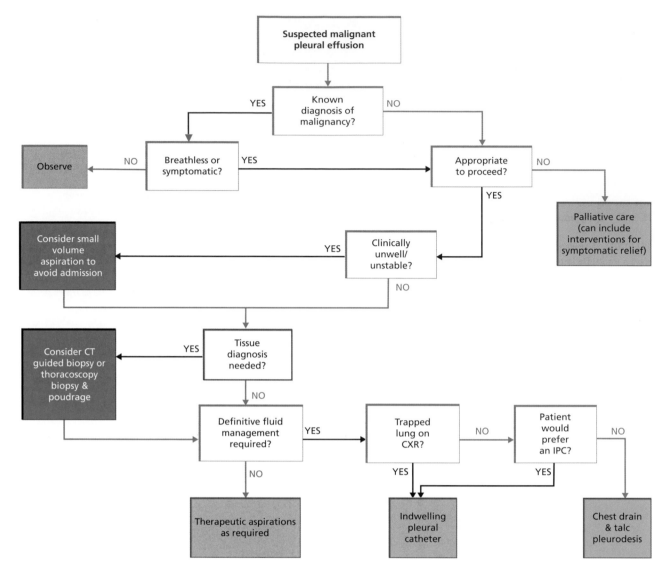

Figure 8.8 An approach to the management of malignant pleural effusions. CXR, chest X-ray; IPC, indwelling pleural catheter.

understanding of this heterogeneous and unpredictable process, and will allow us to provide ongoing improvements in patient care. Novel therapies, including intrapleural monoclonal antibodies, immunotherapy with bacterial proteins and anti-angiogenic agents, are being studied for their anti-tumour effects. Additionally, the technology of IPCs is progressing, with research on silver nitrate-coated catheters to reduce infection, and the use of automated drainage devices to divert pleural fluid into the bladder to be excreted in the urine.

Conclusions

Malignant pleural effusions are common and can cause significant symptoms in patients with serious comorbidity and limited life expectancy. Initial interventions should be aimed at achieving a tissue diagnosis, unless the patient is too frail for active treatment, in which case symptom management should be prioritised. Simple aspiration is frequently the first step, undertaken with the aim of

obtaining cytological samples and temporarily relieving breathlessness. Alternately, in suitable patients, thoracoscopy can be performed to obtain biopsies, drain fluid and perform pleurodesis in one intervention.

Once a diagnosis of malignancy is confirmed, attention focuses on symptom management. Some patients will be asymptomatic from their effusions and a conservative 'watch and wait' policy is appropriate. In symptomatic patients, however, a definitive procedure to remove fluid and prevent re-accumulation is necessary. Rarely, repeat pleural aspirations may be the right choice, but only in the context of extremely short life expectancy. Otherwise, the decision is between an intercostal chest drain with talc pleurodesis or insertion of an IPC. Both are effective at reducing symptoms and improving quality of life, but both have disadvantages; an inpatient hospital stay and risk of pleural infection, respectively. Each patient will view these issues differently, and the final decision will be a result of individual personal preference.

Further reading

Bhatnagar R and Maskell NA. (2014) Indwelling pleural catheters. *Respiration* **88** (1), 74–85.

Clive AO, Kahan BC, Hooper CE, Bhatnagar R, Morley AJ, Zahan-Evans N *et al.* (2014) Predicting survival in malignant pleural effusion: development and validation of the LENT prognostic score. *Thorax* **69** (12), 1098–1104.

Davies HE, Mishra EK, Kahan BC, Wrightson JM, Stanton AE, Guhan A *et al.* (2012) Effect of an indwelling pleural catheter vs chest tube and talc pleurodesis for relieving dyspnea in patients with malignant pleural effusion: the TIME2 randomized controlled trial. *JAMA* **307** (22), 2383–2389.

Huggins JT, Doelken P and Sahn SA. (2011) Intra-pleural therapy. *Respirology* **16**, 891–899.

Roberts ME, Neville E, Berrisford RG, Antunes G and Ali NJ. (2010) Management of a malignant pleural effusion: British Thoracic Society pleural disease guideline 2010. *Thorax* **65** (Suppl 2), ii32–ii40.

CHAPTER 9

Malignant Mesothelioma

Carol Tan[1], Fergus V. Gleeson[2] and Y.C. Gary Lee[3]

[1] St George's Hospital, London, UK
[2] Churchill Hospital, Oxford, UK
[3] University of Western Australia, Perth, Australia

OVERVIEW

- Diffuse pleural malignant mesothelioma is an uncommon tumour, but the incidence is expected to continue to rise in the UK and Europe over the next decade.

- The majority of cases are caused by amphibole asbestos exposure, usually more than 20 years prior to the development of the tumour.

- Diagnosis is complex, requiring the integration of clinical, radiological and, ultimately, histopathological findings.

- The most common subtype is epithelioid malignant mesothelioma, followed by biphasic and sarcomatoid subtypes, all of which may mimic a variety of benign and malignant conditions.

- The outlook is universally poor, especially for desmoplastic variants of sarcomatoid mesothelioma, with no reliable definitive therapy available.

Diffuse malignant mesothelioma (MM) is the most common primary tumour of the pleura, and also occurs less frequently in the peritoneum (6–10%), pericardium, tunica vaginalis and ovary. There is a well-established link between asbestos exposure and MM, as demonstrated by Wagner *et al.*, who investigated asbestos miners dying with pleural tumours in the North West Cape province of South Africa in 1960. Although still a rare tumour, MM has become increasingly common over the last few decades (the number of deaths from MM in the UK increased from 153 in 1968 to 2249 in 2008; Health and Safety Executive statistics 2009/2010). The annual incidence in the UK is expected to peak around the year 2016, with just over 2000 deaths from MM expected in males alone. The rising incidence is a result of the long latency period between exposure to asbestos and the development of MM, which is greater than 20 years in 96% of cases. Despite causing a relatively small number of cancer-related deaths, MM receives a considerable amount of attention because of the legal implications of asbestos-related occupational exposure and the not infrequent difficulties in confirming the diagnosis. MM needs to be distinguished from reactive mesothelial proliferations and is a well-known mimic of other tumours, necessitating the use of immunohistochemical staining of appropriate surgical biopsy material and careful correlation with the clinical and radiological findings. As the prognosis of patients diagnosed with diffuse pleural MM remains universally poor (median survival from diagnosis of 6–12 months) with no reliable definitive therapy, it is paramount that the diagnosis is made correctly.

Epidemiology and aetiology

Because of its fire-resistant properties (the word 'asbestos' is derived from a Greek word meaning 'unquenchable'), asbestos was widely used in the ship-building and construction industries, and affected individuals include electricians, plumbers and carpenters. Of those diagnosed with MM, most are men (male to female ratio = 9 : 1) in the 50–70 year age group. It is estimated that about 5–10% of individuals with significant prolonged asbestos exposure will develop MM and, conversely, more than 90% of patients with MM have had some form of asbestos exposure. Other potential factors predisposing to MM include exposure to the non-asbestos fibre erionite (found in the Cappadoccia region of Turkey) and possibly simian virus 40 (controversial), thorotrast and radiation.

Pathogenesis

Asbestos probably causes MM through a combination of mechanisms ranging from direct to indirect, and genetic to molecular. Direct mechanisms include the deposition of asbestos fibres in the pleura, which is more likely to occur with long, thin, straight fibres of the amphibole group (e.g. crocidolite and amosite) than with the curly fibres of the serpentine group (mainly chrysotile). Some investigators question the role of chrysotile in the development of MM.

Indirectly, asbestos causes MM through the release of reactive oxygen species from macrophages that have ingested fibres, which result in damage to DNA, possible suppression of the immune system and activation of cell signalling pathways. Chromosomal deletions accumulate in many MM, resulting in loss or inactivation of tumour suppressor genes (e.g. CDKN2A/ARF locus at 9p21).

ABC of Pleural Diseases, First Edition. Edited by Najib M. Rahman, Ian Hunt, Fergus V. Gleeson and Nick A. Maskell.
© 2018 John Wiley & Sons Ltd. Published 2018 by John Wiley & Sons Ltd.

Possible contributing genetic factors are suggested by the occurrence of rare familial cases of MM.

Clinical presentation and investigation

Patients with MM often present with dyspnoea related to pleural effusion and/or chest wall pain, but may have associated constitutional symptoms (weight loss, sweats, malaise and anorexia) and, less commonly, symptoms related to invasion of thoracic viscera or vital structures (e.g. dysphagia, hoarseness or superior venal caval obstruction). Physical examination may show signs of a pleural effusion (reduced chest expansion, dull percussion note and decreased breath sounds), chest wall mass, finger clubbing (30%) or signs related to local infiltration (e.g. cardiac tamponade). Patients with MM may present with an incidental finding on chest X-ray, with focal pleural disease in the absence of symptoms. Lymphadenopathy is less commonly present.

Although cytological examination of pleural fluid reveals malignant cells in only about one-third of cases, a pleural biopsy to obtain tissue for diagnosis is recommended, by means of image guided (ultrasound or computed tomography) biopsy, medical thoracoscopy or video-assisted thoracoscopic surgery (VATS).

Radiological investigation, which is mainly with CT, is vital for diagnosis and staging purposes. Various serum markers (e.g. serum osteopontin, soluble mesothelin-related protein and megakaryocyte potentiating factor) are proposed as possible indicators of pleural MM in at-risk patients, but these have not been accepted into routine clinical practice, and may have more of a role in monitoring response to therapy.

Pathological features

Grossly, early MM usually develops in the pleura as multiple small nodules which later coalesce, resulting in fusion of the visceral and parietal pleura with extension of tumour along pulmonary fissures. Later, the tumour encases and invades the lung and other thoracic structures. This pattern of involvement is not unique to MM and other primary or secondary pleural malignancies may demonstrate a similar growth pattern.

MM characteristically invades the chest wall and after biopsy procedures readily spreads along needle tracks and surgical biopsy sites. The presence of pleural plaques, which are usually bilateral, discrete, slightly raised areas of cream-coloured pleural thickening arranged parallel to the ribs and often on the diaphragmatic surfaces, indicates previous exposure to asbestos only. Pleural plaques are not pre-malignant and act as a marker for asbestos exposure only. They do not 'turn into' MM and their presence does not mean that MM will develop in the future.

MM may be rich in hyaluronic acid or proteoglycans, which imparts a slimy, gelatinous appearance to the cut surface of the tumour. The underlying lung may show features of interstitial fibrosis (asbestosis) depending on the duration and level of exposure to asbestos.

The ultimate diagnosis of MM is essentially histological, requiring an adequate biopsy in an appropriate clinical and radiological context with the final diagnosis often resting on the demonstration

Table 9.1 Causes of benign reactive mesothelial hyperplasia and organising pleuritis and histological features mimicking or indicating malignancy. Source: Modified from Cagle and Churg (2005), with permission of College of American Pathologists.

Causes of reactive mesothelial hyperplasia and organising pleuritis	Features of reactive mesothelial proliferations that may mimic malignancy
Infections	High cellularity
Collagen vascular disease	Cytological atypia
Pulmonary infarction	Mitotic activity
Drug reactions	Necrosis
Pneumothorax	Papillary excrescences or lumina
Subpleural lung cancer	Mesothelial
Surgery	entrapment (pseudo-invasion)
Trauma	
Radiation therapy	**Features favouring a diagnosis of**
Other	**malignancy rather than reactive**
	mesothelial hyperplasia
	Unequivocal invasion of fat or skeletal muscle
	Cellular nodules with stromal expansion
	Lack of zonation
	Severe nuclear pleomorphism
	Atypical mitotic figures
	Bland necrosis

of invasion into deep tissues of the pleura, usually fat or skeletal muscle. If the radiological and clinical features are definite, but the histological appearances are equivocal, then definitive diagnosis should be deferred until additional material is obtained (if clinically appropriate). Immunohistochemistry is an important adjunct in the diagnosis of MM in view of the wide differential diagnosis. The importance of an adequate, well-oriented biopsy cannot be understated, as immunohistochemistry is unhelpful in distinguishing between reactive entrapped mesothelium and superficially invasive malignant mesothelioma (Table 9.1).

MM is classified histologically into epithelioid, sarcomatoid and mixed (biphasic) types (WHO 2004 classification).

Epithelioid malignant mesothelioma

Epithelioid malignant mesothelioma (EMM) is the most common histological variant (50–70% of cases). The tumour cells in EMM have a rounded appearance (hence 'epithelial-like') and are arranged in a variety of patterns including tubulopapillary, solid, glandular, microcystic (or adenomatoid) and myxoid. The cytomorphology is also variable: the cuboidal cells may be exceptionally bland with little to no mitotic activity, or show clear cell change (sometimes with a signet ring-like appearance), while others show marked pleomorphism with tumour giant cells or, very rarely, have small cell features (Figure 9.1).

A deciduoid variant where the cells resemble hormonally altered endometrial stromal cells is also described. As a result of this diverse range of cytological and architectural appearances, EMM can mimic a variety of other tumours, and thus may need to be distinguished from metastatic adenocarcinoma (especially from lung, breast and ovary), metastatic renal cell carcinoma (clear cell type; Figure 9.2), metastatic lobular carcinoma of the breast, metastatic squamous cell carcinoma (solid pattern), pleural

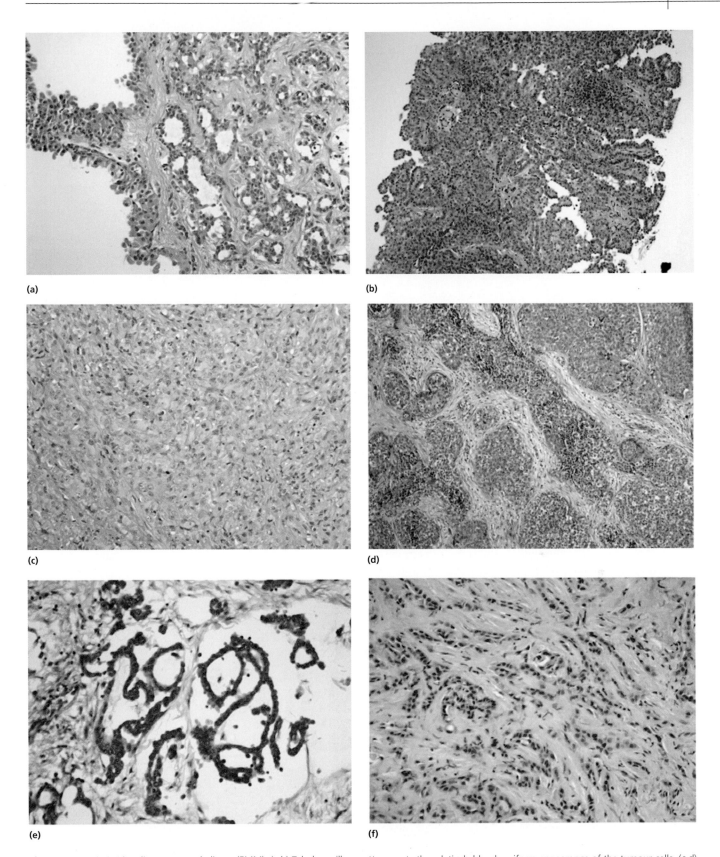

Figure 9.1 Epithelioid malignant mesothelioma (EMM). (a,b) Tubulopapillary pattern: note the relatively bland, uniform appearance of the tumour cells. (c,d) Solid pattern: sheets of large, rounded cells with abundant cytoplasm (c) and nested arrangement (d). (e,f) Lattice-like strands of bland epithelioid cells 'floating' within myxoid stroma (e) and lobular carcinoma-like growth pattern associated with desmoplastic stroma (f).

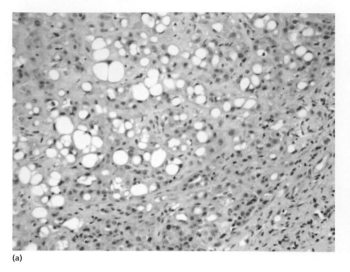
(a)

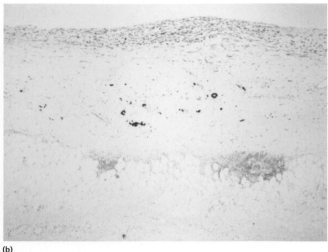
(b)

Figure 9.2 EMM: clear cell change imparting signet ring-like appearance (a) and cytokeratin immunostain (b) demonstrating tubules and cords of mesothelial cells within fibrous tissue beneath the pleural surface: early invasive mesothelioma or entrapped reactive mesothelium? (b) This case subsequently evolved into biphasic diffuse pleural malignant mesothelioma (re-biopsied after 6 months).

thymoma, epithelioid haemangioendothelioma, metastatic melanoma, lymphoma and metastatic germ cell tumours.

It is also worth noting that metastatic pulmonary adenocarcinoma may grow in a 'pseudomesotheliomatous' fashion, causing confusion clinically and pathologically. Reactive mesothelial proliferations with or without entrapped mesothelium need to be distinguished from superficially invasive EMM. EMM tumour cells may shed readily into pleural fluid, in contrast to sarcomatoid tumours which tend to not yield positive pleural fluid cytology.

Sarcomatoid malignant mesothelioma

Sarcomatoid malignant mesothelioma (SMM) is the least common subtype, probably accounting for about 15–20% of mesotheliomas (in its pure form), and is only rarely reported outside the pleura. In SMM, the tumour cells have an elongated, spindle-shaped appearance resembling soft tissue sarcomas seen elsewhere and are arranged in fascicular, storiform or sometimes whorled patterns (Figure 9.3). Within this mesothelioma subtype, distinctive growth patterns may be recognised, the most important of which is the desmoplastic variant, as this has a particularly poor prognosis and may be easily confused with reactive fibrous pleuritis.

The desmoplastic variant of SMM is diagnosed when at least 50% of the tumour comprises atypical hyperchromatic spindle cells set within dense collagenous stroma and arranged in a storiform (or 'patternless') pattern (if 10–50% shows this pattern, then the phrase 'SMM with desmoplastic features' may be used).

Histological clues separating this from organising pleural fibrosis include cellular atypia, necrosis and invasion of adipose tissue or skeletal muscle, and cytokeratin immunostains are particularly helpful at identifying the latter.

Other SMM show significant nuclear pleomorphism or anaplasia, resembling malignant fibrous histiocytoma.

An important consideration for the pathologist is that many SMM are negative for traditional mesothelial markers, but a high percentage are cytokeratin positive which, in the right clinical and

radiological context, is entirely supportive of the diagnosis. Caution needs to be exercised in the context of a mass-forming lung lesion, when metastatic sarcomatoid carcinoma is a possibility.

The differential diagnosis also includes malignant fibrous tumour, monophasic synovial sarcoma, spindle cell melanoma, fibrosarcoma, angiosarcoma, endometrial stromal sarcoma and malignant gastrointestinal stromal tumour, and therefore an appropriate panel of immunohistochemical stains is employed.

The lymphohistiocytoid variant of SMM is characterised by round to ovoid, histiocyte-like cells admixed with an abundant lymphocytic inflammatory infiltrate, which may be confused with malignant lymphoma. Rare cases of SMM contain heterologous elements, for example osteosarcoma, chondrosarcoma, rhabdomyosarcoma or liposarcoma, which may lead to misclassification as metastatic sarcoma.

Biphasic malignant mesothelioma

Biphasic malignant mesothelioma (BMM) contains at least 10% of both epithelioid and sarcomatoid components and comprises approximately 30% of mesothelioma subtypes. BMM sometimes has to be differentiated histologically from other tumours with a mixed epithelial and sarcomatous appearance, for example synovial sarcoma, carcinosarcoma and pulmonary blastoma (Figure 9.4).

Well-differentiated papillary mesothelioma

Well-differentiated papillary mesothelioma is a rare, distinctive mesothelial tumour characterised by bland cytological features, papillary growth pattern and a tendency towards superficial spread without invasion of the underlying soft tissues. It is primarily seen in the peritoneum of women or tunica vaginalis of men. Great caution should be exercised when considering this diagnosis in small biopsies, as unlike diffuse pleural (or peritoneal) MM, these tumours are associated with indolent behaviour and prolonged survival.

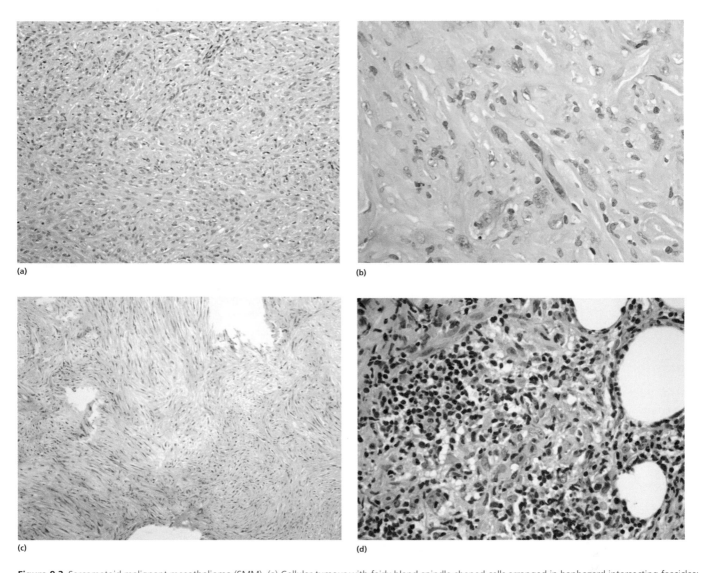

Figure 9.3 Sarcomatoid malignant mesothelioma (SMM). (a) Cellular tumour with fairly bland spindle-shaped cells arranged in haphazard intersecting fascicles; (b) an example demonstrating more pronounced nuclear pleomorphism; (c) desmoplastic variant demonstrating dense collagenous stroma and a storiform arrangement of hyperchromatic spindle cells; and (d) histiocytoid cells partly obscured by a dense lymphoid infiltrate.

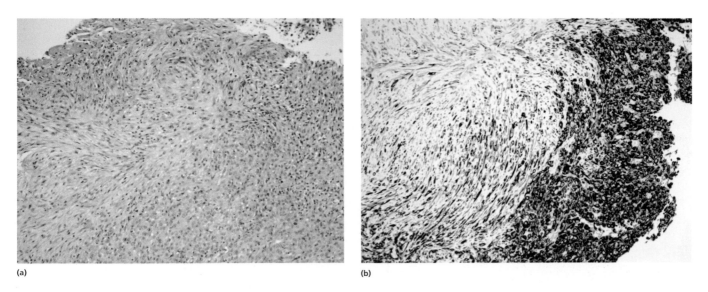

Figure 9.4 Biphasic malignant mesothelioma (BMM). Sarcomatoid pattern in upper left field merging with rounded, epithelioid tumour cells on the lower right (a) and biphasic appearance emphasised by cytokeratin immunohistochemistry (b).

Localised malignant mesothelioma

Localised malignant mesothelioma is a rare, circumscribed, invasive mesothelial lesion which has the same range of histological, immunohistochemical and ultrastructural appearances as diffuse MM, but lacks the diffuse pattern of pleural spread seen with this tumour. The role of asbestos exposure in the pathogenesis of this tumour type is unclear. Localised malignant mesothelioma may be cured by surgical excision. However, patients may die from local recurrence or metastases, but diffuse pleural spread is not seen.

Diagnosis

Diagnosis of MM is based on histology. However, in a substantial number of cases, repeated biopsies (including large surgical biopsies) may not be definitive. In these cases, close clinical and radiological follow-up is required. The presence of a progressing malignant tumour on radiology with appropriate clinical progression in the absence of another cause may be sufficient to give a 'clinical' diagnosis of mesothelioma, especially in the contex of asbestos exposure.

Treatment and prognosis

MM should be considered to be an incurable malignancy. Treatment is based on symptom management (control of pleural fluid, pain management, treatment of breathlessness, nutrition) using 'active symptom control', and the use of chemotherapy in some cases.

Combined chemotherapy with a platinum-based agent and pemetrexed has been demonstrated in a randomised trial to improve quality of life and modestly prolong survival (by around 3 months). A recently announced study suggests improved survival to around 18 months with combined chemotherapy and bevacizumab therapy, compared with platinum and pemetrexed alone. This is likely to be the new standard of treatment, but assessment of costs to healthcare services are awaited to address which patients will be provided with this therapy. There is no randomised evidence currently in support of second line chemotherapy for MM.

Surgical treatment with curative intent has been advocated for MM in certain specialist centres. The operation (extrapleural pnuemonectomy (EPP)) involves a complete parietal pleurectomy, resection of the hemidiaphragm and pericardium, and a pneumonectomy, and is a significant undertaking with risks. Although case series suggested prolonged survival with EPP, the randomised MARS trial demonstrated reduced survival and reduced quality of life with EPP compared with palliative chemotherapy and best supportive care, and EPP is therefore no longer recommended for the treatment of MM.

Increasingly, surgeons have focused on less aggressive surgical interventions, such as radical pleurectomy, involving resection of all macroscopic disease including the parietal and visceral pleura and, if necessary, hemidiaphragm, pericardium, chest wall and parts of the lung but without a pneuomonectomy. For surgery with the intent of prolonging survival or with curative intent, there are there are no randomised trials using these more focused operative strategies and thus these procedures cannot currently be recommended as standard treatment outside of a trial. In the UK, the MARS2 trial (now recruiting) will directly address this question.

A randomised trial has directly addressed the relative benefits of surgical intervention (via thoracoscopic partial pleurectomy) versus talc pleurodesis either via slurry or thorocoscopic poudrage in the treatment of mesothelioma. The MESOVATS trial demonstrated that there is no survival benefit associated with surgery, and that pleural fluid control was not convincingly better using VATs than 'medical' pleurodesis. The only outcome that showed benefit for surgery was one aspect of quality of life at 6 months post randomisation, and because of the small number of patients included in this analysis, and the negative other outcomes, VATS surgery cannot be currently recommended as a first line palliative treatment in mesothelioma.

Prognosis in mesothelioma is poor – epithelioid subtypes have a better prognosis than sarcomatoid. Median survival is between 9 and 18 months for epithelioid mesothelioma.

Further reading

Cagle PT and Churg A. (2005) Differential diagnosis of benign and malignant mesothelial proliferations on pleural biopsies. *Archives of Pathology and Laboratory Medicine* **129**, 1421–1427

Rintoul RC, Ritchie AJ, Edwards JG, Waller DA, Coonar AS, Bennett M *et al*; MesoVATS Collaborators. (2014) Efficacy and cost of video-assisted thoracoscopic partial pleurectomy versus talc pleurodesis in patients with malignant pleural mesothelioma (MesoVATS): an open-label, randomised, controlled trial. *Lancet* **384**, 1118–1127.

Travis WD, Brambilla E, Muller-Hermelink HK and Harris CC (eds). (2004) *World Health Organisation Classification of Tumours: Pathology and Genetics of Tumours of the Lung, Pleura, Thymus and Heart*, IARC Press, Lyon.

Treasure T, Lang-Lazdunski L, Waller D, Bliss JM, Tan C, Entwisle J *et al*; MARS trialists. (2011) Extra-pleural pneumonectomy versus no extra-pleural pneumonectomy for patients with malignant pleural mesothelioma: clinical outcomes of the Mesothelioma and Radical Surgery (MARS) randomised feasibility study. *Lancet Oncology* **12** (8), 763–772.

Zalcman G, Mazieres J, Margery J, Grellier L, Audigier-Valette C, Moro-Sibilot D *et al*; French Cooperative Thoracic Intergroup (FCT). (2016) Bevacizumab for newly diagnosed pleural mesothelioma in the Mesothelioma Avastin Cisplatin Pemetrexed Study (MAPS): a randomised, controlled, open-label, phase 3 trial. *Lancet* **387**, 1405–1414.

CHAPTER 10

Pleural Interventions
Section A: Pleural Aspiration

Ambika Talwar[1], Ahmed Yousuf[2] and Najib M. Rahman[3]

[1] Churchill Hospital, Oxford, UK
[2] Glenfield Hospital, Leicester, UK
[3] Oxford Centre for Respiratory Medicine, Churchill Hospital, Oxford, UK

OVERVIEW

- The main indications for diagnostic and therapeutic thoracocentesis.
- A step-by-step illustrated approach to thoracocentesis.
- The complications of thoracocentesis.

Thoracocentesis is indicated in the diagnosis of pleural effusion and can provide symptomatic relief of breathlessness caused by pleural effusion.

Diagnostic thoracocentesis

Step-by-step approach

1 Obtain written and verbal consent.
2 Check full blood count (FBC), coagulation profile, renal function and glucose.
3 Obtain up-to-date chest X-ray (CXR) and any other available imaging.
4 Check the site of the procedure just prior to starting; the site of the procedure should be drawn on the patient.
5 Position patients sitting forward, leaning on a pillow over a table with their arms folded in front of them (see Figure 10.8).
6 Aspiration site should be chosen by an experienced operator using thoracic ultrasound at the time of the procedure and ultrasound should be available for use throughout the procedure if required.
7 Sterile skin preparation and aseptic technique, using sterile drapes to cover the patient.
8 Infiltrate skin, intercostal muscle and parietal pleura with 10–20 mL 1% lidocaine (Figures 10.1 and 10.2).
9 The needle should be aimed above the upper border of the rib, avoiding the neurovascular bundle.
10 Aspirate pleural fluid with a green (21 G) needle and 50 mL syringe (Figure 10.3).

11 After the diagnostic tap, note the appearance of the pleural fluid. The sample should be sent for analysis in three sterile pots (Table 10.1).
12 A routine CXR is not indicated after thoracocentesis in asymptomatic non-ventilated patients. Ultrasound by an experienced clinician has a diagnostic sensitivity for pneumothorax similar to CXR.
13 Direct (also known as 'real-time') ultrasound guidance may be required for small or loculated effusions, or to distinguish fluid from pleural thickening.

Avoidance of the intercostal arteries

Intercostal arteries can follow a tortuous course, particularly in the elderly, and collateral arteries can traverse the intercostal space. This places them in danger of puncture, even when the operator passes the needle over the upper edge of the rib. To reduce the risk of this, a puncture site 9–10 cm lateral to the spine (assuming that the fluid collection is accessible) should be chosen. Alternatively, colour Doppler can be used to identify intercostal and collateral arteries before performing the procedure.

Therapeutic thoracocentesis

Step-by-step approach

1 The initial procedure is identical to that for diagnostic thoracocentesis (steps 1–8).
2 It is important to confirm that the insertion site is correct by aspirating pleural fluid with a green (21 G) needle.
3 After infiltrating with lidocaine, make a small (0.5 cm) incision with a scalpel at the site of insertion to allow the catheter to pass smoothly.
4 The equipment needed using the Rocket therapeutic thoracocentesis kit is shown in Figure 10.4.
5 Carefully advance the thoracocentesis catheter (e.g. 6 or 8 Fr) along the anaesthetised track. As the needle is advanced, the catheter is passed through the needle into the pleural space and the needle withdrawn from the skin (Figures 10.5 and 10.6).

ABC of Pleural Diseases, First Edition. Edited by Najib M. Rahman, Ian Hunt, Fergus V. Gleeson and Nick A. Maskell.
© 2018 John Wiley & Sons Ltd. Published 2018 by John Wiley & Sons Ltd.

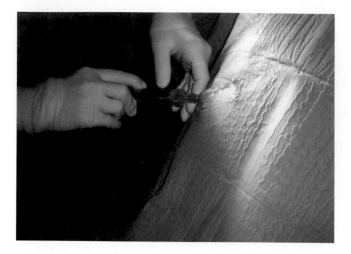

Figure 10.1 Local anaesthetic insertion into subcutaneous tissue.

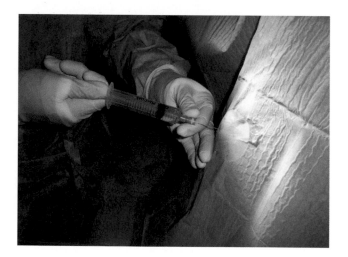

Figure 10.2 Local anaesthetic insertion into intercostal muscles and parietal pleura.

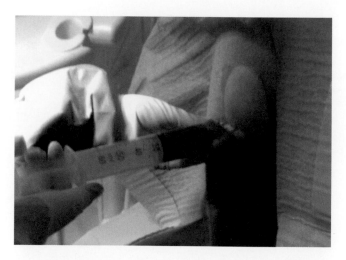

Figure 10.3 Pleural aspiration with 50 mL syringe.

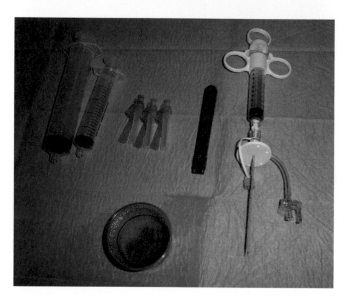

Figure 10.4 Equipment for therapeutic aspiration with 6 Fr aspiration catheter.

Table 10.1 Recommended routine pleural fluid tests after diagnostic pleural aspiration.

Biochemistry	Protein, LDH, glucose
	pH: if pleural infection is suspected (processed by biochemistry or local ABG analyser etc)
	Cholesterol and triglycerides if chylothorax is suspected
Microbiology (send in sterile pot and blood culture bottles)	Gram stain, microscopy, culture and AFB stain and culture
Cytology	Examination of malignant cells and differential cell count if applicable

ABG, arterial blood gas; AFB, acid-fast bacteria; LDH, lactate dehydrogenase.

6 A temporary dressing is used to secure the catheter in place.
7 The fluid is drained using a fluid collection bag, which is attached to the catheter via a three-way tap (Figure 10.7).
8 A sample of 50–60 mL pleural fluid is obtained if needed for diagnostic samples.

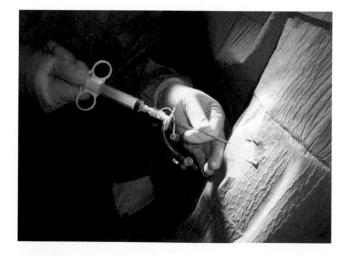

Figure 10.5 Insertion of aspiration catheter.

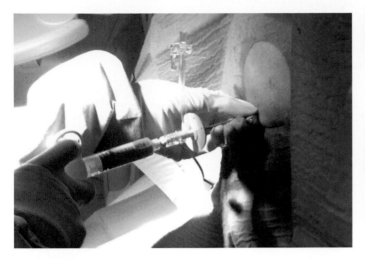

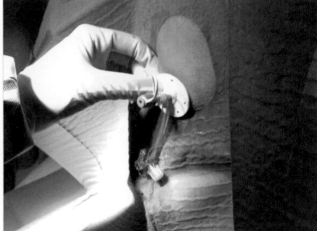

Figure 10.6 Advancing aspiration catheter.

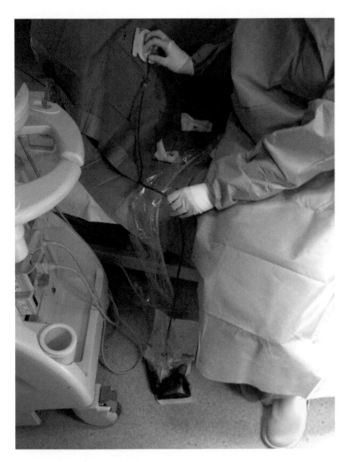

Figure 10.7 Fluid drainage bag collecting pleural fluid.

9 Drain a maximum of 1.5 L of fluid in one sitting to avoid re-expansion pulmonary oedema.

10 The procedure should be stopped if the patient experiences discomfort or severe coughing.

11 Once the fluid has drained, the three-way tap should be closed.

12 The catheter should be removed during full expiration and a small dressing applied to the aspiration site.

13 CXR should be carried out to visualise improvement in effusion size and to exclude pneumothorax or trapped lung. However, post procedure thoracic ultrasound performed by an experienced operator can also be used to assess this.

Complications of diagnostic and therapeutic thoracocentesis

1 Pain;
2 Cough;
3 Bleeding;
4 Infection, occasionally empyema;
5 Pneumothorax;
6 Puncture to organs such as liver or spleen;
7 Malignant seeding down aspiration site (especially in mesothelioma).

Further reading

Rahman NM, Ali NJ, Brown G, Chapman SJ, Davies RJ, Downer NJ *et al.* (2010) Local anaesthetic thoracoscopy: British Thoracic Society Pleural Disease Guideline 2010. *Thorax* **65** (Suppl 2), ii54–ii60.

Section B: Chest Drain Insertion

Ahmed Yousuf [1] and Najib M. Rahman [2]

[1] Glenfield Hospital, Leicester, UK
[2] Oxford Centre for Respiratory Medicine, Churchill Hospital, Oxford, UK

A chest drain is a tube inserted through the chest wall into the pleural space to remove air (pneumothorax), pus (empyema), blood (haemothorax) or fluid (effusion). The drains can be small (8–18 Fr) or large bore (20–28 Fr, also known as a surgical drain). For large-bore chest drain insertion see Chapter 11.

Use of ultrasound-guided drain insertion for pleural effusion allows accurate detection of pleural effusion and reduces the incidence of failed procedures and complications (Box 10.1).

Chest drain insertion (Seldinger technique)

The technique was first described in 1953 by Sven-Ivar Seldinger, a Swedish radiologist. It is an over-wire technique for percutaneous insertion of catheters (e.g. chest drain, vascular access).

Pre-drain insertion

Before insertion of a chest drain, all operators should have adequate training and supervision. The following points should be noted before drain insertion:

1 Confirm side of effusion clinically and radiologically (latest CXR/CT scan/ultrasound scan for pleural effusion – if trained in chest ultrasound).
2 Ensure there are no absolute contraindications to drain insertion (Box 10.2).
3 Obtain informed written consent after explaining the indication and risks (bleeding, infection, pneumothorax in case of pleural effusion, damage to vital organs).
4 Position the patient appropriately (Figures 10.8 and 10.9).
5 Ensure all the necessary equipment is available (Box 10.3).

Box 10.1 Indications for chest drain insertion

- Tension pneumothorax
- Primary spontaneous pneumothorax >2 cm in size or patient symptomatic or that failed to resolve after one attempt at aspiration
- Secondary spontaneous pneumothorax >2 cm in size or patient symptomatic
- Haemothorax
- Empyema
- Large symptomatic pleural effusion (malignant or non-malignant effusion)
- To facilitate talc pleurodesis

Box 10.2 Contraindications to drain insertion

- Coagulopathy* [INR >1.5, patient on novel oral anticoagulant (e.g. apixaban, rivaroxban) and has not stopped it for ≥48 hours; patient on clopidogrel and has not stopped it for 5–7 days]
- Lack of experienced staff to perform or supervise the procedure
- Patient refusal to consent

*These are not absolute contraindications, as each case has to be assessed individually and it is up to the operator to balance the risks and benefits of the procedure.

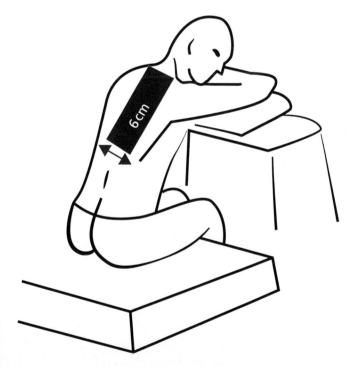

Figure 10.8 The patient is sitting up and leaning over a table. The red shaded area is the 'no fly zone' for chest drain insertion which should be avoided in most cases. A study showed that intercostal arteries are exposed within the intercostal space in the first 6 cm lateral to the spine.

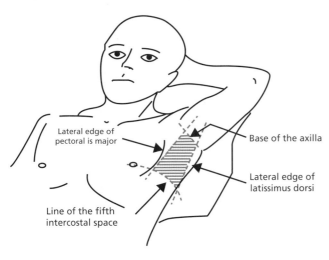

Figure 10.9 Decubitus position; the safety triangle is shaded blue. Source: Havelock (2010). Reproduced with permission of BMJ Publishing Group Ltd.

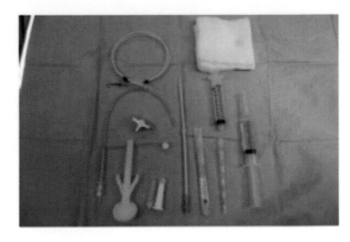

Figure 10.10 Equipment for insertion of a Seldinger chest drain.

Box 10.3 **Equipment for chest drain insertion**

- Sterile gloves and gown
- Antiseptic solution [chlorhexidine in alcohol (ChloraPrep) or iodine]
- Sterile drapes
- Seldinger drain pack (12–18 Fr)
- 2 × green needles (21 gauge), 1 orange needle (25 gauge)
- 1 × 20 mL syringe
- 20 mL local anaesthetic (1% lidocaine)
- Scalpel and sutures (if not included with the drain pack)
- Drain bottle and tubing
- Bio-occlusive dressing

---

6 Check the patient's observations (blood pressure, heart rate, oxygen saturations). If the patient is hypoxic or haemodynamically unstable (unless resulting from the condition that requires chest drain insertion), postpone the procedure until the patient's condition has stabilised.

7 For pleural effusion, identify the side and safe site of drain insertion with ultrasound (if the operator or supervising doctor is trained to do so).

8 Ensure the patient has a working cannula in case he/she requires emergency intravenous medications.

9 Ensure there is another person to act as assistant to help with the procedure or, in case of emergency, to call for help.

Drain insertion technique

- Wear a surgical mask, hat and eye protection.
- Wash your hands and don sterile gown and gloves.
- Ask your assistant to unpack the equipment on a sterile field (Figure 10.10).
- Clean the skin with antiseptic solution (e.g. ChloraPrep, chlorhexidine 2% and alcohol 70%).

- Cover the chest wall with sterile drapes to create a sterile field.
  - Infiltrate the skin with 1% lidocaine using an orange (25 G) needle (Figure 10.11).
  - Infiltrate the subcutaneous tissue, intercostal muscles and parietal pleural with local anaesthetic (approximately 20 mL of 1% lidocaine) using a green needle. Insert the needle above the upper border of the chosen rib to avoid the neurovascular bundle.
  - Aspirate first before injecting to ensure local anaesthetic is not injected into the vein. The length of green needle at which air or fluid is aspirated can be used as a guide to the thickness of the chest wall. Add 0.5 cm to this measurement when using the introducing needle and 1.5 cm when using the dilator to ensure clearance of parietal pleural. (NB If air or fluid is not aspirated, stop the procedure and arrange ultrasound-guided drain insertion by a radiologist or respiratory physician trained in real-time ultrasound-guided drain insertion.)
  - Assemble the equipment while waiting for the local anaesthetic to take effect. It is good practice to have all the equipment within easy reach and in the order to be used.
  - Make a small incision in the skin to allow easy insertion of the introducing needle.
  - Gently insert the introducing needle through the incision into the anaesthetised tract until you have reached the desired depth or until fluid or air is aspirated.
  - Remove the syringe, hold the needle firmly so it does not move and cover the hub of the needle with your thumb to avoid air entering the pleural cavity.
  - Insert the guidewire through the needle hub. Do not force the wire or needle if you feel resistance.
  - Remove the needle while holding on to the guidewire. (NB *Never* let go of the guidewire during the procedure.)
  - Make a small incision (0.5 cm) parallel to the rib with the scalpel blade facing away from the guidewire.
  - Insert the dilator over the guidewire and gently push over the wire in a rotating movement to a depth that is sufficient for the chest wall to be dilated. Avoid over-insertion of the dilator as it has the potential to damage intrathoracic structures.
  - Insert the drain over the guidewire into the pleural cavity. For most people, 10–12 cm at the skin level is sufficient to ensure all

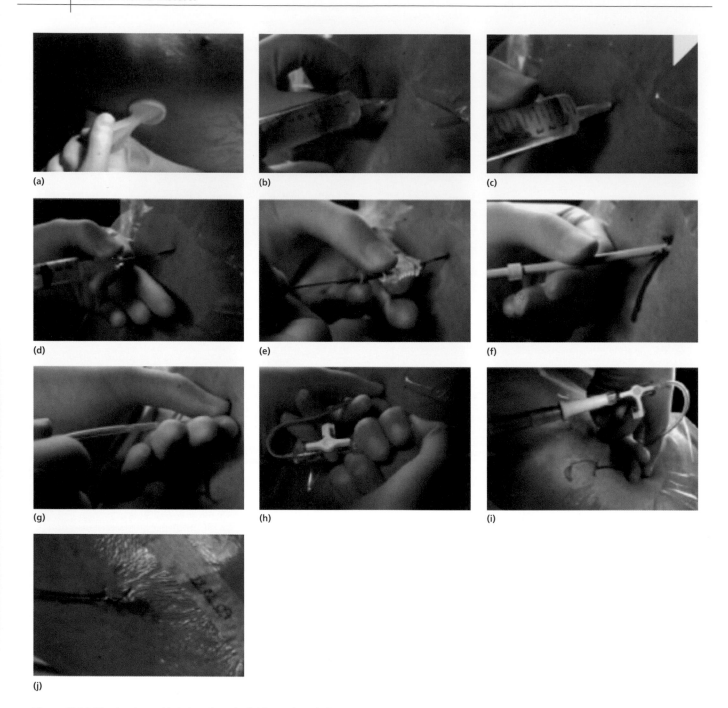

Figure 10.11 Step-by-step guide to insertion of a Seldinger chest drain.

drainage holes are within the pleural cavity to reduce the risk of subcutaneous emphysema.

- Remove the guidewire and drain stiffener and attach a three-way tap, with the tap closed to the chest drain. (NB In pneumothorax, never close the tap to chest drain and always connect the drain to the underwater seal bottle before suturing the drain to skin.)
- Suture the drain to skin using 1.0 or 2.0 silk suture. Avoid tying knots that will pinch the skin or occlude the drain.
- Cover the wound with transparent bio-occlusive dressing.

Post drain insertion

- Dispose your sharps safely in a sharps bin.
- Request a CXR to check drain position.

- Document the procedure in the patient's notes and write clear instructions for nursing staff (e.g. observation every 30 minutes for 2 hours, then hourly for 4 hours, and details of speed of drainage of fluid, e.g. 500 mL per hour maximum drainage).
- Advise the patient to hold the bottle below the waist and to get into and out of bed from the same side as the chest drain.

Drain removal

Remove the drain when the patient takes a deep breath and performs a Valsalva manoeuvre (i.e. on expiration). Cover the wound with a dressing and advise the patient on wound care. There is, in general, no need to close the wound with sutures for smaller drains (12 Fr and smaller).

Tips

- Drain insertion should be avoided, where possible, out of hours (except for tension pneumothorax and confirmed empyema). This will ensure drain is inserted during working hours when there is an appropriate skill mix available.
- Never clamp a drain that is bubbling.

Troubleshooting

1 The drain is not swinging or bubbling. It could be because the drain is either blocked, kinked or has come out of the pleural space:
   - Check the patient first to make sure he/she is well and stable;
   - Make sure the chest drain or tubes are not kinked;
   - Flush the drain with 20 mL normal saline to see if the drain is blocked;
   - Order CXR to check drain position.

2 The drain tube has fallen out:
   - Clamp the drain and connect the drain to a new tube and bottle;
   - Order CXR.

Further reading

Diacon AH, Brutsche MH and Soler M. (2003) Accuracy of pleural puncture sites: a prospective comparison of clinical examination with ultrasound. *Chest* **123**(2), 436–441.

Havelock T, Teoh R, Laws D, Gleeson F; BTS Pleural Disease Guideline Group. (2010) Pleural procedures and thoracic ultrasound: British Thoracic Society Pleural Disease Guideline 2010. *Thorax* **65** (Suppl 2), ii61–ii76.

Helm EJ, Rahman NM, Talakoub O, Fox DL and Gleeson FV. (2013) Course and variation of the intercostal artery by CT scan. *Chest* **143** (3), 634–639.

O'Moore PV, Mueller PR, Simeone JF, Saini S, Butch RJ, Hahn PF *et al.* (1987) Sonographic guidance in diagnostic and therapeutic interventions in the pleural space. *American Journal of Roentgenology* **149** (1), 1–5.

Section C: Insertion of an Indwelling Pleural Catheter

Anna C. Bibby and Nick A. Maskell

Academic Respiratory Unit, University of Bristol, UK

Indwelling pleural catheters (IPCs) can be inserted in awake, non-sedated patients using local anaesthetic. The procedure should be performed in a clean environment such as an operating theatre or dedicated procedure room.

A step-by-step guide to IPC insertion

1 The patient is positioned in the lateral decubitus position (pleural effusion side up) and a thoracic ultrasound performed to confirm the presence of fluid. A suitable insertion site for the drain is chosen and marked. A second site is marked, anteriorly and inferiorly, where the catheter will exit the skin. This is usually approximately 7 cm from the insertion site. Patient comfort and ease of access to the drain should be considered when choosing the exit site. In females, the position of the catheter in relation to their bra straps should also be considered.

2 The skin is sterilised, drapes are positioned and local anaesthesia infiltrated (Figure 10.12).

3 A small incision, measuring 1–2 cm laterally, is made at the insertion and exit sites. The introducer needle is inserted into the pleural space at the insertion site, entering the pleural cavity by travelling directly over the top of a rib. Pleural fluid should then be aspirated freely before proceeding with the next part of the procedure (Figure 10.13).

4 The syringe is removed from the introducer needle and a guidewire passed through the needle into the pleural space. The guidewire remains in situ as the introducer needle is removed (Figure 10.14).

5 Using a blunt tunnelling device (or dissection forceps), the catheter is passed under the skin between the drain exit site and drain insertion site. The catheter is pulled through the tunnel until the polyester cuff is positioned under the skin, 1–2 cm from the drain exit point. The tunnelling device is removed from the proximal end of the catheter (Figures 10.15 and 10.16).

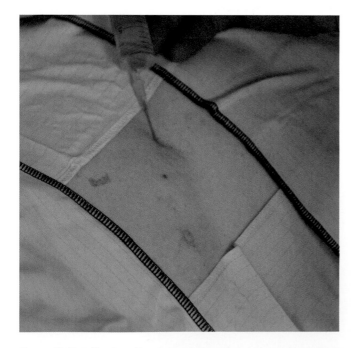

Figure 10.12 Infiltration of local anaesthetic at drain insertion site. A mark is visible inferiorly where the drain will exit the skin.

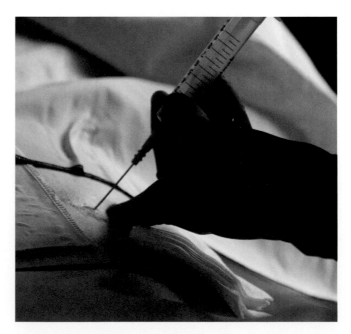

Figure 10.13 Aspiration of pleural fluid via the introducer needle.

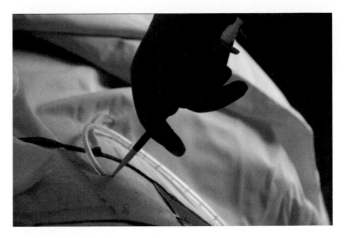

Figure 10.17 Insertion of a blunt dilator and introducer into the pleural space. The proximal end of the catheter is seen exiting the skin at this point.

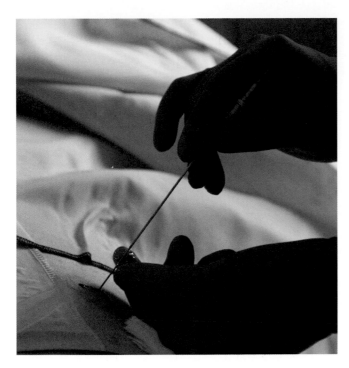

Figure 10.14 Removal of the introducer needle with the guidewire left in situ.

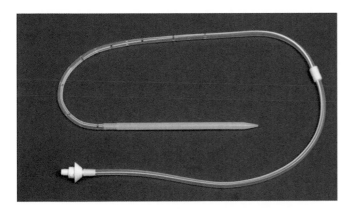

Figure 10.15 Indwelling pleural catheter with plastic tunnelling device attached to the proximal end. A polyester cuff is visible halfway along the catheter.

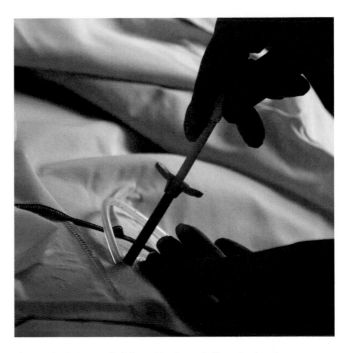

Figure 10.18 Removal of the guidewire and dilator, leaving the introducer in situ.

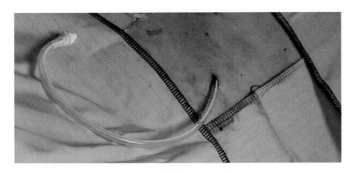

Figure 10.16 Catheter tunnelled under the skin with the distal end visible externally (the proximal end is not visible).

6 A tract is created into the pleural space by passing a dilator within a peel-away introducer over the guidewire (Figure 10.17).
7 The guidewire and dilator are removed, leaving the introducer in situ (Figure 10.18).
8 The proximal end of the catheter is passed through the introducer into the pleural space. The introducer is peeled away from the catheter and removed from the pleural cavity, whilst the catheter is simultaneously advanced until it runs smoothly from the subcutaneous tunnel into the pleural space (Figures 10.19, 10.20 and 10.21).

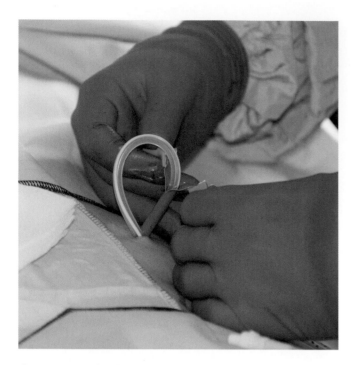

Figure 10.19 Peeling the introducer away from the catheter.

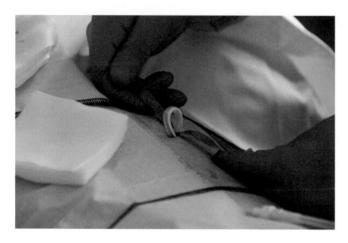

Figure 10.20 Advancing the catheter into the pleural space, as the peel-away introducer is removed.

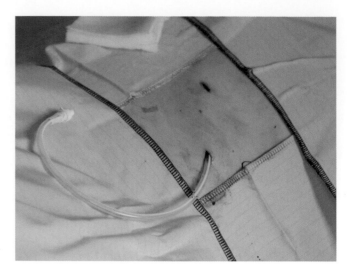

Figure 10.21 Indwelling pleural catheter running smoothly through the subcutaneous tunnel into the pleural space.

9 The incisions are closed and dressings are placed, covering the catheter to maintain sterility.

10 Normally, 1–1.5 L of pleural fluid will be removed from the catheter at the end of the procedure to relieve the patient's immediate symptoms.

11 After a period of observation, a check CXR is performed before the patient is discharged.

CHAPTER 11

Medical Thoracoscopy

Section A: Rigid Thoracoscopy

Matthew Evison[1], Ambika Talwar[2], Ahmed Yousuf[3] and Mohammed Munavvar[4]

[1] Wythenshaw Hospital, Manchester, UK
[2] Churchill Hospital, Oxford, UK
[3] Glenfield Hospital, Leicester, UK
[4] Royal Preston Hospital, Preston, UK

OVERVIEW

- The role of medical thoracoscopy in the diagnosis and management of pleural disease, particularly malignant pleural effusion.
- Which patients should undergo medical thoracoscopy.
- A step-by-step illustrated guide to medical thoracoscopy using both semi-rigid and rigid thoracoscopy approaches.
- The diagnostic accuracy and complication rate of medical thoracoscopy.

The diagnosis and management of pleural disease is a frequent challenge for general and respiratory physicians. A common clinical scenario is the unilateral undiagnosed exudative pleural effusion, which is caused by malignancy in a large number of cases (42–77%). The burden of pleural disease is increasing with an estimated 50 000 new cases of malignant pleural effusion in the UK each year. This equates to 250 new cases per year in an average district general hospital.

Role of medical thoracoscopy

Medical thoracoscopy refers to the percutaneous insertion of a camera into the pleural cavity (usually into pleural fluid), under local anaesthetic and conscious sedation. It is minimally invasive and, once the pleural fluid has been drained, allows the operator to directly visualise the pleura and identify any abnormal areas suitable for biopsy. These biopsies can then be taken under direct visualisation. It is simultaneously a therapeutic procedure, allowing drainage of the fluid, and talc poudrage pleurodesis if appropriate. Direct visualisation of the pleural cavity also allows identification of any intrapleural adhesions that may be broken down and removed to aid complete expansion of the lung.

In undiagnosed exudative pleural effusions, pleural aspiration will yield a diagnosis in less than half of all cases. Blind percutaneous pleural biopsy only increases this yield by a small fraction,

leaving a large proportion without a definitive diagnosis. Medical thoracoscopy dramatically increases the diagnostic yield to 96%. It is also the most effective procedure to achieve complete drainage of pleural fluid and to prevent recurrence of the effusion (84% pleurodesis success rate at 1 month, compared with 60% success rate with talc slurry via a chest drain), although current randomised data do not suggest an advantage for talc poudrage over talc slurry.

Medical thoracoscopy is also effective in the diagnosis and management of tuberculous pleurisy (and sometimes pleural infection). In addition, specialist thoracoscopic practitioners utilise medical thoracoscopy for the management of pneumothorax, lung biopsies and sympathectomy.

Who should undergo a thoracoscopy?

Medical thoracoscopy should be considered in any patient with an undiagnosed exudative pleural effusion. This procedure avoids the risks of general anaesthetic and single lung ventilation required for surgical diagnostic strategies (VATS). It is also a possible option for patients for whom video-assisted thoracic surgery (VATS) is precluded because of comorbidity or poor prognosis.

A summary of the indications and contraindications for medical thoracoscopy is shown in Table 11.1.

Types of medical thoracoscopy

Medical thoracoscopy can be performed using the rigid and semi-rigid thoracoscope. The choice of instrument depends on operator experience and preference.

Rigid thoracoscopes allow a wide field of view of the thoracic cavity and permit larger sized pleural biopsies. The semi-rigid thoracoscope has a similar design to a bronchoscope and therefore may be more 'familiar' to respiratory physicians. However, the working channel is narrower than the rigid scope, allowing smaller biopsies to be obtained and a narrower field of view. Nonetheless, good diagnostic yields have been reported using both instruments (see Section B).

ABC of Pleural Diseases, First Edition. Edited by Najib M. Rahman, Ian Hunt, Fergus V. Gleeson and Nick A. Maskell.
© 2018 John Wiley & Sons Ltd. Published 2018 by John Wiley & Sons Ltd.

Table 11.1 A summary of the indications and contraindications for medical thoracoscopy.

Indications	Relative contraindications
Undiagnosed exudative pleural effusion	Obliterated pleural space
Suspected mesothelioma	Extensive pleural adhesions
Staging of pleural effusion in lung cancer	Bleeding disorder
Treatment of recurrent pleural effusions with pleurodesis	Hypoxia (O2 sats <92% on air)
Pneumothorax requiring chemical pleurodesis as an alternative if patient unfit for surgery	Unstable cardiovascular disease
	Persistent uncontrollable cough

Medical thoracoscopy is performed with local anaesthesia and conscious sedation by operators with the appropriate level of expertise. The procedure should be performed in an operating theatre, endoscopy suite or clean treatment room depending upon the resources available. Full patient resuscitation facilities should be available.

A step-by-step guide to medical thoracoscopy

An illustrated guide to the procedure is described. The differences in semi-rigid and rigid thoracoscopy are highlighted in the text and figures. Much of this guide is based on expert opinion in the UK and is therefore not always evidenced based.

Patient preparation and consent

It is good practice to use the WHO checklist just before commencing the procedure. These are the principal elements to check:

- Patient should have written information >24 hours before the procedure and written consent prior to the procedure by a doctor with the appropriate level of expertise.
- Full blood count (FBC), coagulation profile, renal function and glucose (where indicated).
- Up-to-date chest radiograph and any CT scans available.
- Check the site of the procedure just prior to starting; the site of procedure should be drawn with a skin marker on the patient.
- Preprocedure thoracic ultrasound to confirm the presence of pleural fluid is advisable.
- Nil by mouth for at least 4 hours pre-procedure.
- An intravenous cannula in the arm on the same side as the thoracoscopy to make repeated administration of sedation during the procedure easier.
- Pre-medication with analgesia, such as paracetamol or ibuprofen.
- Prophylactic antibiotics such as 1.2 g IV co-amoxiclav are used by some centres, although this has not been subject to formal study.
- Baseline oxygen saturations, pulse, BP, temperature.
- The patient should be monitored with pulse oximetry, BP and three-lead ECG throughout the procedure.

Procedure

Full aseptic technique should be observed throughout the procedure.

- The patient is positioned in the lateral decubitus position (disease side up) and a thoracic ultrasound performed to confirm the presence of fluid and a suitable puncture site (usually in the mid axillary line).
- Sedation is administered with dose titration and allowed time to take effect.
- Oxygen (2–4 L/min) is administered via nasal cannulae.
- Skin is cleaned with an alcohol-based skin sterilising solution over the whole hemithorax including the axilla. A sterile drape should be placed over the patient, leaving a small exposed area through which the procedure is performed.
- Local anaesthesia infiltration and confirmation of the presence of pleural fluid with needle aspiration.
- A 1 cm incision is performed, following the orientation of the ribs at the thoracoscope insertion point.
- Modified horizontal mattress suture should be inserted; this will act as a closing suture when the post procedure chest drain is removed.
- Blunt dissection through the intercostal space into the pleural cavity (Figure 11.1).
- Once the pleural space is entered, a 7 mm trocar or introducer should be gently eased into the pleural cavity to create a port of entry (Figure 11.2).
- Pleural fluid is then aspirated with a soft suction catheter (Figure 11.3).
- As pleural fluid is removed, air can enter the pleural space through the port to keep the lung deflated, preventing rapid re-expansion of the lung.
- The pleural cavity is then inspected by passing the semi-rigid thoracoscope (Figure 11.4a) or rigid scope (Figure 11.4b) through the port. Images from a rigid scope are shown in Figure 11.5.
- Parietal pleural biopsies are then taken at appropriate sites under direct vision using the optical biopsy forceps (Figure 11.6).
- Talc poudrage can be performed if malignant aetiology is strongly suspected. In semi-rigid thoracoscopy, this can be performed under direct visualisation. With the rigid approach, the thoracoscope is removed from the port and the talc is delivered into the pleural cavity if a one-port technique is used (Figures 11.7 and 11.8).
- The thoracoscope is then removed and a chest drain (at least 20 Fr) is inserted through the tract and sutured in place. This allows removal of air from the pleural space and complete re-expansion of the underlying lung (Figures 11.9 and 11.10).

Other considerations
Induction of pneumothorax

Safe thoracoscopy requires there to be a large pleural space between the lung and chest wall. In cases where there is little pleural fluid, a pneumothorax can be induced to increase the size of the pleural cavity. This procedure requires advanced expertise.

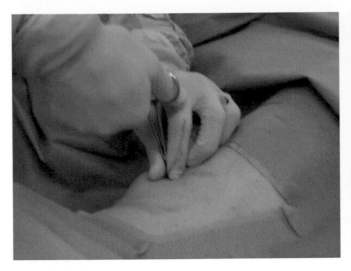

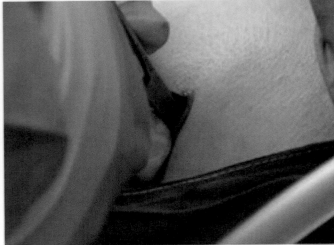

Figure 11.1 Blunt dissection into the pleural cavity.

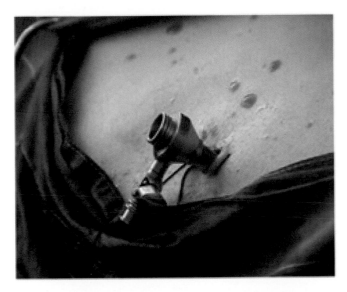

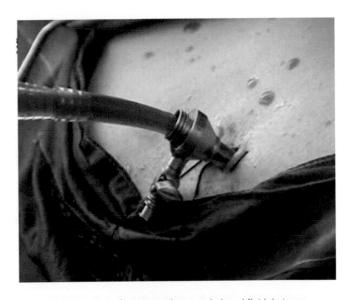

Figure 11.2 Trocar insertion.

Figure 11.3 Insertion of suction catheter and pleural fluid drainage.

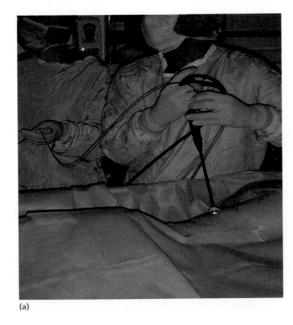

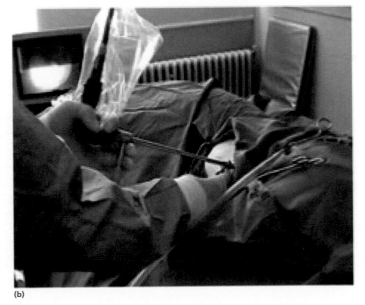

(a)

(b)

Figure 11.4 Insertion of (a) semi-rigid scope; (b) rigid scope.

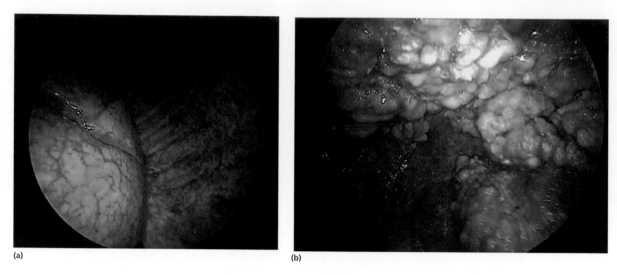

(a)   (b)

Figure 11.5 Inspection of pleural surface using rigid scope: (a) normal pleura; (b) diffuse pleural nodularity seen in malignancy.

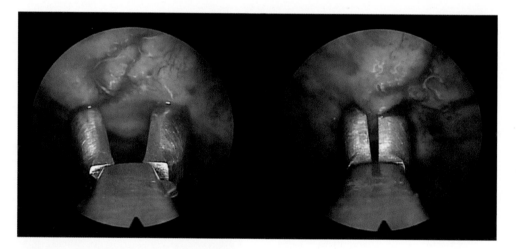

Figure 11.6 Taking pleural biopsies (rigid approach, single port).

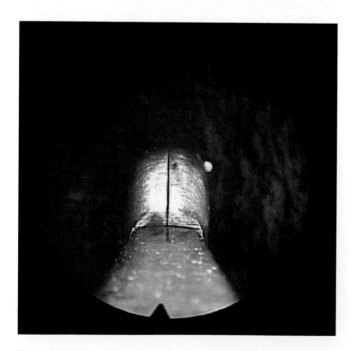

Figure 11.7 Talc poudrage. Image from rigid scope approach, post poudrage.

Second entry port

A second entry port may be required in cases where it may be technically challenging to obtain pleural biopsies via a single port.

Post procedure care

Medical thoracoscopy can be performed as a day case procedure when talc poudrage is not conducted, with discharge after 4 hours of observation for procedures that do not involve talc pleurodesis. However, the decision for overnight stay should be evaluated on a case-by-case basis.

- Monitor oxygen saturations, pulse, BP and temperature every 15 minutes for the first hour after the procedure.
- The chest drain should be on free drainage initially, but continuous suction may be required when the drain stops bubbling and if the lung has not re-expanded.
- Analgesia with opioids and/or non-steroidals is frequently required.
- Deep venous thrombosis (DVT) prophylaxis (increased coagulopathy with talc pleurodesis).
- Mobile chest radiograph on the day of and day after procedure if the chest drain is kept in situ.
- Remove the chest drain when the lung is re-inflated on chest radiograph and there is no evidence of ongoing air leak from the chest tube.

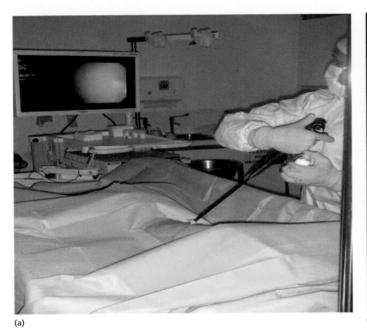
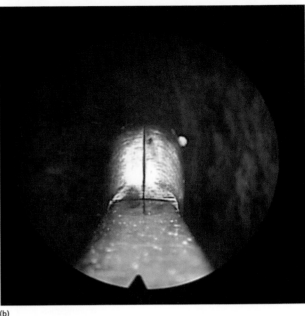

(a)   (b)

Figure 11.8 Talc poudrage: (a) under direct vision using semi-rigid approach; (b) image taken from rigid scope approach.

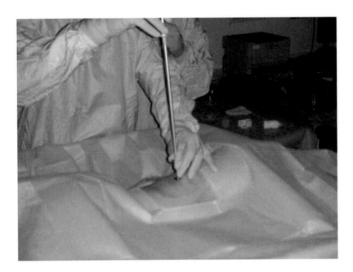

Figure 11.9 Chest drain insertion.

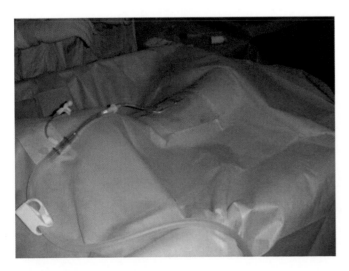

Figure 11.10 End of the procedure.

Diagnostic accuracy of medical thoracoscopy

The diagnostic accuracy of medical and surgical thoracoscopic biopsy in malignant pleural effusion is approximately 93%.

There are two randomised controlled trials comparing rigid thoracoscopy with semi-rigid thoracoscopy, and they concluded that the diagnostic accuracy of the two techniques was comparable. In 2006, two centres in the UK compared the two types of scope (27 patients undergoing rigid thoracoscopy and 41 patients undergoing semi-rigid thoracoscopy). The diagnostic accuracy was found to be 26/27 patients in the rigid thoracoscopy group (96.2%) and 38/41 (92.6%) in the semi-rigid thoracoscopy group.

Complications and adverse events with medical thoracoscopy

Mortality rates are low (<0.01% of cases). Box 11.1 lists the potential minor and major complications.

Complications and adverse events: rigid thoracoscopy versus semi-rigid thoracoscopy

A randomised trial comparing rigid with semi-rigid thoracoscopy showed that the two techniques were safe, and had very similar, low complication rates. Combining data from 47 studies, the BTS Guidelines on Medical Thoracoscopy reported 16 deaths in 4736 rigid thoracoscopy procedures (0.34%). All 16 cases involved talc poudrage and 9 out of the 16 cases involved the use of non-graded talc. This form of talc is known to cause acute respiratory distress syndrome (ARDS) and is now not recommended for use. In a separate case series of 8000 patients undergoing rigid thoracoscopy there was only one reported fatality. Using the same 47 studies (4736 patients), the incidence of minor and major complications are reported as 5.6% and 1.9%, respectively.

Box 11.1 **Complications of thoracoscopy**

Potential minor complications of thoracoscopy

Intra-operative

Tachycardia

Benign cardiac arrhythmias (e.g. atrial fibrillation)

Hypotension (often secondary to sedation)

Hypoxaemia (requiring correction with administration of oxygen)

Chest pain (often during biopsy and talc poudrage)

Minor bleeding

Postoperative

Chest pain and/or discomfort at drain site

Transient fever (often post talc poudrage)

Subcutaneous emphysema

Wound infection

Potential major complications of thoracoscopy

Intra-operative

Major haemorrhage secondary to blood vessel (intercostal artery or major vessel) trauma

Traumatic damage to the lung

Cardiac arrhythmias causing cardiac decompensation

Re-expansion pulmonary oedema

Postoperative

Empyema

Pneumonia

Failure of the lung to re-expand

Malignant seeding and tumour growth at puncture site

Death

Conclusions

Medical thoracoscopy is a highly valuable tool for the diagnosis and management of pleural disease, particularly malignant pleural disease. It has a very high diagnostic accuracy and high success rate for therapeutic interventions. As the burden of pleural disease continues to rise, the role of medical thoracoscopy is likely to become even more important.

Further reading

Dhooria S, Singh N, Aggarwal AN, Gupta D and Agarwal R. (2014) A randomized trial comparing the diagnostic yield of rigid and semirigid thoracoscopy in undiagnosed pleural effusions. *Respir Care* **59** (5), 756–764.

Mohan A, Chandra S, Agarwal D, Naik S and Munavvar M. (2010) Utility of semirigid thoracoscopy in the diagnosis of pleural effusions: a systematic review. *Journal of Bronchology and Interventional Pulmonology* **17** (3), 195–201.

Munavvar M, Khan MA, Edwards J, Wagaruddin Z and Mills J. (2007) The autoclavable semirigid thoracoscope: the way forward in pleural disease? *European Respiratory Journal* **29**, 571–574.

Rahman NM, Ali NJ, Brown G, Chapman SJ, Davies RJ, Downer NJ *et al.* (2010) Local anaesthetic thoracoscopy: British Thoracic Society pleural disease guideline 2010. *Thorax* **65** (Suppl 2), ii54–ii60.

Rozman A, Camlek L, Marc-Malovrh M, Triller N and Kern I. (2013) Rigid versus semi-rigid thoracoscopy for the diagnosis of pleural disease: a randomized pilot study. *Respirology* **18** (4), 704–710.

Wang Z, Tong ZH, Li HJ, Zhao TT, Xu LL, Luo J *et al.* (2008) Semi-rigid thoracoscopy for undiagnosed exudative pleural effusions: a comparative study. *Chinese Medical Journal* **121** (15), 1384–1389.

Section B: Semi-Rigid Thoracoscopy

Matthew Evison[1] and Mohammed Munavvar[2]

[1] Wythenshaw Hospital, Manchester, UK
[2] Royal Preston Hospital, Preston, UK

OVERVIEW

- A step-by-step illustrated guide to medical thoracoscopy using a semi-rigid thoracoscope.
- The advantages of the semi-rigid thoracoscope over the traditional rigid scope and fully flexible scope.
- The diagnostic accuracy and complication rate of semi-rigid thoracoscopy.

Role of medical thoracoscopy

The use of thoracoscopy is not widespread in the UK despite its clear benefits. A survey in 2004 showed only 6% of respiratory physicians had performed more than 10 procedures. Alternatives to the traditional rigid scope have recently been developed to try to improve the utility of this valuable tool. This chapter focuses on the semi-rigid thoracosocpe.

A step-by-step guide to semi-rigid thoracoscopy

Semi-rigid medical thoracoscopy refers to the inspection of the pleural cavity through a semi-rigid camera similar in design to the well-known bronchoscope, including the bi-directional tip. It is performed in a non-intubated patient under conscious sedation without the need for general anaesthesia. An illustrated guide to the procedure is described:

- The patient is positioned in the lateral decubitus position (disease side up) and a thoracic ultrasound performed to confirm the presence of fluid and a suitable puncture site (usually in the mid axillary line).
- Following local anaesthesia infiltration and confirmation of the presence of pleural fluid with needle aspiration, blunt dissection through the intercostal space into the pleural cavity is performed (Figure 11.11).
- Once the pleural space is entered a trocar and/or cannula is inserted into the tract (Figure 11.12).
- The semi-rigid thoracoscope is inserted into the pleural cavity through the cannula and the pleural fluid suctioned under continual direct visualisation.
- As pleural fluid is removed air can enter the pleural space through the port to keep the lung deflated, preventing rapid re-expansion of the lung.
- The pleural surfaces are inspected and biopsies taken at appropriate sites (Figures 11.13, 11.14, 11.15 and 11.16).

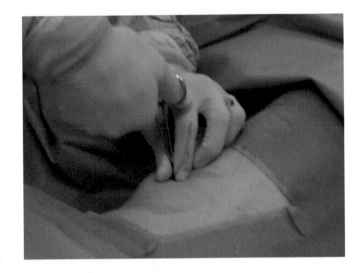

Figure 11.11 Blunt dissection into the pleural cavity.

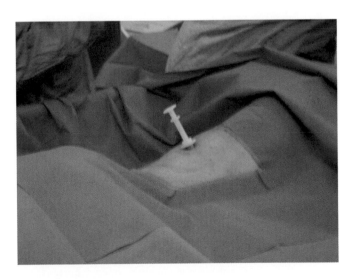

Figure 11.12 Trocar insertion.

- Talc poudrage is performed if malignant aetiology is strongly suspected (Figures 11.17, 11.18 and 11.19).
- The thoracoscope is removed and a chest drain inserted through the tract and sutured in place. This allows removal of air from the pleural space and complete re-expansion of the underlying lung (Figures 11.20 and 11.21).

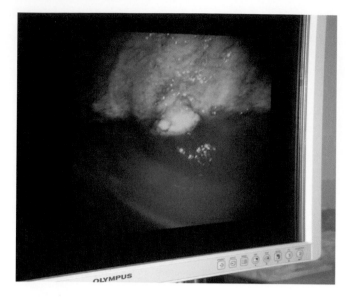

Figure 11.13 Inspection of pleural surface (pleural nodule and thickening seen).

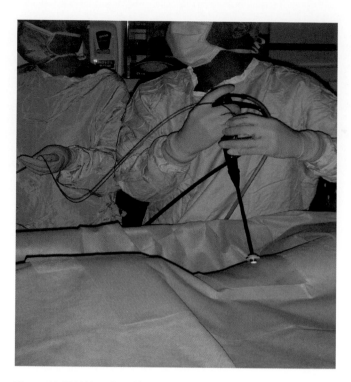

Figure 11.15 Taking pleural biopsies.

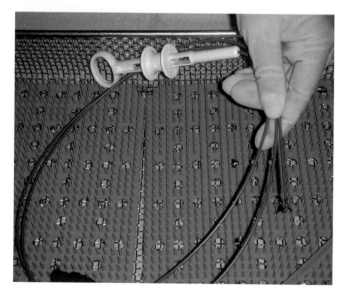

Figure 11.14 Biopsy forceps.

Advantages of the semi-rigid thoracoscope

It has been suggested that respiratory physicians are not familiar with the instruments of rigid thoracoscopy, as it requires the use of a specialised camera and light source equipment. This may be why rigid thoracoscopy is not more widely performed. Thoracoscopy has therefore been attempted with the familiar flexible broncho-scope but it was reported as being difficult to manipulate within the pleural cavity (the flexibility of the instrument made steering diffi-cult) and it produced inferior results compared to rigid thoracos-copy. In addition, full sterilisation of the bronchoscope is not usual, and is required when entering instruments in to the sterile pleural cavity. The semi-rigid thoracoscope aims to combine the best fea-tures of rigid and flexible scopes:

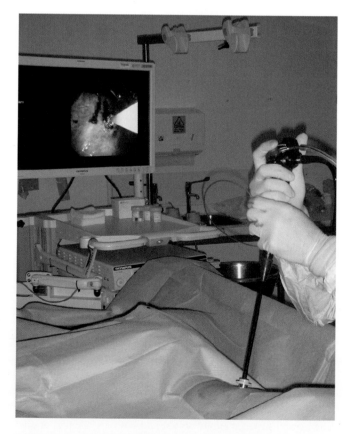

Figure 11.16 Taking pleural biopsies under direct visualisation.

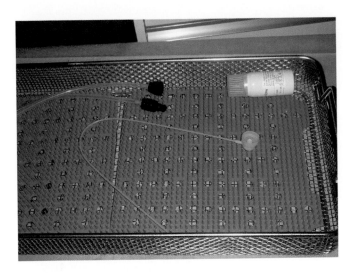

Figure 11.17 Talc poudrage kit.

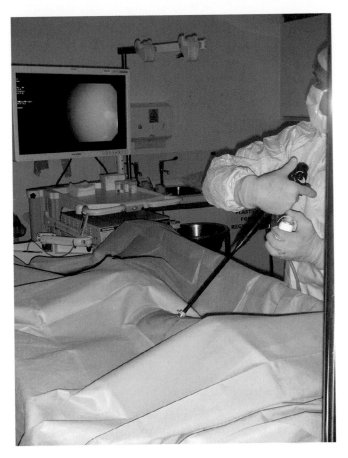

Figure 11.19 Talc poudrage.

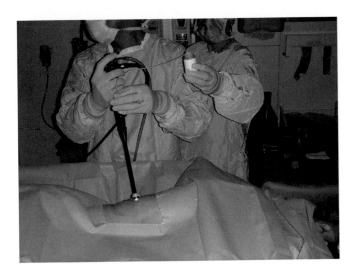

Figure 11.18 Talc poudrage.

- Similarity to the controls of a flexible bronchoscope;
- Compatible with existing video processors and light sources available in most endoscopy suites;
- Autoclavable instrument also allows easy integration into already functioning endoscopy suites;
- Compatible with standard biopsy forceps;
- Maintains ease of movement and control within the pleural cavity;
- All-in-one instrument with no need to change instruments for visual inspection, biopsy and talc poudrage;
- Always a single puncture technique;
- Simplistic talc poudrage technique under direct visualisation.

Disadvantages of the semi-rigid thoracoscope

Semi-rigid thoracosocpy produces smaller size biopsies than rigid thoracoscopy although there is no statistical difference in the diagnostic rate between the two.

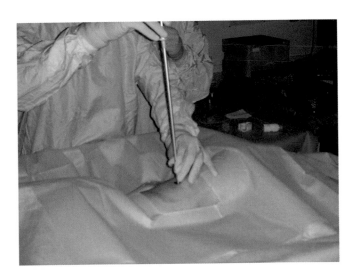

Figure 11.20 Chest drain insertion.

Diagnostic accuracy of semi-rigid thoracoscopy

In 2010, the British Thoracic Society (BTS) published guidelines on medical thoracoscopy. This guideline details four studies that report on the diagnostic rate for semi-rigid thoracoscopy between 1988 and 2007. These four studies give a combined diagnostic sensitivity for malignancy of 96/113 (85%).

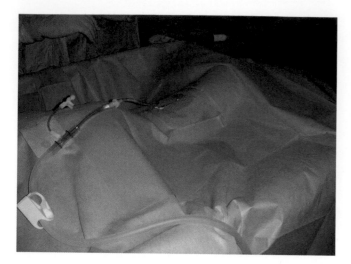

Figure 11.21 End of the procedure.

Within the last year there have two further publications on semi-rigid thoracoscopy. First, a comparative study in China reported a diagnostic accuracy of 93% (23/25 cases). Secondly, a systematic review has been completed on the diagnostic accuracy of semi-rigid thoracoscopy. Five studies met the inclusion criteria, encompassing 154 patients. The results included a pooled sensitivity of 0.97, specificity of 1.0, positive likelihood ratio of 5.47 and negative likelihood ratio of 0.08.

Diagnostic accuracy: rigid thoracoscopy versus semi-rigid thoracoscopy

The BTS guideline reviewed 22 studies of rigid thoracoscopy and reports a diagnostic accuracy of 96.2% for malignant disease. In 2006, two centres in the UK compared the two types of scope: 27 patients undergoing rigid thoracoscopy versus 41 patients undergoing semi-rigid thoracoscopy. The diagnostic accuracy was found to be 26/27 patients in the rigid thoracoscopy group (96.2%) and 38/41 (92.6%) in the semi-rigid thoracoscopy group.

Semi-rigid thoracoscopy is an effective procedure for the diagnosis of pleural disease. Two randomised controlled trials have shown that there is no significant difference in diagnostic accuracy when compared with rigid thoracoscopy.

Complications and adverse events with semi-rigid thoracoscopy

Semi-rigid thoracoscopy is a very safe procedure. In all of the above-mentioned research on semi-rigid thoracoscopy, totalling 375 patients, there were no reported major complications or fatalities. There were a small number of minor adverse events reported: transient pain at the chest drain site (6%) controlled with simple analgesia, asymptomatic subcutaneous emphysema (<1%) and asymptomatic transient fever (<1%). Box 11.1 lists the potential minor and major complications found for semi-rigid thoracoscopy.

Conclusions

Semi-rigid thoracoscopy is a very safe procedure with only minor, benign complications reported in the limited literature to this point. Rigid thoracoscopy has a sizeable bank of data that confirms its safety and low complication rate. The semi-rigid thoracoscope, with its similarity to the bronchoscope and easy integration into functioning endoscopy suites, may encourage a significant increase in the uptake of the vital procedure of medical thoracoscopy.

CHAPTER 12

Surgical Management of Pleural Disease

Stephanie Fraser[1] and Ian Hunt[2]

[1] Guy's Hospital, London, UK
[2] St. George's Hospital, London, UK

OVERVIEW

- Thoracic surgical and anaesthetic advances have allowed increasingly frail patients to undergo pleural procedures performed keyhole (thorascopically).

- Surgical pleural operations including simple diagnostic procedures such as pleural biopsies and drainage of pleural effusions can be performed but alternative interventions such as medical thorascopy are increasingly offered.

- More complex therapeutic operations including decortications for pleural infection and excision of pleura-based tumours are increasingly performed thorascopically.

Historical developments

Thoracic surgery has an integral role in the management of pleural disease, augmented by significant advancements in both thoracic anaesthesia and operative techniques over the last century. Minimally invasive techniques, in particular, have evolved significantly since they were first performed in 1910 by H.C. Jacobeus using a modified cystoscope. At the turn of the twentieth century, this technique for intrapleural pneumolysis transformed operative treatment for tuberculosis (TB). However, over the following decades, advancements in the medical treatment for TB resulted in a decline in the number of procedures performed. This continued to decline until the advent of video-assisted devices vastly widened applications in the management of pleural disease and developed into the current video-assisted thoracic surgery (VATS). Increasingly, such keyhole advancements have allowed interventional pleural procedures to be carried out by chest physicians who perform such procedures under sedation in selected patients.

Thoracic surgery has evolved alongside the development of aseptic techniques, advancements in radiology, transfusion and monitoring techniques. However, the most profound changes to practice have resulted from developments in thoracic anaesthesia.

Thoracic anaesthetic

Thoracic anaesthesia has altered almost unrecognisably from the early days of ether and chloroform. At the time, surgery was time-limited, because of the physiological effects of the iatrogenic pneumothorax caused when the thoracic cavity is first entered. This posed significant risk, together with the potential for contaminating the contralateral healthy lung in procedures which were largely performed for infection. The ability to secure the airway with a cuffed endotracheal (ET) tube allowed deeper anaesthesia and periods of apnoea during which a more effective procedure could be performed. Further strides were made in the 1930s with the introduction of bronchial blockers which facilitated single-lung ventilation. A pivotal leap in the management of thoracic patients occurred with the introduction of double lumen ET tubes, in particular the Robertshaw, introduced in 1962, with its wide lumen and moulded curvature which is still widely used today. Safe surgery for pleural disease was further optimised thanks to advances in multi-modal pain management, mechanical ventilation and novel anaesthetic agents.

Additional advancements in anaesthesia have also influenced the groups now considered for thoracic surgery, including patients who may have previously been seen as poor surgical candidates such as elderly frail patients with multiple comorbidities or complex anatomy. The accurate placement of double lumen ET tubes to enable good lung isolation in patients with difficult airways is now possible with the use of fibreoptic bronchoscopy. Patients with poor preoperative lung function can have their oxygenation maximised during surgery with positive pressure ventilation and patients with multiple comorbidities or at high risk for general anaesthesia can now have complex thoracic intervention performed safely as awake non-intubated procedures.

Thoracic surgery

The current operative techniques for thoracic surgery have largely been guided by technological advancement. The key pieces of equipment are under a constant process of revision and refinement but, at present, include a rigid 5 or 10 mm diameter thoracoscope

---

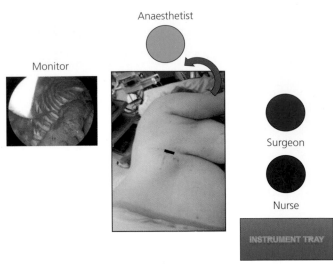

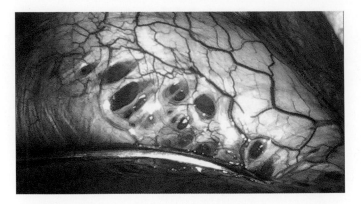

Figure 12.2 Diaphragmatic fenestrations (whorles) in a young woman who has multiple episodes of pneumothoraxes.

Figure 12.1 Theatre set up for a video-assisted thoracic surgery (VATS) procedure.

with either a 0 or 30 degree angle. A light source and cable are essential, and higher light output is required than with other scopes as blood in the operative field absorbs 50% of the light, darkening the picture. An image processor and camera complete the set up and most recently 3D cameras, which increase the surgical depth of field, have been trialled.

Refinements in this equipment have led to a reduction in the size and number of incisions, with most simple pleural procedures requiring only a single small (10–20 mm) incision. Minimally invasive techniques have been demonstrated to benefit the patient with regards to postoperative pain and length of inpatient stay. Additionally, the practicability of simulation training on VATS techniques can minimise the exposure of patients to the learning curves of new surgeons (Figure 12.1).

Although there are a plethora of applications for thoracic surgery in pleural disease, here we discuss the most common indications and techniques.

Primary and secondary pneumothoraces

Patients with spontaneous pneumothoraces are frequently referred for consideration of surgical intervention. These include, but are not limited to: recurrent ipsilateral pneumothoraces, bilateral pneumothoraces, tension pneumothoraces, haemopneumothoraces, catamenial pneumothoraces, pneumothoraces occurring in pregnancy or with severe underlying disease (including AIDS and cystic fibrosis) and prolonged pneumothoraces (3–5 days). Definitive surgical intervention in adults has been demonstrated to reduce the risk of recurrence and potentially reduce costs. Talc pleurodesis performed intra-operatively has been shown to be potentially more effective than talc slurry via an intercostal drain. Additionally, management of the underlying cause of a pneumothorax including resection of sub-pleural bullae (bullectomy) or patching diaphragmatic fenestrations seen in catamenial pneumothoraces can be performed surgically (Figure 12.2).

Malignant pleural effusions

These pose a huge burden of disease with an ever-increasing prevalence and incidence. Not only are they commonly seen in current medical practice, but they carry a poor prognosis, and interventions to guide cancer treatment and control symptoms should be expedited. A Cochrane Review demonstrated increased efficacy of pleurodesis with thoracoscopy compared to medical pleurodesis with no increase in mortality. Surgical VATS (with or without general anaesthetic) or medical thoracoscopy can provide an accurate tissue diagnosis as well as effective pleurodesis using a single small incision and should be considered in all patients presenting with either recurrent pleural effusions or those with no cytological diagnosis.

Empyema

Pleural infections are a common reason for referral to thoracic surgeons. In this case, a failure of medical management including ongoing evidence of sepsis or a persistent pleural collection following tube drainage are the main indications for surgical intervention. The approach to surgical intervention should vary on both patient factors and stage of the empyema. Both traditional thoracotomy and VATS debridement have been shown to be effective treatment options with the aim of decontaminating the pleural space and evacuating infected debris. Earlier referral for intervention is recommended as VATS drainage and debridement is more likely to be effective when performed in the fibrinopurulent stage (Figure 12.3), whereas a chronic organising empyema is more likely to require decortication (removing restricting pleural cortex around the lung) to facilitate lung expansion (Figure 12.4). As referral practices change, the need for thoracotomy decortication as opposed to VATS debridement has dramatically deceased in the UK over the last 5 years.

Pleural tumour

Patients with mesothelioma commonly present with pleural thickening and effusion. Surgery to diagnose this should be considered early, as VATS pleural biopsies carry the highest diagnostic yield when compared with CT-guided fine needle aspiration or cytological

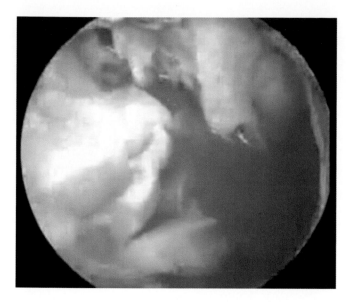

Figure 12.3 VATS images of early empyema at fibrinopurulent stage.

analysis, and the life expectancy from the time of presentation is short (commonly 6–12 months). Additionally, early pleurodesis via VATS may reduce the potential number of sites for tumour seeding resulting from multiple drains or needle aspirations. The surgical technique is the same as for malignant pleural effusions and is performed with a single VATS port site for drainage, pleural biopsy and instillation of talc.

The role of surgery for treatment of mesothelioma (and not just the symptoms, such as pleural effusion) remains controversial with previously extensive resections of the entire pleural cavity including lung, diaphragm and pericardium as well as both pleurae (extra-pleural pneumonectomy) being increasingly questioned regarding

whether it increases survival. Alternative surgical procedures to remove both pleurae alone, with or without diaphragm and pericardium (radical pleurectomy), remain unproven and are currently the subject of several surgical trials including the randomised MARS2 trial.

Trauma

Thoracic surgery has an essential role in the management of trauma. VATS can assist the treatment of traumatic haemothoraces and pneumothoraces in addition to diagnosing and managing significant injuries to major intrathoracic structures. A thoracotomy is indicated to control haemorrhage if the patient is haemodynamically unstable or if single-lung ventilation is not possible.

Conclusions

The evolution of thoracic surgery to its current practice has been heavily influenced by technological advancements over the last century. In particular, minimally invasive techniques have an important role in the management of pleural disease and should be considered early to maximise the potential benefits for patients.

Further reading

Baltayiannis N, Michail C, Lazaridis G, Anagnostopoulos D, Baka S, Mpoukovinas I *et al.* (2015) Minimally invasive procedures. *Annals of Translational Medicine* **3** (4), 55.

Brodsky JB and Lemmens HJ. (2007) The history of anesthesia for thoracic surgery. *Minerva Anestesiologica* **73** (10), 513–524.

Casós SR and Richardson JD. (2006) Role of thoracoscopy in acute management of chest injury. *Current Opinion in Critical Care* **12** (6), 584–589. [Review.]

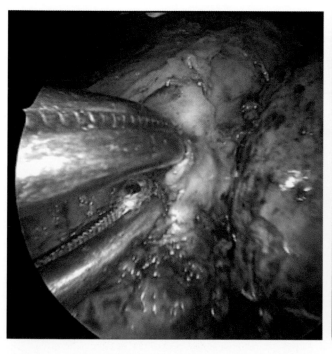
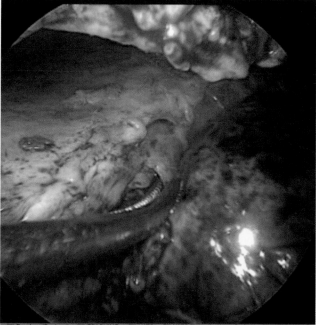

Figure 12.4 Decortication of thickened visceral pleura in a chronic organising empyema.

Chambers A and Scarci M. (2009) In patients with first-episode primary spontaneous pneumothorax is video-assisted thoracoscopic surgery superior to tube thoracostomy alone in terms of time to resolution of pneumothorax and incidence of recurrence? *Interactive Cardiovascular and Thoracic Surgery* **9** (6), 1003–1008.

Clive AO, Kahan BC, Hooper CE, Bhatnagar R, Morley AJ, Zahan-Evans N *et al.* (2014) Predicting survival in malignant pleural effusion: development and validation of the LENT prognostic score. *Thorax* **69** (12), 1098–1104.

Gonzalez-Rivas D. (2015) Recent advances in uniportal video-assisted thoracoscopic surgery. *Chinese Journal of Cancer Research* **27** (1), 90–93.

Guedel A and Waters R. (1928) A new intratracheal catheter. *Current Research in Anesthesia and Analgesia* **7** (4), 238–239.

Jenkins AV. (1956) Carlens catheter: a simple method of intubation. *British Journal of Anaesthesia* **28** (2), 85–86.

Luh S and Liu H. (2006) Video-assisted thoracic surgery: the past, present status and the future. *Journal of Zhejiang University Science B* **7** (2), 118–128.

Macduff A, Arnold A and Harvey J. (2010) Management of spontaneous pneumothorax: British Thoracic Society Pleural Disease Guideline 2010. A Quick Reference Guide. https://www.brit-thoracic.org.uk/document-library/clinical-information/pleural-disease/pleural-disease-guidelines-2010/pleural-disease-guideline-quick-reference-guide/ (accessed 20 September 2017).

Molnar TF. (2007) Current surgical treatment of thoracic empyema in adults. *European Journal of Cardiothoracic Surgery* **32** (3), 422–430. [Epub 2007 Jul 23. Review.]

Mott FE. (2012) Mesothelioma: a review. *Ochsner Journal* **12** (1), 70–79.

Pompeo E, Rogliani P, Palombi L, Orlandi A, Cristino B, Dauri M; Awake Thoracic Surgery Research Group (ATSRG). (2015) The complex care of severe emphysema: role of awake lung volume reduction surgery. *Annals of Translational Medicine* **3** (8), 108.

Shaw P and Agarwal R. (2004) Pleurodesis for malignant pleural effusions. *Cochrane Database Systematic Review* **1**, CD002916. [Review. Update in: *Cochrane Database Systematic Review* (2013) **11**, CD002916.]

Trehan K, Kemp CD and Yang SC. (2014) Simulation in cardiothoracic surgical training: where do we stand? *Journal of Thoracic and Cardiovascular Surgery* **147** (1), 18–24.

Index

ABC of Pleural Diseases, First Edition. Edited by Najib M. Rahman, Ian Hunt, Fergus V. Gleeson and Nick A. Maskell.
© 2018 John Wiley & Sons Ltd. Published 2018 by John Wiley & Sons Ltd.

Imaging in Endocrinology

Imaging in Endocrinology

Paolo Pozzilli MD

Professor of Endocrinology
Chair, Department of Endocrinology and Diabetes
University Campus Bio-Medico
Rome, Italy;
Professor of Diabetes Research
Centre of Diabetes
The Blizard Institute
St. Bartholomew's and the London School of Medicine
Queen Mary University of London
London, UK

Andrea Lenzi MD

Professor of Endocrinology
Chair, Section of Medical Pathophysiology, Food Science, and Endocrinology
Department of Experimental Medicine
Sapienza University of Rome
Policlinico Umberto I
Rome, Italy

Bart L Clarke MD

Associate Professor of Medicine
Division of Endocrinology, Diabetes, Metabolism, and Nutrition
Department of Internal Medicine
Mayo Clinic College of Medicine
Rochester, MN, USA

William F Young Jr MD, MSC

Chair, Division of Endocrinology, Diabetes, Metabolism, and Nutrition
Tyson Family Endocrinology Clinical Professor
Professor of Medicine
Mayo Clinic College of Medicine
Rochester, MN, USA

WILEY Blackwell

Registered office: John Wiley & Sons, Ltd, The Atrium, Southern Gate, Chichester, West Sussex,
PO19 8SQ, UK

Editorial offices: 9600 Garsington Road, Oxford, OX4 2DQ, UK
The Atrium, Southern Gate, Chichester, West Sussex, PO19 8SQ, UK
111 River Street, Hoboken, NJ 07030-5774, USA

For details of our global editorial offices, for customer services and for information about how to apply
for permission to reuse the copyright material in this book please see our website at
www.wiley.com/wiley-blackwell

Library of Congress Cataloging-in-Publication Data

Pozzilli, Paolo, author.
   Imaging in endocrinology / Paolo Pozzilli, Andrea Lenzi, Bart L. Clarke, William
F. Young Jr.
       p. ; cm.
     Includes bibliographical references and index.
     ISBN 978-0-470-65627-3 (cloth : alk. paper) – ISBN 978-1-118-74907-4 (epub) – ISBN
978-1-118-74908-1 – ISBN 978-1-118-74930-2 (emobi) – ISBN 978-1-118-74931-9 (epdf)
   I. Lenzi, Andrea, author.   II. Clarke, Bart, author.   III. Young, William F., Jr., 1951- author.   IV.
Title.
     [DNLM: 1. Endocrine System Diseases–Atlases.   2. Diagnostic Imaging–methods–Atlases.
3. Metabolic Diseases–Atlases.   WK 17]
     RC649
     616.40022′3–dc23
                                                                                          2013029209

A catalogue record for this book is available from the British Library.

Contents

Contents

Contents

Chapter 6 Gonads, 155

Contents

About the Companion Website

This book is accompanied by a companion website:
www.wiley.com\go\Pozzilli\endocrinemetabolicdisease

The website includes:

• Powerpoints of all figures from the book for downloading

Preface

No medical discipline requires such a precise phenotypic classification and careful consideration of the "image" as does endocrinology. Indeed, it is from "observation" that the endocrinologist extrapolates the elements upon which he or she bases clinical reasoning in the identification of a medical condition.

This atlas aims to be a valuable guide in endocrine diagnosis – suitable for both specialists and physicians in training, as well as physicians in other disciplines with an interest in endocrine disorders. Using the image as a unifying theme, we address the most salient themes of the science of endocrinology – including thyroid, pituitary, adrenal, endocrine pancreas, bone and mineral metabolism, and gonads. Each section provides iconographic support for the pathologies examined.

The universal character of this atlas guarantees a high standard of quality. The work was carried out in both Italy and the USA and has the added benefit of combining the rigor and scientific integrity belonging to the cradle of modern endocrinology (Rome) and the clinical resources of a major quaternary endocrine referral center (Mayo Clinic).

We would like to express our gratitude to all those who collaborated on this project. Their passion and enthusiasm toward the completion of this work has been exceptional. Without their hard work and dedication, this publication would have not seen the light.

We would also like to thank Wiley and its editors, who have demonstrated, once again, the high level of professionalism and special attention to detail needed to successfully bring to fruition this type of publication. We hope you enjoy consulting the Atlas.

Paolo Pozzilli, Andrea Lenzi, Bart L Clarke
and William F Young Jr
July 2013

Collaborators

Giusy Beretta
(collaborator for Thyroid and Pancreas chapters)
Senior Investigator
Dept of Endocrinology and Diabetes
University Campus Bio-Medico
Rome, Italy

Daniele Gianfrilli
(collaborator for Gonads and Mucocutaneous Manifestations of Endocrine Disorders chapters)
Senior Investigator in Endocrinology
Dept of Experimental Medicine
Section of Medical Pathophysiology, Food Science, and Endocrinology
Sapienza University of Rome
Rome, Italy

Elisa Giannetta
(collaborator for Gonads and Mucocutaneous Manifestations of Endocrine Disorders chapters)
Senior Investigator in Endocrinology
Dept of Experimental Medicine
Section of Medical Pathophysiology, Food Science, and Endocrinology
Sapienza University of Rome
Rome, Italy

Andrea M. Isidori
(collaborator for Gonads and Mucocutaneous Manifestations of Endocrine Disorders chapters)
Assistant Professor of Endocrinology
Dept of Experimental Medicine
Section of Medical Pathophysiology, Food Science, and Endocrinology
Sapienza University of Rome
Rome, Italy

Angelo Lauria
(collaborator for Thyroid and Pancreas chapters)
Senior Investigator
Dept of Endocrinology and Diabetes
University Campus Bio-Medico
Rome, Italy

Andrea Palermo
(collaborator for Thyroid and Pancreas chapters)
Senior Investigator
Dept of Endocrinology and Diabetes
University Campus Bio-Medico
Rome, Italy

Alberto Signore
(collaborator for Thyroid and Pancreas chapters)
Professor, Dept of Nuclear Medicine
Sapienza University II Medical Faculty
Rome, Italy; and
Dept of Nuclear Medicine
University of Groningen,
The Netherlands

1 Thyroid

Hashimoto's thyroiditis (chronic autoimmune thyroiditis)

Definition and epidemiology

Hashimoto's thyroiditis (HT), or chronic lymphocytic thyroiditis, is an autoimmune disease in which the thyroid gland is attacked by a variety of cell and antibody-mediated immune processes. The name "Hashimoto's thyroiditis" is derived from the 1912 original report by Hashimoto describing patients with both goiter and intense lymphocytic infiltration of the thyroid (Figs 1.1 & 1.2) as "struma lymphomatosa."

Hashimoto's thyroiditis is the most common cause of primary hypothyroidism in iodine-sufficient areas of the world; it is among the most common causes of nonendemic goiter. On average 1.0–1.5/1000 people suffer from this disease. It occurs far more often in women than in men (incidence of 10 : 1 to 20 : 1, respectively), and it is most prevalent between 45 and 65 years of age. Occurrence in children is also uncommon, especially in populations where iodine is not a dietary scarcity.

Etiology and pathogenesis

Autoantibodies may be present against thyroid peroxidase, thyroglobulin, and thyroid-stimulating hormone (TSH) receptors, although a small percentage of patients may have none of these antibodies present. Antibody-dependent cell-mediated cytotoxicity is a substantial factor behind the apoptotic fallout of HT. Activation of cytotoxic T lymphocytes (CD8$^+$ T cells) in response to cell-mediated immune response affected by helper T lymphocytes (CD4$^+$ T cells) is central to thyrocyte destruction. Recruitment of macrophages is another effect of helper T-lymphocyte activation, with Th1-axis lymphocytes producing inflammatory cytokines within the thyroid tissue to further macrophage activation and migration into the thyroid gland for a direct effect. Infection, stress, sex steroids, pregnancy, iodine intake, and radiation exposure are known possible precipitating factors for HT. Fetal microchimerism within the maternal thyroid is also a possibility.

Signs and symptoms

Hashimoto's thyroiditis very often results in hypothyroidism with bouts of hyperthyroidism. Symptoms of HT include weight gain, depression, mania, sensitivity to heat and cold, paresthesia, fatigue, panic attacks, bradycardia, tachycardia, high cholesterol, reactive hypoglycemia, constipation, migraine, muscle weakness, cramps, memory loss, infertility, hair loss, and myxedematous psychosis.

Diagnosis

Laboratory findings

Laboratory tests for HT include:
- Antithyroid peroxidase antibodies (TPOAbs) and thyroglobulin antibodies (TgAbs)
- TSH, free thyroxine (FT$_4$)
- Total cholesterol, high density lipoprotein (HDL), and triglycerides

Imaging tests

Imaging tests for HT include:
- Neck ultrasound (Fig. 1.3)
- Computed tomography (CT) scan (rare)
- ^{99m}TcO$_4$ thyroid scintigraphy (Fig. 1.4)

Treatment

In patients with primary hypothyroidism, the main treatment is levothyroxine.

Imaging in Endocrinology, First Edition. Paolo Pozzilli, Andrea Lenzi, Bart L Clarke and William F Young Jr.
© 2014 John Wiley & Sons, Ltd. Published 2014 by John Wiley & Sons, Ltd.

Illustrations (Figs 1.1–1.4)

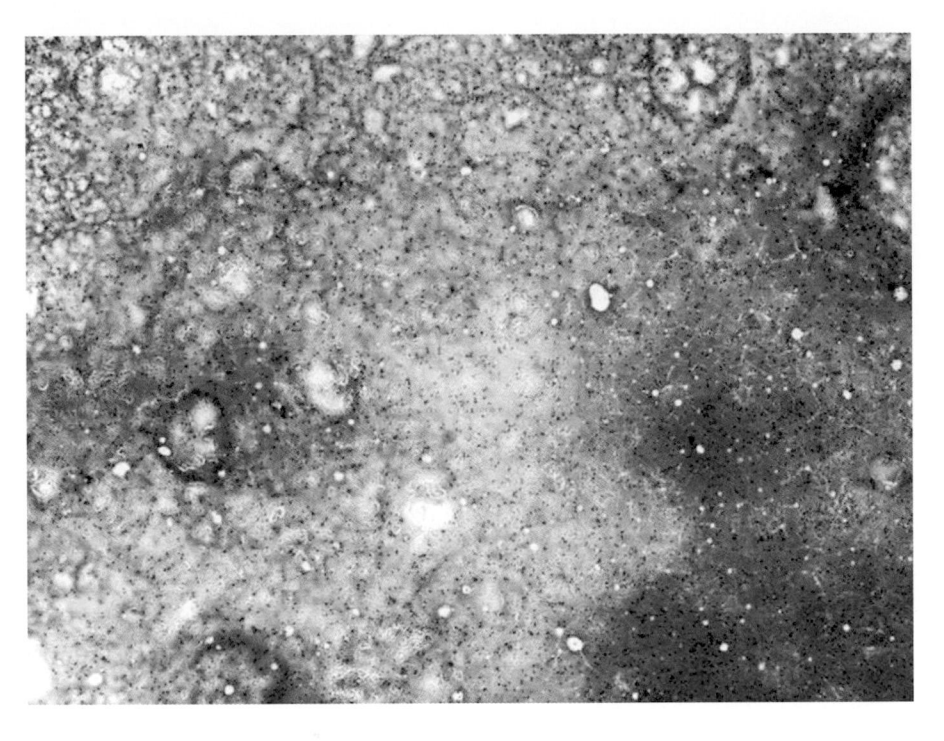

Figure 1.1 Cytology of thyroiditis. This figure shows rare and normal thyrocytes associated with numerous lymphocytes (Papanicolau, 10 ×).

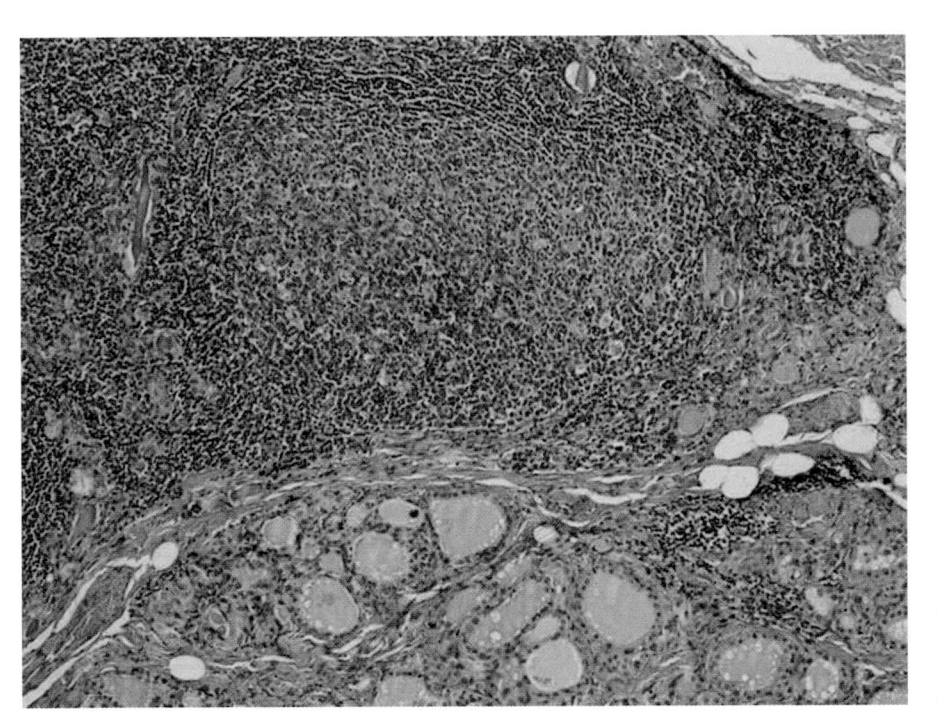

Figure 1.2 Histology of thyroiditis. Hashimoto thyroiditis is characterized by Hürthle cells associated with follicular lymphoid structures (HE, 10 ×).

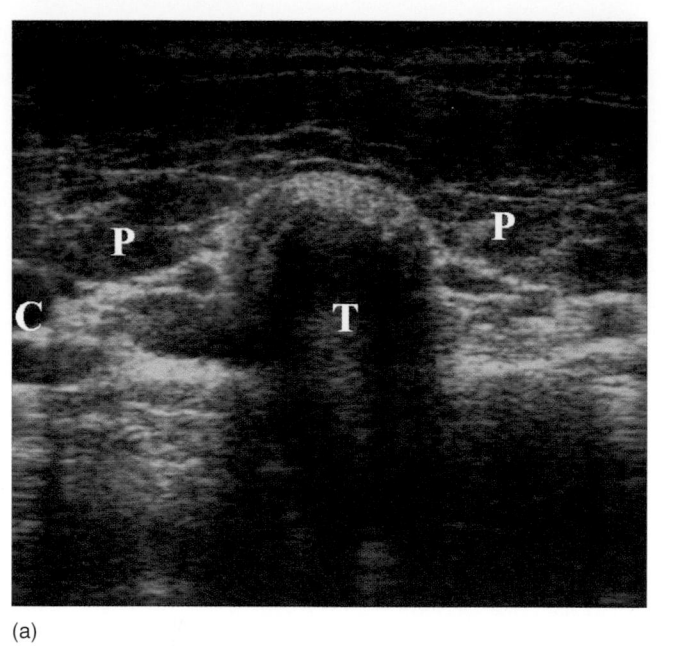

(a)

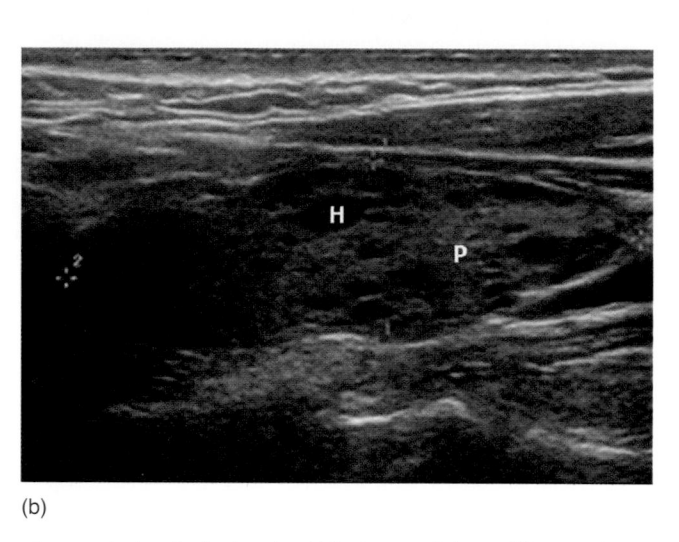

(b)

Figure 1.3 A 46-year-old woman with a recent episode of cervical tenderness and a familiar history of thyroid disease. The patient complained of fatigue and reported a weight gain of about 10 kg in the last 2 months. (a) Thyroid ultrasound – cross section. This ultrasound shows a thyroid with a slight increase in volume, globular shape, and homogeneous structure, and less echogenic than normal. (b) Thyroid ultrasound – longitudinal section. This ultrasound shows diffuse patchy hypoechoic lesions throughout the gland. This sonographic appearance is called a "leopard skin" pattern and is seen in lymphocytic infiltration of the thyroid in Hashimoto's thyroiditis. The hypoechoic lesions within the thyroid are areas of lymphocytic infiltration of the thyroid tissue. C, carotid artery; H, hypoechoic lesions; P, thyroid parenchyma; T, trachea.

Figure 1.4 The same patient as in Fig. 1.3: $^{99m}TcO_4$ thyroid scintigraphy with iodine uptake curve. Iodine uptake was 2% at 4 hours (a) and 2% at 24 hours (b). The scan showed no uptake in the thyroid bed. The free triiodothyronine (FT_3) and free thyroxine (FT_4) levels were low with elevated thyroid stimulating hormone (TSH) and antibodies against thyroperoxidase (TPOAb) values. The patient started levothyroxine treatment.

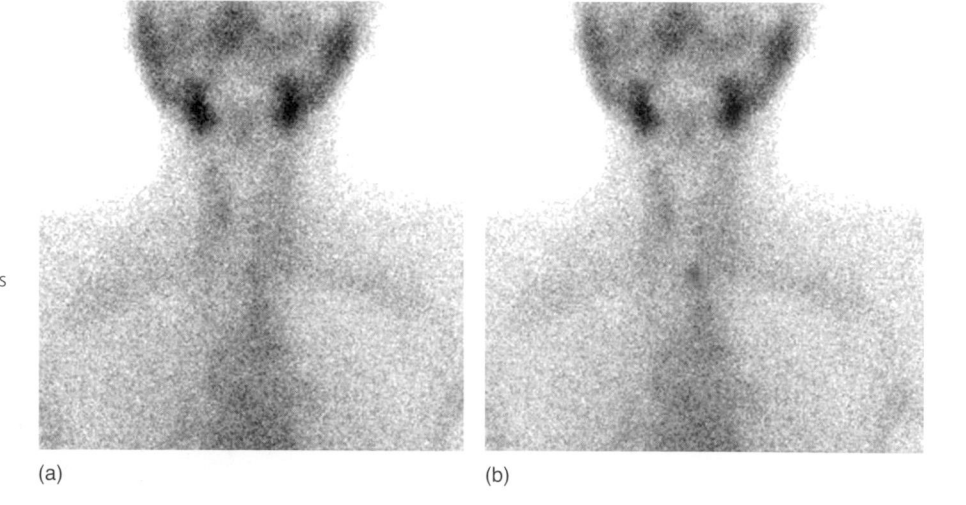

(a)

(b)

Graves' disease (Basedow's disease)

Definition and epidemiology

Graves' disease (GD) is an autoimmune disease representing the most common cause of hyperthyroidism (60–90% of all cases).

Graves' disease has a powerful hereditary component, affecting up to 2% of the female population, and is between five and ten times more common in females than in males (incidence of 5 : 1 to 10 : 1, respectively). It is also the most common cause of severe hyperthyroidism, which is accompanied by extended clinical signs and symptoms and laboratory abnormalities compared with milder forms of hyperthyroidism. About 30–50% of patients with GD will also suffer from Graves' ophthalmopathy, which is caused by inflammation of the eye muscles mediated by an inflammatory immune process.

Etiology and pathogenesis

Graves' disease is an autoimmune disorder in which the body produces antibodies to the receptor for thyroid stimulating hormone (TSHrAb). (Antibodies to thyroglobulin and thyroperoxidase may also be produced.) TSHrAb bind to the thyroid stimulating hormone (TSH) receptors, which are located on cells producing thyroid hormone in the thyroid gland (follicular cells), and chronically stimulate them, resulting in an abnormally high production of triiodothyronine (T_3) and thyroxine (T_4). There are several factors that predispose to GD and Graves' ophthalmopathy; in particular, genetic susceptibility, infection, smoking, pregnancy, iodine, and iodine-containing drugs.

Signs and symptoms

Signs and symptoms of GD all result from the direct and indirect effects of hyperthyroidism, with the main exceptions being Graves' ophthalmopathy, goiter, and pretibial myxedema.

Diagnosis

Laboratory findings
Laboratory tests for GD include:
- Thyroid stimulating hormone (TSH), free triiodothyronine (FT_3), and free thyroxine (FT_4)
- TSHrAb
- Total cholesterol, high density lipoprotein (HDL), triglycerides

Imaging tests
Imaging tests for GD include:
- Thyroid ultrasound (Fig. 1.5)
- $^{99m}TcO_4$ thyroid scintigraphy (Fig. 1.6)
- Computed tomography (CT) neck scan
- Orbital nuclear magnetic resonance (NMR)

Treatment
Treatment options for GD are:
- Beta blockers (rapid amelioration of symptoms)
- Thionamide
- Radioiodine ablation
- Surgery
- Glucocorticoid (for Graves' ophthalmopathy)
- Orbital irradiation (for Graves' ophthalmopathy)
- Orbital decompression surgery (for Graves' ophthalmopathy)

Illustrations (Figs 1.5 & 1.6)

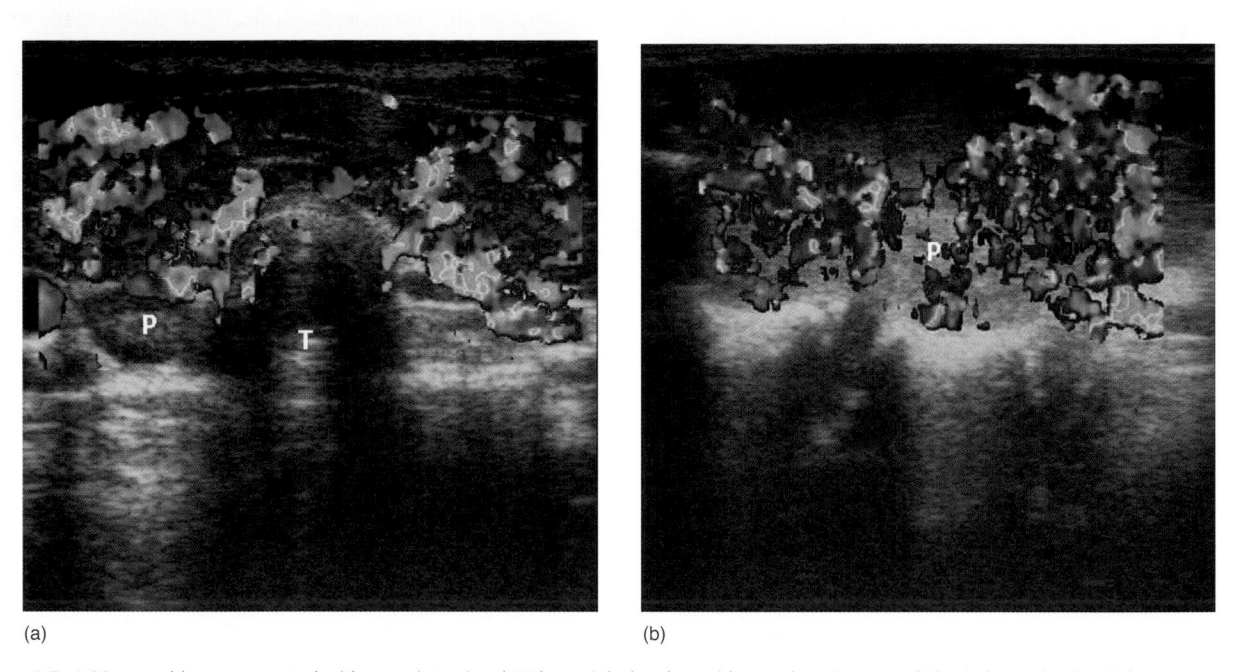

(a)   (b)

Figure 1.5 A 32-year-old man presented with an unintentional 15 kg weight loss but with an otherwise normal physical examination. Laboratory studies revealed a suppressed thyroid stimulating hormone (TSH) concentration and an elevated thyroxine level, which are consistent with hyperthyroidism. Thyroid ultrasound – (a) cross section and (b) longitudinal section. These ultrasound/color Doppler images reveal markedly increased vascularity throughout the thyroid gland ("thyroid hell"). P, thyroid parenchyma; T, trachea.

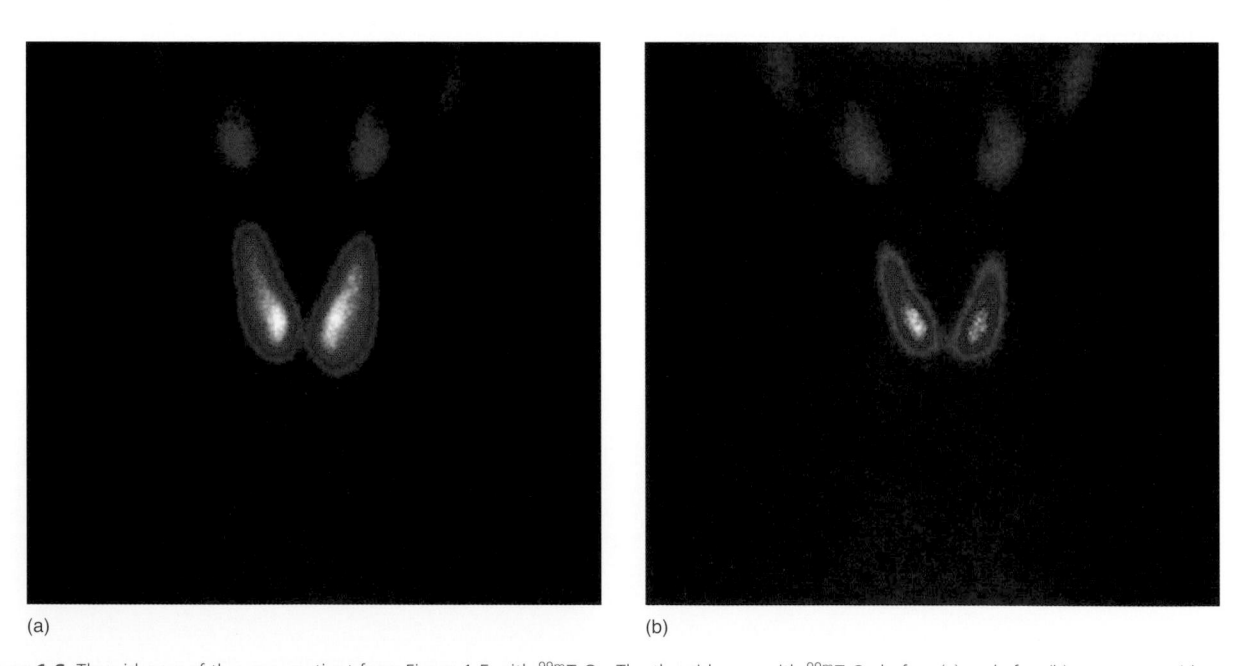

(a)   (b)

Figure 1.6 Thyroid scan of the same patient from Figure 1.5 with $^{99m}TcO_4$. The thyroid scan with $^{99m}TcO_4$ before (a) and after (b) treatment with methimazole. Intense and homogeneous uptake of the radiopharmaceutical in both lobes of thyroid gland is seen before therapy. The post-therapy scan was performed 6 months after therapy and shows a reduction of thyroid size and uptake.

Subacute thyroiditis (de Quervain's thyroiditis)

Definition and epidemiology

Subacute thyroiditis (ST) is a subacute granulomatous thyroiditis that belongs to a group of thyroiditis conditions known as resolving thyroiditis. Other names for this disorder are de Quervain's thyroiditis, subacute nonsuppurative thyroiditis, giant cell thyroiditis, and painful thyroiditis. It has an incidence of 12.1/100 000 per year with a higher incidence in females than in males (19.1 and 4.1/100 000 per year, respectively). It is most common in young adulthood (24/100 000 per year) and middle age (35/100 000 per year), and decreases with increased age.

Etiology and pathogenesis

Subacute thyroiditis is presumed to be caused by a viral infection or a postviral inflammatory process. The majority of patients have a history of an upper respiratory infection prior to the onset of thyroiditis (typically 2–8 weeks beforehand). The disease was thought to have a seasonal incidence (higher in the summer), and clusters of cases have been reported in association with Coxsackievirus, mumps, measles, adenovirus, and other viral infections. Thyroid autoimmunity does not appear to play a primary role in the disorder, but it is strongly associated with HLA-B35 in many ethnic groups. A unifying hypothesis might be that the disorder results from a common subclinical viral infection that provides an antigen, either of viral origin or resulting from virus-induced host tissue damage, that uniquely binds to HLA-B35 molecules on macrophages. The resulting antigen-HLA-B35 complex activates cytotoxic T lymphocytes that then damage thyroid follicular cells, since the cells have partial structural similarity with the infection-related antigen. Unlike autoimmune thyroid disease, however, the immune reaction is not self-perpetuating, so the process is limited. The resulting thyroid inflammation damages thyroid follicles and activates proteolysis of the thyroglobulin stored within the follicles. The result is an unregulated release of large amounts of thyroxine (T_4) and triiodothyronine (T_3) into the circulation resulting in clinical and biochemical hyperthyroidism.

Signs and symptoms

Subacute thyroiditis is a self-limiting thyroid condition associated with a triphasic clinical course of hyperthyroidism, hypothyroidism, and return to normal thyroid function. In particular, ST may be responsible for 15–20% of patients with thyrotoxicosis and 10% of patients presenting with hypothyroidism. Pain is the main symptom and it may be limited to the thyroid region or it may radiate to the upper neck, jaw, throat, upper chest, or ears. It can be exacerbated by coughing or turning the head. Fever, fatigue, malaise, anorexia, and myalgia are common.

Diagnosis

Laboratory findings

Laboratory tests for ST include:
- Thyroid stimulating hormone (TSH), free triiodothyronine (FT_3), and free thyroxine (FT_4)
- Erythrocyte sedimentation rate (ESR)
- Polymerase chain reaction (PCR) for C-reactive protein
- Hemochrome

Imaging tests

A neck ultrasound is needed (Fig. 1.7).

Treatment

Subacute thyroiditis is a self-limiting condition and so in most patients no specific therapy, such as antithyroid or thyroid hormone replacement therapy, is necessary. Treatment of patients with ST should be directed at providing relief for thyroid pain (e.g. prednisone) and tenderness, and ameliorating symptoms of hyperthyroidism (e.g. with a beta blocker such as propranolol).

Illustration (Fig. 1.7)

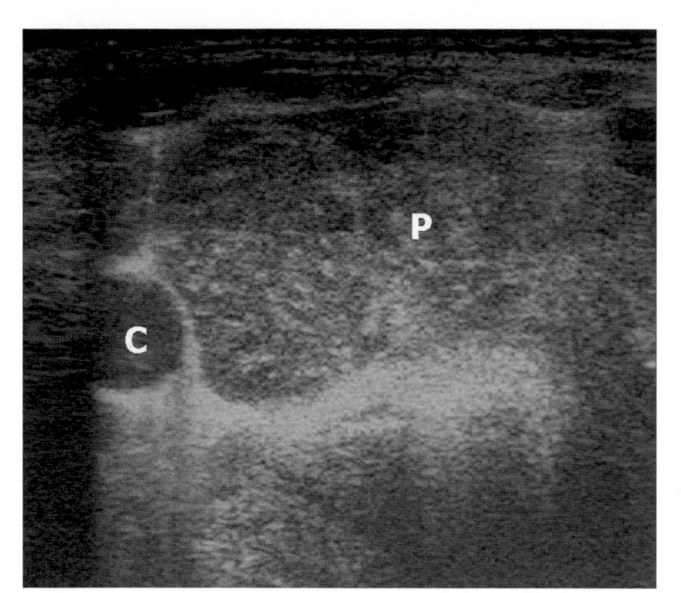

(a)

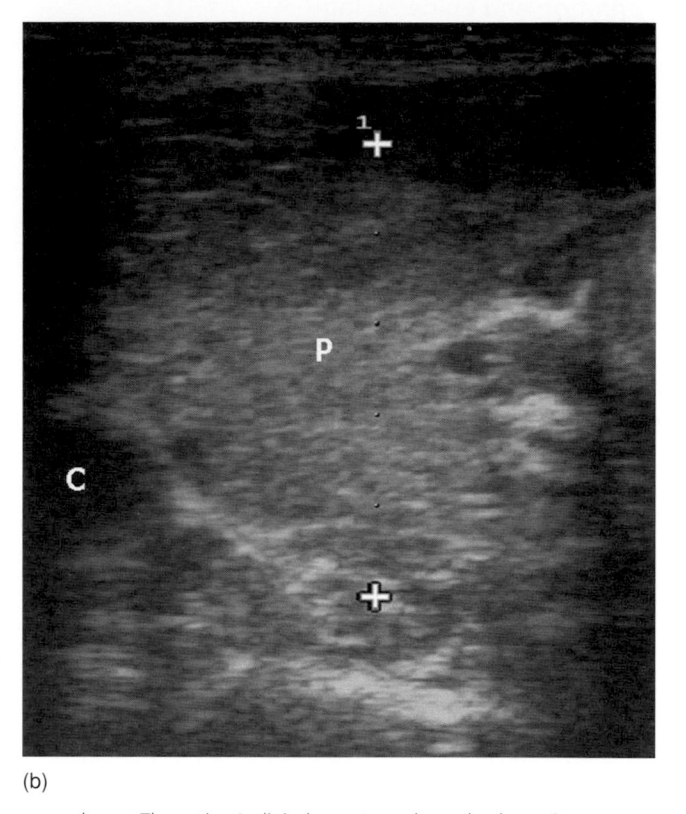

(b)

Figure 1.7 A 47-year-old woman presents with pain and tenderness on her right side due to a chronic goiter. Her erythrocyte sedimentation rate was elevated and her thyroid laboratory tests suggested subclinical hypothyroidism. Two weeks previously, she had a fever and now her ^{99m}Tc pertechnetate uptake is markedly decreased. (a) Thyroid ultrasound – cross section (before treatment). Focal hypoechogenicity in the painful area with decreased vascular flow by Doppler scan. C, carotid artery; P, thyroid parenchyma. The patient's clinical symptoms showed a dramatic response to glucocorticoid treatment. She became hypothyroid and began levothyroxine therapy. (b) Thyroid ultrasound – cross section (after treatment). The focal hypoechogenicity is reduced and the thyroid parenchyma has become more homogeneous. C, carotid artery; P, thyroid parenchyma.

Benign thyroid nodules

Definition and epidemiology

Thyroid nodules are the most common of thyroid diseases. They affect up to 5% of the general population and are more frequent in iodine deficient areas and in women (female to male ratio, 5 : 1). Thyroid nodules are mostly benign (adenoma, cysti, focal hyperplasia) and the incidence of malignant neoplasia is very low (4/100 000 per year).

Thyroid nodules are abnormal cell growths in the thyroid gland. The thyroid can be uninodular when a single nodule is present or multinodular when multiple nodules are present.

Thyroid nodules are mostly nonfunctioning but can be hyperfunctioning (toxic multinodular goiter, Plummer's disease) leading to symptoms of hyperthyroidism.

Etiology and pathogenesis

The etiology of thyroid nodules is unknown. There are several factors that predispose to these nodules; in particular, genetic susceptibility, iodine deficiency, neck irradiation, and unknown environmental agents.

Signs and symptoms

Usually thyroid nodules are asymptomatic and they are occasionally discovered during physical examination or an ultrasound neck scan.

Signs and symptoms of large nodules or multinodular goiter mainly result from thyroid increased volume and neck compression. The signs and symptoms include:
• Neck lump
• Neck pain, dyspnea, dysphagia, dysphonia
• Symptoms due to hyperthyroidism (in toxic multinodular goiter or Plummer's adenoma)

Diagnosis

The gold standard for diagnosing thyroid nodules consists of both a neck ultrasound scan (evaluating nodules size and eventually suspicious features) and fine needle cytology (FNC) to diagnose malignant neoplasia.

Laboratory and cytology tests

The laboratory and cytology tests for thyroid nodules include:
• Calcitonin (in nodules suspicious for medullary carcinoma)
• Thyroid stimulating hormone (TSH), free triiodothyronine (FT_3), free thyroxine (FT_4)
• Cytology (fine needle cytology)

Imaging tests

Imaging tests for thyroid nodules include:
• Thyroid ultrasounds (Figs 1.8a, 1.9a & 1.10a): Relevant ultrasound scan features of thyroid nodules are: echostructure (solid, cystic, or mist nodules), echogenicity (ipo-, iso-, or anechogen nodules), vascular pattern, presence of microcalcifications (regular or irregular), and defined or undefined margins
• Computed tomography (CT) neck scan (Fig. 1.11)
• Neck X-ray
• Scintigraphy thyroid scans (Figs 1.8b, 1.9b & 1.10b)

Treatment

Treatment options for thyroid nodules are:
• Clinical and ultrasound scan follow-up
• Surgery (for compressive symptoms, tracheal or neck vessel compression or dislocation, mediastinal thyroid)
• Treatment of hyperthyroidism (toxic multinodular goiter, Plummer's adenoma)

Illustrations (Figs 1.8–1.11)

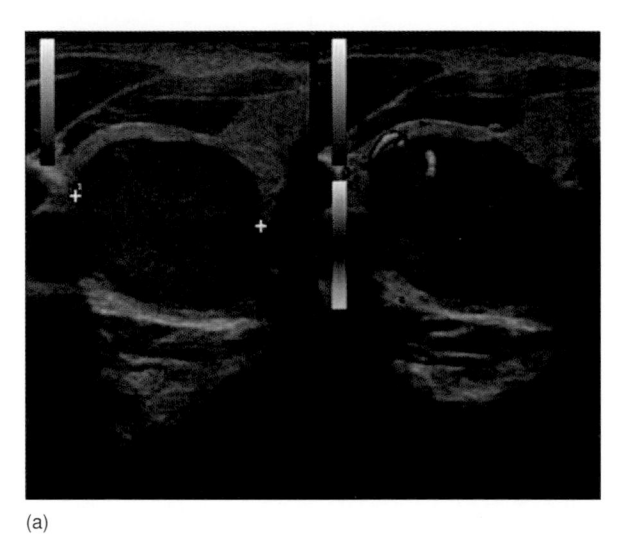

(a)

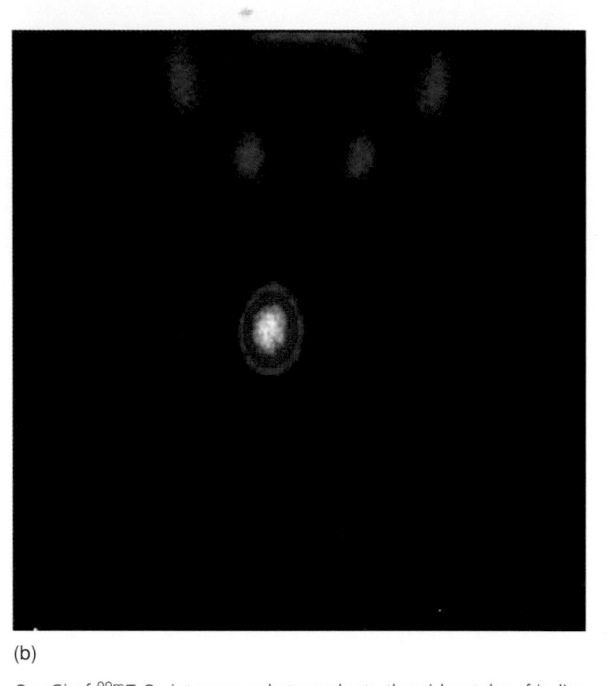

(b)

Figure 1.8 A case of thyroid toxic adenoma. A 56-year-old female patient with symptoms of hyperthyroidism. Hormonal blood levels showed increased free triiodothyronine (FT_3), free thyroxine (FT_4), and suppressed thyroid stimulating hormone (TSH). (a) Thyroid ultrasound showed a hypoechoic solid nodule of 14 × 15 mm with intra- and perinodular vascularization in the lower third of the right thyroid lobe. (b) The thyroid morpho-functional study was performed with 50 μCi of ^{131}I orally and 3 mCi of $^{99m}TcO_4$ intravenously to evaluate thyroid uptake of iodine and scintigraphic distribution of Tc, respectively. Thyroid uptake was 17% at 6 hours, 29% at 24 hours, and 22% at 48 hours (data relevant for dosimetric calculations). The thyroid scan confirmed the clinical suspicion of Plummer's adenoma and showed complete functional inhibition of extranodular glandular tissue (inhibiting adenoma), which is the ideal condition for performing ^{131}I therapy.

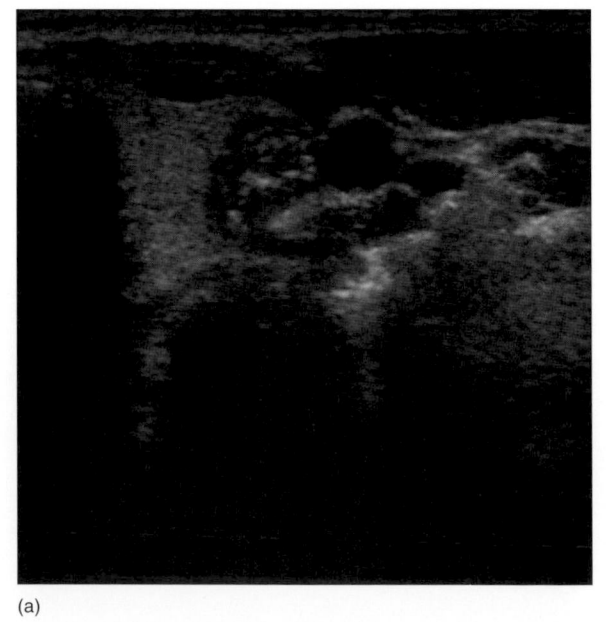

(a)

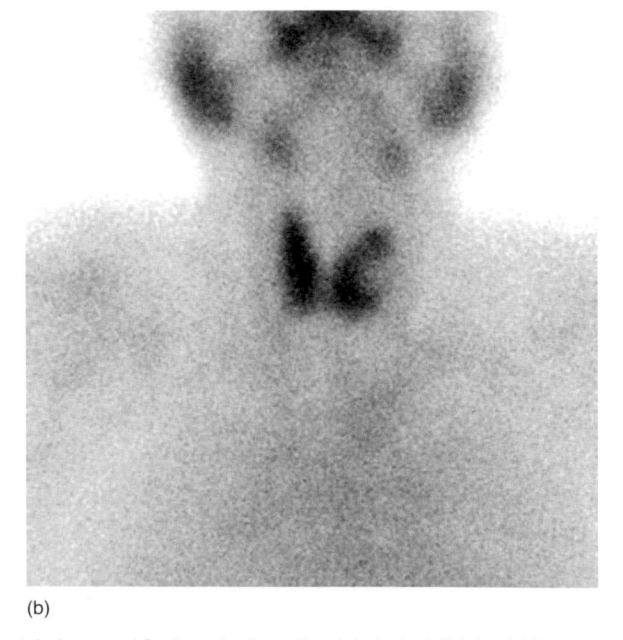

(b)

Figure 1.9 A case of single thyroid nodule. A 25-year-old patient with incidental ultrasound finding of a thyroid nodule in the left lobe. (a) Thyroid ultrasound shows a solid hypoechoic nodule, with microcalcifications. (b) Thyroid scintigraphy shows the "cold" nodule with no detectable $^{99m}TcO_4$ uptake. The patient underwent fine needle cytology and the cytology was suspicious for papillary carcinoma.

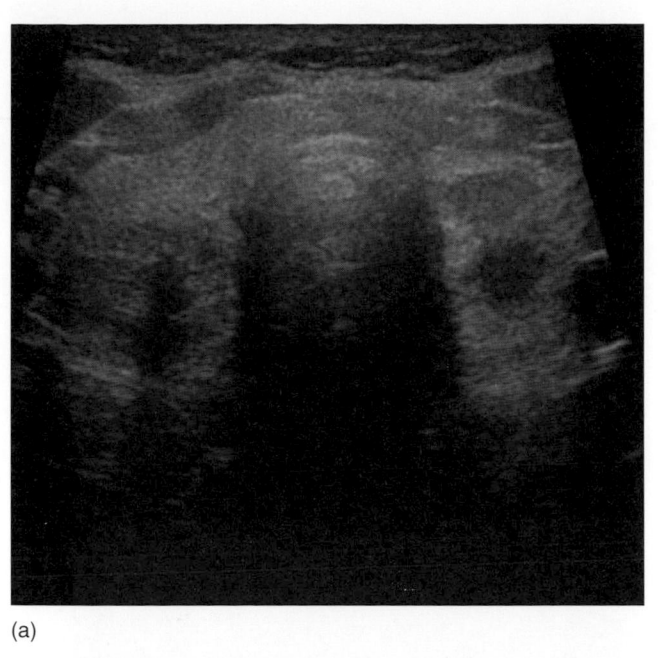

(a)

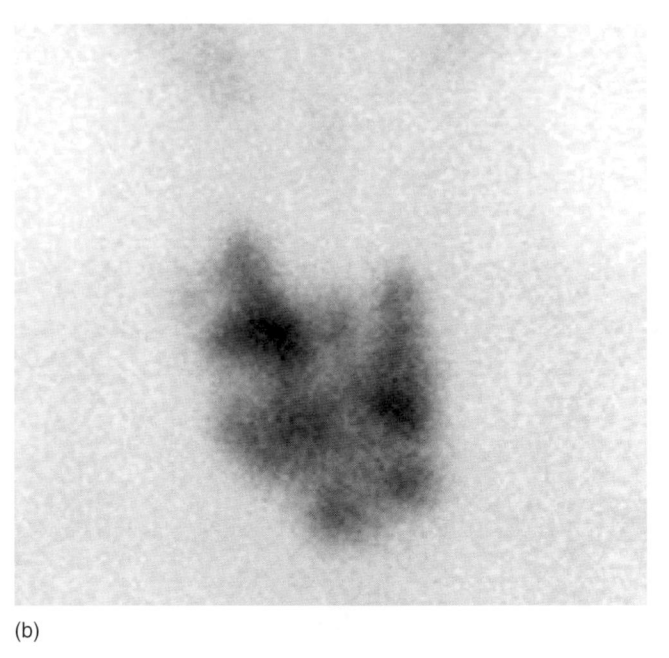

(b)

Figure 1.10 A case of multinodular toxic thyroid. A hyperthyroid 46-year-old woman with a palpable multinodular thyroid. (a) Ultrasound scan shows an enlarged thyroid with multiple nodules in both right and left lobe. The gland seems to extend in the mediastinum. (b) Thyroid scan with $^{99m}TcO_4$. The scan shows intense uptake in the glandular parenchima with multiple "cold" areas in correspondence to the major nodules seen at ultrasound. This finding is consistent with the diagnosis of a "multinodular toxic thyroid." The patient underwent surgery.

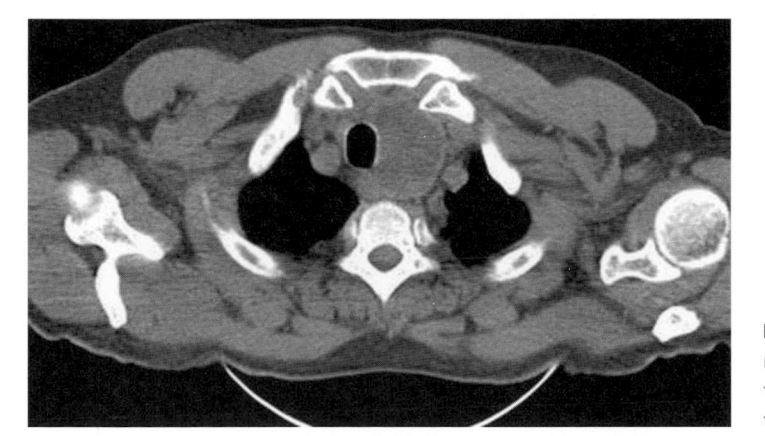

Figure 1.11 A case of goiter. A 70-year-old man with a palpable multinodular goiter. The axial contrast-enhanced computed tomography (CT) image shows increased thyroid volume compressing the tracheal and esophageal lumen.

Thyroid cancer

Definition and epidemiology

Carcinoma of the thyroid is an uncommon cancer but it is the most common malignancy of the endocrine system (Figs 1.12–1.25). Differentiated tumors (papillary [Figs 1.14–1.17] or follicular [Fig. 1.20]) are highly treatable and are usually curable. Poorly differentiated tumors (medullary [Fig. 1.23] or anaplastic) are much less common, are aggressive, metastasize early, and have a much poorer prognosis. Thyroid cancer affects women more often than men and usually occurs in people between the ages of 25 and 65. The incidence of this malignancy has been increasing over the last decade.

The World Health Organization 2004 classification is shown in Table 1.1. The prognosis for differentiated carcinoma is better for patients aged below 40 without extracapsular extension or vascular invasion. Age appears to be

Table 1.1 World Health Organization 2004 classification of neoplasms of the thyroid

I Adenomas
  A Follicular
    1. Colloid variant
    2. Embryonal
    3. Fetal
    4. Hürthle cell variant
  B Papillary (probably malignant)
  C Teratoma
II Malignant tumors
  A Differentiated
    1. Papillary adenocarcinoma
      1. Pure papillary adenocarcinoma
      2. Mixed papillary and follicular carcinoma (variants including tall cell, follicular, oxyphyl, solid)
    2. Follicular adenocarcinomas (variants: "malignant adenoma," Hürthle cell carcinoma or oxyphil carcinoma, clear-cell carcinoma, insular carcinoma)
  B Medullary carcinoma
  C Undifferentiated
    1. Small cell (to be differentiated from lymphoma)
    2. Giant cell
    3. Carcinosarcoma
  D Miscellaneous
    1. Lymphoma, sarcoma
    2. Squamous cell epidermoid carcinoma
    3. Fibrosarcoma
    4. Mucoepithelial carcinoma
    5. Metastatic tumor

Courtesy of Delellis RA, Lloyd RV, Heitx PU & Eng C. (2004) Pathology and genetics of tumours of endocrine organs. *WHO Classification of Tumours*, IARC, Lyon, France.

the single most important prognostic factor. The prognostic significance of lymph node status is controversial. Adverse factors include: Older than 45 years; follicular histology; primary tumor > 4 cm (T2–T3); extrathyroid extension (T4); and distant metastases.

Etiology and pathogenesis

Risk factors for thyroid cancer
The risk factors for thyroid cancer are:
- External radiation and thyroid cancer
- History of goiter
- Family history of thyroid disease
- Female gender
- Asian ethnicity

While an increased incidence of thyroid cancer in patients with Hashimoto's thyroiditis has been reported, clinical experience does not suggest a strong relationship between this relatively common disease and thyroid cancer.

Signs and symptoms
Most frequently the tumor is discovered accidentally as a finding during an ultrasound of the neck. It may appear as a gradually enlarging, painful mass with associated symptoms of hoarseness, dysphagia, or dysphonia, or there may be difficulty breathing. Occasionally a patient arrives with metastatic nodules in the neck, pulmonary symptoms from metastases, or a pathologic fracture of the spine or hip. Usually there are no symptoms of hyper- or hypothyroidism.

Upon examination of the neck, carcinoma of the thyroid characteristically appears as an asymmetrical lump in the gland. If it is still within the confines of the gland, it will move with the gland when the patient swallows and may be moveable within the gland. If it has invaded the trachea or neighboring structures, it may be fixed in place. Lymph nodes containing metastases may be found in the supraclavicular triangles, in the carotid chain, along the thyroid isthmus, and rarely in the axillary nodes. Although carcinoma of the thyroid is typically firm or hard, rapidly growing lesions may sometimes be soft or even fluctuant.

Diagnosis
Most patients with thyroid carcinoma are recognized because of the observation of a neck mass and the result of fine needle aspiration cytology.

Laboratory findings
Laboratory tests for thyroid carcinoma:
- Thyroid stimulating hormone (TSH), and free thyroxine (FT_4) are usually measured to verify metabolic status.
- Antithyroid peroxidase antibodies (TPOAbs) and thyroglobulin antibodies (TgAbs).

• Thyroglobulin (Tg) assay: Although Tg assay has been suggested as an important marker for thyroid cancer, practice shows that elevated Tg levels can be caused by adenoma, multinodular goiter, and other diseases; thus, the determination is of little value before operating.
• Calcitonin immunoassay: Some groups recommend this on all patients with nodules to allow preoperative diagnosis of medullary thyroid carcinoma.

Imaging tests

Imaging tests for thyroid carcinoma include:
• Ultrasound studies, which are the most basic and useful test.
• Isotope scans (Figs 1.18a&f, 1.19, 1.21 & 1.24) have a limited role in the initial diagnosis.
• Chest X-rays may be informative but are often omitted.
• Computed tomography (CT) (Figs 1.12, 1.13, 1.22–1.25) and TC-18F-FDG positron emission tomography (PET) (Fig. 1.18d&g) scanning of the lungs and magnetic resonance imaging (MRI) of the neck can provide useful information prior to surgery in lesions that extend outside the thyroid or have metastasis.

Treatment

In differentiated cancers contemporary medical and surgical practice depends mainly on the clinical stage of the disease rather than on the exact histologic status. The classification can be conveniently reduced to four categories that have prognostic significance and clear therapeutic relevance (Table 1.2).
• Thyroid cancer may require surgery. The possible surgical approaches range from a simple removal of the nodule to total thyroidectomy with bilateral radical neck dissection.
• Radioactive iodine-131 is used in patients with papillary or follicular thyroid cancer for ablation of residual thyroid tissue after surgery and for the treatment of thyroid cancer.

Table 1.2 Thyroid cancer: Classification

Clinical stage	Comparable TNM classification
I. Intrathyroidal	T0, T1, T2, N0, M0
II. Cervical adenopathy	T0–T2, N0, N1a, N1b, M0
III. Locally invasive disease	T3, T4a, T4b, M0
IV. Distant metastases	M1

Courtesy of Edge SB, Byrd DR, Compton CC, et al. (eds) (2010) *AJCC Cancer Staging Manual*, 7th edn. Springer, New York, NY.

Table 1.3 Thyroid cancer: 5-year survival rates

Thyroid cancer type	5-year survival (%) Stage I	Stage II	Stage III	Stage IV
Papillary	100	100	93	51
Follicular	100	100	71	50
Medullary	100	98	81	28
Anaplastic	(Always Stage IV)			7

Courtesy of Edge SB, Byrd DR, Compton CC, et al. (eds) (2010) *AJCC Cancer Staging Manual*, 7th edn. Springer, New York, NY.

Patients with medullary, anaplastic, and most Hürthle cell cancers do not benefit from this therapy.

External irradiation may be used when the cancer is unresectable, when it recurs after resection, or to relieve pain from bone metastasis.

Sorafenib and sunitinib, approved for other indications, show promise as treatments for thyroid cancer and are being used by some patients who do not qualify for clinical trials.

Survival rate for thyroid cancer is related to both type of cancer and stage at time of diagnosis (Table 1.3).

Illustrations (Figs 1.12–1.25)

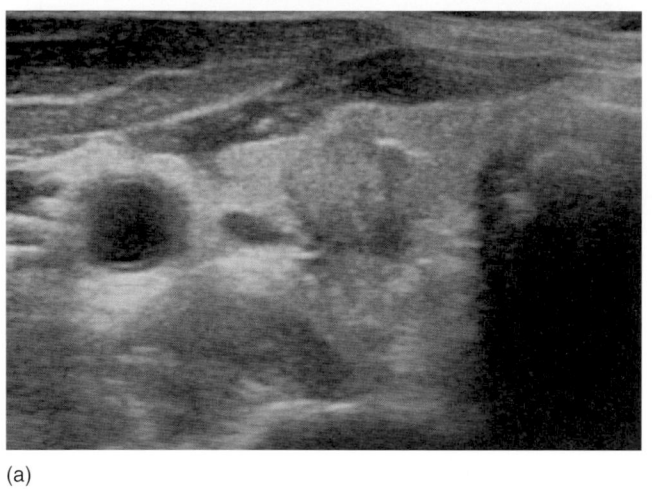

(a)

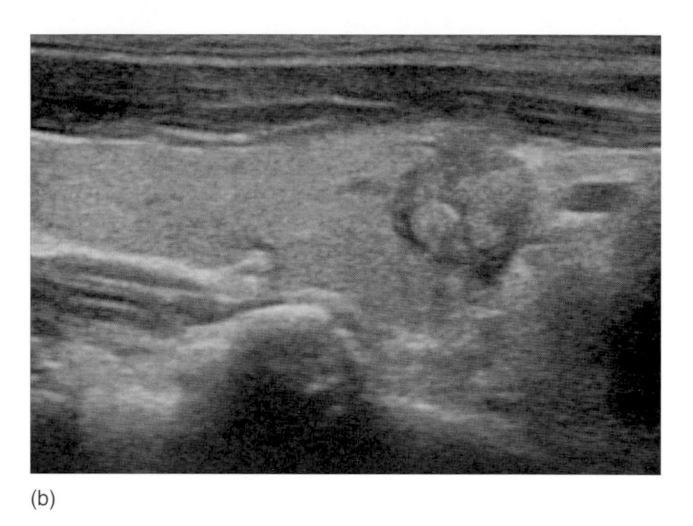

(b)

Figure 1.12 Papillary thyroid carcinoma and cystic lymph node metastasis in a 57-year-old man. (a) Transverse sonogram of the right lobe of the thyroid shows a solitary, isoechoic, inhomogenous nodule with irregular margin. (b) Longitudinal sonogram of the same thyroid nodule.

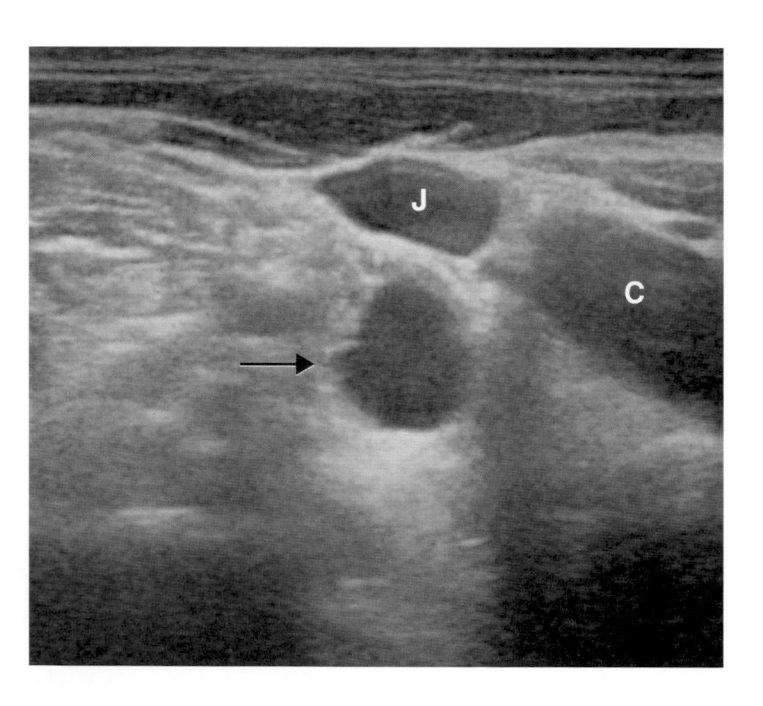

Figure 1.13 Transverse sonogram of the right neck shows a cystic level 4 nodal (red arrow). C: carotid artery; J, jugular vein.

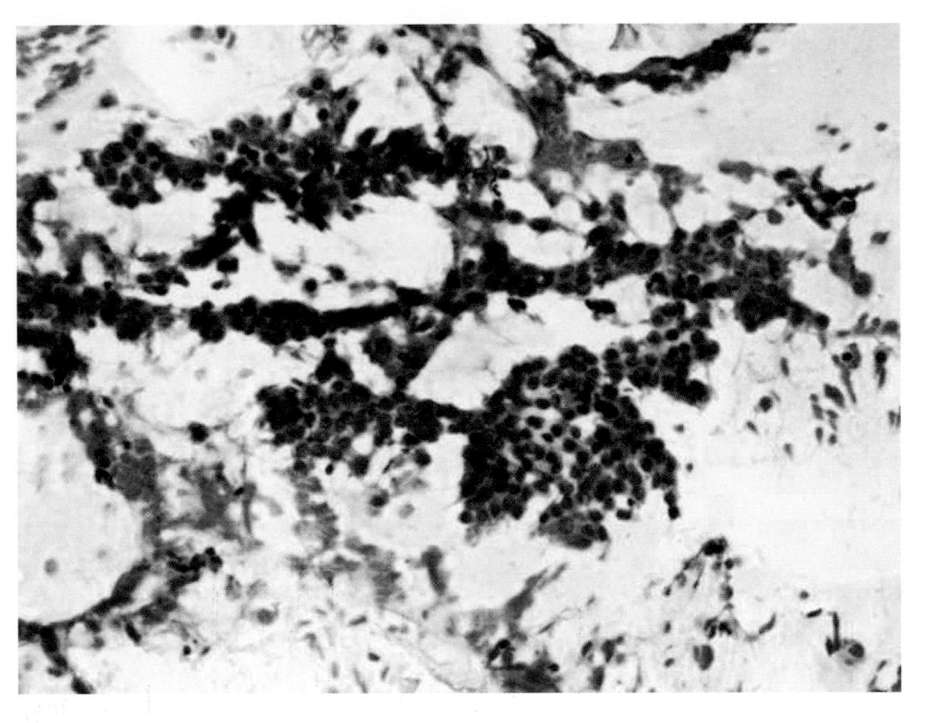

Figure 1.14 Cytology of papillary carcinoma (Papanicolau, 20 ×). Thyrocytes are arranged in a pseudopapillary structure with nuclear irregularity.

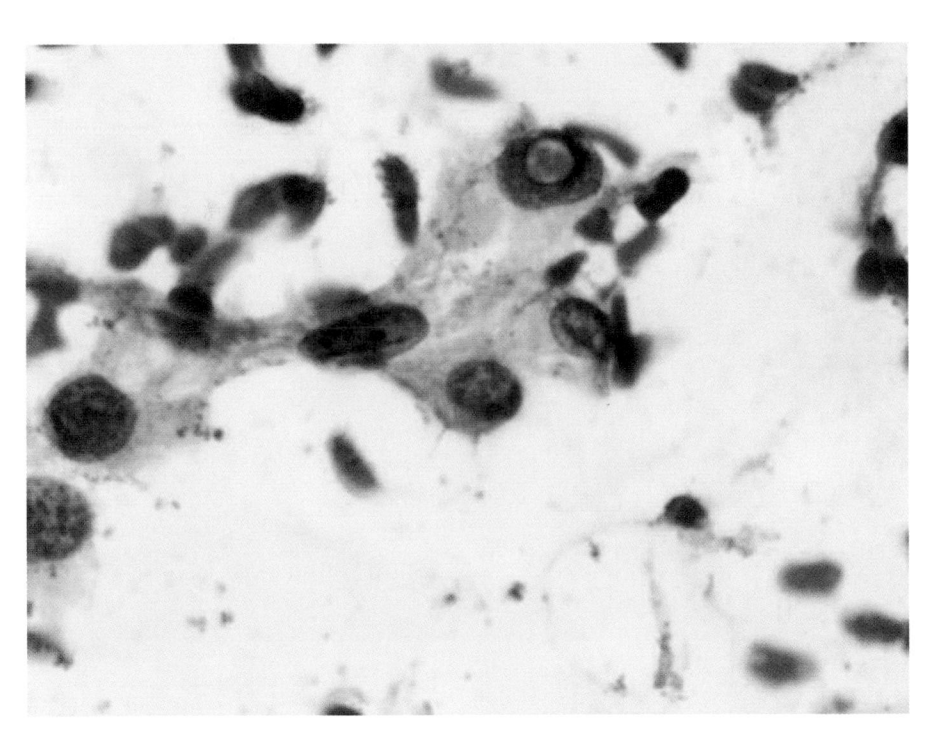

Figure 1.15 Cytology of papillary carcinoma (Papanicolau, 40 ×). Thyrocytes with evidence of little nucleus, nuclear pseudoinclusion, and nuclear incision.

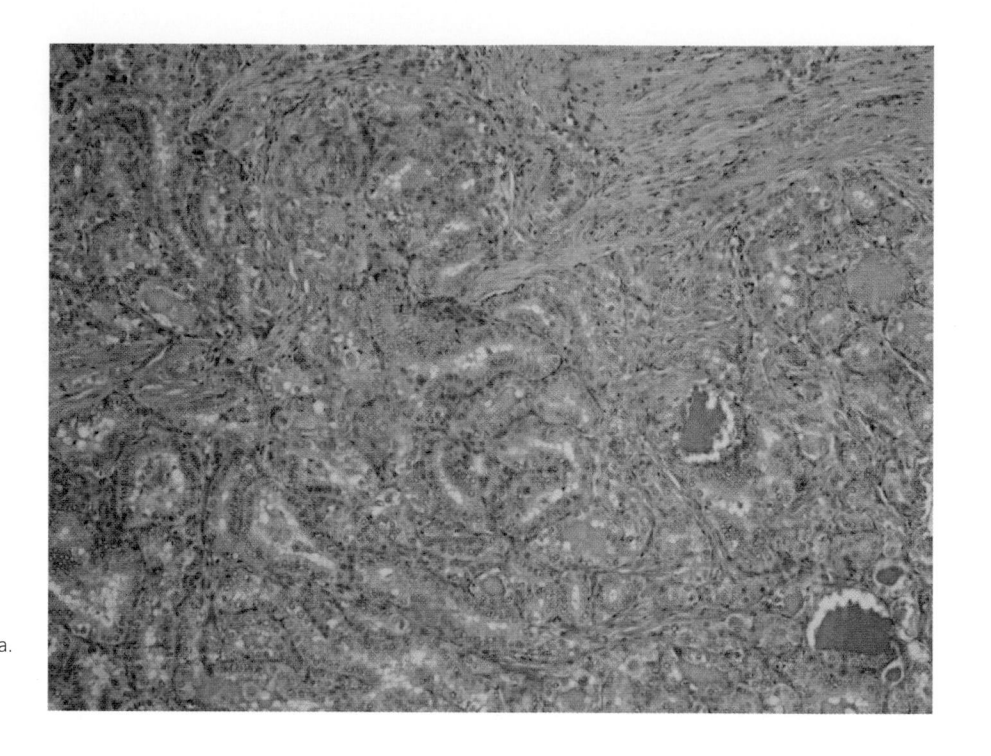

Figure 1.16 Histology of papillary carcinoma. Papillary carcinoma with ground glass nuclei (HE, 10 ×).

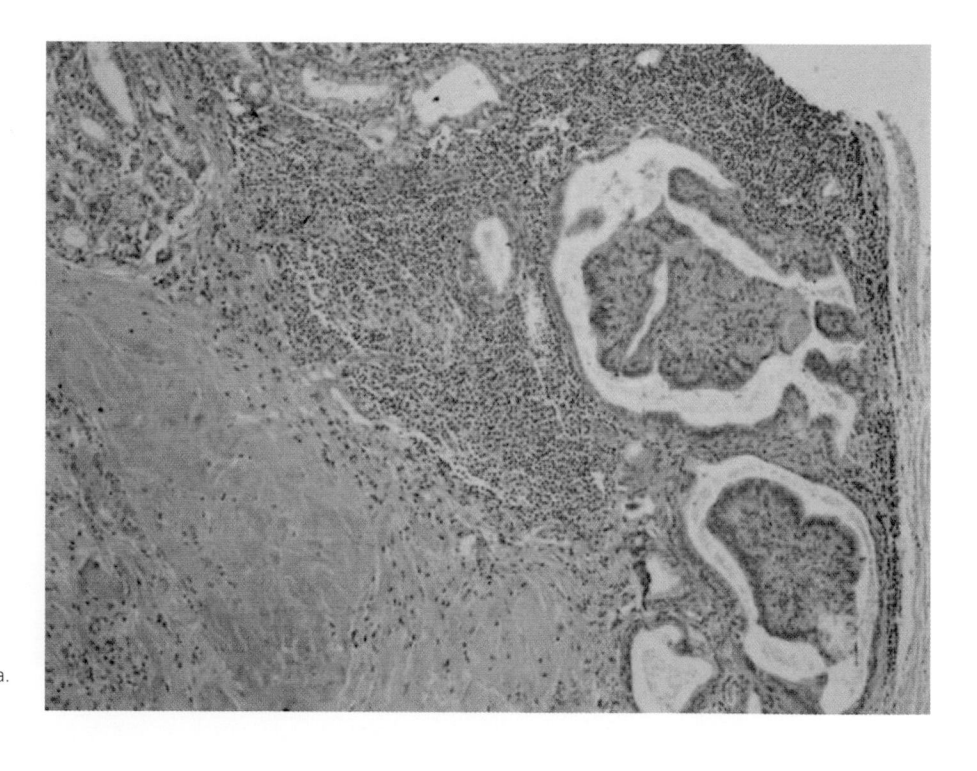

Figure 1.17 Histology of papillary carcinoma. Metastasis in neck node (HE, 10 ×).

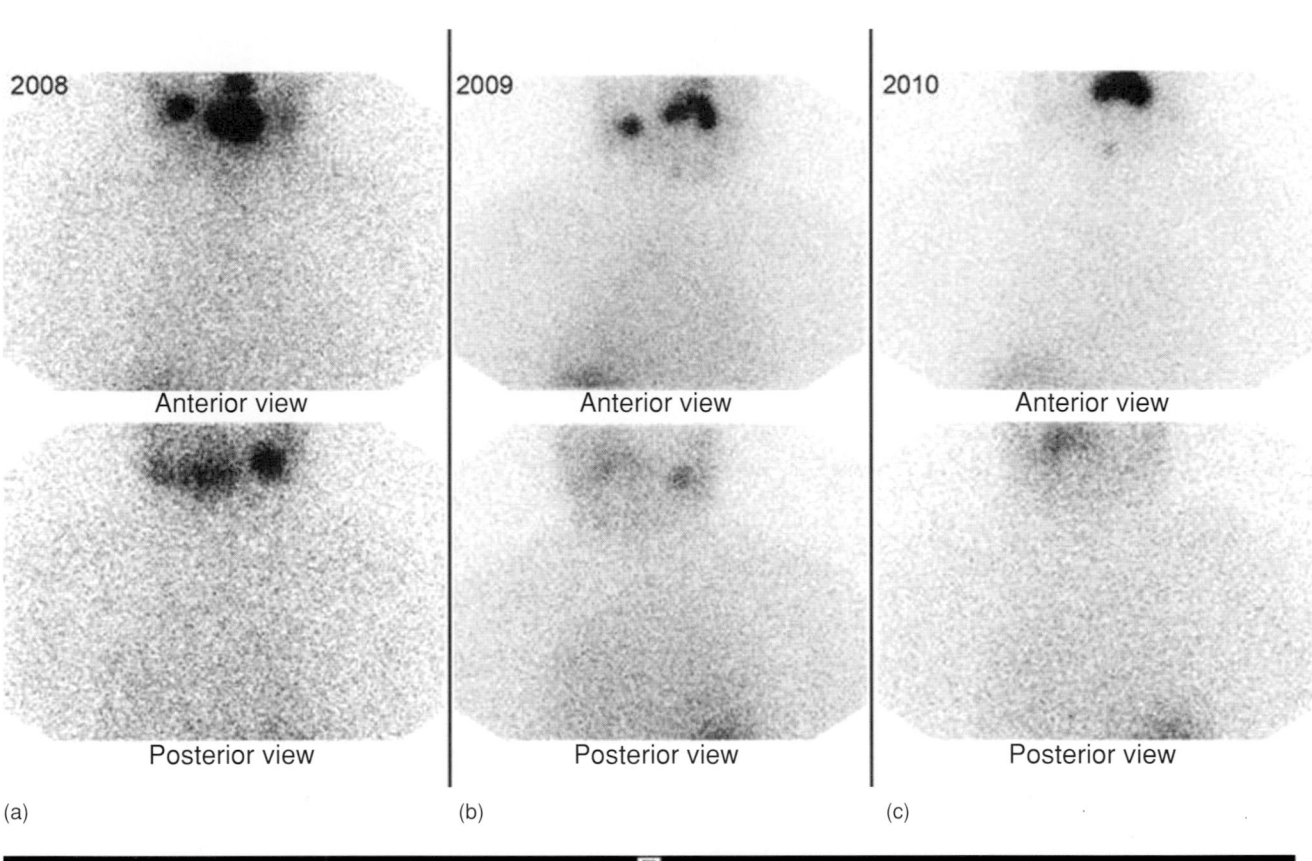

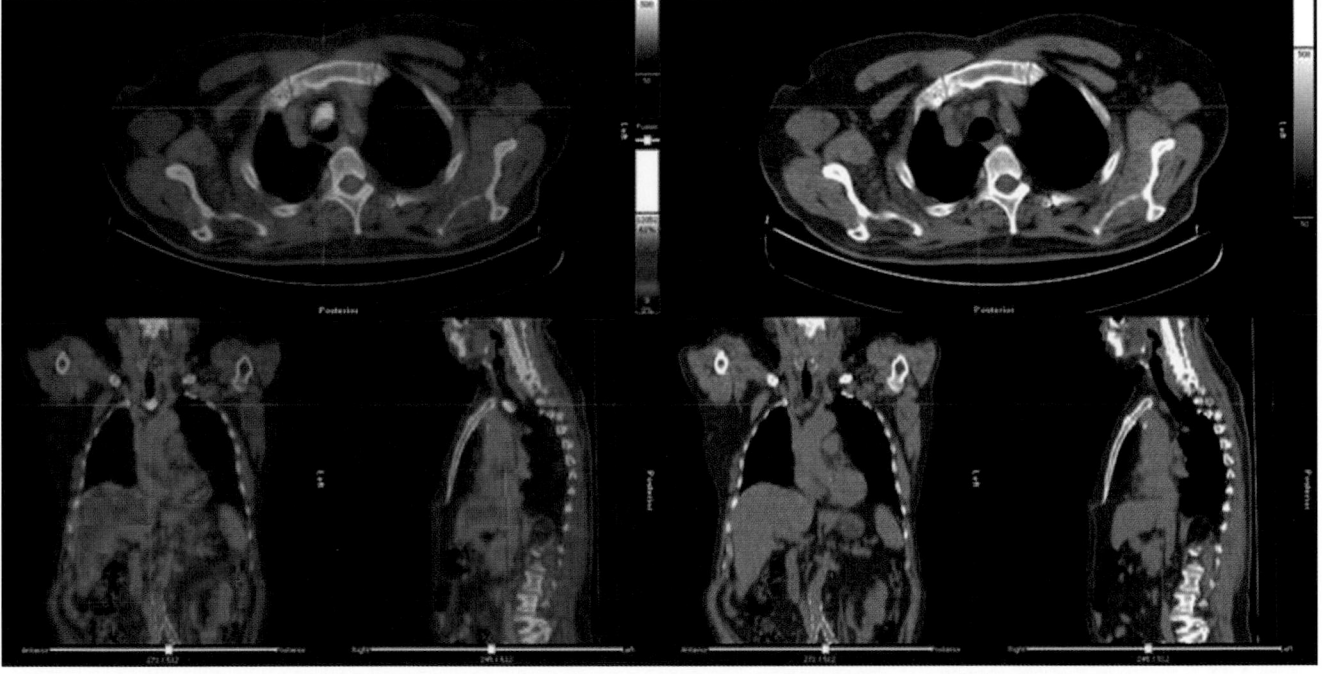

(d)

Figure 1.18 A case of differentiated thyroid cancer: Papillary thyroid cancer infiltrating the periglandular soft tissues with lymph node metastases (pT4 N1a Mx). After several cycles of ^{131}I therapy (a–c) the patient still had residual disease in the paratracheal lymph nodes unaffected by the iodine therapy and clearly detected by ^{18}F-FDG positron emission tomography (PET) performed in 2008 (d) during ^{131}I therapy and in 2009 (e) after the last ^{131}I treatment. An increase in the size of the metastases was observed despite the iodine therapy. Iodine therapy was therefore discontinued and the patient performed an ^{111}In-Octreoscan to verify if metastases had somatostatin receptors. The scan showed high density of somatostatin receptors (f). The patient started treatment with long-acting somatostatin analogs, with stable disease after 2 years as shown by the ^{18}F-FDG PET scan performed for restaging 2 years after (g).

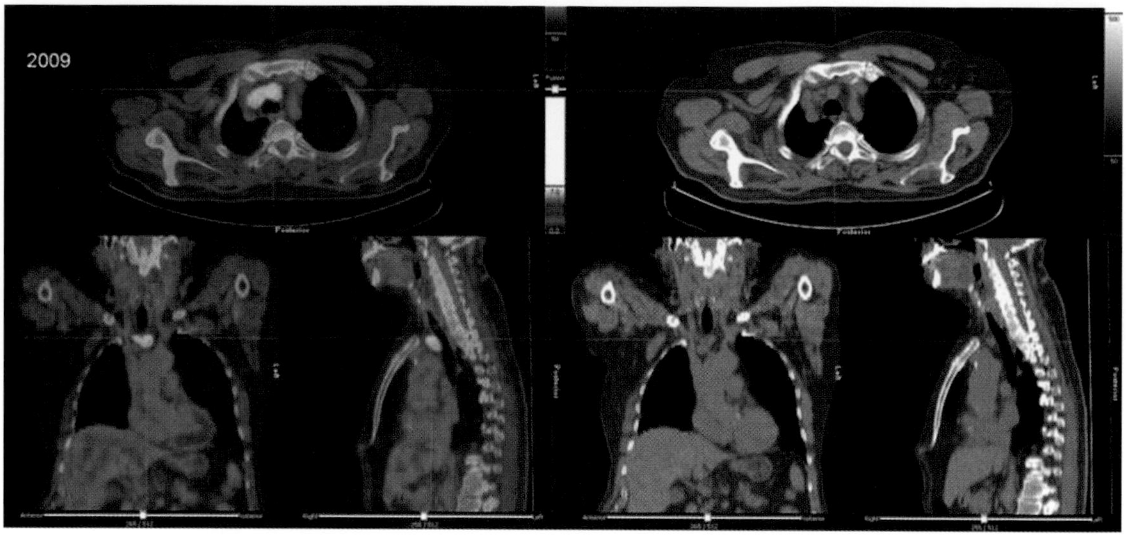
2009

(e)

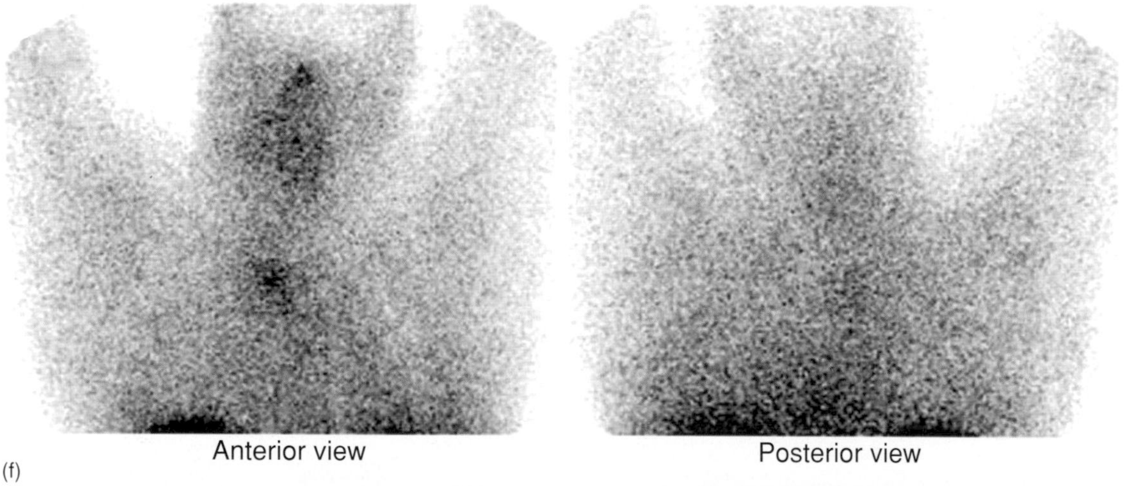
Anterior view
Posterior view

(f)

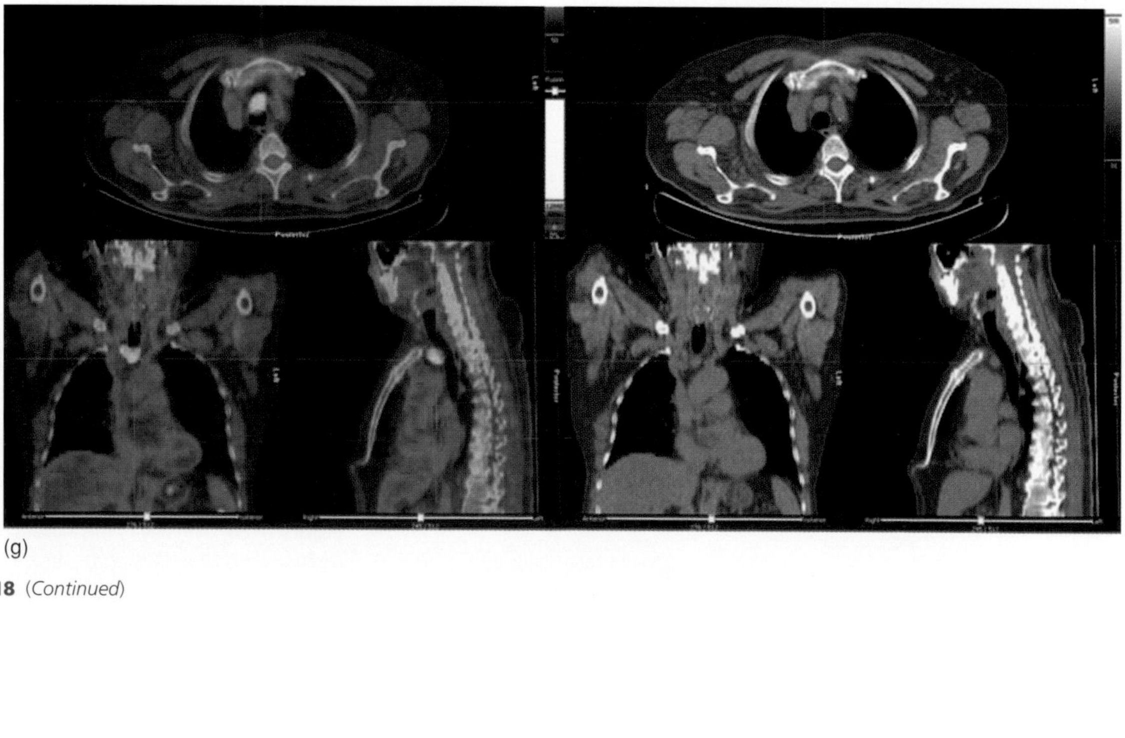

(g)

Figure 1.18 (*Continued*)

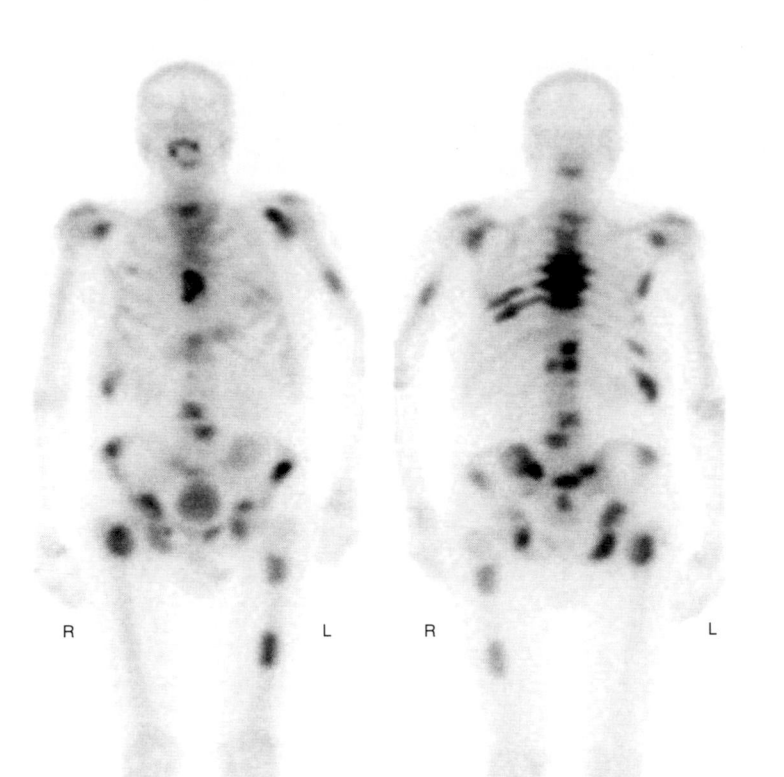

R   L   R   L

Anterior   Posterior

Figure 1.19 A case of follicular thyroid cancer with bone metastases. Bone metastases is rare in differentiated thyroid cancer but may occur with or without ^{131}I uptake and variable thyroglobulin (Tg) production. These metastases can be detected with ^{18}F-FDG positron emission tomography (PET) when metabolically active, but the diagnostic exam of choice is a bone scan with ^{99m}Tc-hydroxymethylene-diphosphonate (HDP) or ^{99m}Tc-methyl-diphosphate (MDP) as shown in this figure. An avid bone uptake offers the treatment option with a beta-emitting isotope (^{188}Re-HEDP, ^{153}Sm-EDTMP, ^{89}Sr-Chloride, etc.).

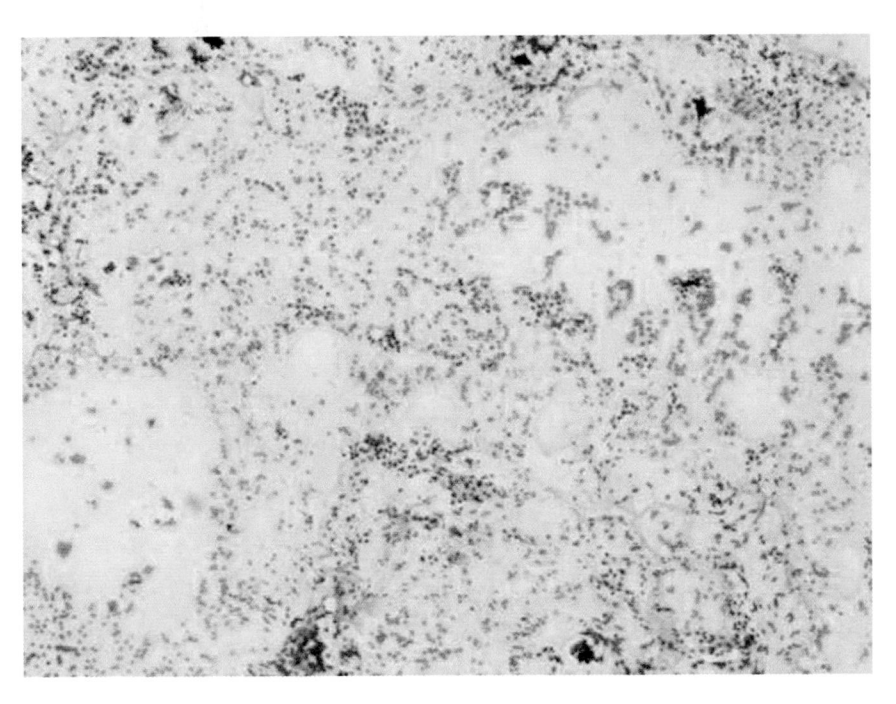

Figure 1.20 Cytology of follicular lesion (Papanicolau, 10 ×). Thyrocytes arranged in microfollicular structure, with scant colloid.

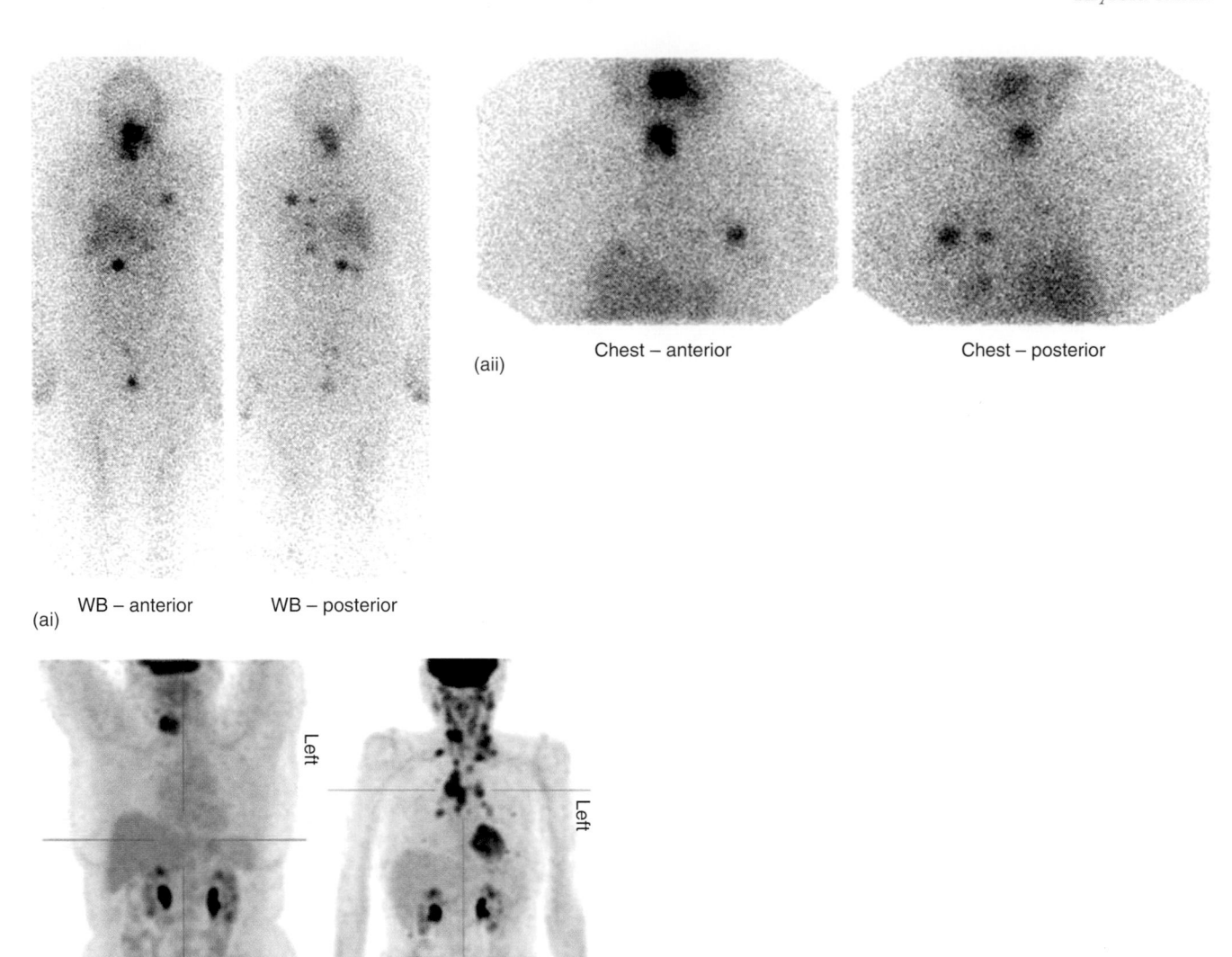

(aii)   Chest – anterior   Chest – posterior

(ai)   WB – anterior   WB – posterior

(b)   (c)

Figure 1.21 A case of undifferentiated thyroid cancer: These images show the case of a 64-year-old woman who underwent several surgeries for primary and recurrent undifferentiated thyroid cancer. She also performed ^{131}I therapy and the whole body scan post-therapy showed disease recurrence in the neck and lungs (ai & aii). At the same time an ^{18}F-FDG positron emission tomography (PET) scan showed high glucose metabolism in the neck metastasis (a negative prognostic factor) but not in the other metastases (b). The patient therefore performed a salvage radiotherapy with external beam, but the following ^{18}F-FDG PET scan showed progression of the disease with multiple focal areas of increased uptake in the laterocervical lymph nodes, the mediastinum, the pulmonary parenchima, and the hilum (c).

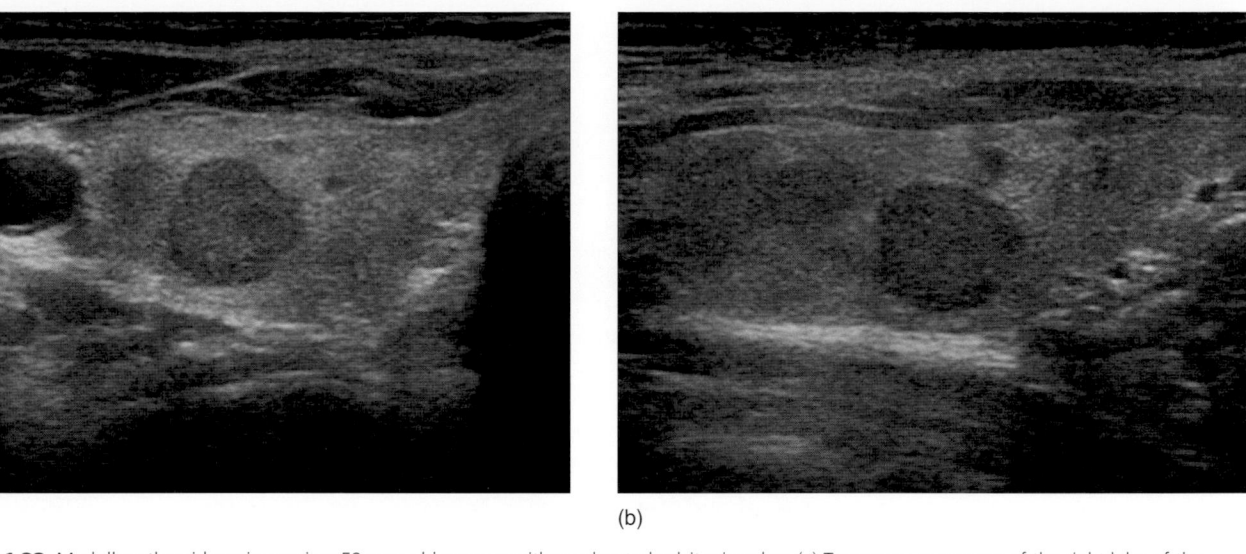

(a)   (b)

Figure 1.22 Medullary thyroid carcinoma in a 52-year-old woman with an elevated calcitonin value. (a) Transverse sonogram of the right lobe of the thyroid shows a solitary, hypoechoic, nodule with an irregular margin. (b) Longitudinal sonogram of the same thyroid nodule.

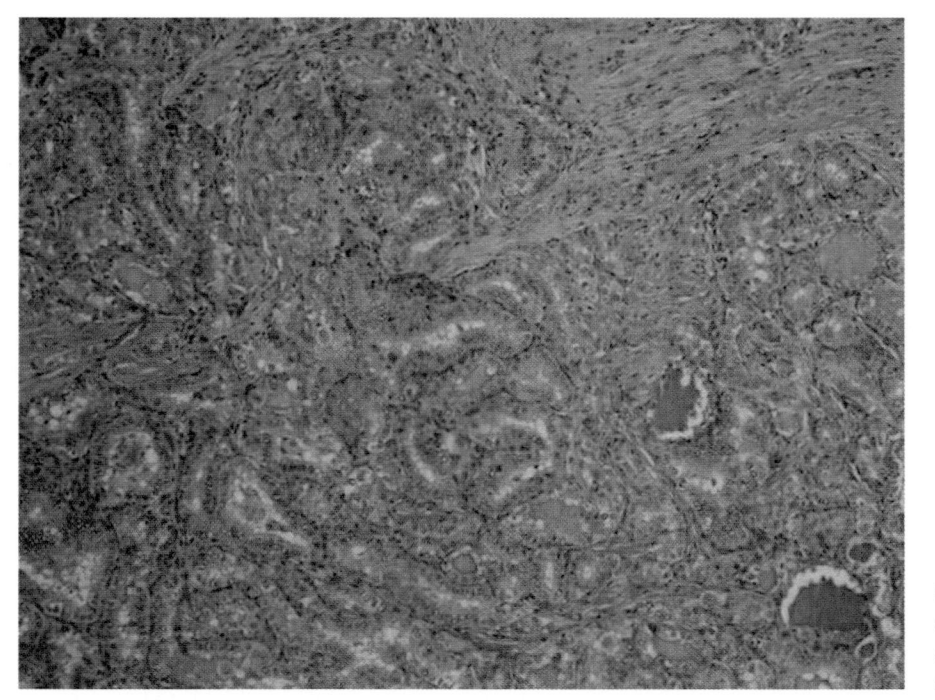

Figure 1.23 Histology of medullary carcinoma: Solid nests of polygonal cells associated to amyloid deposits within the stroma (HE, 20 ×).

Figure 1.24 A case of medullary thyroid cancer (MTC): Gamma camera images of the chest of a patient with metastatic MTC. Images were acquired 1 hour after the intravenous administration of 15 mCi of ^{99m}Tc-HYNICTOC (a somatostatin analog that binds to type 3 receptors) before (a) and after (b) therapy with 60 mCi of ^{90}Y-DOTATOC (the same somatostatin analog radiolabeled with a beta-emitting isotope). In MTC primary and metastatic lesions can express somatostatin receptors (SSTRs). The scintigraphic demonstration of SSTRs is therefore mandatory for both correct staging and therapy decision making. In this patient the treatment of choice was with radiolabeled somatostatin analogs, and after just one cycle of therapy the scan (b) shows large necrosis and reduction in size of all metastasis.

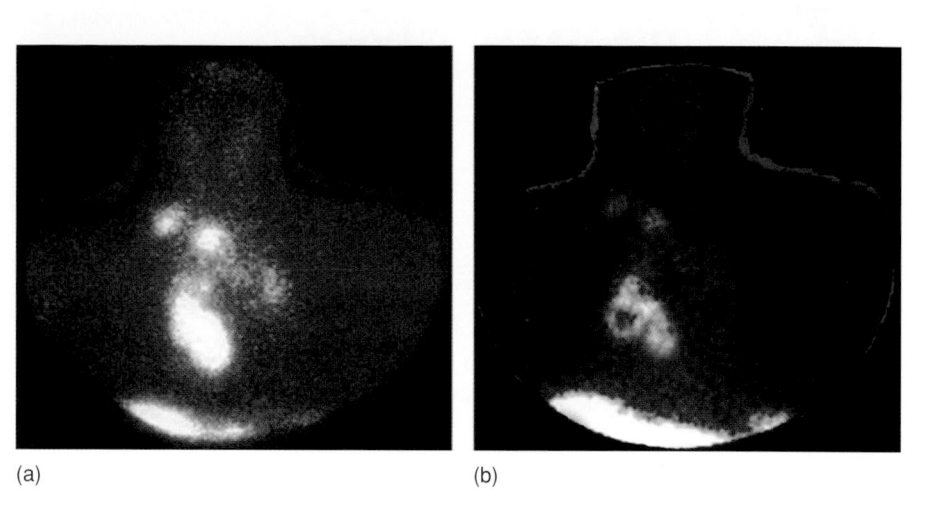

(a) (b)

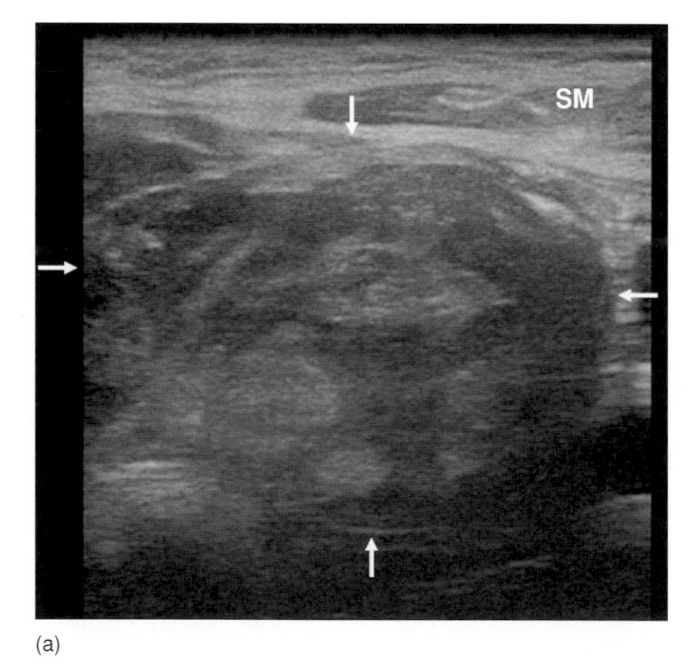

(a)

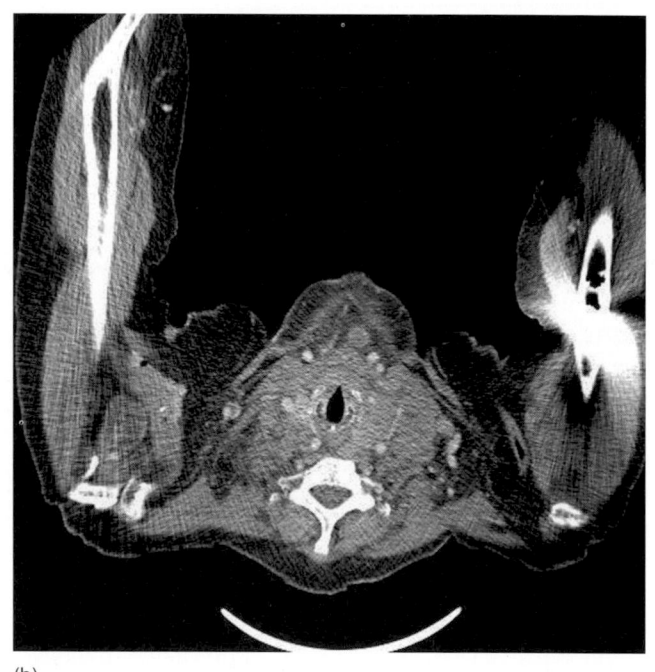

(b)

Figure 1.25 B-cell non-Hodgkin lymphoma of the thyroid in a 77-year-old woman with Hashimoto thyroiditis. (a) Transverse sonogram of the left lobe of the thyroid shows a large heterogeneous mass with marked hypoechogenicity when compared with the strap muscles (SM). (b) Axial contrast-enhanced computed tomography (CT) imaging shows widespread morphostructural disruption of the thyroid left lobe, replaced by hypodense solid tissue, invading adjacent muscle planes and extending to the posterior mediastinum, compressing the tracheal and esophageal lumen, and to the origin of neck vessels, significantly reducing the size of the internal jugular vein. Lymphadenopathies in the right side of the neck and in the superior mediastinum are also evident.

2 Pituitary Gland

Craniopharyngioma

Definition
Craniopharyngiomas may be large and invade the third ventricle and associated brain structures. This tumorous process is usually located above the sella turcica, depressing the optic chiasm and extending up into the third ventricle (Fig. 2.1).

Etiology
Craniopharyngioma is a benign epithelioid tumor arising from embryonic squamous remnants of Rathke's pouch and it is the most common tumor found in the region of the pituitary gland in children and adolescents – constituting about 3% of all intracranial tumors and up to 10% of all childhood brain tumors.

Signs and symptoms
Signs and symptoms are primarily due to mass effect and typically occur in the adolescent years and rarely after age 40. The mass effect symptoms include: vision loss by compression of the optic chiasm; diabetes insipidus by invasion or disruption of the hypothalamus or pituitary stalk; hypothalamic dysfunction (e.g. obesity with hyperphagia, hypersomnolence, disturbance in temperature regulation); various degrees of anterior pituitary insufficiency (e.g. growth hormone deficiency with short stature in childhood, hypogonadism, adrenal insufficiency, hypothyroidism); hyperprolactinemia due to compression of the pituitary stalk or damage to the dopaminergic neurons in the hypothalamus; signs and symptoms of increased intracranial pressure (e.g. headache, projectile emesis, papilledema, optic atrophy); symptoms of hydrocephalus (e.g. mental dullness and confusion); and cranial nerve palsies caused by cavernous sinus invasion.

Diagnosis

Imaging tests
The findings on radiologic imaging are quite characteristic. Plain skull roentgenograms and computed tomography (CT) show irregular calcification in the suprasellar region. Magnetic resonance imaging (MRI) typically shows a multilobulated cystic structure – usually suprasellar in location, but it may also appear to arise from the sella (Fig. 2.2). The cystic regions are usually filled with a turbid, cholesterol-rich, viscous fluid (Fig. 2.3).

Laboratory findings
There is no specific laboratory test for craniopharyngioma. Hypothalamic–pituitary function may be intact, or testing may demonstrate varying degrees of hormonal deficiencies.

Treatment
Treatment options for patients with craniopharyngiomas include observation, transsphenoidal surgery for smaller intrasellar tumors, craniotomy for larger suprasellar tumors, stereotactic radiotherapy, or a combination of these modalities.

Imaging in Endocrinology, First Edition. Paolo Pozzilli, Andrea Lenzi, Bart L Clarke and William F Young Jr.
© 2014 John Wiley & Sons, Ltd. Published 2014 by John Wiley & Sons, Ltd.

Illustrations (Figs 2.1–2.3)

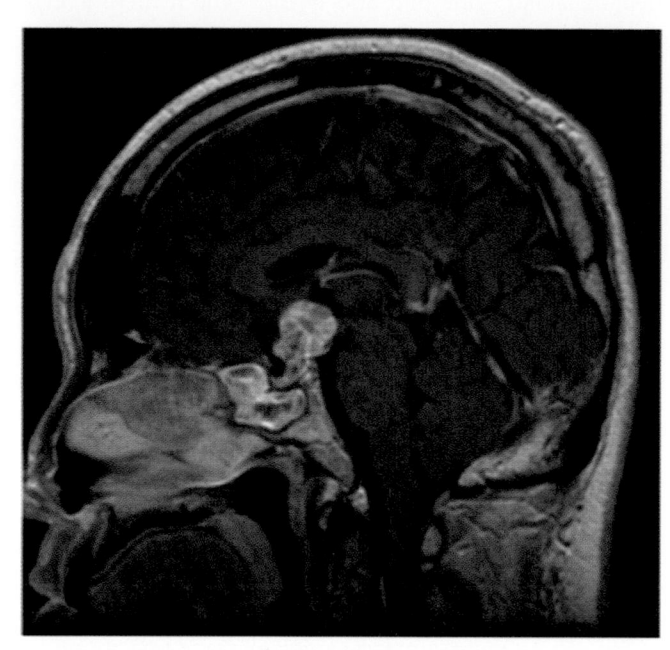

Figure 2.1 Magnetic resonance imaging (MRI) (sagittal view) showing cystic suprasellar craniopharyngioma.

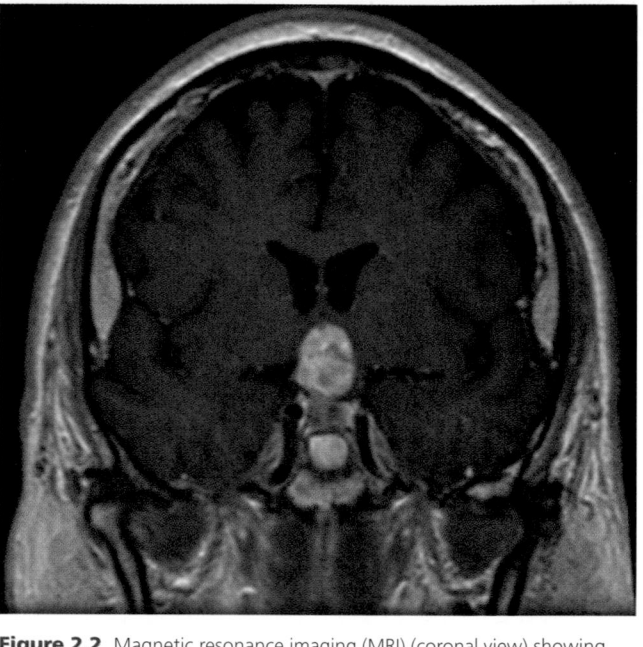

Figure 2.2 Magnetic resonance imaging (MRI) (coronal view) showing suprasellar craniopharyngioma.

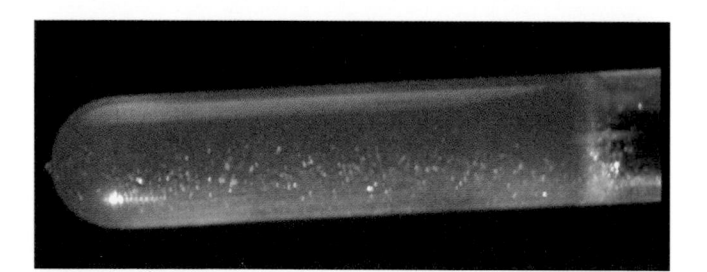

Figure 2.3 Turbid, cholesterol-rich, viscous fluid from a craniopharyngioma.

Hypothalamic dysgerminoma

Definition
Hypothalamic dysgerminomas are germ cell tumors.

Etiology
The locations of central nervous system germ cell tumors include the diencephalic area, pineal region, and hypothalamus. Germ cell tumors primarily affect young people and represent 5% of intracranial neoplasms in children.

Signs and symptoms
Due to the proximity to the optic chiasm, hypothalamic lesions are frequently associated with vision loss. An enlarging hypothalamic mass may also cause headaches and recurrent emesis. The hypothalamus is responsible for many homeostatic functions such as appetite control, the sleep–wake cycle, water metabolism, temperature regulation, anterior pituitary function, circadian rhythms, and inputs to the parasympathetic and sympathetic nervous systems. The clinical presentation is dependent on the location of the dysgerminoma within the hypothalamus and patients may present with a constellation of symptoms including: hypersomnolence; hyperactivity and insomnia; alterations in the sleep–wake cycle (e.g. nighttime hyperactivity and daytime sleepiness); dysthermia (acute hyperthermia or chronic hypothermia); hyperphagia and obesity; hypophagia with weight loss and cachexia; central diabetes insipidus; polydipsia or hypodipsia; and varying degrees of anterior pituitary dysfunction.

Hypothalamic germ cell tumors may produce peptides normally secreted by the hypothalamus. For example, children may present with precocious puberty when beta-human chorionic gonadotropin (β-hCG) is hypersecreted by suprasellar germ cell tumors.

Diagnosis
Although hypothalamic dysgerminoma may be diagnosed based on measurement of cerebral spinal fluid β-hCG, α-fetoprotein, or cytology, the diagnosis typically requires tissue confirmation with a biopsy.

Magnetic resonance imaging (MRI) typically reveals a gadolinium-enhancing hypothalamic mass extending into the pituitary stalk in a "V-shape" (Figs 2.4 & 2.5). Occasionally the dysgerminoma may appear to be primarily located in the pituitary stalk or it may extend into the sella.

In patients with disease that extends beyond the hypothalamus, the cerebrospinal fluid analysis may show increased concentrations of β-hCG, α-fetoprotein, or abnormal cytology.

Treatment
Treatment typically involves radiation therapy to the hypothalamic region and also to the spine if there is evidence of drop metastases. Systemic chemotherapy may be indicated in patients with more primitive tumor types.

Illustrations (Figs 2.4 & 2.5)

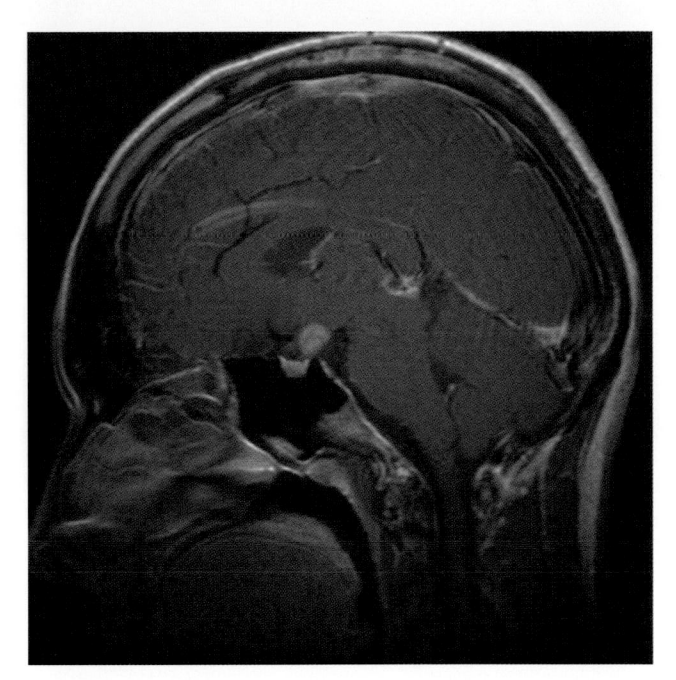

Figure 2.4 Magnetic resonance imaging (MRI) (sagittal view) showing suprasellar dysgerminoma.

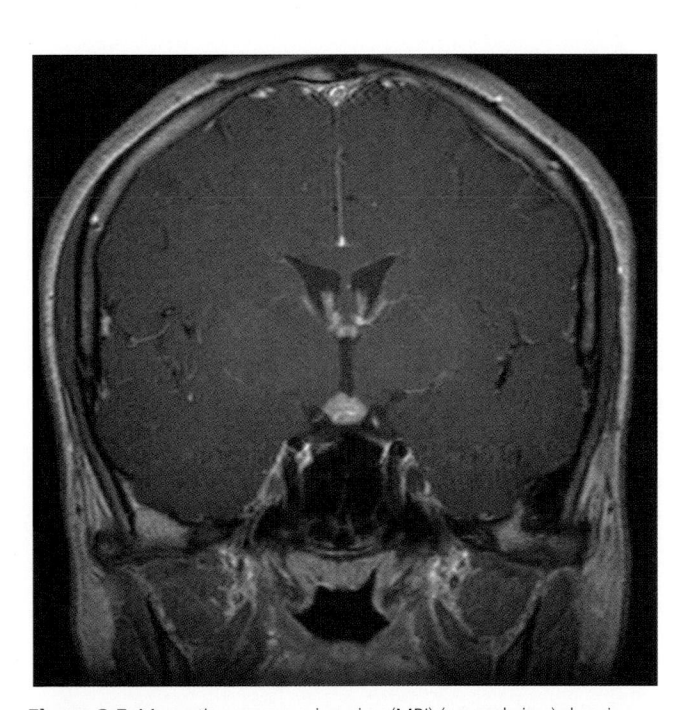

Figure 2.5 Magnetic resonance imaging (MRI) (coronal view) showing suprasellar dysgerminoma.

Growth hormone-secreting pituitary tumor

Definition

Chronic growth hormone (GH) excess from a GH-producing pituitary tumor results in the clinical syndrome of acromegaly in adults and gigantism in children or adolescents (before the epiphyses fuse).

Etiology

Growth hormone-secreting pituitary tumors are monoclonal somatotroph cell adenomas that appear to result from sporadic mutations. Although the annual incidence is estimated to be only 3 per 1 million persons in the general population, a GH-secreting pituitary adenoma is the second most common hormone-secreting pituitary tumor.

Signs and symptoms

The effects of the chronic GH excess include acral and soft-tissue overgrowth, expansion of the frontal sinuses – termed "frontal bossing" (Fig. 2.6), increased tissue on the plantar surfaces of the feet leading to plantar grooves (Fig. 2.7), progressive dental malocclusion (underbite), widening of the nose and thick lips (Fig. 2.8), degenerative arthritis related to chondral and synovial tissue overgrowth within joints, low-pitched sonorous voice, headaches, malodorous hyperhidrosis, oily skin, increased numbers of skin tags (Fig. 2.9), perineural hypertrophy leading to nerve entrapment (e.g. carpal tunnel syndrome), proximal muscle weakness, carbohydrate intolerance (initial presentation may be diabetes mellitus), hypertension, colonic neoplasia, obstructive sleep apnea, and cardiac dysfunction. The mass effects of GH-producing pituitary macroadenomas (> 10 mm in diameter) are similar to those of other pituitary macroadenomas – they include visual field defects, oculomotor pareses, headaches, and pituitary insufficiency.

The patient with acromegaly has a characteristic appearance with coarsening of facial features (Fig. 2.8), prognathism, frontal bossing (Fig. 2.6), spade-like hands, and wide feet. Often there is a history of progressive increase in shoe, glove, ring, or hat size. These changes may occur slowly and may go unrecognized by the patient, family, and physician. The average delay in diagnosis from the onset of the first symptoms to the eventual diagnosis is 8.5 years. Comparison with earlier photographs of the patient is helpful in confirming the clinical suspicion of acromegaly.

When a GH-secreting tumor develops in infancy, it may lead to exceptional height. The tallest well-documented person with pituitary gigantism measured 8 ft 11 in (2.72 m).

Diagnosis

Laboratory findings

The diagnosis of acromegaly or gigantism depends on two criteria: a GH level that is not suppressed to < 1 ng/dL after an oral glucose load (75–100 g) and an increased serum concentration (based on reference range adjusted for age and sex) of insulinlike growth factor 1 (IGF-1).

Imaging tests

The laboratory assessment of acromegaly is supplemented with magnetic resonance imaging (MRI) of the pituitary (Fig. 2.10) and with visual field examination by quantitative perimetry. If imaging of the pituitary fails to detect an adenoma, then plasma GH-releasing hormone (GHRH) concentration and computed tomography (CT) of the chest and abdomen are indicated in search of an ectopic GHRH-producing tumor (e.g. pancreatic or small cell lung neoplasms).

Treatment

Treatment is indicated for all patients with acromegaly or gigantism. The goals of treatment are to prevent the long-term consequences of GH excess, to remove the sellar mass, and to preserve normal pituitary tissue and function. Treatment options include surgery, irradiation, and medical therapy. Surgery is the treatment of choice and should be supplemented, if necessary, with irradiation or pharmacotherapy or both.

Illustrations (Figs 2.6–2.10)

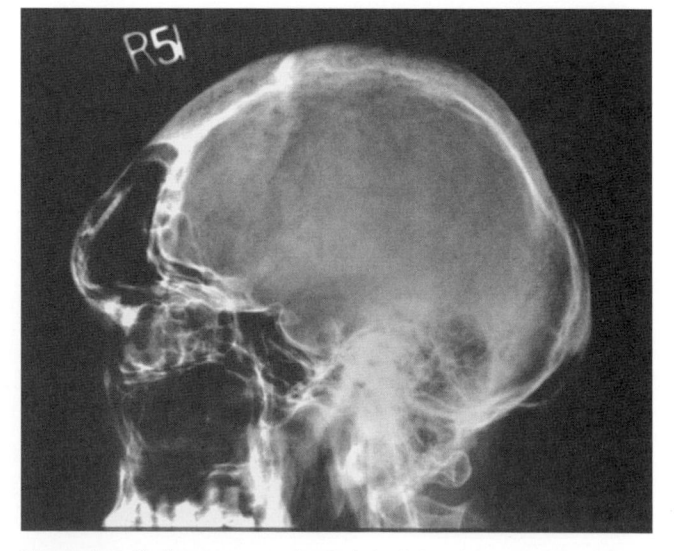

Figure 2.6 Skull roetenogram (sagittal view) showing expansion of the frontal sinuses (frontal bossing).

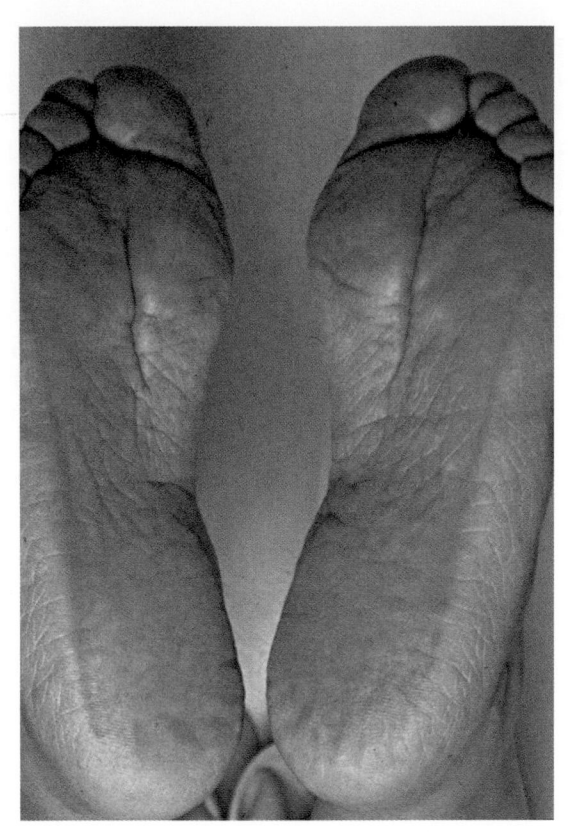

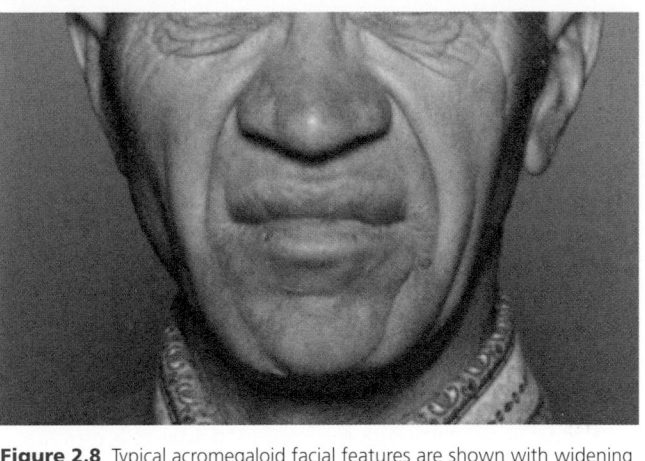

Figure 2.8 Typical acromegaloid facial features are shown with widening of the nose and thick lips.

Figure 2.7 Increased soft tissue build up on the plantar surfaces of the feet leading to plantar grooves.

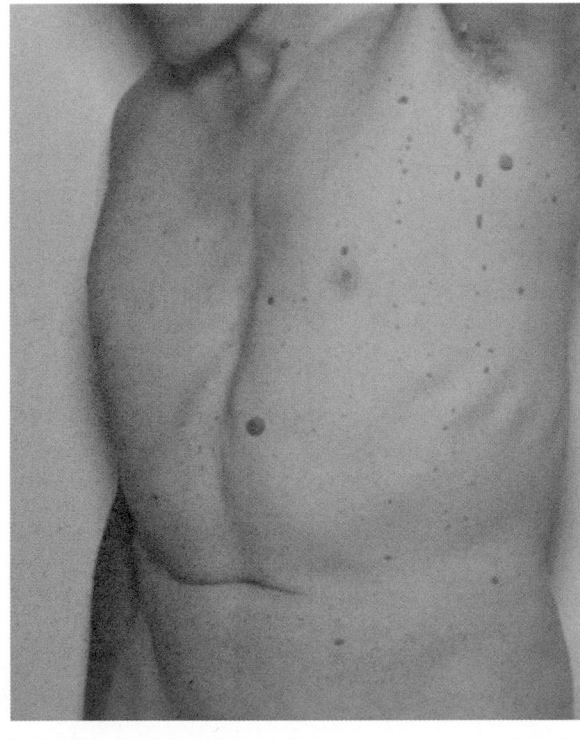

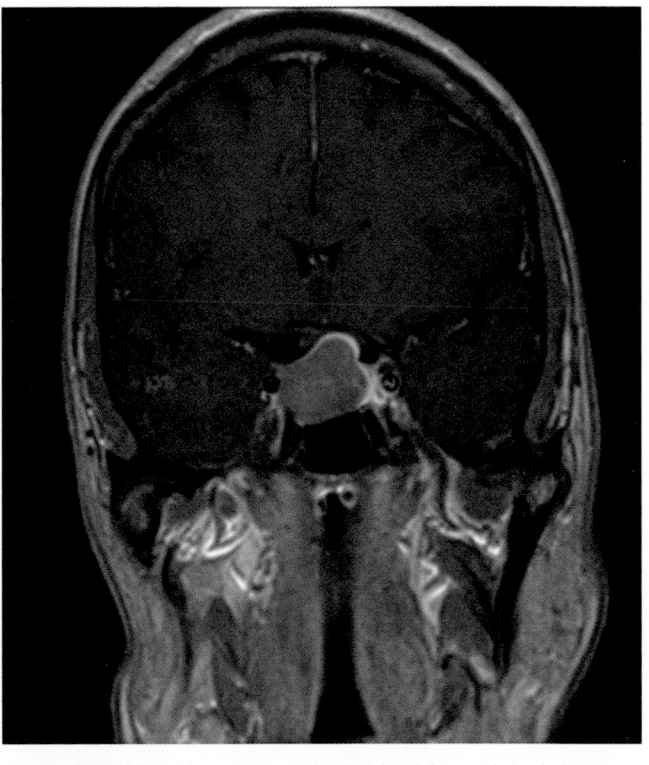

Figure 2.9 Increased numbers of skin tags are very common in patients with acromegaly.

Figure 2.10 Magnetic resonance imaging (MRI) (coronal view) showing a 2.2 cm pituitary tumor extending into the right cavernous sinus and suprasellar extension to left side of the optic chiasm.

Prolactin-secreting pituitary tumor

Definition
Prolactin-secreting pituitary tumors (prolactinomas) are the most common hormone-secreting pituitary tumor.

Etiology
Prolactinomas are monoclonal lactotroph cell adenomas that appear to result from sporadic mutations.

Signs and symptoms
In women, the typical clinical presentation of a prolactin-secreting microadenoma ($\leq$ 10 mm in largest diameter) is secondary amenorrhea with or without galactorrhea. In men, because of the lack of symptoms related to small prolactinomas, a prolactinoma is not usually diagnosed until the tumor has enlarged enough to cause mass-effect symptoms. This late diagnosis is also the typical clinical scenario in postmenopausal women. Mass-effect symptoms of prolactin-secreting macroadenomas include visual field defects with suprasellar extension, cranial nerve palsies with lateral (cavernous sinus) extension (e.g. diplopia, ptosis), headaches, and varying degrees of hypopituitarism with compression of the normal pituitary tissue.

Hyperprolactinemia results in decreased gonadotropin secretion in men and women. In men, hypogonadotropic hypogonadism causes testicular atrophy, low serum testosterone concentrations, decreased libido, sexual dysfunction, decreased facial hair growth, and decreased muscle mass. Because men lack the estrogen needed to prepare breast glandular tissues, they rarely present with galactorrhea. In premenopausal women, however, hyperprolactinemia may cause bilateral spontaneous or expressible galactorrhea. In addition, prolactin-dependent hypogonadotropic hypogonadism in women results in secondary amenorrhea and estrogen deficiency symptoms. Long-standing hypogonadism in both men and women may lead to osteopenia and osteoporosis.

Diagnosis
A serum prolactin concentration > 250 ng/mL (reference range, 4–30 ng/mL) is diagnostic of a prolactin-secreting pituitary tumor. Mild hyperprolactinemia may be associated with very small pituitary tumors (Fig. 2.11). Whereas, serum prolactin concentrations > 500 ng/mL are usually associated with pituitary macroadenomas (Figs 2.12 & 2.13).

Treatment
Treatment decisions in patients with prolactin-secreting pituitary tumors are guided by the signs and symptoms related to hyperprolactinemia and mass-effect symptoms related to the sellar mass. For example, a 4-mm prolactin-secreting microadenoma detected incidentally in an asymptomatic postmenopausal woman may be observed without treatment. However, because prolactin-secreting pituitary macroadenomas grow over time, treatment is almost always indicated for macroprolactinomas, even if the patient lacks tumor-related symptomatology. When treatment is indicated (e.g. if secondary hypogonadism is present in men or in premenopausal women or if a macroadenoma is present), an orally administered dopamine agonist (e.g. cabergoline or bromocriptine) is the treatment of choice. Prolactin-secreting pituitary macroadenomas typically show marked shrinkage in response to dopamine agonist therapy.

Illustrations (Figs 2.11–2.13)

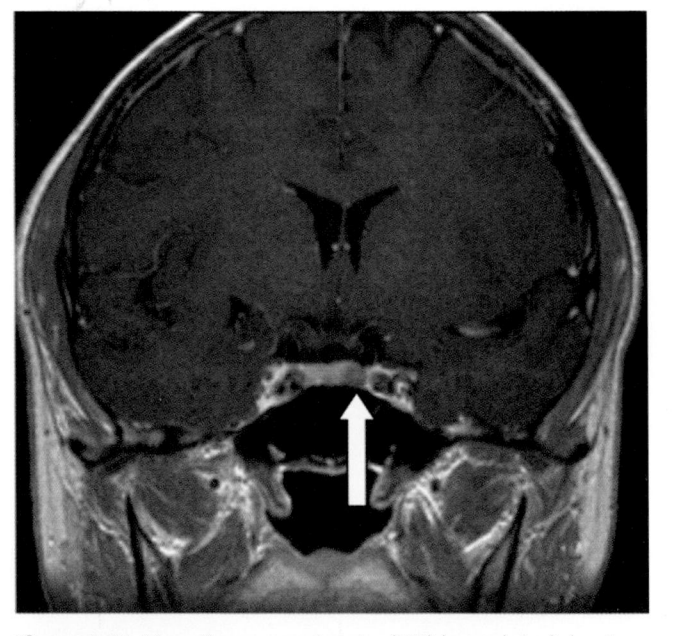

Figure 2.11 Magnetic resonance imaging (MRI) (coronal view) showing a 4-mm left sellar prolactin-secreting microadenoma (arrow).

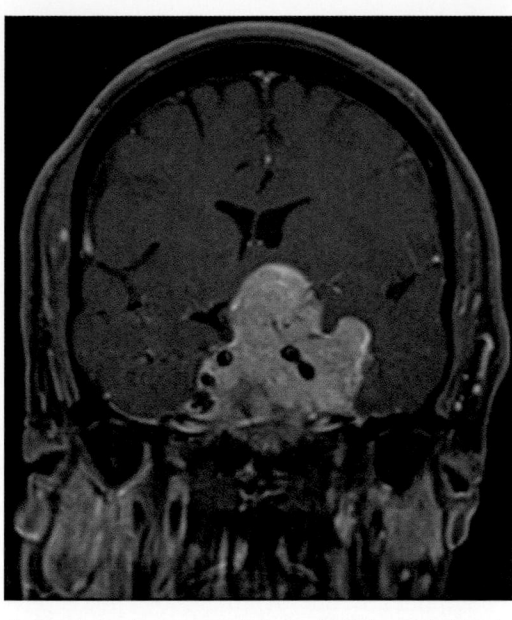

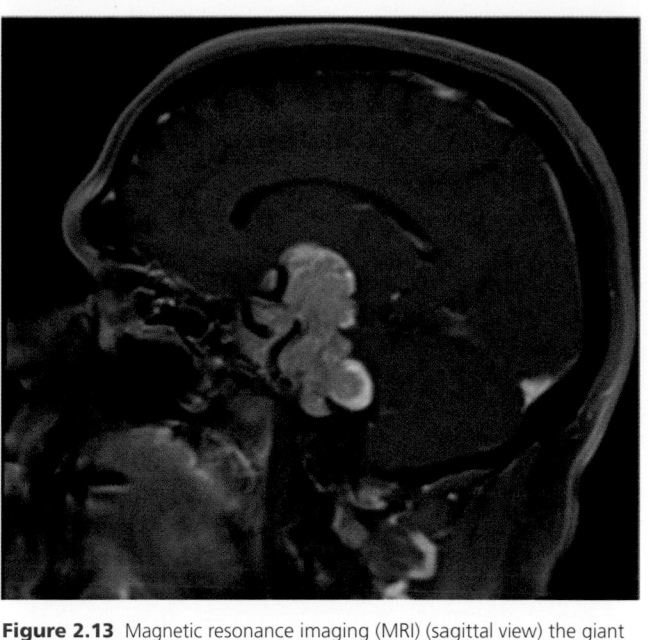

Figure 2.12 Magnetic resonance imaging (MRI) (coronal view) showing a 6-cm multiobulated and enhancing prolactin-secreting pituitary macroadenoma with marked suprasellar and left temporal lobe extension.

Figure 2.13 Magnetic resonance imaging (MRI) (sagittal view) the giant prolactin-secreting pituitary tumor encasing the intracavernous left carotid artery and invasion of brain tissue.

Corticotropin-secreting pituitary tumor (Cushing syndrome)

Definition
Corticotropin (ACTH)-secreting pituitary adenomas stimulate excess adrenal secretion of cortisol, resulting in the signs and symptoms characteristic of Cushing syndrome.

Etiology
Secreting pituitary tumors are typically benign microadenomas (≤ 10 mm in largest diameter); occasionally they are macroadenomas; and very rarely they are carcinomas.

Signs and symptoms
Cushing syndrome is a symptom complex that results from prolonged exposure to supraphysiologic concentrations of glucocorticoids.

Typical signs and symptoms of Cushing syndrome include weight gain with central obesity; facial rounding with fat deposition in the temporal fossae and cheeks ("moon face") and plethora (Fig. 2.14); supraclavicular fat pads (Fig. 2.14); dorsocervical fat pad ("buffalo hump") (Fig. 2.14); easy ("spontaneous") bruising (ecchymoses); fine "cigarette paper–thin skin" that tears easily; poor wound healing; red-purple striae (usually > 1 cm in thickness located over abdomen, flanks, axilla, breasts, hips, and inner thighs) (Fig. 2.15); scalp hair thinning; proximal muscle weakness associated with muscle loss and resulting in thin extremities (Fig. 2.16); emotional and cognitive changes (e.g. irritability, crying, depression, insomnia, restlessness); hirsutism and acne; hypertension; osteopenia and osteoporosis; renal lithiasis; glucose intolerance and diabetes mellitus; hyperlipidemia; opportunistic and fungal infections (e.g. mucocutaneous candidiasis, tinea versicolor, pityriasis); menstrual dysfunction and infertility.

The clinical features of Cushing syndrome may occur slowly over time; thus, comparison of the patient's current appearance with his or her appearance in old photographs is invaluable.

Diagnosis

Laboratory findings
Case detection testing should start with measurements of 24-hour urinary free cortisol (UFC), 11 PM salivary cortisol, and serum cortisol concentrations measured at 8 AM and 4 PM. The 1-mg overnight dexamethasone suppression test (DST) is an additional case-detection test. Additional confirmatory studies are not needed if the baseline 24-hour UFC excretion is > 300 μg/24 h (> 828 nmol/24 h) and the clinical picture is consistent with Cushing syndrome. The plasma ACTH concentration classifies the subtype of hypercortisolism as ACTH-dependent (normal to high levels of ACTH) or ACTH-independent (undetectable ACTH).

Imaging tests
A pituitary-dedicated magnetic resonance imaging (MRI) is indicated in all patients with ACTH-dependent Cushing syndrome. If a definite pituitary tumor is found (e.g. ≥ 4 mm in diameter) and the clinical scenario is consistent with pituitary disease (e.g. woman, slow onset of disease, and baseline 24-hour UFC < 5-fold increase above the reference range), then additional studies are usually not required before definitive treatment. Smaller apparent pituitary lesions (e.g. < 4 mm) are common in healthy persons and should be considered nonspecific and in this setting inferior petrosal sinus sampling (IPSS) should be considered. Also, if the pituitary MRI findings are normal (seen in approximately 50% of patients with pituitary-dependent Cushing syndrome) IPSS should be considered.

Treatment
Transsphenoidal pituitary surgery is the treatment of choice. Cure rates are 80–90% when a microadenoma can be localized preoperatively with either MRI or IPSS. When transsphenoidal surgery fails to cure pituitary-dependent Cushing syndrome, the two main treatment options are to perform another transsphenoidal surgery or to perform bilateral laparoscopic adrenalectomy. The third and less frequently used option is radiation therapy to the sella.

Illustrations (Figs 2.14–2.16)

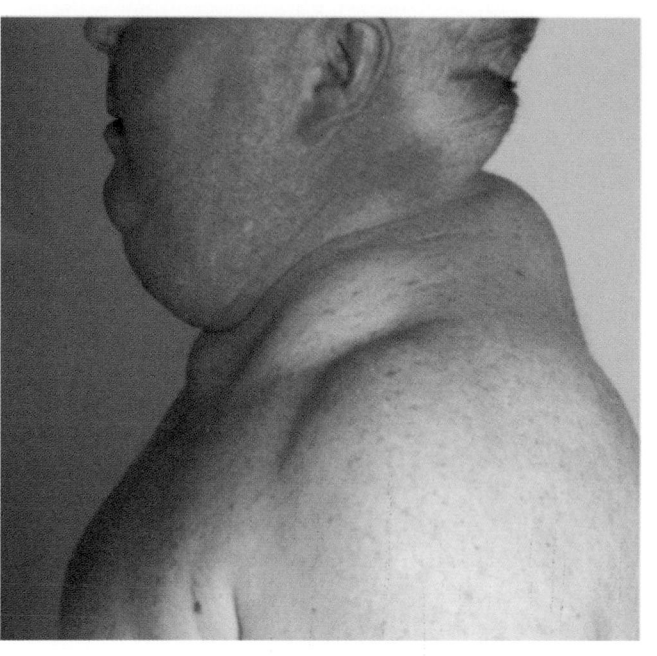

Figure 2.14 Photo of a man with Cushing syndrome showing full and plethoric face, dorsocervical fat pad, and supraclavicular fat pad.

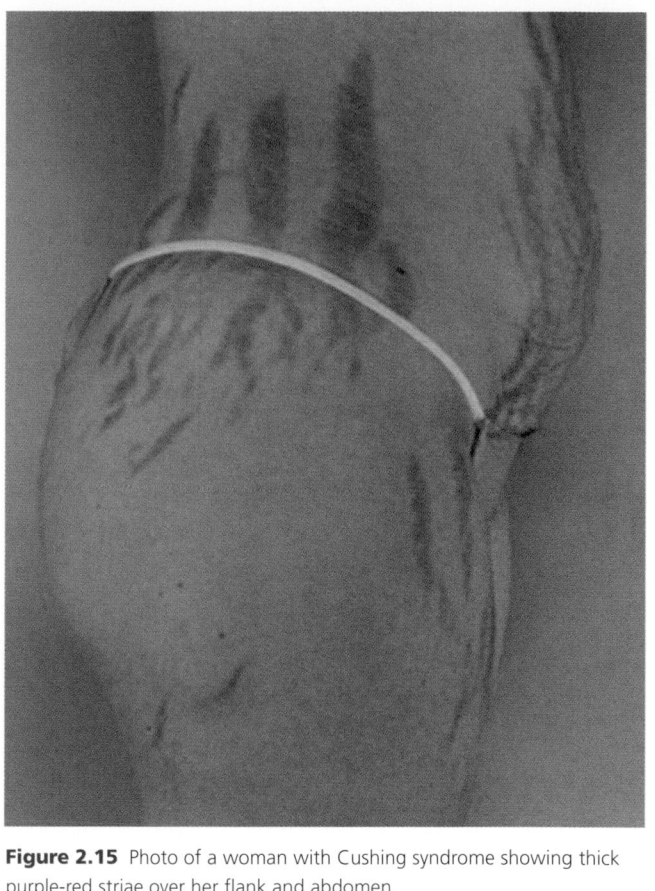

Figure 2.15 Photo of a woman with Cushing syndrome showing thick purple-red striae over her flank and abdomen.

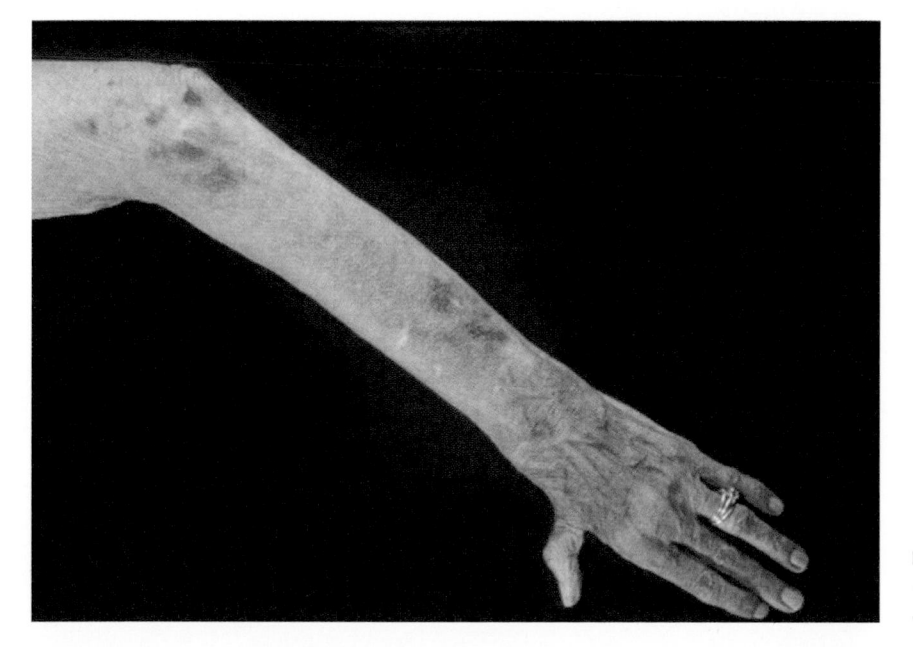

Figure 2.16 Photo of an arm from a patient with Cushing syndrome showing muscular atrophy and ecchymoses.

Nelson syndrome

Definition

Nelson syndrome refers to progressive pituitary corticotroph tumor enlargement after bilateral adrenalectomy is performed for the treatment of pituitary-dependent Cushing syndrome.

Etiology

Although the treatment of choice for a corticotroph adenoma is selective adenectomy at the time of transsphenoidal surgery, bilateral adrenalectomy is indicated when pituitary surgery is not successful. While bilateral adrenalectomy cures hypercortisolism, there is less negative feedback on the corticotroph tumor cells with the postoperative physiologic glucocorticoid replacement, and the pituitary adenoma may grow. Nelson syndrome occurs in a minority of patients who follow the treatment sequence of failed transsphenoidal surgery and bilateral adrenalectomy. Most corticotroph microadenomas do not enlarge over time in this setting. However, when pituitary-dependent Cushing syndrome is caused by a corticotroph macroadenoma (> 10 mm in largest diameter), the risk of tumor enlargement after bilateral adrenalectomy is high.

Signs and symptoms

The clinical features of Nelson syndrome are skin hyperpigmentation (related to the markedly increased blood levels of proopiomelanocortin and corticotropin [ACTH]) and symptoms related to mass effects of an enlarging pituitary tumor (e.g. visual field defects, oculomotor nerve palsies, hypopituitarism, and headaches). As in Addison disease, generalized hyperpigmentation is caused by ACTH-driven increased melanin production in the epidermal melanocytes (Fig. 2.17). The extensor surfaces (e.g. knees, knuckles, elbows) and other friction areas (e.g. belt line, brassier strap) tend to be even more hyperpigmented (Fig. 2.18). Other sites of prominent hyperpigmentation include the inner surface of lips, buccal mucosa, gums, hard palate, recent surgical scars, areolae, freckles, and palmar creases. The fingernails may show linear bands of darkening arising from the nail beds (Fig. 2.17).

Diagnosis

Nelson syndrome can be confirmed by magnetic resonance imaging (MRI) of the sella that demonstrates an enlarging sellar mass (Figs 2.19 & 2.20). In addition, blood ACTH concentrations are markedly increased in this setting (e.g. > 1000 pg/mL; reference range, 10–60 pg/mL). Patients with pituitary-dependent Cushing syndrome that is treated with bilateral adrenalectomy should be monitored annually with pituitary MRI for approximately 10 years.

Treatment

Tumor-directed radiation therapy should be considered if tumor growth is documented on serial MRI. If feasible, focused radiotherapy (e.g. gamma knife radiosurgery) is the treatment of choice for Nelson corticotroph tumors. However, unlike most pituitary adenomas, these neoplasms may demonstrate aggressive growth despite radiotherapy. Extensive cavernous sinus involvement may result in multiple cranial nerve palsies. Despite the concern about potential development of Nelson syndrome, clinicians should never hesitate to cure Cushing syndrome with bilateral laparoscopic adrenalectomy when transsphenoidal surgery has not been curative. Untreated Cushing syndrome can be fatal; Nelson syndrome is usually manageable.

Illustrations (Figs 2.17–2.20)

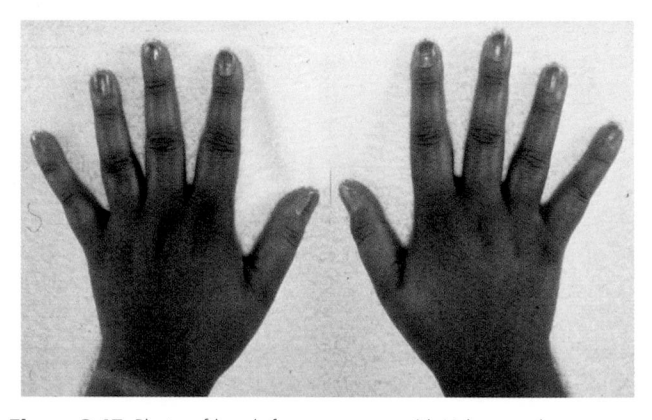

Figure 2.17 Photo of hands from a woman with Nelson syndrome. Hyperpigmentation is seen over the knuckles and fingernail beds.

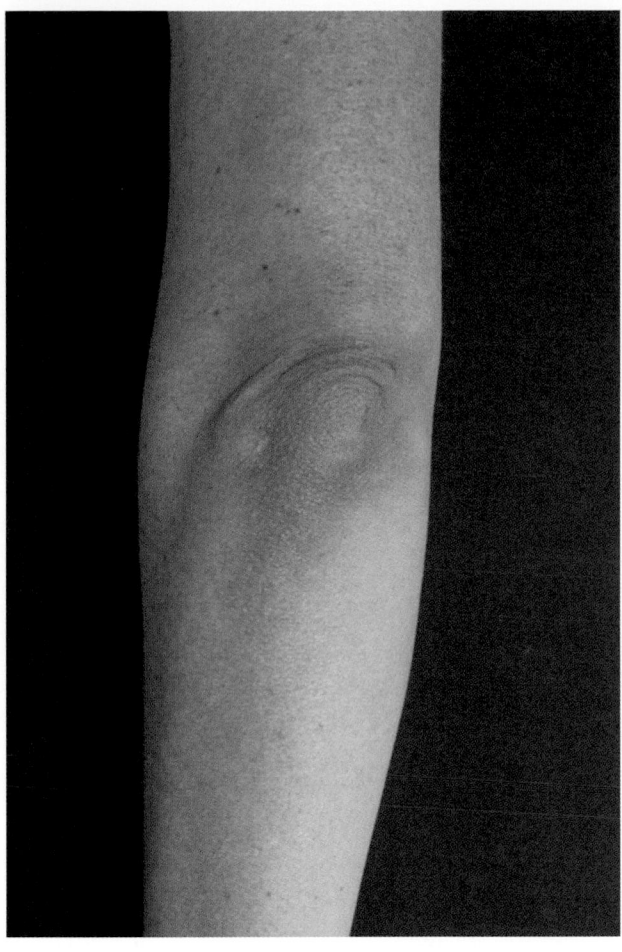

Figure 2.18 Photo of an elbow from a woman with Nelson syndrome showing hyperpigmentation.

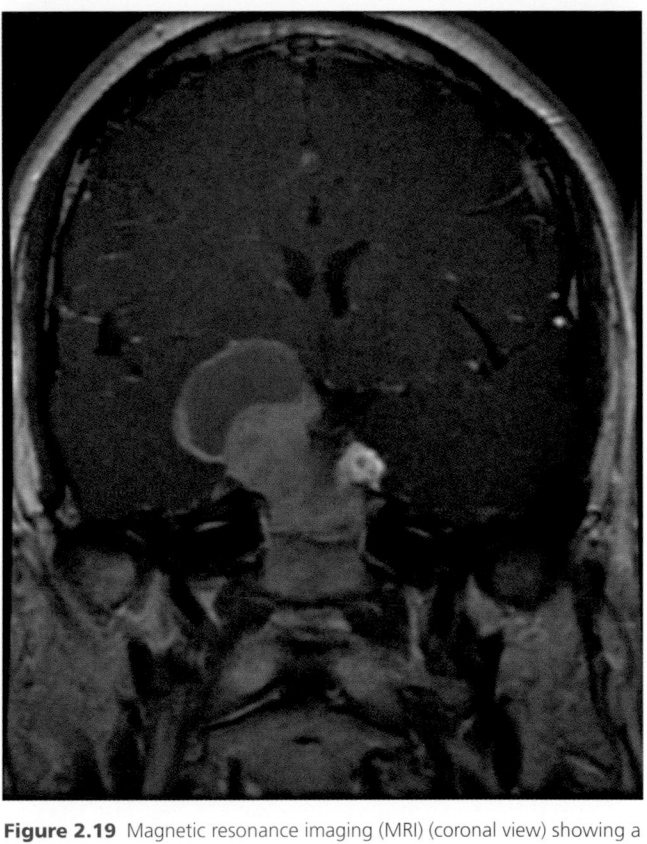

Figure 2.19 Magnetic resonance imaging (MRI) (coronal view) showing a large invasive multilobulated and enhancing ACTH-secreting pituitary macroadenoma with marked suprasellar and right temporal lobe extension.

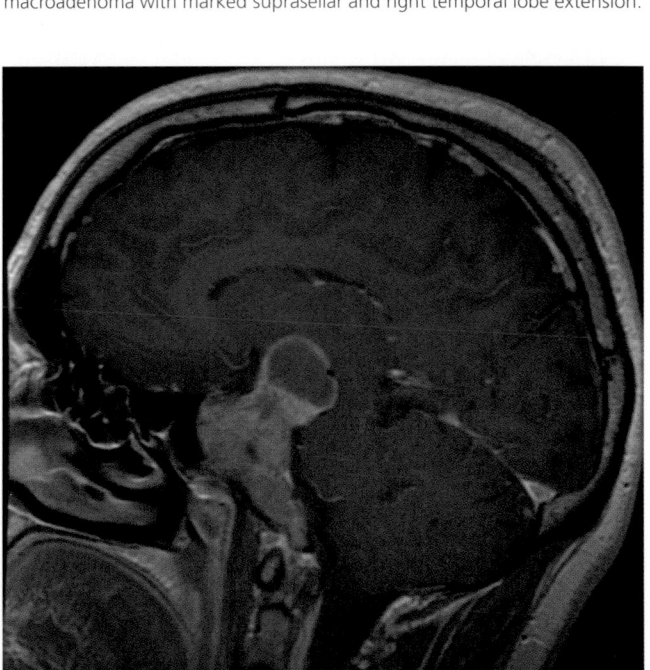

Figure 2.20 Magnetic resonance imaging (MRI) (sagittal view) of the large ACTH-secreting pituitary tumor showing cystic degeneration and suprasellar and posterior extension.

Clinically nonfunctioning pituitary tumors

Definition
Clinically nonfunctioning pituitary tumors are identified either incidentally or because of sellar mass-related symptoms.

Etiology
On the basis of autopsy studies, pituitary microadenomas (≤ 10 mm in largest dimension) are relatively common, found in approximately 10% of all pituitary glands examined. However, pituitary macroadenomas (> 10 mm in largest dimension) are uncommon. The most frequent type of pituitary macroadenoma is the gonadotroph cell adenoma; most do not hypersecrete gonadotropins, and thus, affected patients do not present with a hormone excess syndrome. The second most common clinically nonfunctioning pituitary macroadenoma is the null cell adenoma – a benign neoplasm of adenohypophyseal cells that stains negatively for any anterior pituitary hormone on immunohistochemistry. Rarely, lactotroph, somatotroph, and corticotroph pituitary adenomas may be clinically silent.

Signs and symptoms
The mass-effect symptoms in patients with clinically nonfunctioning pituitary macroadenomas usually prompt evaluation with head magnetic resonance imaging (MRI). Suprasellar extension of the pituitary adenoma causes compression of the optic chiasm, resulting in the gradual onset of superior bitemporal quadrantopia (Fig. 2.21) that may progress to complete bitemporal hemianopsia. Because the onset is gradual, patients may not recognize vision loss until it becomes marked. Additional mass-effect symptoms from an enlarging sellar mass include diplopia (with cavernous sinus extension and oculomotor nerve compression), varying degrees of pituitary insufficiency (related to compression of the normal pituitary gland by the macroadenoma), and headaches.

Diagnosis
Imaging tests
Magnetic resonance imaging clearly shows the degree of suprasellar and parasellar extension of pituitary macroadenomas (Figs 2.22 & 2.23).

Laboratory findings
All patients with pituitary macroadenomas should be assessed for tumoral hyperfunction, compression-related hypopituitarism, and visual field defects. Nonfunctioning pituitary macroadenomas are usually associated with mild hyperprolactinemia (e.g. serum prolactin concentration between 30 and 200 ng/mL) because of pituitary stalk compression and prevention of hypothalamic dopamine from reaching all of the anterior pituitary lactotrophs.

Additional pituitary-related hormones that should be measured in all patients with pituitary macroadenomas include luteinizing hormone, follicle-stimulating hormone, α-subunit of glycoprotein hormones, target gonadal hormone (estrogen in women and testosterone in men), insulin-like growth factor 1, corticotropin, cortisol, thyrotropin, and free thyroxine.

Diabetes insipidus is rare in patients with benign tumors of the adenohypophysis.

Treatment
The goals of treatment are to correct mass-effect symptoms (e.g. vision loss) and to preserve pituitary function. Currently, no effective pharmacologic options are available to treat patients with clinically nonfunctioning pituitary tumors. Observation is a reasonable management approach in elderly patients who have normal visual fields. However, intervention should be considered in all patients with vision loss. Transsphenoidal surgery can provide prompt resolution of visual field defects and permanent cure.

Illustrations (Figs 2.21–2.23)

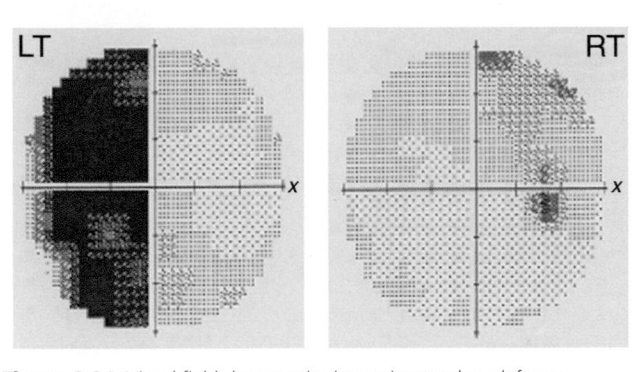

Figure 2.21 Visual fields by quantitative perimetry show left eye temporal hemianopsia and some mild vision loss in the superior temporal quadrant of the right eye.

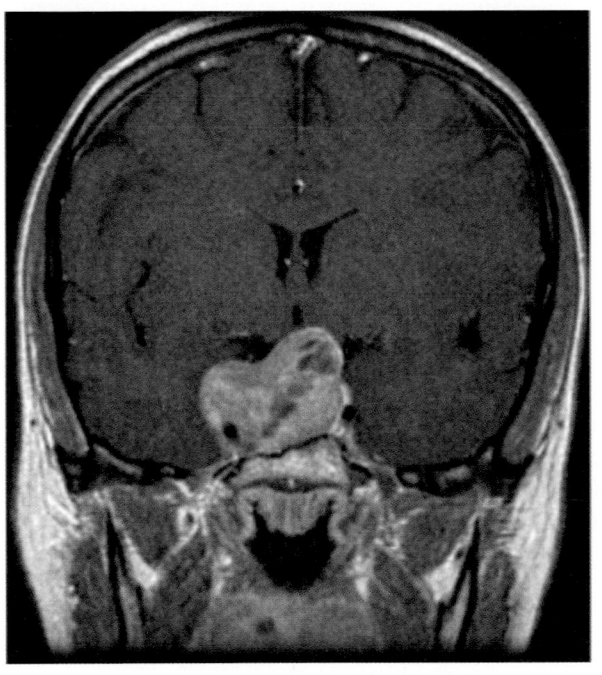

Figure 2.22 Magnetic resonance imaging (MRI) (coronal view) showing a 4.0 × 2.5-cm gadolinium-enhancing sellar and suprasellar mass with associated right cavernous sinus extension.

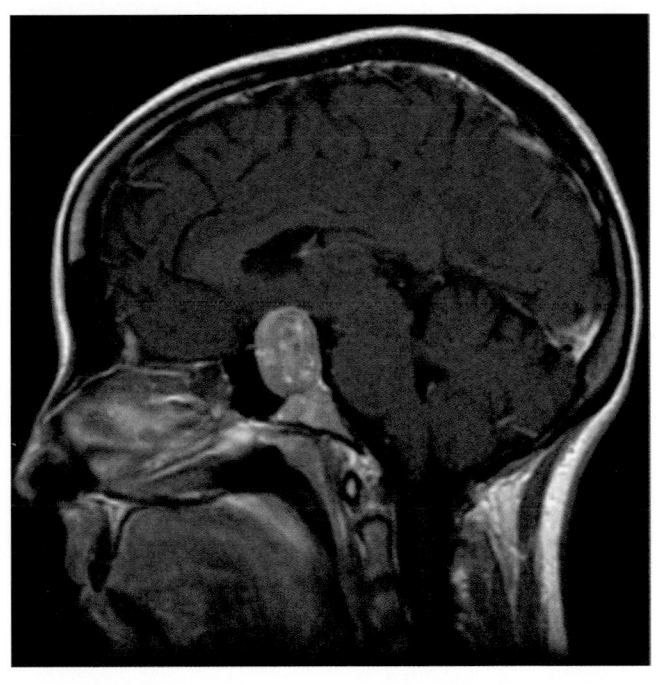

Figure 2.23 Magnetic resonance imaging (MRI) (sagittal view) showing the large sellar mass from Fig. 2.22 with suprasellar extension. The optic chiasm is stretched and thinned by this nonfunctioning pituitary tumor and resulting in visual field defects (see Figure 2.21).

Primary pituitary carcinoma

Definition
Pituitary carcinoma is defined as a primary pituitary tumor with cerebrospinal and/or systemic metastasis. Pituitary carcinomas are rare tumors – there are < 200 well-documented cases reported to date. These tumors are aggressive and associated with a high mortality rate.

Etiology
Pituitary carcinomas represent approximately 0.2% of all operated pituitary neoplasms. The pathogenesis of pituitary carcinomas is poorly understood. It appears that pituitary carcinomas transform by genetic events from adenomas rather than arise de novo.

Signs and symptoms
The latency period between presentation of the primary pituitary tumor and recognition of metastases can range from a mean of 5 years for lactotroph carcinomas to 20 years for gonadotroph carcinomas. Pituitary carcinomas are usually endocrinologically active – most often hypersecreting prolactin or corticotropin (ACTH). The clinical presentation is dominated by the mass effect symptoms of the primary tumor, metastatic sites, and hormone hypersecretion. Hyperprolactinemia results in galactorrhea and amenorrhea in women and hypogonadism in men. Hypersecretion of ACTH results in Cushing syndrome in patients with intact adrenal glands and in Nelson syndrome in patients who have undergone bilateral adrenalectomy. The hypersecreted hormone is typically 10 to 100-fold higher than that seen with typical pituitary tumors (Fig. 2.24).

Diagnosis

Imaging tests
Magnetic resonance imaging (MRI) usually demonstrates a contrast-enhancing macroadenoma with invasion of the cavernous sinuses, bone, and adjacent brain tissue (Figs 2.24 & 2.25). The metastases are indistinguishable from secondary deposits of other carcinomas (Figs 2.26 & 2.27). Positron emission tomography (PET) may be helpful in documenting number and locations of the metastatic disease.

Treatment
The prognosis of pituitary carcinomas is poor. In one series, 66% of the patients died within 1 year of the recognition of metastatic disease. Treatment options include debulking of the sellar primary and resection of central nervous system metastases. Radiation therapy may provide modest and temporary tumor regression. High doses of dopamine agonists such as bromocriptine and cabergoline are used in patients with prolactin cell carcinomas. Temozolomide is an alkylating agent that has been used in some with benefit.

Illustrations (Figs 2.24–2.27)

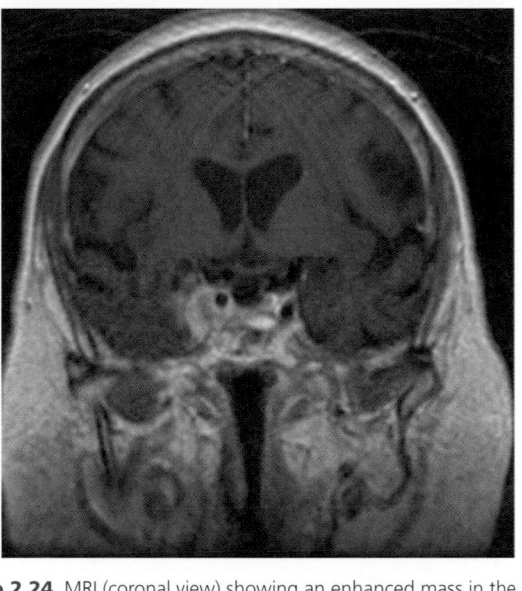

Figure 2.24 MRI (coronal view) showing an enhanced mass in the right cavernous sinus and engulfment of the intracavernous carotid artery. This patient had noncurative pituitary surgery 4 years previously for the treatment of Cushing syndrome. She was subsequently treated with bilateral adrenalectomy and she then developed Nelson syndrome, which was treated with sellar-directed radiation therapy. Six years after her pituitary surgery, she presented with marked hyperpigmentation and the serum ACTH was 33 000 pg/mL (normal < 60 pg/mL). Abdominal pain led to CT imaging of the abdomen (see Fig. 2.26).

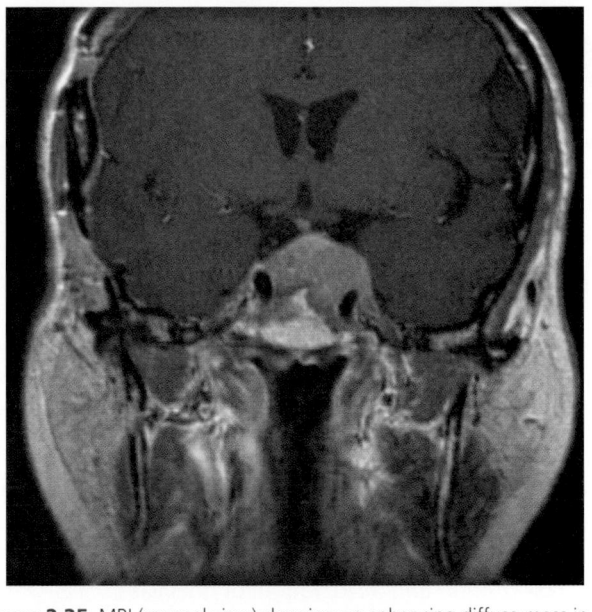

Figure 2.25 MRI (coronal view) showing an enhancing diffuse mass in with invasion of the left cavernous sinus. Twenty years previously this patient presented with a clinically nonfunctioning tumor and underwent transsphenoidal surgery for incomplete resection of a gonadotroph tumor. The patient was treated with sellar-directed radiation therapy 9 years after the pituitary surgery to treat an enlarging sellar mass. Nineteen years after her initial surgery, head imaging showed a 10 cm recurrent tumor, which was partially resected by the transcranial approach. The current MRI shows the sellar tumor regrowing. The patient also complained of back pain (see Fig. 2.27).

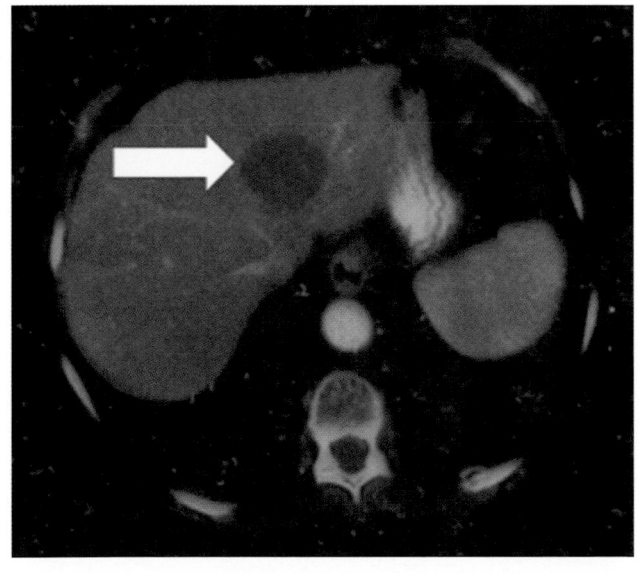

Figure 2.26 CT scan of the abdomen (axial view) of the patient described in Figure 2.24 showed a solitary 3.5-cm liver lesion (arrow), which proved to be ACTH-secreting pituitary carcinoma. The serum ACTH concentration fell to 1800 pg/mL following partial hepatectomy.

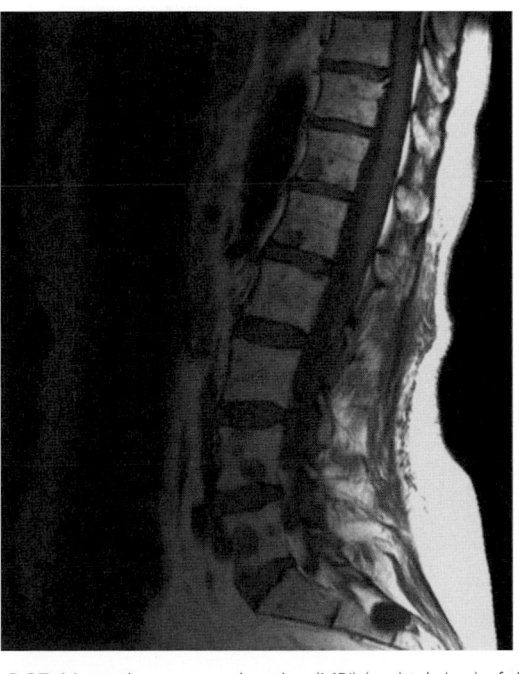

Figure 2.27 Magnetic resonance imaging (MRI) (sagittal view) of the spine from the patient in Figure 2.25 shows multiple metastases. Biopsy confirmed metastatic gonadotroph pituitary tumor.

Pituitary cyst

Definition

Pituitary cysts are defined as fluid-filled structures within the pituitary gland.

Etiology

Developmental failure of the Rathke pouch obliteration may lead to Rathke cysts, which are usually small (e.g. < 5 mm) cysts entrapped by squamous epithelium. Rathke cysts are found in about 20% of individuals at autopsy.

Signs and symptoms

Rathke cleft cysts do not usually grow and are often diagnosed incidentally on head MRI performed for other reasons (Fig. 2.28). However, some Rathke cleft cysts do enlarge and can present in adulthood with mass-effect symptoms and hyperprolactinemia due to stalk effect (Fig. 2.29). Suprasellar extension of a pituitary cyst may compress the optic chiasm (Fig. 2.30), resulting in the gradual onset of superior bitemporal quadrantopia, which may progress to complete bitemporal hemianopsia. Additional mass-effect symptoms from an enlarging pituitary cyst include diplopia (with cavernous sinus extension and oculomotor nerve compression), varying degrees of pituitary insufficiency (related to compression of the normal pituitary gland by the macroadenoma), and headaches.

Diagnosis

Imaging tests

The diagnosis of a pituitary cyst is suggested by the typical appearance on magnetic resonance imaging (MRI) (Figs 2.28–2.30). Cyst contents range from CSF-like fluid to mucoid material. Arachnoid cysts are much less common than Rathke cysts and generate an MRI image isointense with cerebrospinal fluid (Fig. 2.31).

Treatment

Treatment directed at pituitary cysts should be avoided unless they are causing vision loss due to optic chiasm compression. It is difficult to prevent pituitary cyst recurrence following surgery because the entire cyst wall must be removed – a procedure that carries a high risk of varying degrees of hypopituitarism.

Illustrations (Figs 2.28–2.31)

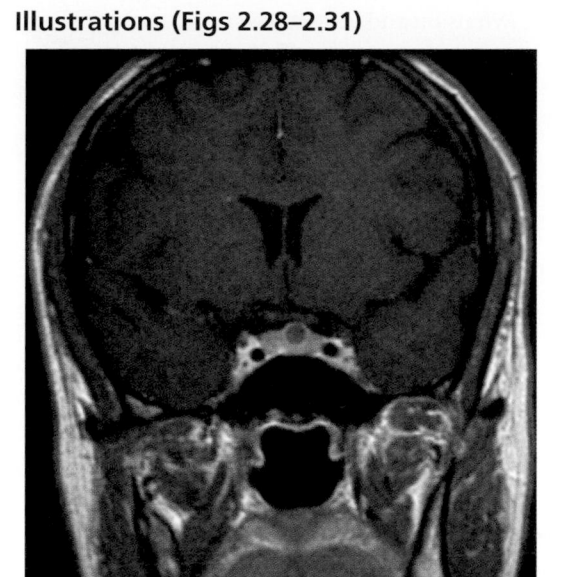

(a)

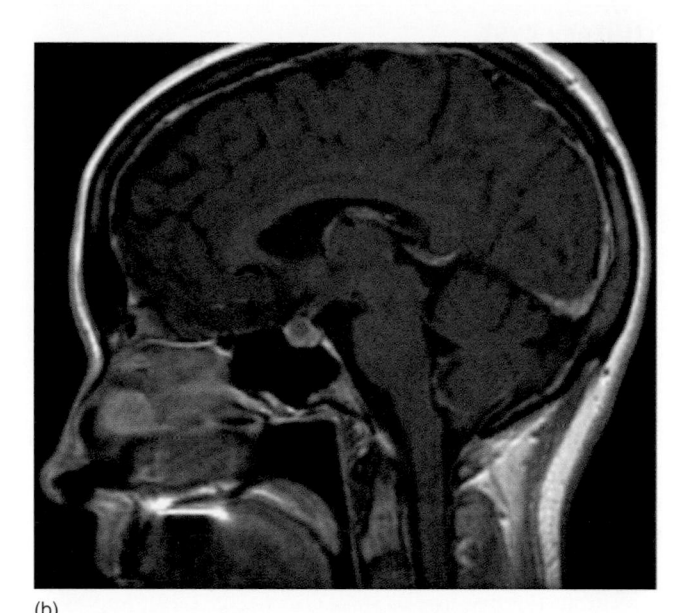

(b)

Figure 2.28 Magnetic resonance imaging (MRI) showing a 4-mm Rathke cleft cyst discovered incidentally on a scan done to investigate headaches. (a) Coronal view; (b) sagittal view.

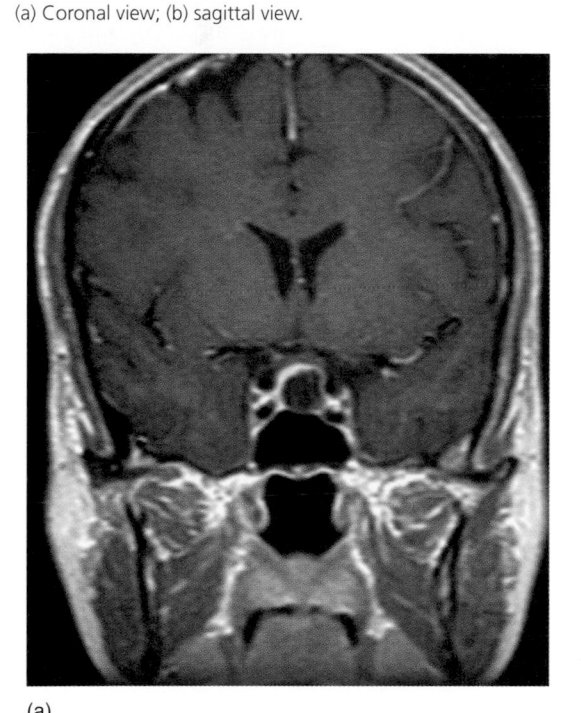

(a)

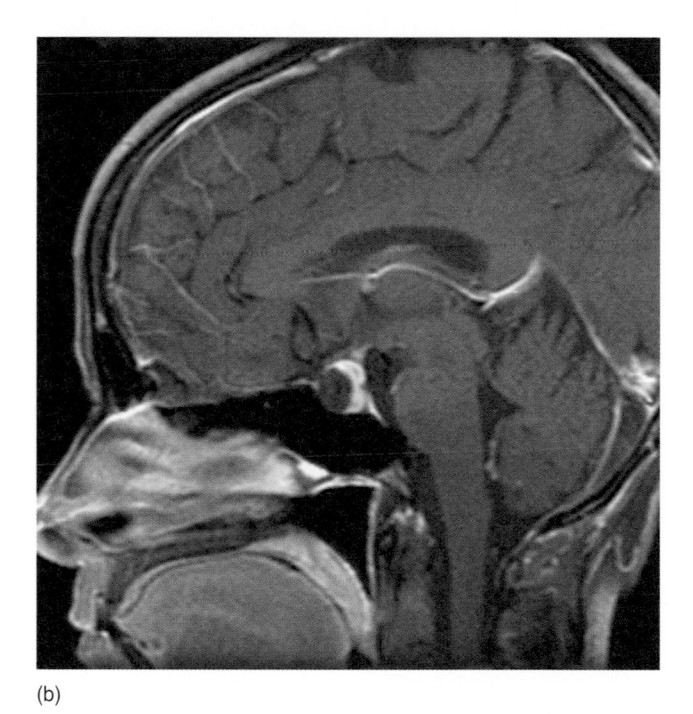

(b)

Figure 2.29 Magnetic resonance imaging (MRI) showing a 10-mm Rathke cleft cyst in the anterior aspect of the sella discovered during and evaluation of hyperprolactinemia. (a) Coronal view; (b) sagittal view.

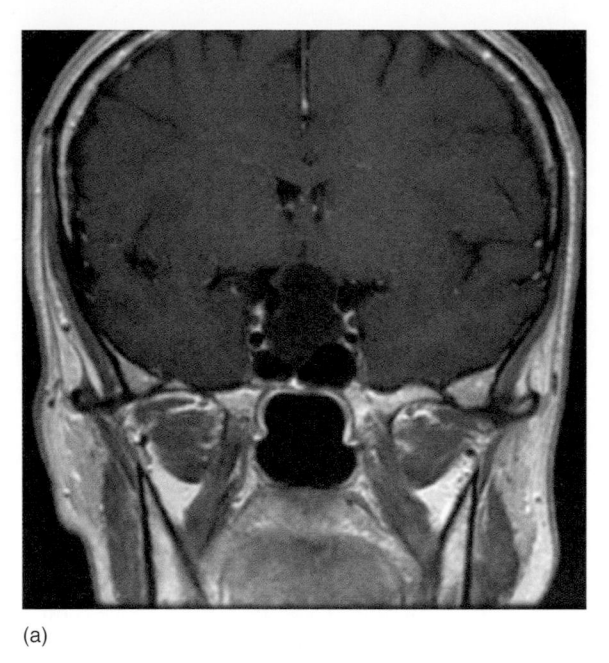
(a)

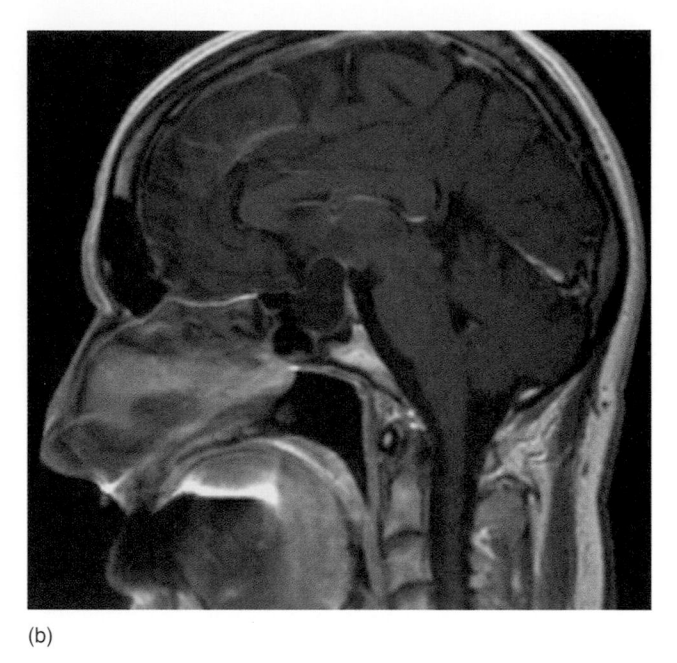
(b)

Figure 2.30 Magnetic resonance imaging (MRI) showing a large Rathke cleft cyst discovered during an evaluation for vision loss. This patient had visual field defects due to optic chiasm compression. (a) Coronal view; (b) sagittal view.

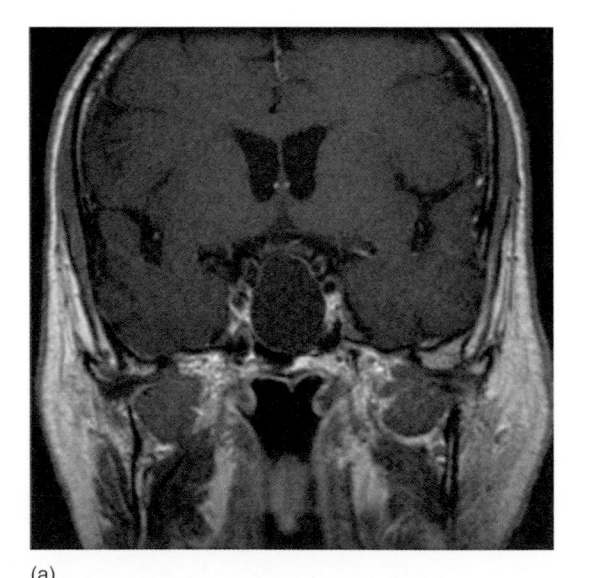
(a)

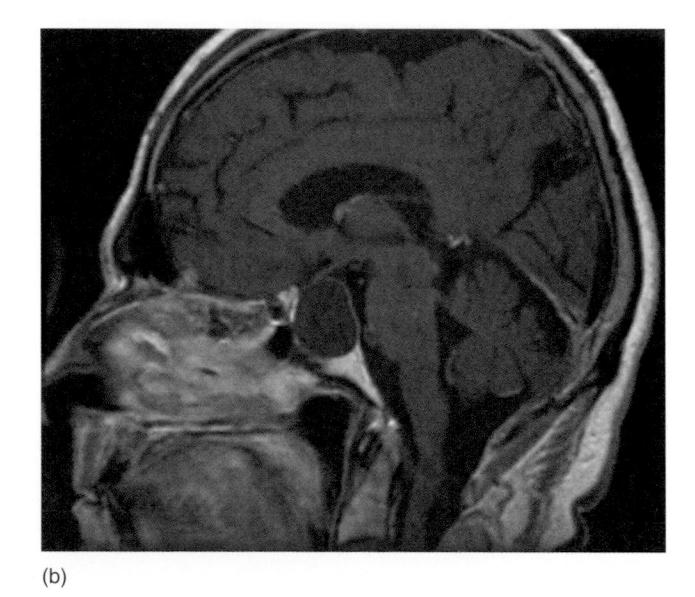
(b)

Figure 2.31 Magnetic resonance imaging (MRI) showing a large arachnoid cyst. (a) Coronal view; (b) sagittal view.

Nontumorous lesions of the pituitary gland and pituitary stalk

Definition

Nontumorous lesions of the pituitary gland include all of those disorders that are not tumors but occupy pituitary space or directly (anatomically) impact pituitary function.

Etiology

Nontumorous lesions of the pituitary gland include inflammatory disorders, head trauma with skull base fracture, iron overload states, intrasellar carotid artery aneurysm, primary empty sella, infection, mutations in genes encoding pituitary transcription factors, and developmental midline anomalies.

Signs and symptoms

Nontumorous lesions of the pituitary gland can affect pituitary function and impact surrounding structures. For example, suprasellar extension of the nontumorous process causes compression of the optic chiasm, resulting in vision loss. Additional mass-effect symptoms from an enlarging sellar mass include diplopia (with cavernous sinus extension and oculomotor nerve compression), varying degrees of pituitary insufficiency (related to compression of the normal pituitary gland by the macroadenoma), and headaches.

Lymphocytic hypophysitis (Fig. 2.32) is an autoimmune disorder characterized by lymphocytic infiltration and enlargement of the pituitary gland, pituitary stalk, and base of the hypothalamus. The most common clinical setting is in late pregnancy or in the postpartum period. Patients typically present with headaches and signs and symptoms of deficiency of one or more pituitary hormones.

Granulomatous hypophysitis can be caused by sarcoidosis, tuberculosis, Langerhans cell histiocytosis (Fig. 2.33), or Wegener's granulomatosis. The granulomatous inflammation can involve the hypothalamus, pituitary stalk, and pituitary gland and cause hypopituitarism, including diabetes insipidus.

Head trauma that results in a skull base fracture can cause hypothalamic hormone deficiencies, resulting in deficient secretion of anterior and posterior pituitary hormones.

Iron overload states of hemochromatosis and hemosiderosis of thalassemia may involve the pituitary, resulting in iron deposition (siderosis) in pituitary cells. Iron overload most commonly results in selective gonadotropin deficiency.

The term *empty sella* refers to an enlarged sella turcica that is not filled with pituitary tissue (Fig. 2.34). In a primary empty sella, a defect in the sellar diaphragm allows cerebrospinal fluid to enter and enlarge the sella. With a primary empty sella, pituitary function is usually intact. On magnetic resonance imaging (MRI), demonstrable pituitary tissue is usually compressed against the sellar floor (Fig. 2.34).

Hypopituitarism is also associated with mutations in genes that encode the transcription factors whose expression is necessary for the differentiation of anterior pituitary cells. Mutations in *PROP1* are the most common cause of familial and sporadic congenital hypopituitarism.

Diagnosis

The diagnosis of nontumorous sellar lesion is usually suggested by findings on MRI (Figs 2.32–2.34). Laboratory findings vary from intact pituitary function to panhypopituitarism.

Treatment

Many of these nontumorous lesions require no direct therapy. For example, lymphocytic hypophysitis usually runs a self-limited course and surgery is not needed. Granulomatous hypophysitis may require a course of corticosteroids. Typically the treatment for patients with nontumorous sellar lesions relates to hormone replacement for hypopituitarism.

Illustrations (Figs 2.32–2.34)

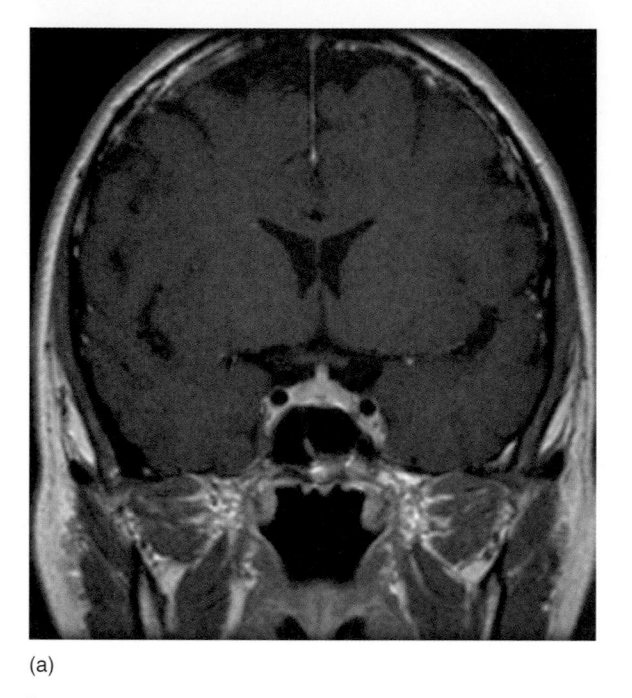

(a)

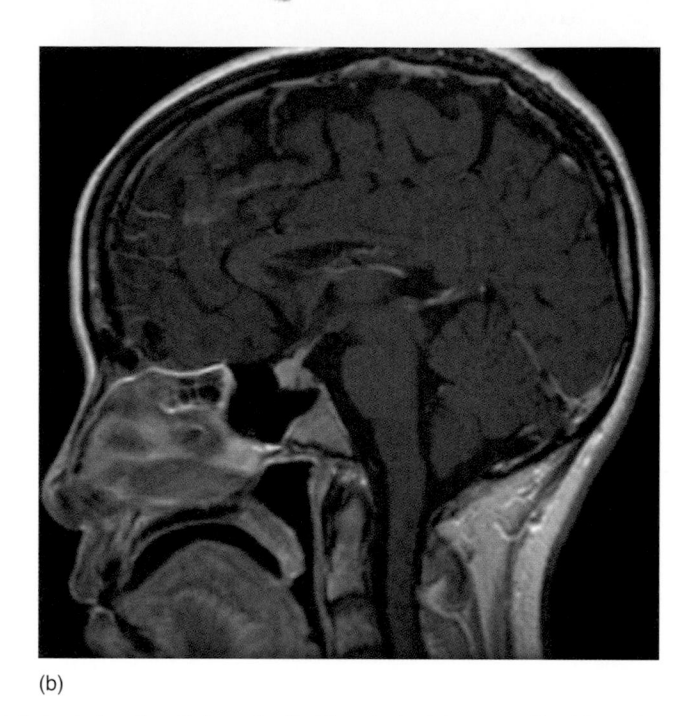

(b)

Figure 2.32 Magnetic resonance imaging (MRI) showing a thick pituitary stalk due to lymphocytic hypophysitis. There is also inhomogeneity of the sellar contents due to lymphocytic involvement of the anterior pituitary gland. (a) Coronal view; (b) sagittal view.

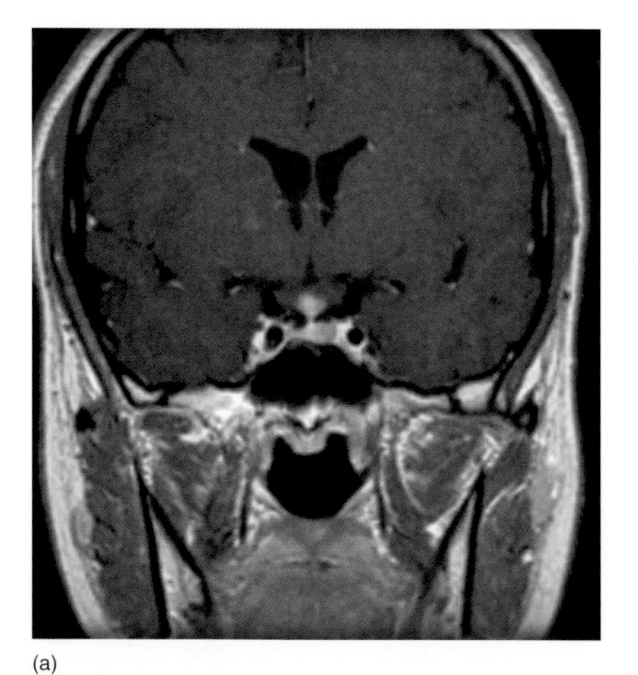

(a)

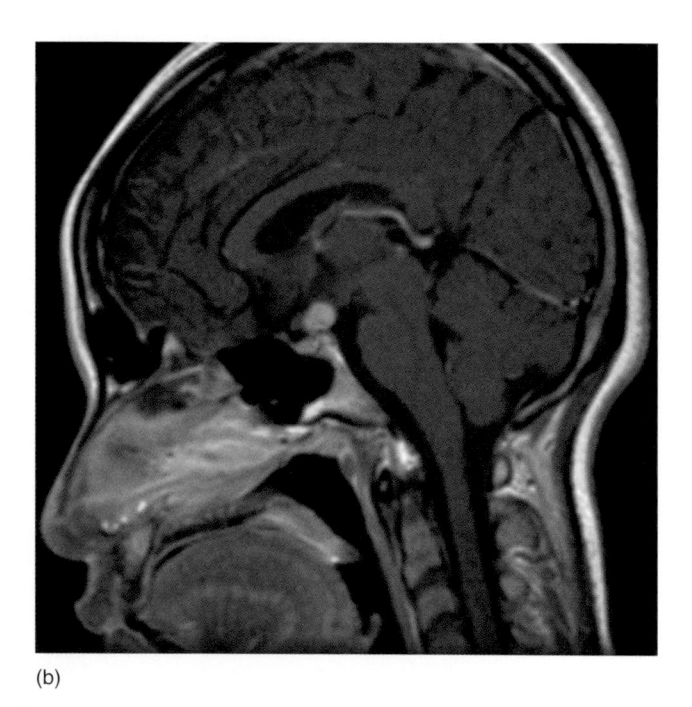

(b)

Figure 2.33 Magnetic resonance imaging (MRI) showing an enhancing hypothalamic mass with left sellar involvement due to Langerhans cell histiocytosis. (a) Coronal view; (b) sagittal view.

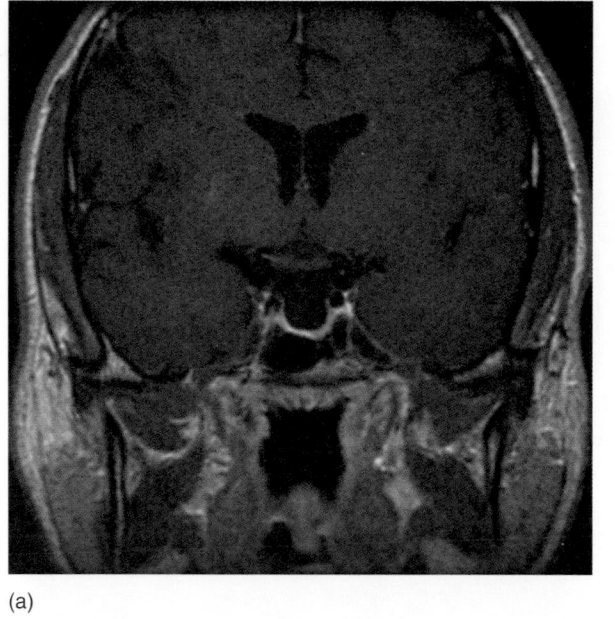
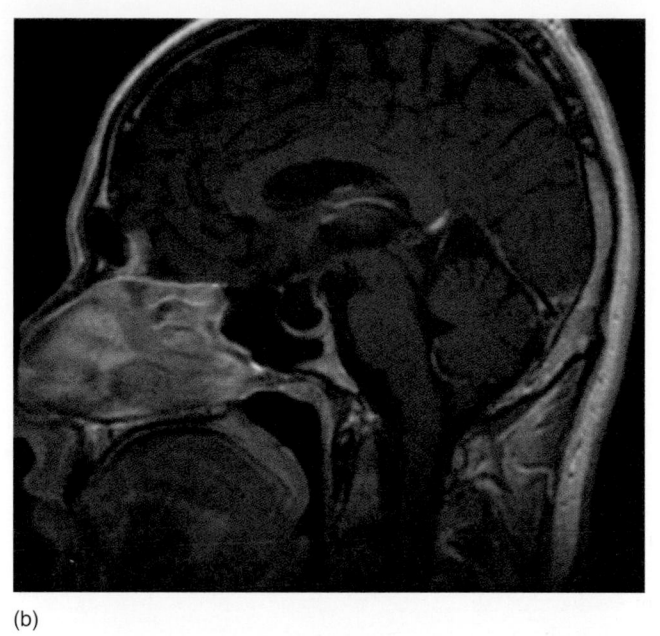

(a) (b)

Figure 2.34 Magnetic resonance imaging (MRI) showing a primary empty sella with the normal pituitary gland compressed inferiorly and posteriorly. (a) Coronal view; (b) sagittal view.

Pituitary apoplexy

Definition

Pituitary apoplexy is the acute hemorrhage of the pituitary gland, typically related to an underlying pituitary adenoma.

Etiology

Pituitary apoplexy occurs most often in the setting of a pre-existing pituitary macroadenoma or cyst, and the hemorrhage may be spontaneous or triggered by head trauma, coagulation disorders (e.g. idiopathic thrombocytopenic purpura), or anticoagulant (e.g. heparin, warfarin) administration. In addition, pituitary tumor apoplexy may be induced by the administration of a hypothalamic-releasing hormone (e.g. gonadotropin-releasing hormone agonist in a patient with a gonadotropin-secreting adenoma) or by the administration of an agent used to treat the pituitary tumor (e.g. bromocriptine for a prolactin-secreting pituitary tumor). In more than half the cases of pituitary apoplexy, the apoplectic event is the initial clinical presentation of a pituitary tumor. It is important to note that necrosis and hemorrhage within a pituitary tumor occur much more frequently than the clinical syndrome of pituitary apoplexy – especially in silent corticotroph adenomas, where hemorrhage occurs in more than 50% of the tumors. Overall, hemorrhage occurs in 10–15% of pituitary adenomas, and it is usually clinically silent.

Signs and symptoms

The typical presentation of pituitary apoplexy is acute onset of severe headache, vision loss, facial pain, nausea and vomiting, or ocular nerve palsies caused by impingement of the third, fourth, and sixth cranial nerves in the cavernous sinuses. In addition, patients may have signs of meningeal irritation and an altered level of consciousness. The most immediate hormonal deficiency is secondary adrenal insufficiency, which may lead to hypotension and adrenal crisis.

Diagnosis

Pituitary imaging with magnetic resonance imaging (MRI) is diagnostic and typically shows signs of intrapituitary or intra-adenoma hemorrhage (Fig. 2.35), fluid–fluid level (Fig. 2.36), and compression of normal pituitary tissue. Hormonal evaluation typically shows complete anterior pituitary failure. Because of the anatomy of the pituitary circulation and the sparing of the infundibular circulation the posterior pituitary is usually spared and diabetes insipidus is rare in patients with pituitary apoplexy.

Treatment

Pituitary apoplexy is an endocrine emergency and prompt diagnosis and treatment are critical. The clinical course of pituitary apoplexy varies widely in duration and severity. Treatment is aimed at alleviating or relieving local compression that compromises adjacent structures such as the optic chiasm. In addition, the endocrine status of the patient must be considered and treated accordingly. Neurosurgical intervention is often the most rapid and effective method of decompressing the sella turcica and the surrounding structures and is indicated in the event of mental status changes and other symptoms attributable to increased intracranial pressure.

In patients with normal visual fields who lack cranial nerve palsies, observation is a reasonable treatment approach – the hemorrhage typically is reabsorbed and total mass size regresses (Fig. 2.37). Stress dosages of glucocorticoids should be initiated in all patients with pituitary apoplexy. Pituitary function does not usually recover, and long-term pituitary target gland hormone replacement therapy is needed.

Illustrations (Figs 2.35–2.37)

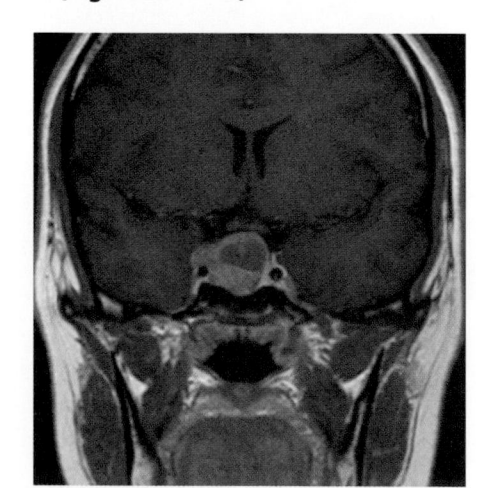

(a) (b)

Figure 2.35 Magnetic resonance imaging (MRI) showing an area of cystic hemorrhage in the superior aspect of this pituitary macroadenoma, which extends into the right cavernous sinus. (a) Coronal view; (b) sagittal view.

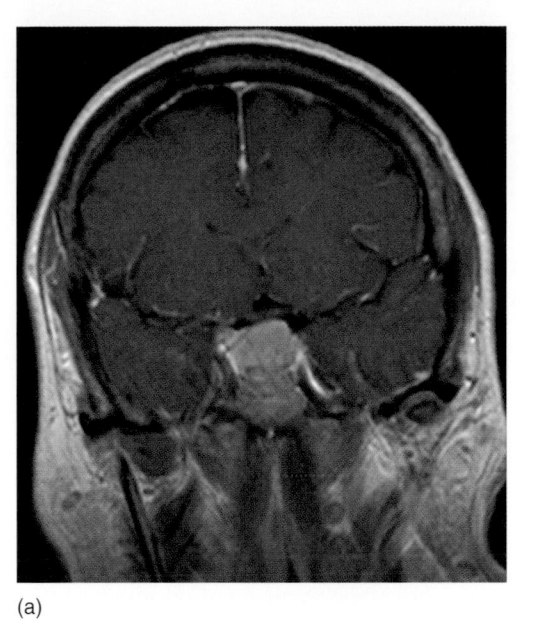

(a)

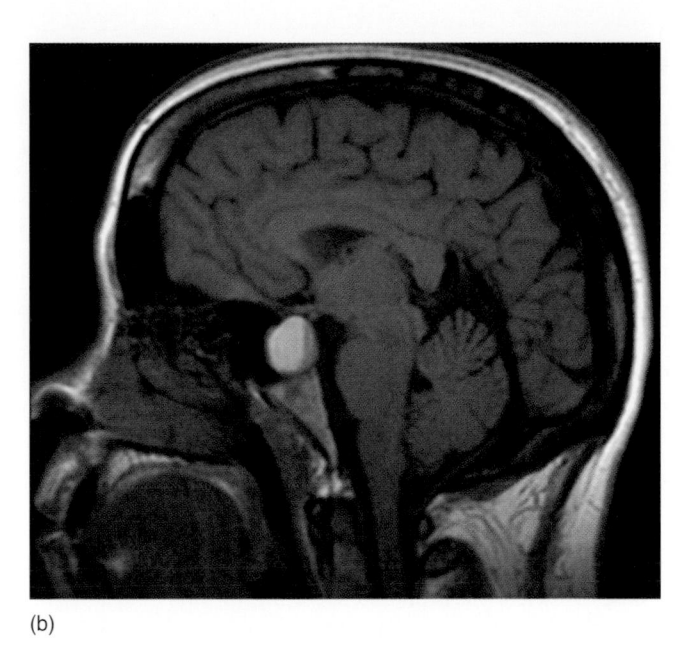

(b)

Figure 2.36 Magnetic resonance imaging (MRI) showing hemorrhage completely replacing the pituitary macroadenoma. (a) Coronal view; (b) sagittal view. Note fluid–fluid level on sagittal view (b).

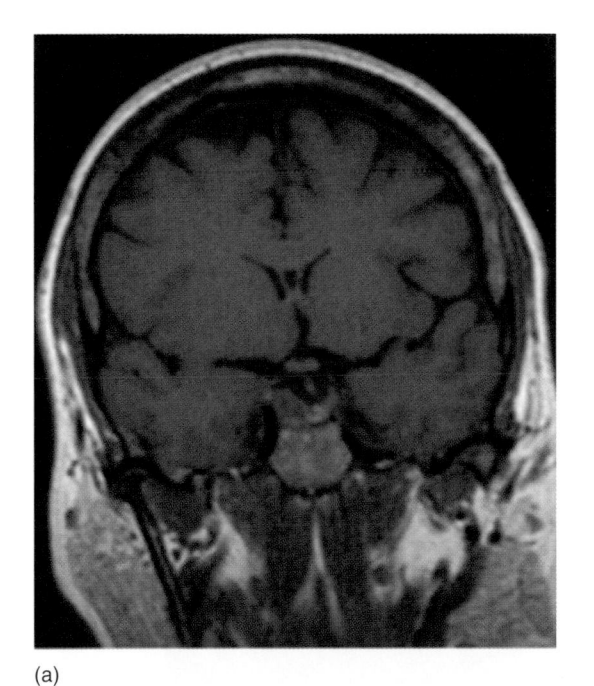

(a)

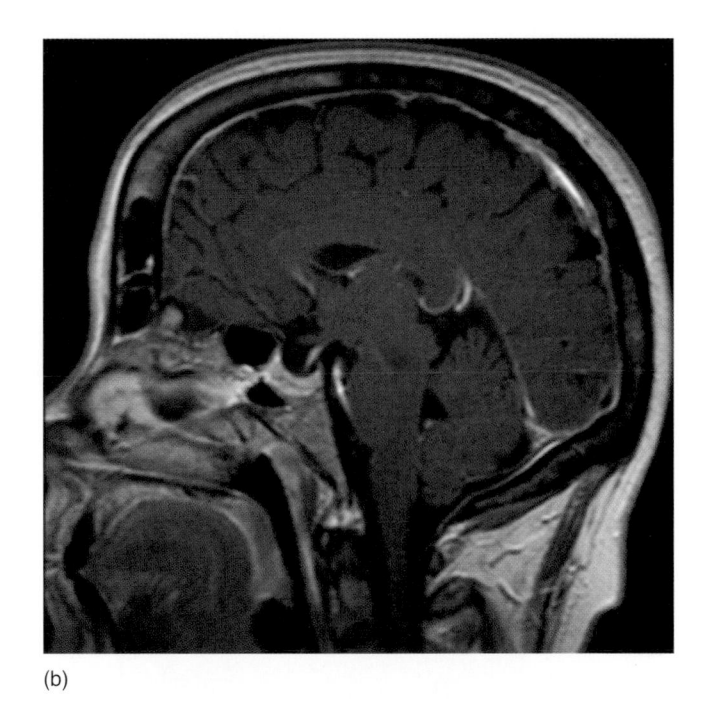

(b)

Figure 2.37 Magnetic resonance imaging (MRI) 9 months later of the patient from Figure 2.36. The hemorrhage has resolved and residual pituitary tumor can be seen on the right side of the sella. (a) Coronal view; (b) sagittal view.

Tumors metastatic to the pituitary

Definition
A tumor metastatic to the pituitary gland occurs when there is spread of a malignant tumor from elsewhere in the body (e.g. breast, lung, kidney).

Etiology
When the pituitary gland of patients with cancer is examined at autopsy, pituitary metastases are found in about 3.5%. Most metastases to the pituitary are clinically silent and may be too small to be detected on computed imaging. The most common organ locations for the primary malignancy (in order of frequency) are: breast, lung, kidney, colon, skin (melanoma), prostate, thyroid, stomach, pancreas, nasopharynx, lymphoma, uterine, and liver. Breast and lung cancer account for most metastases to the pituitary. The routes by which metastases reach the pituitary include: hematogenous spread; spread from a hypothalamo–hypophyseal metastasis though the portal vessels; direct extension from parasellar sites or skull base; or meningeal spread from the suprasellar cistern. Most metastases involve the posterior lobe – presumably because of its direct arterial blood supply from the hypophyseal arteries. Since the anterior lobe does not have a direct arterial supply, metastases that involve the anterior lobe are usually due to direct extension from the posterior lobe nidus.

Signs and symptoms
The most common clinical presentations of pituitary metastases are diabetes insipidus, visual impairment, headaches, cranial nerve deficits, and varying degrees of hypopituitarism. In approximately 80% of cases, the pituitary metastasis is discovered after or concurrent with the primary malignancy – the average interval is 3 years. Since diabetes insipidus is a very unusual (< 1%) component of the presentation of benign pituitary adenomas, sellar metastasis should be highly suspect when patients present with diabetes insipidus and a rapidly growing pituitary mass.

Diagnosis
A pituitary metastasis may closely mimic pituitary adenoma – the clinical presentation and the neuroimaging and endocrinologic data usually suggest a nonfunctioning pituitary adenoma. Magnetic resonance imaging (MRI) may show lesions that involve the pituitary and hypothalamic area (Fig. 2.38) or the metastasis may be limited to the sella (Fig. 2.39). Thus, metastatic disease should always be considered in the differential diagnosis of a pituitary mass. Tissue diagnosis is required to confirm metastatic disease.

Treatment
Metastatic disease to the pituitary is a poor prognostic sign; the 1-year mortality is 70%. Because of the poor prognosis associated with sellar metastases, the most reasonable therapeutic approaches are palliative radiotherapy, pituitary target hormone replacement therapy when indicated, and primary tumor-directed chemotherapy. Total resection is usually not possible because metastases are usually diffuse, invasive, vascular, and hemorrhagic. Surgical debulking of the sellar metastasis may be beneficial in patients with visual field defects caused by compression of the optic chiasm.

Illustrations (Figs 2.38 & 2.39)

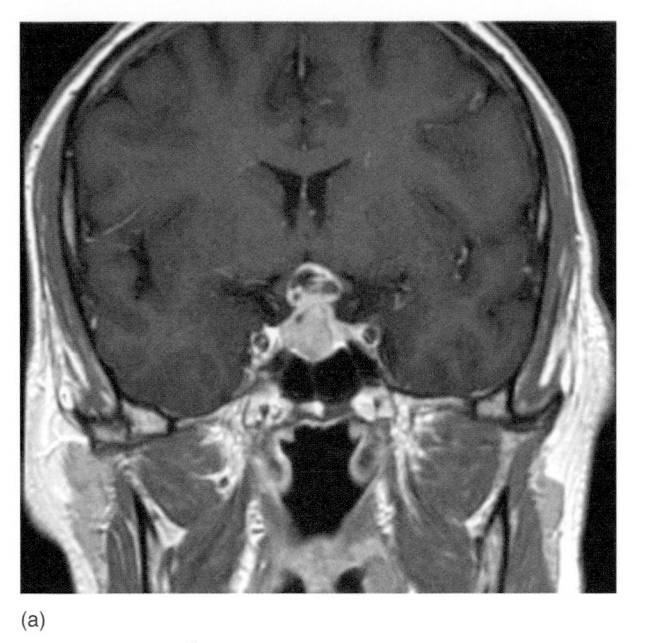

(a)

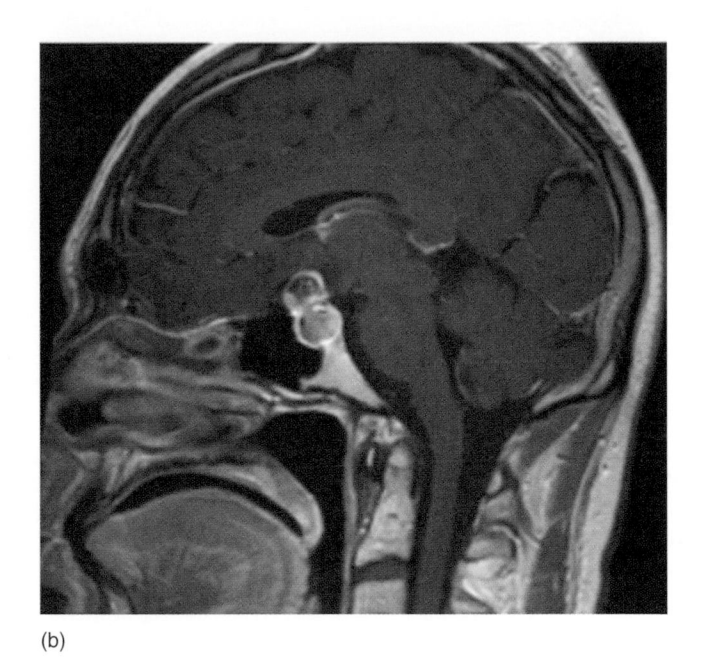

(b)

Figure 2.38 Magnetic resonance imaging (MRI) showing an inhomogenous mass with suprasellar extension. This lesion is metastatic disease from an adenoid cystic carcinoma from a submandibular gland. (a) Coronal view; (b) sagittal view.

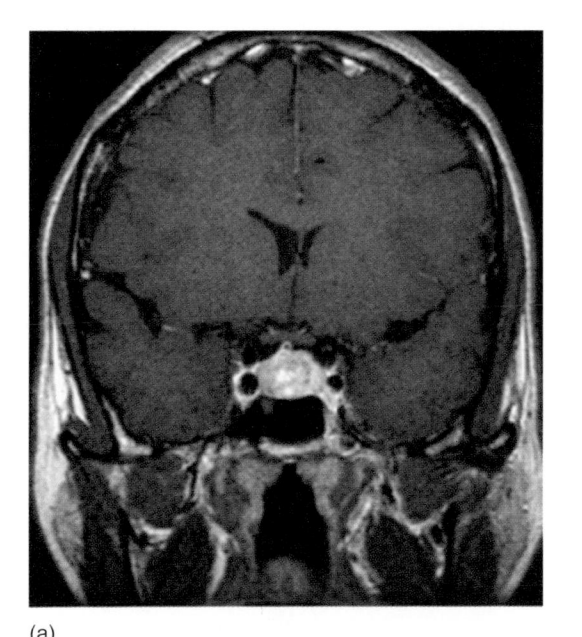

(a)

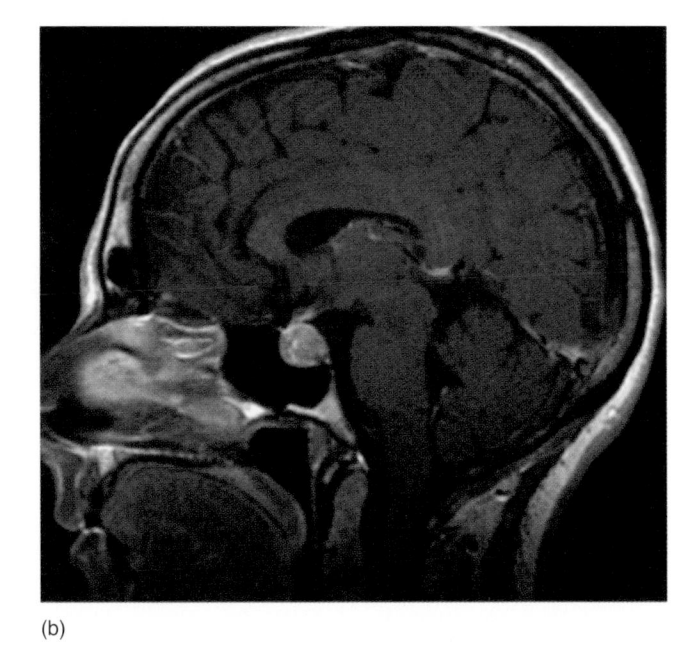

(b)

Figure 2.39 Magnetic resonance imaging (MRI) showing an intrasellar tumor caused by a metastatic carcinoid tumor. The patient presented with diabetes insipidus and this was the clue that the tumor might represent metastatic disease. (a) Coronal view; (b) sagittal view.

Adrenal Gland

Adrenal incidentaloma

Definition

An adrenal incidentaloma is an adrenal mass > 1 cm in diameter, serendipitously discovered by radiologic examination in patients without adrenal-related symptomatology.

Etiology

Adrenal incidentalomas are a product of technological advances in imaging – computed tomography (CT) and magnetic resonance imaging (MRI). The prevalence of adrenal incidentalomas on abdominal CT is approximately 4% and this percentage increases with age. The prevalence of primary malignancy in patients with adrenal incidentalomas is approximately 2–5% and in metastatic malignancy is approximately 1%. Bilateral adrenal masses are found in 10–15% of adrenal incidentaloma cases and raise the possibilities of metastatic disease, congenital adrenal hyperplasia, cortical adenomas, infection (e.g. tuberculosis, fungal), hemorrhage, Cushing syndrome, pheochromocytoma, and infiltrative disease of the adrenal glands.

Signs and symptoms

Because the definition of an adrenal incidentaloma includes patients without adrenal-related symptomatology, most patients are asymptomatic. However, some adrenal incidentaloma patients may have signs and symptoms of glucocorticoid secretory autonomy detected with a careful interview and examination.

Diagnosis

Laboratory findings

Although most adrenal incidentalomas are nonfunctional, 10–15% secrete excess cortical or medullary hormones. Appropriate case-detection tests should be performed if the patient has clinical features that are suggestive of increased adrenal function. However, subclinical Cushing syndrome and pheochromocytoma are sufficiently common in the clinical setting of incidentally discovered adrenal masses that all of these patients should be tested for these disorders. In addition, hypertensive patients should be evaluated for an aldosteronoma even if the serum potassium concentration is normal.

Imaging tests

On CT scanning, the density of the image is attributed to X-ray attenuation. The intracytoplasmic fat in adenomas results in low attenuation on nonenhanced CT (Fig. 3.1); nonadenomas have higher attenuation in nonenhanced CT (Fig. 3.2). The Hounsfield scale is a semiquantitative method of measuring X-ray attenuation. Typical precontrast Hounsfield unit (HU) values are adipose tissue = –20 to –150 HU and kidney = 20 to 150 HU. If an adrenal mass measures < 10 HU on unenhanced CT (i.e. has the density of fat), the likelihood that it is a benign adenoma is nearly 100%. On delayed contrast-enhanced CT, adenomas typically show rapid contrast medium washout (> 50% at 10 min), whereas nonadenomas have delayed contrast material washout.

Pheochromocytomas have increased attenuation on nonenhanced CT (> 20 HU), increased vascularity, cystic and hemorrhage changes, delay in contrast medium washout, and high signal intensity on T-2 weighted MRI. Adrenocortical carcinoma can appear very similar to pheochromocytoma on CT, but tend to be larger, have an irregular shape, and tumor calcification. Adrenal cysts (Fig. 3.3), adrenal hemorrhage, and myelolipoma (Fig. 3.4) have distinctive imaging characteristics.

Treatment

All patients with documented pheochromocytoma and adrenocortical cancer should undergo prompt surgical intervention. Patients with aldosterone-producing adenomas should be offered surgery to cure aldosterone excess. Patients with documented subclinical Cushing syndrome

Imaging in Endocrinology, First Edition. Paolo Pozzilli, Andrea Lenzi, Bart L Clarke and William F Young Jr.
© 2014 John Wiley & Sons, Ltd. Published 2014 by John Wiley & Sons, Ltd.

should be considered for surgery. Adrenal masses with either suspicious imaging phenotype or size larger than 4 cm should be considered for resection because a substantial fraction will be adrenocortical carcinomas.

Illustrations (Figs 3.1–3.4)

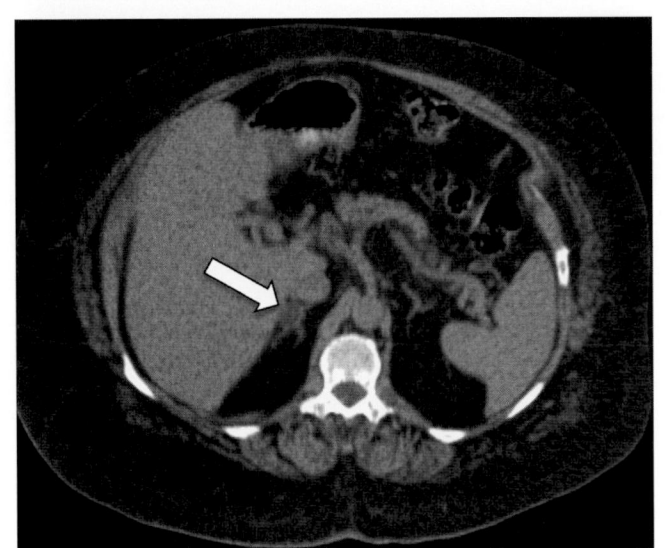

(a)

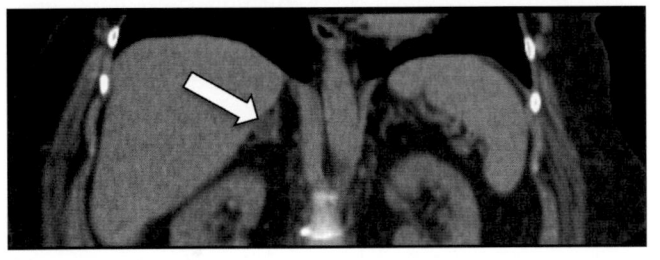

(b)

Figure 3.1 Computed tomography (CT) showing a 1 cm homogenous and hypodense right adrenal cortical adenoma (arrows). The nonenhanced CT showed a density of < 10 HU and there was more than 50% contrast washout at 10 minutes. (a) Axial view; (b) coronal view.

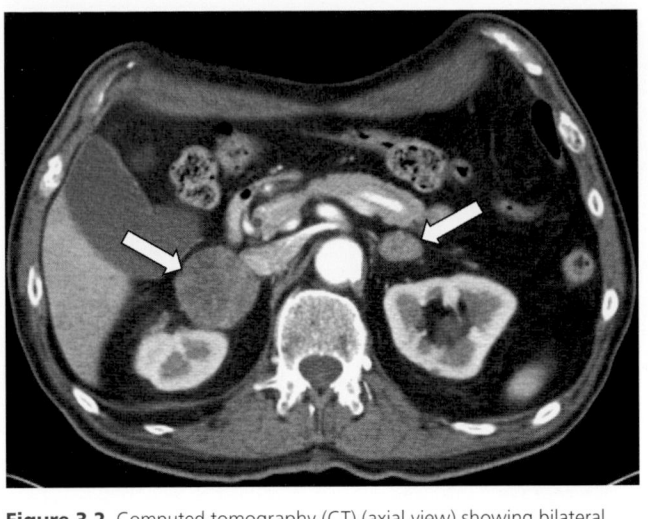

Figure 3.2 Computed tomography (CT) (axial view) showing bilateral dense and peripherally enhancing adrenal masses due to metastatic disease in a patient with small cell lung cancer. The right adrenal mass measures 4.6 × 4.5 × 5.2 cm (arrow) and the left adrenal mass measures 1.8 × 2.2 × 2.0 cm (arrow). The nonenhanced CT showed a density of > 10 HU and there was < 50% contrast washout at 10 minutes.

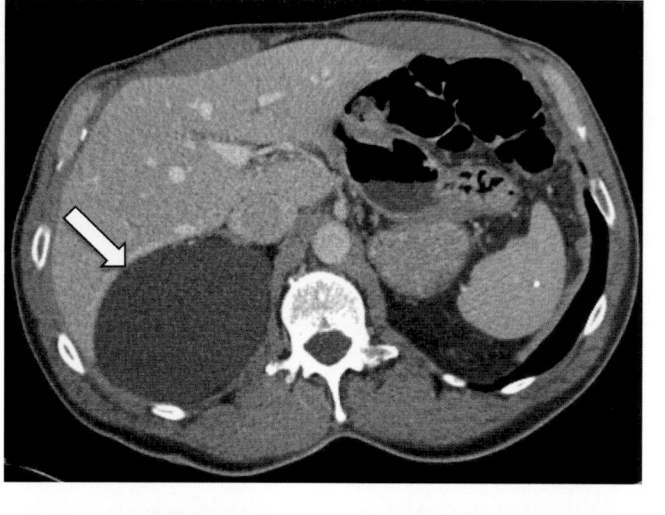

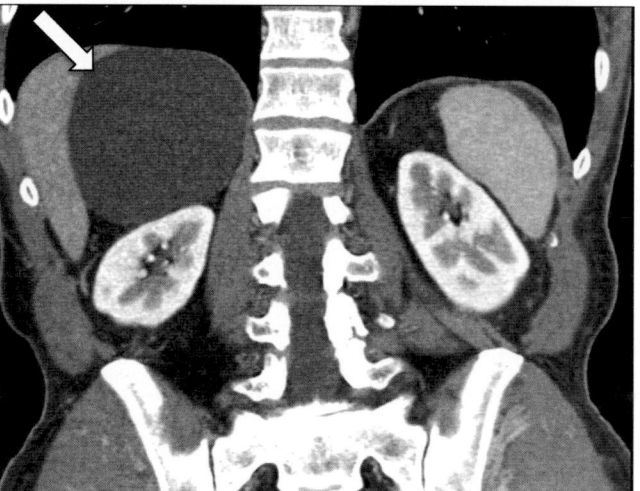

Figure 3.3 Computed tomography (CT) showing a 10 × 8.5 × 8.5 cm homogenous and hypodense right adrenal cyst (arrows). (top) Axial view; (bottom) coronal view.

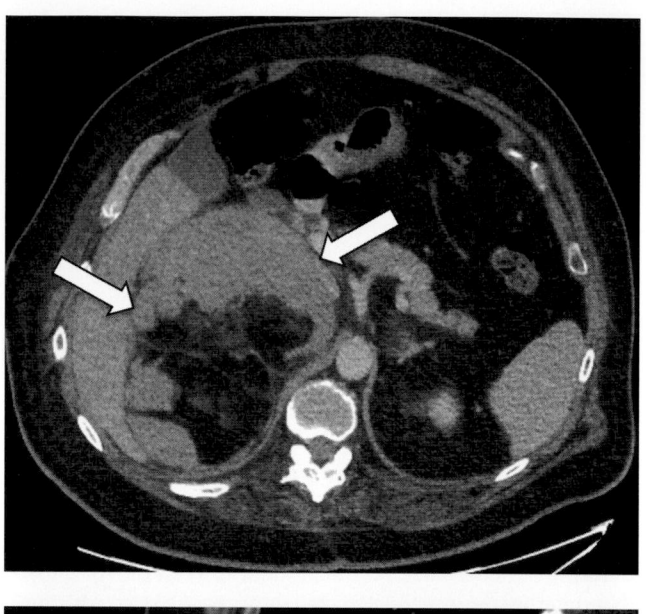

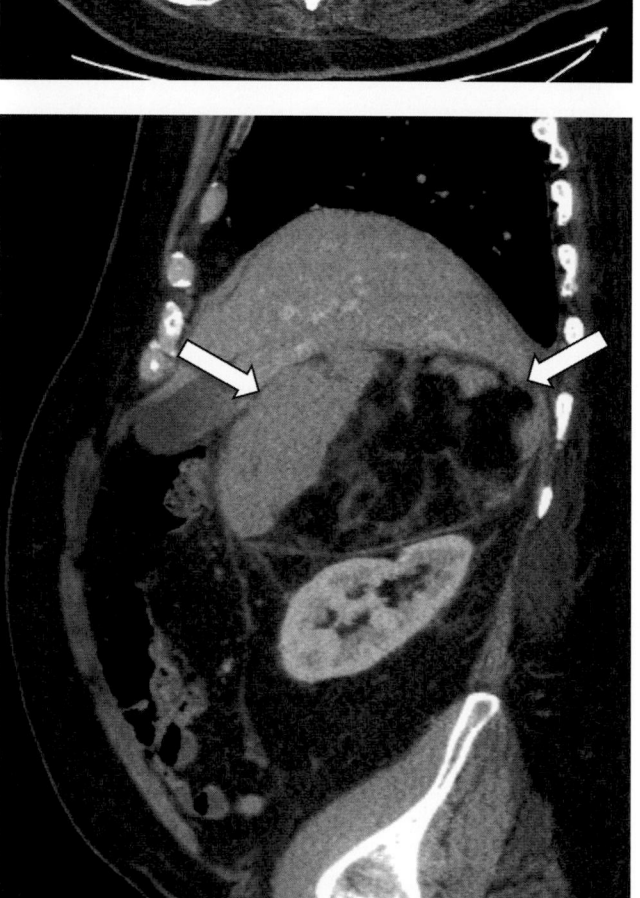

Figure 3.4 Computed tomography (CT) shows an 19 × 14 × 14 cm mixed signal intensity right adrenal mass (arrow) with large amounts of macroscopic fat consistent with adrenal myelolipoma. (top) Axial view; (bottom) coronal view.

Adrenocortical carcinoma

Definition

Adrenocortical carcinoma (ACC) is a rare cortical neoplasm that may hypersecrete cortical hormones (e.g. glucocorticoids, gonadal steroids, or mineralocorticoids) or may be biochemically nonfunctional.

Etiology

Adrenocortical carcinoma is rare with an annual incidence of 2 per million people; peak ages are < 5 years and 30–50 years. Men are more likely to have nonfunctional ACC. Although most ACCs are sporadic, they can be associated with Li–Fraumeni syndrome (breast cancer, sarcoma, brain tumors, and ACC caused by inactivating mutations of the *TP53* tumor suppressor gene) and Beckwith–Wiedemann syndrome (neuroblastoma, hepatoblastoma, and ACC associated with abnormalities on chromosome 11p15). Although the molecular basis for sporadic ACC is unclear, a unique germline *TP53* mutation (*R337H*) has been identified in more than 90% of children with ACC in Southern Brazil.

Signs and symptoms

Approximately 60% of ACCs hypersecrete adrenocortical hormones – most commonly glucocorticoids, followed by adrenal androgens. Thus, the clinical presentation in patients with functional ACC is usually that of Cushing syndrome or virilization in women. Estrogen and aldosterone hypersecretion affect < 10% of patients with ACC. The clinical presentation may be dominated by mass-effect symptoms (e.g. flank pain, inferior vena cava obstruction). Also, patients with ACC may present as an incidentally discovered adrenal mass.

Diagnosis

Laboratory findings

The hormonal evaluation of patients with suspected ACC should include testing for pheochromocytoma (e.g. 24 h urinary fractionated metanephrines and catecholamines), Cushing syndrome (e.g. 24 h urine cortisol and 1 mg overnight dexamethasone suppression test), and androgen excess (e.g. dehydroepiandrosterone sulfate [DHEA-S] and testosterone). Additional testing should be obtained if there is clinical suspicion for aldosterone or estrogen hypersecretion.

Imaging tests

The imaging phenotype is key to suspecting that an adrenal mass may be ACC. Adrenocortical carcinomas are large irregularly shaped adrenal masses (e.g. > 5 cm in diameter) that have increased attenuation on nonenhanced computed tomography (CT) (> 20 HU), increased vascularity, cystic and hemorrhagic changes, and delay in contrast medium washout (Fig. 3.5). If obtained, positron emission tomography (PET) scanning with ^{18}F-fluorodeoxyglucose (FDG) typically shows high uptake in the ACC and may also show associated metastatic disease (Fig. 3.6). The most common sites of metastatic disease include the lungs (Fig. 3.7), liver, lymph nodes, and bone. The gross pathology typically shows a large brown to yellow tumor with hemorrhagic areas (Fig. 3.8). The pathologic confirmation of ACC includes distant metastasis or local tumor invasion. For adrenal-limited ACC, the Weiss histopathologic criteria are used and they include: > 6 mitoses/50 high power fields, ≤ 25% clear tumor cells in cytoplasm, abnormal mitoses, necrosis, and capsular invasion.

Treatment

The optimal treatment is complete surgical resection. However, this may not be possible due to local invasion or distant metastases. Due to the poor 5-year survival rates (see below) adjuvant therapy with mitotane is considered in those patients with apparent complete surgical resections. Combination chemotherapy with etoposide, dacarbazine, and cisplatin (EDP) is considered in those patients with unresectable disease. The stage of ACC correlates with prognosis:
- Stage I ACCs are found in about 5% of patients and are ≤ 5 cm in diameter and confined to the adrenal gland without local invasion or distant metastases. The 5-year survival rate is approximately 80%.
- Stage II ACCs are found in about 45% of patients and are > 5 cm in diameter and confined to the adrenal gland without local invasion or distant metastases. The 5-year survival rate is approximately 60%.
- Stage III ACCs are found in about 15% of patients and the tumor is of any size with at least one of the following factors: tumor infiltration in surrounding tissues; tumor invasion into tumor thrombus in the vena cava or renal vein; positive lymph nodes. But no distant metastases. The 5-year survival rate is approximately 50%.
- Stage IV ACCs are found in about 35% of patients and is defined by distant metastases. The 5-year survival rate is approximately 10%.

Illustrations (Figs 3.5–3.8)

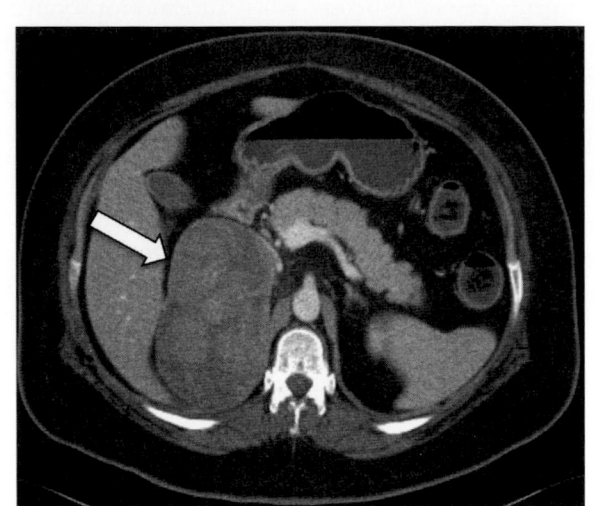

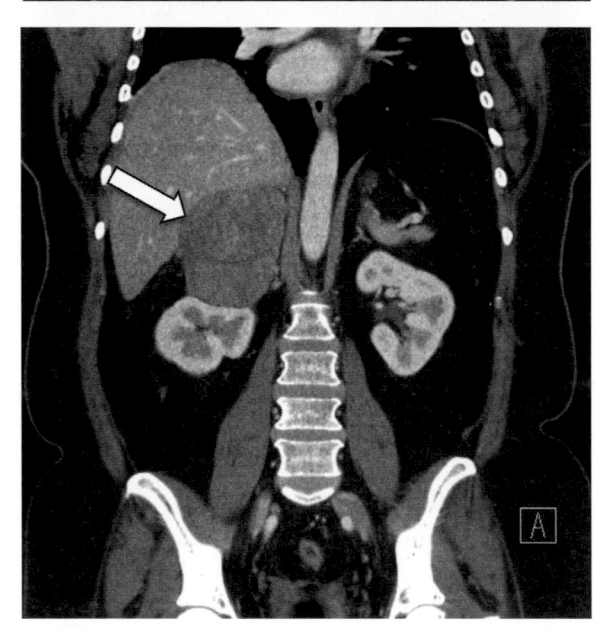

Figure 3.5 Computed tomography (CT) showing a 13 × 7 × 10-cm inhomogenous right adrenal cortical carcinoma (arrows) in a 42-year-old woman with Cushing syndrome. (top) Axial view; (bottom) coronal view.

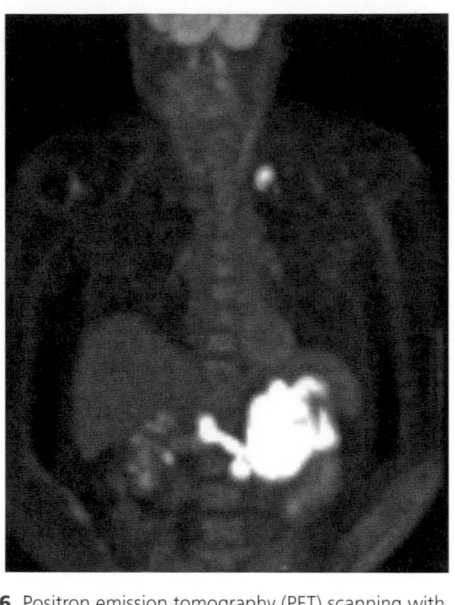

Figure 3.6 Positron emission tomography (PET) scanning with ^{18}F-fluorodeoxyglucose (FDG) (coronal view) shows a 10 × 10 cm intensely hypermetabolic left adrenocortical carcinoma with tumor thrombus extending into the left renal vein and infrahepatic inferior vena cava. Also seen is a 2 cm left apical pulmonary metastasis.

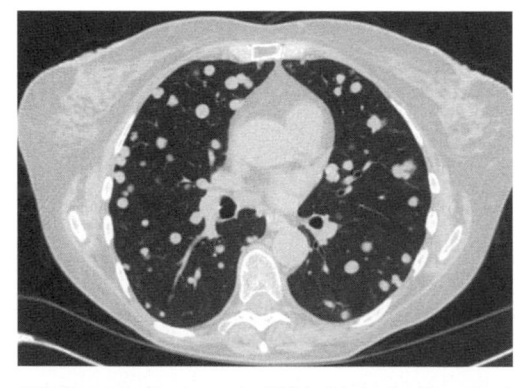

Figure 3.7 Computed tomography (CT) (axial view) with contrast enhancement showing diffuse bilateral pulmonary metastases from an adrenocortical carcinoma.

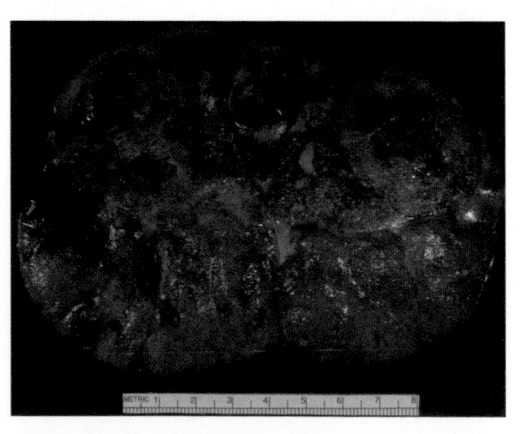

Figure 3.8 Cut section from a gross pathology specimen showing areas of necrosis and hemorrhage in this 12.5 × 8.5 cm adrenocortical carcinoma.

Adrenal-dependent Cushing syndrome

Definition
Primary adrenal hypersecretion of cortisol results in the signs and symptoms characteristic of Cushing syndrome.

Etiology
The causes of adrenal-dependent Cushing syndrome include: benign adrenal cortical adenoma, adrenocortical carcinoma, micronodular hyperplasia, and macronodular hyperplasia.

Signs and symptoms
Cushing syndrome is a symptom complex that results from prolonged exposure to supraphysiologic concentrations of glucocorticoids. Typical signs and symptoms of Cushing syndrome include weight gain with central obesity; facial rounding with fat deposition in the temporal fossae and cheeks ("moon face") and plethora; supraclavicular fat pads; dorsocervical fat pad ("buffalo hump"); easy ("spontaneous") bruising (ecchymoses); fine "cigarette paper-thin skin" that tears easily; poor wound healing; red-purple striae (usually > 1 cm in thickness located over abdomen, flanks, axilla, breasts, hips, and inner thighs); scalp hair thinning; proximal muscle weakness associated with muscle loss and resulting in thin extremities; emotional and cognitive changes (e.g. irritability, crying, depression, insomnia, restlessness); hirsutism and acne; hypertension; osteopenia and osteoporosis; renal lithiasis; glucose intolerance and diabetes mellitus; hyperlipidemia; opportunistic and fungal infections (e.g. mucocutaneous candidiasis, tinea versicolor, pityriasis); menstrual dysfunction and infertility.

Physical examination findings may provide a clue as to the cause of adrenal-dependent Cushing syndrome. For example, the finding of spotty facial pigmentation involving the vermillion borders of the lips and eyelids in a patient with Cushing syndrome is suggestive of Carney complex and primary pigmented nodular adrenal disease (PPNAD) (Fig. 3.9). Benign adrenal cortical adenomas typically secrete only cortisol and thus symptoms of androgen excess (e.g. hirsutism) are usually absent. Whereas, when adrenocortical carcinomas cause Cushing syndrome they also typical secrete excess adrenal androgens resulting in hirsutism and virilization in women.

Diagnosis

Laboratory findings
Case-detection testing should start with measurements of 24 hour urinary free cortisol (UFC), 11 PM salivary cortisol, and serum cortisol concentrations measured at 8 AM and 4 PM. The 1 mg overnight dexamethasone suppression test (DST) is an additional case-detection test. Additional confirmatory studies are not needed if the baseline 24-hour UFC excretion is > 300 μg/24 h (> 828 nmol/24 h) and the clinical picture is consistent with Cushing syndrome. A low or undetectable plasma corticotropin (adrenocorticotropic hormone [ACTH]) concentration confirms adrenal-dependent Cushing syndrome and the subtype is determined by computed adrenal imaging.

Imaging tests
Adrenal computed tomography (CT) provides optimal spatial resolution to detect and differentiate between benign adrenal adenoma (Fig. 3.10), adrenocortical carcinoma (Fig. 3.11), ACTH-independent macronodular adrenocortical hyperplasia (AIMAH) (Fig. 3.12), and PPNAD (Fig. 3.13). In patients with unilateral adrenal Cushing syndrome, the contralateral adrenal is usually atrophic appearing on CT (Fig. 3.10) and due to chronic suppression of ACTH.

Treatment
Treatment of choice for cortical adenoma and adrenocortical carcinoma is complete surgical resection of the culprit adrenal gland. Cure of Cushing syndrome due to AIMAH and PPNAD requires bilateral adrenalectomy. Primary pigmented nodular adrenal disease has a diagnostic appearance on gross pathology (Fig. 3.14).

Illustrations (Figs 3.9–3.14)

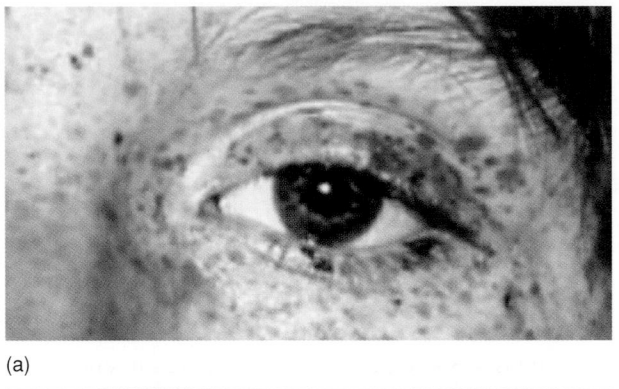

(a)

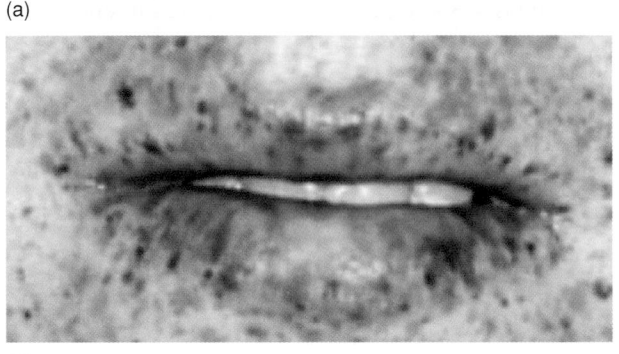

(b)

Figure 3.9 Photographs of a patients left eye (a) and lips (b) showing diffuse lentingines seen in patients with Carney complex.

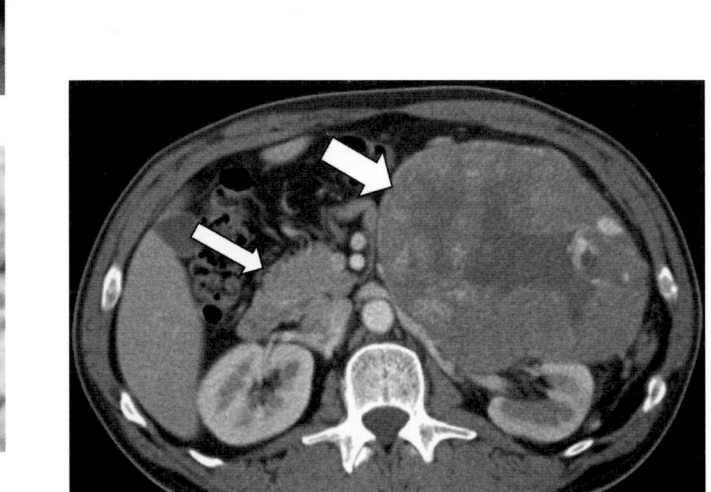

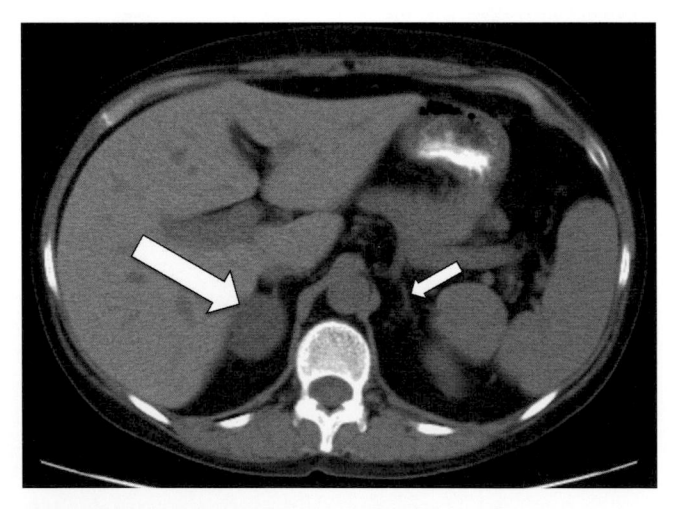

Figure 3.10 Computed tomography (CT) (axial view) shows a 3.5 × 3.0 cm cortisol-secreting right adrenal adenoma (large arrow) and an atrophic left adrenal gland (small arrow).

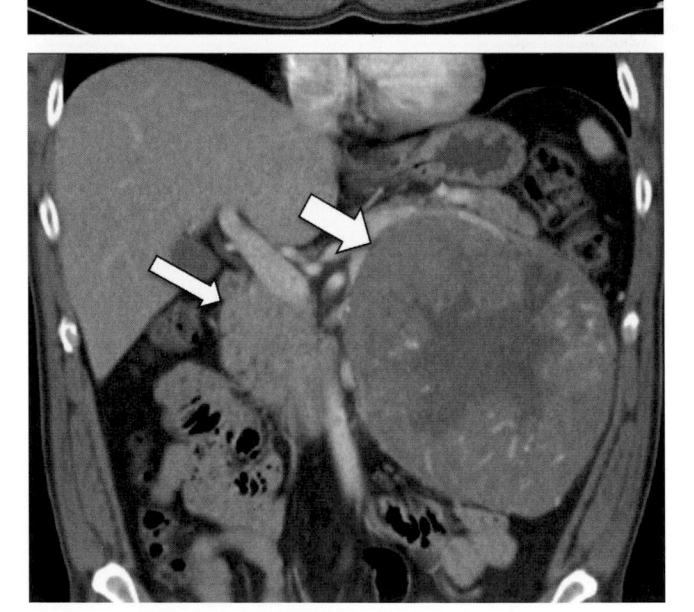

Figure 3.11 Computed tomography (CT) showing a large left adrenocortical carcinoma (large arrows) and metastatic disease (small arrows) along the inferior vena cava. (top) Axial view; (bottom) coronal view.

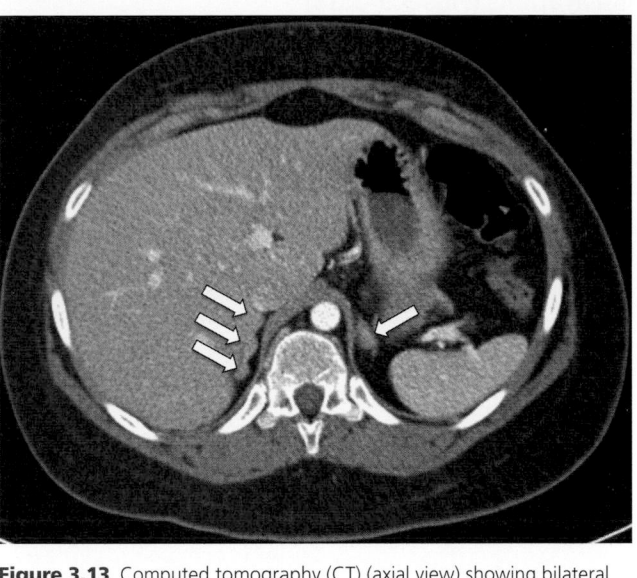

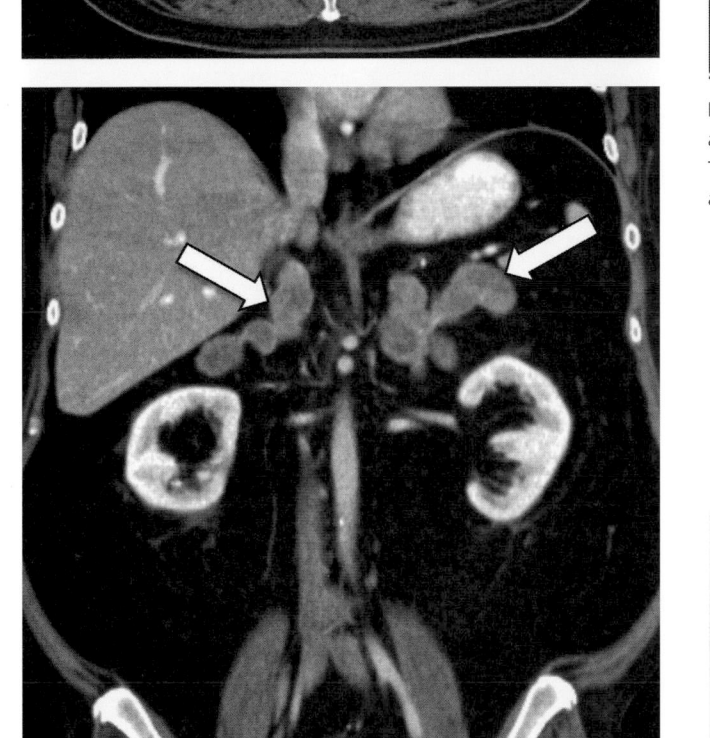

Figure 3.13 Computed tomography (CT) (axial view) showing bilateral adrenal micronodularity of primary pigmented nodular adrenal disease. Three nodules in the right adrenal gland (arrows) and one nodule in the left adrenal gland (arrow) are seen in this axial image.

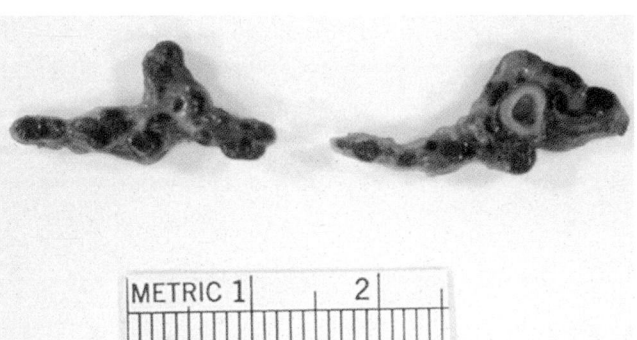

Figure 3.12 Computed tomography (CT) showing bilateral massive nodular hyperplasia (arrows) in a patient with ACTH-independent massive adrenal hyperplasia. (top) Axial view; (bottom) coronal view.

Figure 3.14 Gross pathology specimen showing cut sections of the right and left adrenal glands with pigmented micronodularity found in primary pigmented nodular adrenal disease.

Classic congenital adrenal hyperplasia

Definition
Congenital adrenal hyperplasia (CAH) refers to the clinical disorders associated with the decreased production of cortisol because of deficiencies and inefficiencies in the cortisol synthetic enzyme pathway. The most severe forms of CAH are referred to as *classic*, and the milder forms of CAH are referred to as *late-onset* or *nonclassic*.

Etiology
The causes of CAH include blocks of any of the enzymes in the cortisol synthetic pathway.

Signs and symptoms
With decreased cortisol production, there is a secondary corticotropin (ACTH)-driven buildup of precursor steroids that have activity at the mineralocorticoid or androgen receptors. In addition, dependent on the site of enzymatic deficiency, deficiency of mineralocorticoid or androgen production may occur. Depending on the mutation and resultant degree of protein dysfunction, the deficiency in adrenal enzyme activity may be severe or there may be a more mild degree of signs and symptoms of adrenal insufficiency.

Congenital lipoid adrenal hyperplasia
Mutations in the genes encoding either the steroidogenic acute regulatory protein (StAR) or the steroid side-chain cleavage enzyme (P450scc) result in congenital lipoid adrenal hyperplasia, the most severe form of CAH (Fig. 3.15). This disorder is characterized by a deficiency in all adrenal and gonadal steroid hormones and an ACTH-driven buildup of cholesterol esters in the adrenal cortex. Neonates with congenital lipoid hyperplasia usually present with signs and symptoms of marked adrenocortical insufficiency shortly after birth. Because of the lack of testicular androgen production, infants with a 46,XY karyotype have female external genitalia.

CAH due to 3β-HSD deficiency
Pregnenolone is converted to progesterone by 3β-hydroxysteroid dehydrogenase (3β-HSD) (Fig. 3.15). Mutations in the 3β-HSD2 gene (*HSD3B2*) cause a rare form of CAH associated with deficiency in cortisol, aldosterone, and gonadal steroids. The clinical presentation of CAH due to 3β-HSD deficiency is similar to that of StAR deficiency – infants present with signs and symptoms of both cortisol and aldosterone deficiencies. The excess dehydroepiandrosterone (DHEA) may cause mild virilization in infants with a 46,XX karyotype. The phenotype in infants with a 46,XY karyotype varies from normal to hypospadias to female external genitalia.

CAH due to 17α-hydroxylase deficiency
Progesterone is hydroxylated to 17-hydroxyprogesterone through the activity of 17α-hydroxylase (P450c17) (Fig. 3.15). The 17α-hydroxylase deficiency is a rare form of CAH caused by mutations in *CYP17A1*. It causes ACTH-driven increased production of 11-deoxycorticosterone and corticosterone – both of which have some activity at the mineralocorticoid receptor – leading to hypokalemia and hypertension. The deficiency in 17,20-lyase activity results in decreased androgen and estrogen production. The clinical presentation may not occur until puberty when individuals with a 46,XX karyotype are found to have primary amenorrhea, absent secondary sexual development, hypertension, and hypokalemia. Individuals with a 46,XY karyotype, who are phenotypically female, are usually not evaluated until the lack of pubertal development – they have female external genitalia, intra-abdominal testes, short vagina, absent uterus and fallopian tubes, hypertension, and hypokalemia.

CAH due to 21-hydroxylase deficiency
The 21-hydroxylation of either progesterone in the zona glomerulosa or 17-hydroxyprogesterone in the zona fasciculata is catalyzed by 21-hydroxylase (P450c21) to yield deoxycorticosterone or 11-deoxycortisol, respectively (Fig. 3.15). Deficiency of P450c21 is the most common form of CAH, accounting for more than 90% of all cases. Classic 21-hydroxylase deficiency presents in infancy with typical signs and symptoms of adrenal insufficiency and androgen excess. Ambiguous genitalia are found in infants with a 46,XX karyotype. Depending on the severity of the enzymatic defect and its effect on the mineralocorticoid synthetic pathway, classic 21-hydroxylase deficiency may be referred to as *salt-wasting* or *simple-virilizing*.

CAH due to deficiency of 11β-hydroxylase
Deficiency of 11β-hydroxylase (P450c11β) is the second most common form of CAH. With more severe defects in 11β-hydroxylase function, neonates with a 46,XX karyotype are born with ambiguous genitalia, and neonates with a 46,XY karyotype are born with penile enlargement. With *CYP11B1* mutations that result in decreased, but not absent, 11β-hydroxylase activity, affected individuals may present later in childhood with hypertension and precocious puberty or in young adulthood with hypertension, acne, hirsutism, and oligomenorrhea or amenorrhea.

Diagnosis

Laboratory findings
Laboratory testing shows a build-up of precursors to the enzyme block and deficiencies distal to the enzyme block (Fig. 3.15). For example, with lipoid CAH there are low serum cortisol and plasma aldosterone concentrations and

increased serum ACTH concentration and plasma renin activity.

In 3β-HSD deficiency, in addition to hyperkalemia, hyponatremia, cortisol deficiency, and aldosterone deficiency, laboratory studies show increased blood concentrations of DHEA and DHEA sulfate (DHEA-S).

In 17α-hydroxylase deficiency, laboratory studies show hypokalemia, low plasma renin activity, and low plasma aldosterone concentration.

In classic 21-hydroxylase deficiency, a markedly increased (e.g. > sixfold above the upper limit of the reference range) blood concentration of 17-hydroxyprogresterone is diagnostic. In borderline cases, a cosyntropin-stimulation test may be needed to demonstrate the enzymatic block. Newborn screening for 21-hydroxylase deficiency by measuring 17-hydroxyprogesterone in a dried blood sample is routinely performed in the United States and in many other countries.

Laboratory testing in patients with 11β-hydroxylase deficiency shows increased blood concentrations of 11-deoxycortisol, 11-deoxycorticosterone, DHEA, DHEA-S, androstenedione, and testosterone.

Imaging tests

Dedicated adrenal imaging shows normal-sized adrenal glands in patients with optimally treated CAH and enlarged adrenal glands in patients with suboptimally treated CAH (Fig. 3.16).

Treatment

If not recognized and treated, congenital lipoid hyperplasia is lethal. Treatment consists of glucocorticoid and mineralocorticoid replacement. Patients with 3β-HSD deficiency are treated with glucocorticoid and mineralocorticoid replacement and, at puberty, with gonadal steroid replacement. Treatment for 17α-hydroxylase deficiency includes replacement of glucocorticoid and gonadal steroids. Glucocorticoid replacement is indicated in patients with deficiencies in either 21-hydroxylase or 11β-hydroxylase.

Illustrations (Figs 3.15 & 3.16)

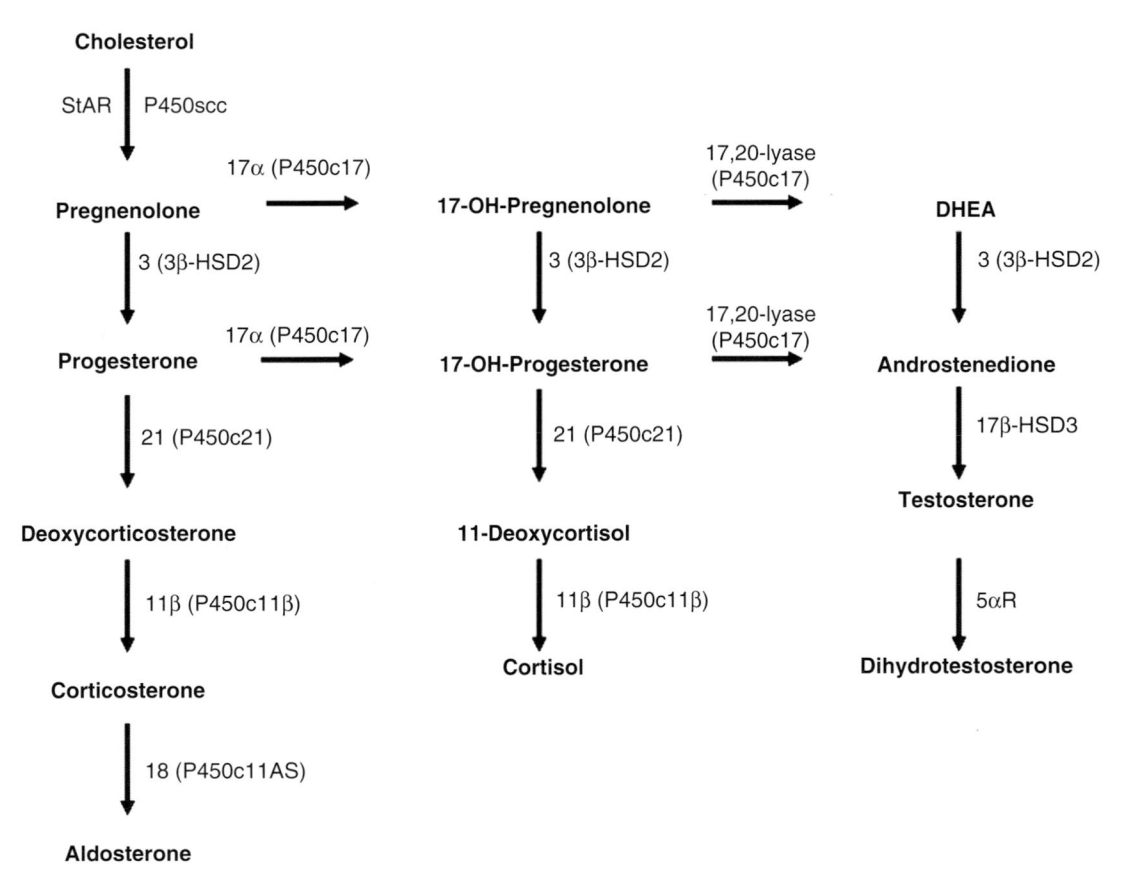

Figure 3.15 Steroid biosynthetic pathway. Abbreviations: 3βHSD, 3β-hydroxysteroid dehydrogenase; 5αR, 5α-reductase; 11β, 11 β-hydroxylase (*CYP11B1*, P450c11); 17α, 17 α-hydroxylase (*CYP17*, P450c17); 17βR, 17β-reductase; 18, aldosterone synthase (*CYP11B2*, P450c11as), addition of a hydroxyl group that is then oxidized to an aldehyde group at the 18-C position; 21, 21-hydroxylase (*CYP21A2*, P450c21); DHEA, dehydroepiandrostenedione; P450$_{SCC}$, side-chain-cleavage enzyme (*CYP11A1*) catalyzes the conversion of cholesterol to pregnenolone in mitochondria in steroidogenic cells.

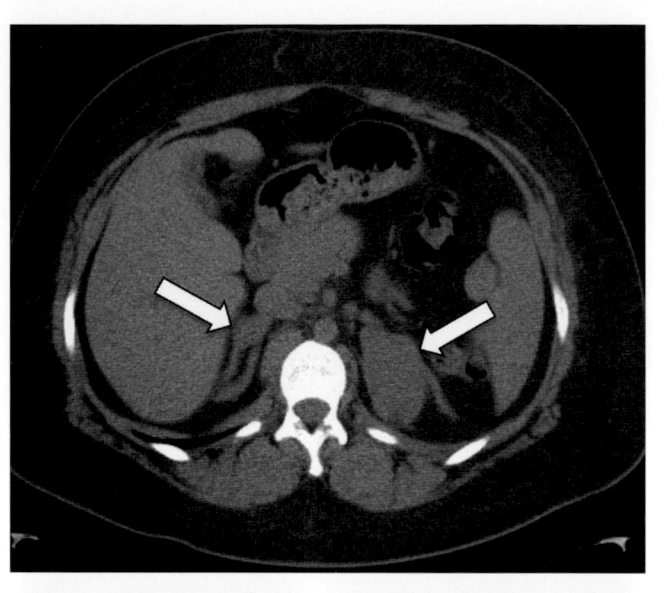

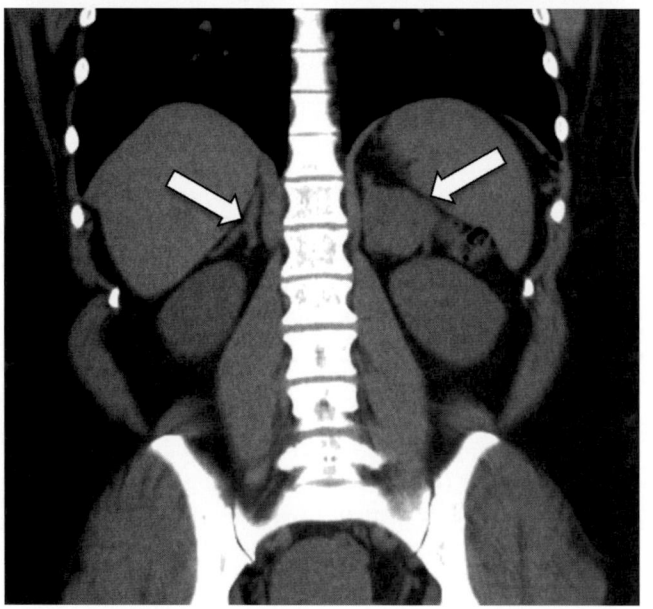

Figure 3.16 Computed tomography (CT) showing bilateral adrenal enlargement due to suboptimally treated congenital adrenal hyperplasia due to 21-hydroxylase deficiency. (top) Axial view; (bottom) coronal view.

Primary aldosteronism

Definition
Primary aldosteronism (PA) is characterized by hypertension, suppressed renin, and increased aldosterone secretion. It is the most common form of secondary hypertension, affecting 5–10% of all patients with hypertension.

Etiology
The two most common subtypes of PA are idiopathic hyperaldosteronism (IHA) and aldosterone-producing adenoma (APA). A much less common form, unilateral adrenal hyperplasia (UAH), is caused by zona glomerulosa hyperplasia of predominantly one adrenal gland.

Three rare forms of familial hyperaldosteronism (FH) have been described: FH type I, or glucocorticoid-remediable aldosteronism (GRA), where aldosterone hypersecretion suppresses with exogenous glucocorticoids; FH type II refers to the familial occurrence of APA or IHA or both; and, FH type III refers to PA caused by germline mutations in the potassium channel subunit *KCNJ5*. Very rarely, excessive aldosterone may be secreted by a neoplasm outside of the adrenal gland (e.g. ovary).

Signs and symptoms
Most patients with PA are not hypokalemic and present with asymptomatic hypertension, which may be mild or severe. Aldosterone excess results in the renal loss of potassium and hydrogen ions. When hypokalemia does occur, it is usually associated with an alkalosis, and patients may present with nocturia and polyuria (caused by hypokalemia-induced failure in renal concentrating ability), palpitations, or muscle cramps.

Diagnosis
Case-detection can be completed with a morning blood test (plasma aldosterone concentration [PAC] to plasma renin activity [PRA] ratio) in a seated, ambulant patient. All patients with an increased PAC : PRA ratio should undergo aldosterone-suppression testing (e.g. oral sodium loading, saline-suppression testing, captopril-stimulation testing, or fludrocortisone-suppression testing). Unilateral adrenalectomy in patients with APA or UAH results in normalization of hypokalemia in all; hypertension is improved in all and is cured in approximately 30–60% of these patients. In IHA, unilateral or bilateral adrenalectomy seldom corrects the hypertension. Both IHA and GRA should be treated medically. Therefore, for those patients who want to pursue a surgical cure, the accurate distinction between the subtypes of PA is a critical step.

Subtype evaluation may require one or more tests, the first of which is imaging the adrenal glands with CT. When a small, solitary, hypodense macroadenoma (> 1 cm and < 2 cm) and normal contralateral adrenal morphology are found on CT in a patient younger than 40 with PA, unilateral adrenalectomy is a reasonable therapeutic option (Fig. 3.17). However, in many cases, adrenal venous sampling (AVS) is essential to direct appropriate therapy in patients with PA who want to pursue the surgical treatment option.

Treatment
The treatment goal is to prevent the morbidity and mortality associated with hypertension, hypokalemia, and cardiovascular damage. The cause of the PA helps to determine the appropriate treatment. Normalization of blood pressure should not be the only goal in managing the patient with PA. Excessive secretion of aldosterone is associated with increased cardiovascular morbidity. Therefore, normalization of circulating aldosterone concentrations or mineralocorticoid receptor (MR) blockade should be part of the management plan for all patients with PA. Unilateral laparoscopic adrenalectomy is an excellent treatment option for patients with APA or UAH (Fig. 3.18). Both IHA and GRA should be treated medically with an MR antagonist.

Illustrations (Figs 3.17 & 3.18)

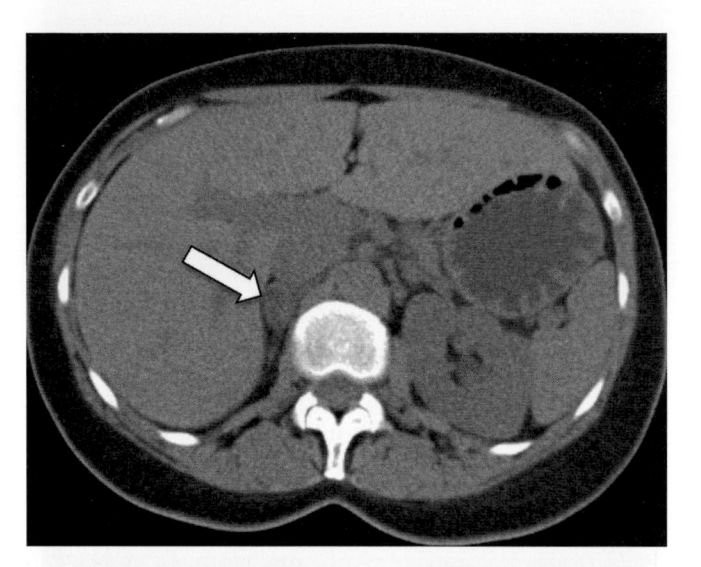

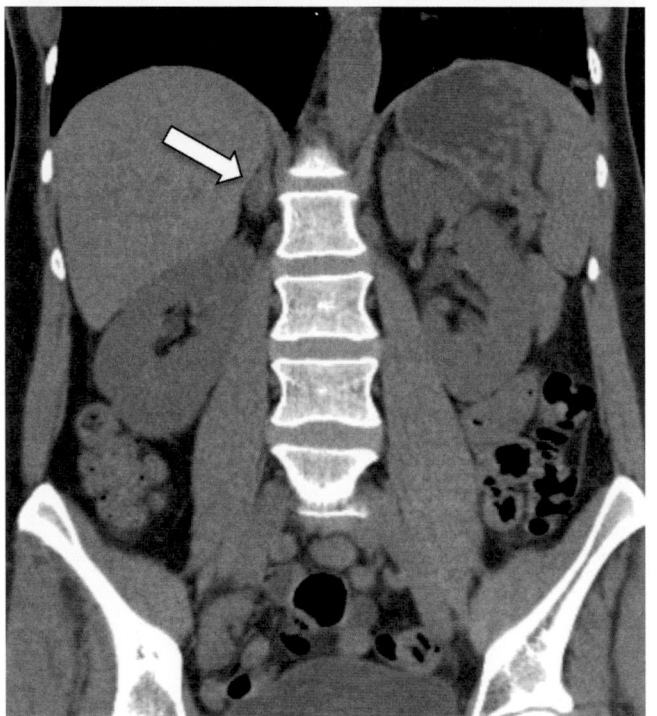

Figure 3.17 Computed tomography (CT) showing a 1.5-cm hypodense right adrenal cortical adenoma in a 27-year-old woman with well-documented primary aldosteronism. (top) Axial view; (bottom) coronal view.

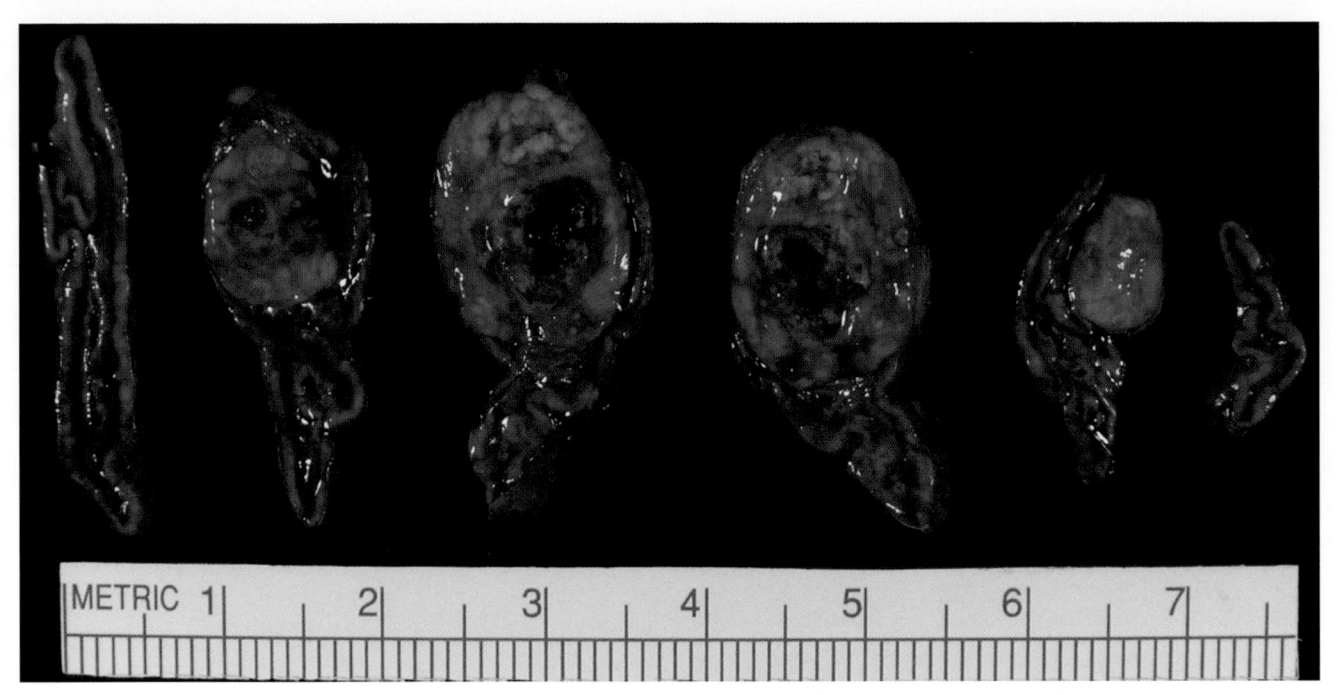

Figure 3.18 Gross pathology specimen from patient with computed tomography (CT) scan in Fig. 3.17. Serial sections show the yellow cortical adenoma that measures 1.8 × 1.7 × 1.3 cm. Postoperatively the plasma aldosterone concentration was undetectable and long-term follow-up documented hypertension cure.

Adrenal venous sampling

Definition

Adrenal venous sampling (AVS) involves catheterizing both adrenal veins and measuring concentrations of aldosterone and cortisol.

Background

Most patients with primary aldosteronism (PA) have either bilateral idiopathic hyperaldosteronism (IHA), treated medically with mineralocorticoid receptor blockade, or a unilateral aldosterone-producing adenoma (APA), treated surgically with unilateral laparoscopic adrenalectomy. The accuracy of adrenal computed tomography (CT) in localizing the source of aldosterone excess is approximately 50%. For example, CT may suggest unilateral disease incorrectly (Fig. 3.19).

Procedure and keys to successful AVS

The keys to successful AVS include appropriate patient selection, careful patient preparation, focused technical expertise, defined protocol, and accurate data interpretation. A center-specific, written protocol is mandatory.

Most centers use a continuous cosyntropin infusion (50 μg/h started 30 min before sampling and continued throughout the procedure) during AVS in an effort to:
• minimize stress-induced fluctuations in aldosterone secretion during nonsimultaneous AVS;
• maximize the gradient in cortisol from adrenal vein to inferior vena cava (IVC); and
• maximize the secretion of aldosterone from an APA

The adrenal veins are sequentially catheterized through the percutaneous femoral vein approach under fluoroscopic guidance – the correct catheter tip location is confirmed with injection of a small amount of contrast medium (Fig. 3.20). Blood is obtained by gentle aspiration from both adrenal veins.

The right adrenal vein enters the IVC posteriorly several centimeters above the right renal vein. It is more difficult to catheterize than the left one for a variety of reasons – it is short, small in caliber, and often has an angulated path causing the catheter tip to impact the intima making blood aspiration problematic. Occasionally it arises in conjunction with a hepatic vein branch and needs to be separately engaged using a specific catheter shape to match the anatomy. In addition, some radiologists confuse the right adrenal vein with adjacent small hepatic vein branches, which are frequently encountered entering the IVC near the adrenal vein region.

The left adrenal vein is a tributary of the inferior phrenic vein, which enters the roof of the left renal vein near the lateral margin of the vertebral column in most patients. The venous sample from the left side is typically obtained from the common inferior phrenic vein close to the junction of the adrenal vein (Fig. 3.20).

The final sample needs to be from a pure background source isolated from any possible contamination from the adrenal venous drainage. Although referred to as the "IVC" sample, it is actually from the external iliac vein to be certain that it is free of contamination from collateral left adrenal venous effluent, which on rare occasions drains through a large left gonadal vein caudally into the internal iliac veins.

Aldosterone and cortisol concentrations are measured in the blood from all three sites (right adrenal vein, left adrenal vein, and IVC). All of the blood samples should be assayed at 1 : 1, 1 : 10, and 1 : 50 dilutions – absolute values are mandatory. At centers with experience with AVS, the complication rate is < 2.5%. Complications can include symptomatic groin hematoma, adrenal hemorrhage, and dissection of an adrenal vein.

Interpretation of AVS

The cortisol concentrations from the adrenal veins and IVC are used to confirm successful catheterization; the adrenal vein to IVC cortisol ratio is typically > 10 : 1 with the continuous cosyntropin infusion protocol (Table 3.1). When cosyntropin infusion is used, an adrenal vein to IVC cortisol gradient of at least 5 : 1 is required to be confident that the adrenal veins were successfully catherterized. However, when cosyntropin infusion is not used, an adrenal vein to IVC cortisol gradient of more than 3 : 1 is recommended.

Dividing the right and left adrenal vein plasma aldosterone concentrations (PAC) by their respective cortisol concentrations corrects for the dilutional effect of the inferior phrenic vein flow into the left adrenal vein; these are termed *cortisol-corrected ratios*. In patients with APA, the mean cortisol-corrected aldosterone ratio (APA–side PAC/cortisol to normal adrenal PAC/cortisol) is 18 : 1. A cutoff for the cortisol-corrected aldosterone ratio from high-side to low-side > 4 : 1 indicates unilateral aldosterone excess (Table 3.1). In patients with IHA, the mean cortisol-corrected aldosterone ratio is 1.8 : 1 (high-side to low-side); a ratio < 3 : 1 is suggestive of bilateral aldosterone hypersecretion. Thus, most patients with unilateral aldosterone hypersecretion will have cortisol-corrected aldosterone lateralization ratios ≥ 4.0; ratios ≥ 3.0 but < 4.0 represent a zone of overlap. A ratio < 3.0 is consistent with bilateral aldosterone hypersecretion.

Centers that perform AVS without the benefit of cosyntropin infusion use lower lateralization cutoff values. In addition, the contralateral aldosterone to cortisol ratio is less than the IVC aldosterone to cortisol ratio in 93% of patients with surgically confirmed APA (Table 3.1). Using the preceding diagnostic cutoffs, the test characteristics of AVS for detecting unilateral aldosterone hypersecretion include a specificity of 100% and an apparent sensitivity of 95%.

Table 3.1 Adrenal venous sampling data from the patient whose CT scan is shown in Fig. 3.19*

Vein	Aldosterone (A), ng/dL	Cortisol (C), μg/dL	A/C ratio	Aldosterone ratio*
Right adrenal vein	5700	600	9.5	7.9
Left adrenal vein	733	597	1.2	–
IVC	39	26	1.5	–

*Right adrenal vein A/C ratio divided by left adrenal vein A/C ratio. CT, computed tomography; IVC, inferior vena cava.

The cortisol-corrected aldosterone ratio from high-side to low-side > 4 : 1 indicates right adrenal aldosterone excess; aldosterone hypersecretion lateralized to the adrenal gland with the small nodule seen on CT. In addition, the left adrenal aldosterone to cortisol ratio is less than the IVC aldosterone to cortisol ratio, which is consistent with a right adrenal aldosterone-producing adenoma.

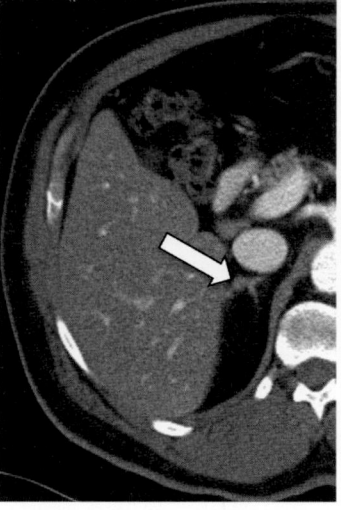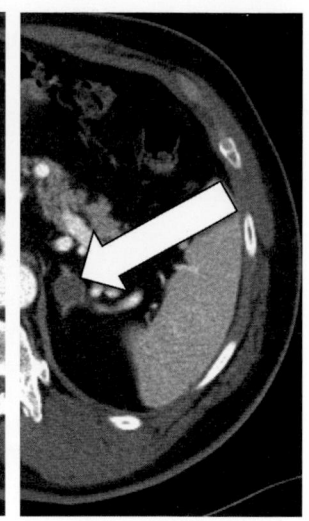

Figure 3.19 Computed tomography (CT) (axial view) showing a 1.7 cm hypodense left adrenal cortical nodule (large arrow) and 0.4 cm nodule in the right adrenal gland (small arrow) in a man with well-documented primary aldosteronism.

Illustrations (Figs 3.19 & 3.20)

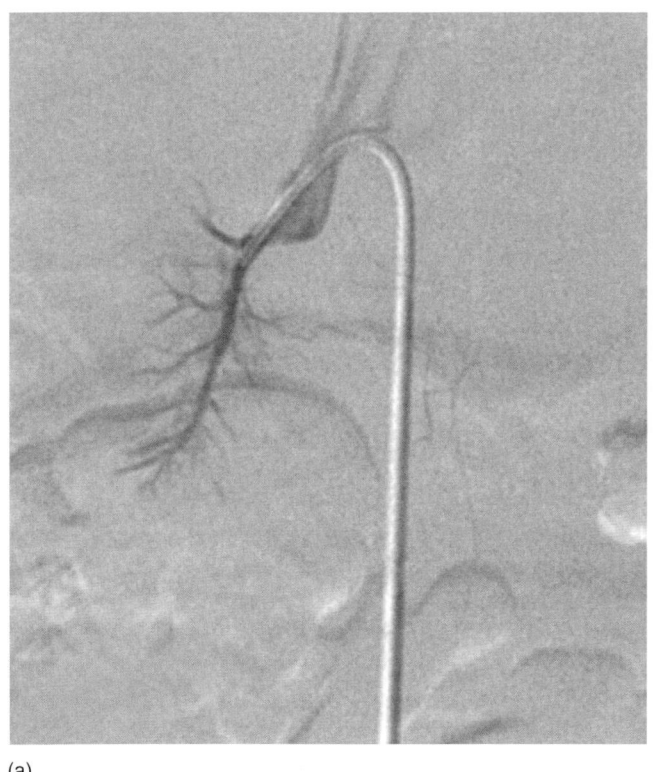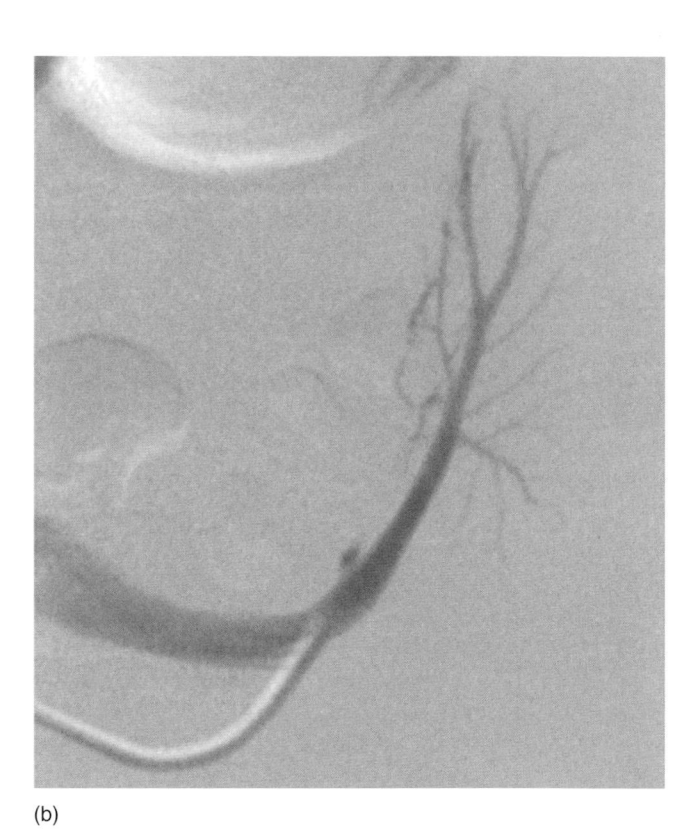

(a)   (b)

Figure 3.20 Adrenal venous sampling fluoroscopy images showing the delicate venous anatomy of the right and left adrenal glands in the patient from Fig. 3.19.

Primary adrenal failure (Addison's disease)

Definition
Primary adrenal failure is the failure of the adrenal cortex to produce physiologic amounts of glucocorticoids and mineralocorticoids.

Etiology
The most common cause of primary adrenal failure has evolved from tuberculosis in 1855 when Thomas Addison described the autopsy findings in 11 patients with the disease that bears his name, to autoimmune disease today (in approximately 80% of cases). Other less common causes of primary adrenal failure include metastatic disease (e.g. lymphoma, lung cancer, breast cancer, melanoma), infections (e.g. fungal, HIV, tuberculosis), adrenal hemorrhage, adrenoleukodystrophies, congenital adrenal hypoplasia, bilateral adrenalectomy, and drug-induced causes (e.g. mitotane, ketoconazole).

Approximately one-half of patients with autoimmune adrenal failure have one or more other autoimmune endocrine disorders. In such patients, the etiology of their findings may be autoimmune polyglandular syndrome type II (APS2). Affected patients typically present between the ages of 20–40 years with primary adrenal failure as the main manifestation. Autoimmune thyroid disease (e.g. Hashimoto's thyroiditis, Graves' disease) and type 1 diabetes mellitus are common in patients with APS2.

Signs and symptoms
The clinical presentation of primary adrenal insufficiency depends on both the rate and extent of adrenocortical destruction. If slowly progressive, the patient may not come to clinical detection until an illness (e.g. infection) or other stress (e.g. trauma, surgery) precipitates an adrenal crisis.

The typical chronic signs and symptoms relate to both glucocorticoid and mineralocorticoid insufficiency, and these include fatigue, generalized weakness, diffuse myalgias and arthralgias, anorexia, weight loss, nausea, emesis, abdominal pain, psychiatric symptoms, postural lightheadedness, hypotension, hyperpigmentation (skin and hair), hyponatremia, hyperkalemia, and anemia. Low blood pressure and postural lightheadedness are both associated with both mineralocorticoid and glucocorticoid deficiencies. Generalized hyperpigmentation is caused by corticotropin (ACTH)-driven increased melanin production in the epidermal melanocytes (Fig. 3.21). The extensor surfaces (e.g. knees, knuckles, elbows) and other friction areas (e.g. belt line, brassier strap) tend to be even more hyperpigmented (Fig. 3.22). Other sites of prominent hyperpigmentation include the inner surface of lips, buccal mucosa, gums, hard palate, recent surgical scars, areolae (Fig. 3.21), freckles, and palmar creases (Fig. 3.23). In women with primary adrenal failure, secondary sex hair (axillary and pubic hair) may be lost and libido decreased because of loss of adrenal androgen secretion.

Diagnosis
Laboratory findings
The typical general laboratory clue to primary adrenal insufficiency is hyponatremia with hyperkalemia. The hyponatremia is associated with an inappropriate increase in vasopressin secretion and a cortisol-related decreased free-water clearance at the kidney. The hyperkalemia is a direct result of lack of aldosterone effect at the mineralocorticoid receptor. In symptomatic patients, all that is needed to confirm the diagnosis is an 8 AM serum ACTH concentration > 500 pg/mL and a simultaneous serum cortisol concentration < 5 μg/dL (138 nmol/L). In this setting, stimulation testing with cosyntropin is not needed.

When the cosyntropin-stimulation test is performed in patients with primary adrenal failure, the serum cortisol concentration does not change from baseline (the baseline value is typically < 5 μg/dL [<138 nmol/L], and the increment after cosyntropin administration is < 7 μg/dL) [193 nmol/L], and the peak value remains < 18 μg/dL (497 nmol/L). Antibodies directed against 21-hydroxylase can be found in nearly all patients with autoimmune primary adrenal failure, and they are absent in patients with other causes of adrenal insufficiency.

Imaging tests
If primary adrenal failure is due to infiltrative disease, adrenal CT may show bilateral adrenal masses.

Treatment
In an attempt to replicate the normal glucocorticoid circadian rhythm, two-thirds of the glucocorticoid dose (hydrocortisone, 10 or 15 mg) is administered in the morning and one-third (hydrocortisone, 5 or 10 mg) is administered before the evening meal. Clinical judgment and lack of symptoms of glucocorticoid deficiency or excess are the primary means for determining dosage adequacy. Patients should be told to:
• Increase the replacement dosage of glucocorticoids twofold to threefold during major physical stress (e.g. fever higher than 101°F, acute illness, tooth extraction).
• Seek medical care if more than 3 days of stress glucocorticoid coverage is required.
• Avoid long-term supraphysiologic dosages because of the potential for iatrogenic Cushing syndrome.
• Be aware that increased glucocorticoid dosage is not required for mental stress, headaches, or minor illness.
• Administer the increased glucocorticoid dose intramuscularly if it cannot be taken orally because of nausea or emesis.

• Carry and wear medical identification (wallet card and bracelet or necklace) that includes the diagnosis ("adrenal insufficiency") and the words "give cortisone," so that appropriate glucocorticoid treatment can be given if the patient is found unconscious.

Fludrocortisone is used to replace aldosterone. Typically, 50–200 μg (100 μg daily is the usual dose) is administered orally in a single dose daily. The dosage is titrated to achieve a normal serum level of potassium. Inade-

quate dosage causes dehydration, hyponatremia, and hyperkalemia. Excessive dosage results in hypertension, weight gain, and hypokalemia. Most patients are advised to maintain a sodium intake of approximately 150 mEq per day.

Illustrations (Figs 3.21–3.23)

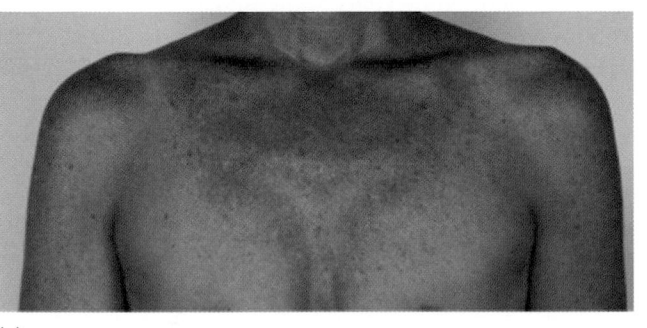

(a)

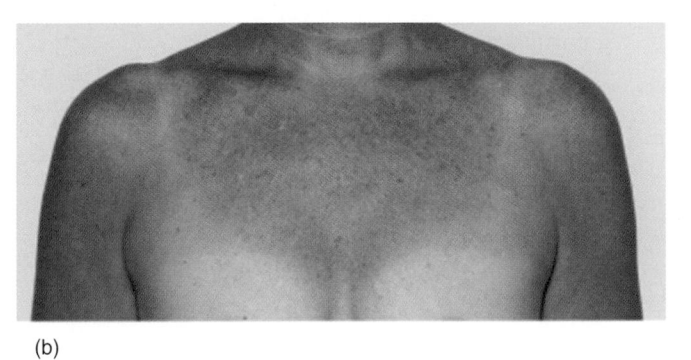

(b)

Figure 3.21 Photographs of a 50-year-old woman who presented with progressive "flu-like" symptoms, weight loss (BMI = 19.5 kg/m^2), hyponatremia, and hyperkalemia. Her baseline serum cortisol was 1.4 μg/dL and the serum ACTH concentration was 716 pg/mL. (a) Patient's ppearance at presentation with diffuse hyperpigmentation, including the areolae. (b) Patient after 14 months of glucocorticoid and mineralocorticoid replacement therapy. The hyperpigmentation has resolved and her BMI increased to 22 kg/m^2.

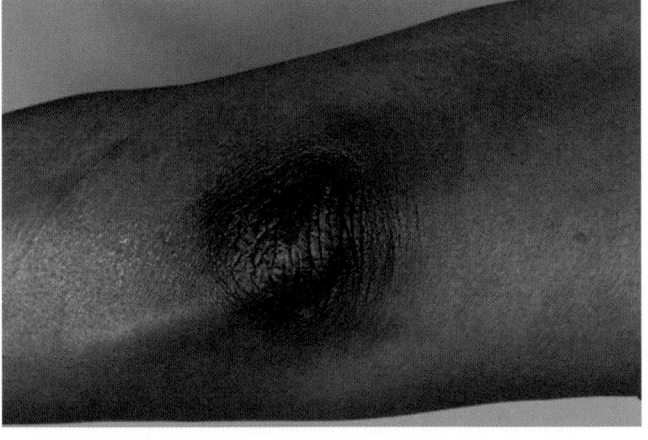

Figure 3.22 Photograph showing the elbow of a patient with Addison's disease showing diffuse hyperpigmentation, especially over the extensor surface.

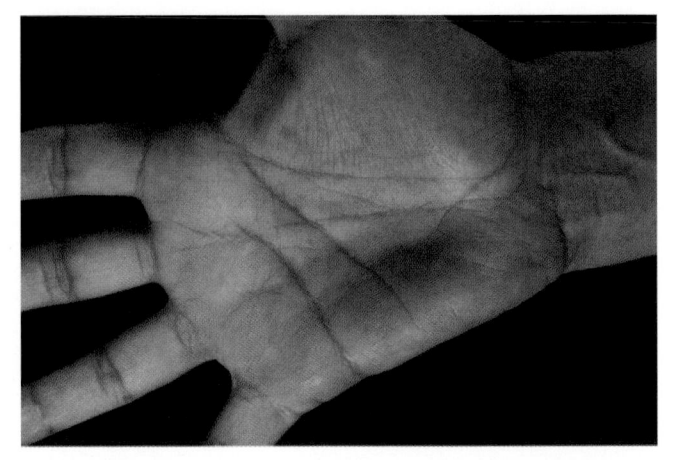

Figure 3.23 Photograph showing hyperpigmented palmar creases in a patient with Addison's disease.

Pheochromocytoma

Definition

Catecholamine-secreting tumors that arise from chromaffin cells of the adrenal medulla and the sympathetic ganglia are referred to as *pheochromocytomas* and *catecholamine-secreting paragangliomas*, respectively. The distinction between pheochromocytoma and paraganglioma is an important one because of implications for associated neoplasms, risk for malignancy, and genetic testing. The term *pheochromocytoma*, proposed by Pick in 1912, comes from the Greek words "phaios" (dusky), "chroma" (color), and "cytoma" (tumor) because of the dark staining reaction that is caused by the oxidation of intracellular catecholamines when exposed to dichromate salts.

Etiology

Pheochromocytomas are rare, with an annual incidence of 2–8 cases per million people. Nevertheless, it is important to suspect, confirm, localize, and resect these tumors because:
• The associated hypertension is curable with surgical removal of the tumor.
• A risk of lethal paroxysm exists.
• At least 10% of the tumors are malignant.
• Ten to twenty percent of the tumors are familial, and detection of this tumor in the proband may result in early diagnosis in other family members.

Pheochromocytomas occur with equal frequency in men and women, primarily in the third, fourth, and fifth decades. These tumors are rare in children, and when discovered, they may be multifocal and associated with a hereditary syndrome. Approximately one-third of pheochromocytomas are genetic and due to germline mutations.

Signs and symptoms

When symptoms are present, they are due to the pharmacologic effects of excess concentrations of circulating catecholamines. The resulting hypertension may be sustained (in approximately half of patients) or paroxysmal (in approximately a one-third of patients). The remaining patients have normal blood pressure. Episodic symptoms may occur in spells, or paroxysms, that can be extremely variable in presentation, but typically include forceful heartbeat, pallor, tremor, headache, and diaphoresis. Spells may be either spontaneous or precipitated by postural change, anxiety, medications (e.g. metoclopramide, anesthetic agents), exercise, or maneuvers that increase intra-abdominal pressure (e.g. change in position, lifting, defecation, exercise, colonoscopy, pregnancy, trauma). Spells may occur multiple times daily or as infrequently as once monthly. The typical duration of a pheochromocytoma-related spell is 15–20 minutes, but it may be much shorter or last several hours.

Additional clinical signs of pheochromocytoma include hypertensive retinopathy, orthostatic hypotension, angina, nausea, constipation (megacolon may be the presenting symptom), hyperglycemia, diabetes mellitus, hypercalcemia, Raynaud's phenomenon, livedo reticularis, erythrocytosis, and mass effects from the tumor. Fasting hyperglycemia and diabetes mellitus are caused in part by the α-adrenergic inhibition of insulin release. Some of the co-secreted hormones that may dominate the clinical presentation include corticotropin (Cushing syndrome), parathyroid hormone-related peptide (hypercalcemia), vasopressin (syndrome of inappropriate antidiuretic hormone secretion), vasoactive intestinal peptide (watery diarrhea), and growth hormone-releasing hormone (acromegaly). Cardiomyopathy, whether dilated or hypertrophic, may be totally reversible with tumor resection. Many physical examination findings are associated with genetic syndromes that predispose to pheochromocytoma; these findings include retinal angiomas (Fig. 3.24), marfanoid body habitus, café-au-lait spots (Fig. 3.25), axillary freckling (Fig. 3.26), subcutaneous neurofibromas, and mucosal neuromas on the eyelids and tongue (Fig. 3.27).

Diagnosis

Laboratory findings

The diagnosis must be confirmed biochemically by the presence of increased concentrations of fractionated catecholamines and fractionated metanephrines in the blood or a 24-hour urine collection. Localization studies should not be initiated until biochemical studies have confirmed the diagnosis of a catecholamine-secreting tumor. Pheochromocytomas are localized to the adrenal glands and have an average diameter of 4.5 cm (Fig 3.28).

Imaging tests

Computed tomography (CT) is the optimal localization test (Fig. 3.29). However, in an effort to avoid radiation exposure, magnetic resonance imaging (MRI) is a suitable alternative (Fig. 3.30). Iodine-123 metaiodobenzylguanidine scintigraphy may be obtained in patients with adrenal pheochromocytoma if there is concern about metastatic disease. For example, there is increased risk with malignancy with pheochromocytomas > 10 cm in diameter.

Treatment

The treatment of choice for pheochromocytoma is complete surgical resection. Surgical survival rates are 98–100% and are highly dependent on the skill of the endocrinologist–endocrine surgeon–anesthesiologist team. Careful preoperative pharmacologic preparation with α- and β-adrenergic blockade is crucial for successful treatment. Most pheochromocytomas are benign and can be totally excised. Tumor excision usually cures hypertension.

Illustrations (Figs 3.24–3.30)

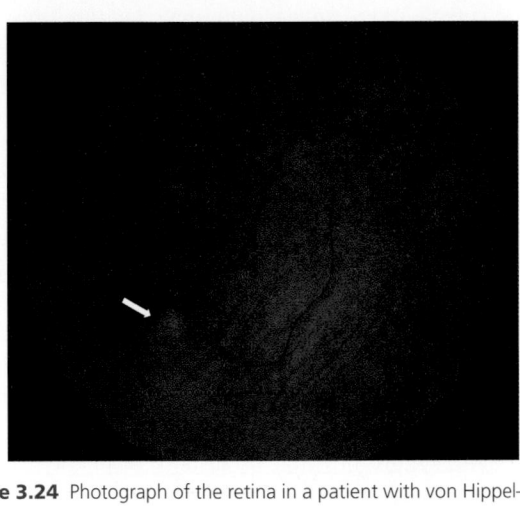

Figure 3.24 Photograph of the retina in a patient with von Hippel–Lindau (VHL) syndrome shows a retinal angioma (arrow). This syndrome is an autosomal dominant disorder that may present with a variety of benign and malignant neoplasms: pheochromocytoma (frequently bilateral), paraganglioma (mediastinal, abdominal, pelvic), hemangioblastoma (involving the cerebellum, spinal cord, or brain stem), retinal angioma, clear cell renal cell carcinoma, pancreatic neuroendocrine tumors, endolymphatic sac tumors of the middle ear, serous cystadenomas of the pancreas, and papillary cystadenomas of the epididymis and broad ligament.

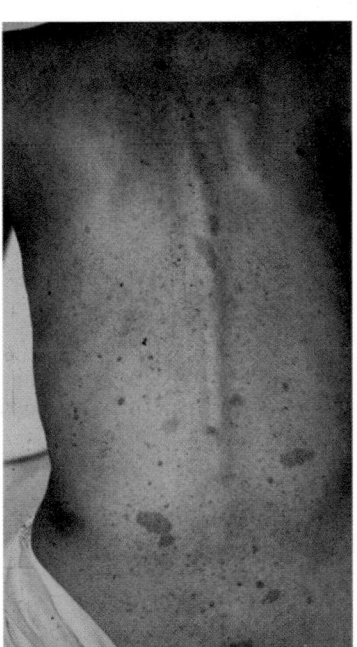

Figure 3.25 Photograph of a patient with neurofibromatosis type 1 (NF1) showing multiple café-au-lait spots over his back. NF1 is an autosomal dominant disorder characterized by neurofibromas, multiple café-au-lait spots, axillary and inguinal freckling, iris hamartomas (Lisch nodules), boney abnormalities, central nervous system gliomas, pheochromocytoma and paraganglioma, macrocephaly, and cognitive deficits. Approximately 2% of patients with NF1 develop catecholamine-secreting tumors.

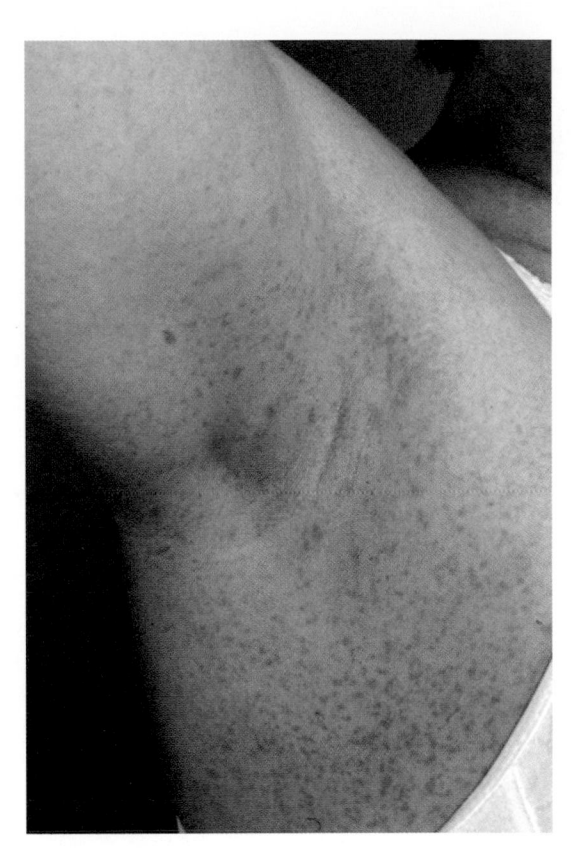

Figure 3.26 Photograph of a patient with neurofibromatosis type 1 (NF1) showing diffuse axillary freckling.

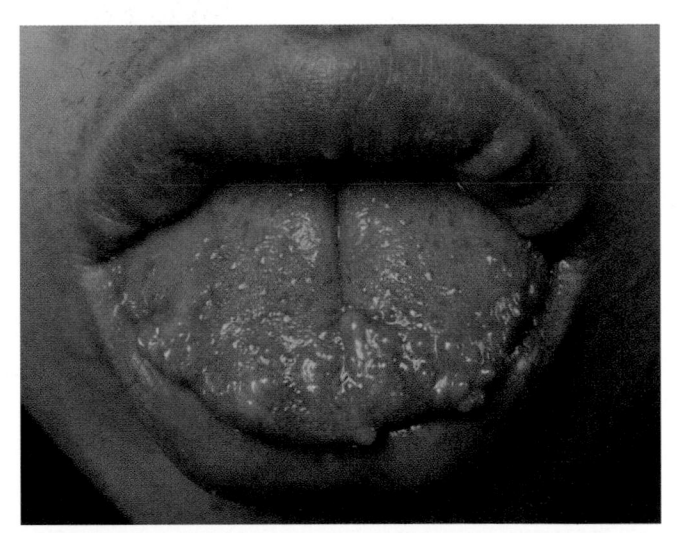

Figure 3.27 Photograph of the tongue and lips of a patient with multiple endocrine neoplasia (MEN) type 2B. MEN 2B is characterized by medullary thyroid carcinoma in all patients, pheochromocytoma in 50%, mucocutaneous neuromas (typically involving the tongue, lips, and eyelids) in most patients, skeletal deformities (e.g. kyphoscoliosis or lordosis), joint laxity, myelinated corneal nerves, and intestinal ganglioneuromas (Hirschsprung's disease).

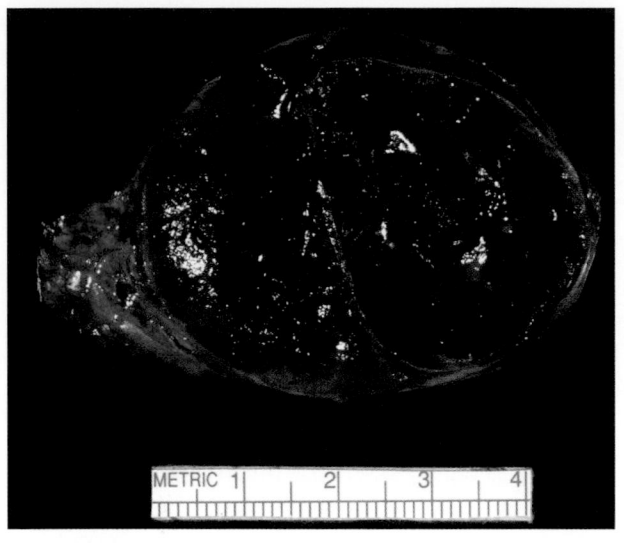

Figure 3.28 Gross pathology cut section of a 4.7 × 3.6 × 3.5 cm pheochromocytoma showing central hemorrhagic cystic degeneration. This is the pathology specimen from the patient whose computed tomographic (CT) scan is shown in Fig. 3.29.

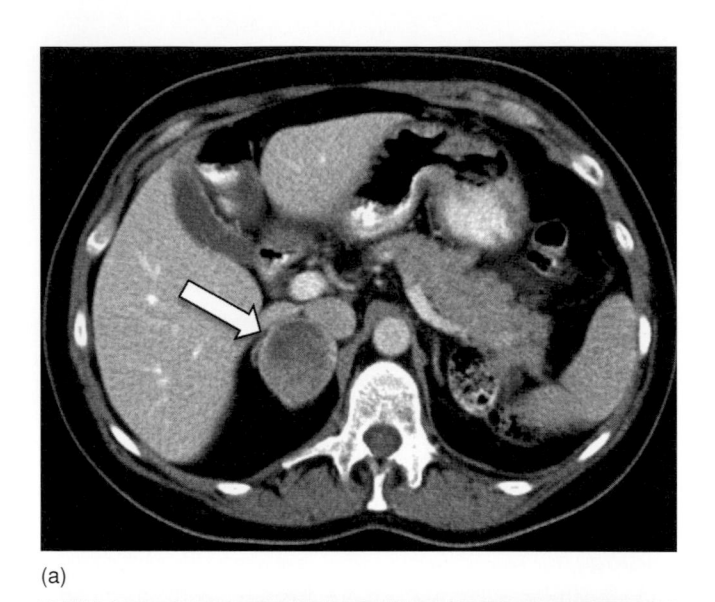

(a)

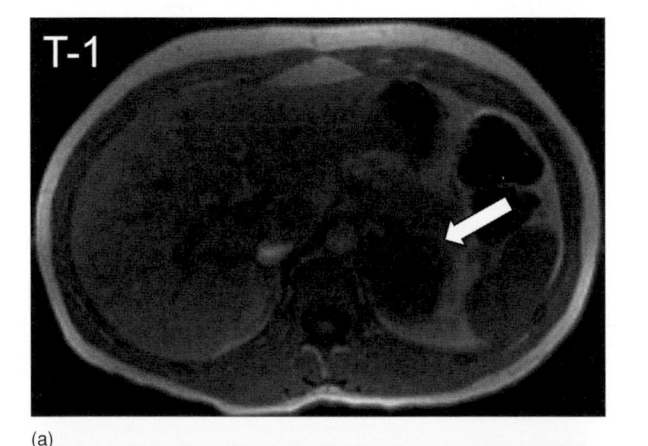

(a)

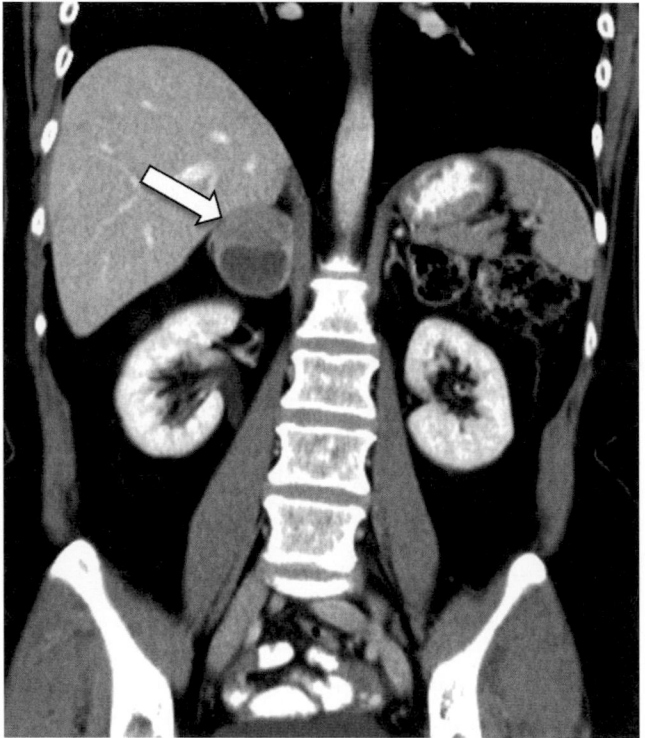

(b)

Figure 3.29 Computed tomography (CT) showing a 4.5 cm right adrenal pheochromocytoma (arrows) with typical area of cystic degeneration in the caudal aspect. This CT scan is from the patient whose gross pathology is shown in Fig. 3.28. (a) Axial view; (b) coronal view.

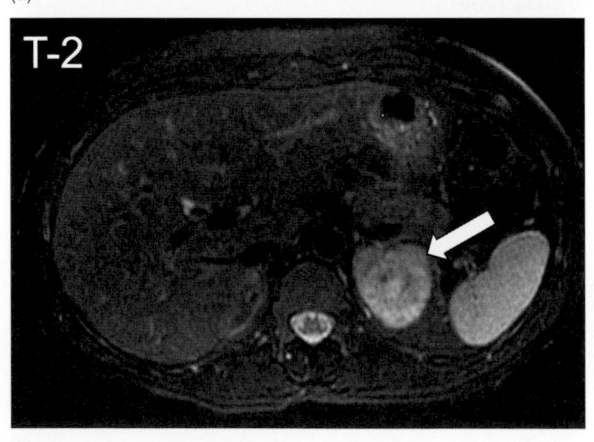

(b)

Figure 3.30 Magnetic resonance imaging (MRI) showing a 4.8 × 4.2 × 6.4 cm left adrenal pheochromocytoma. (a) T-1 weighted image; (b) T-2 weighted image. Note increased signal intensity on T-2 weighted image (b) typically seen in vascular adrenal masses.

Paraganglioma

Definition
Catecholamine-secreting tumors that arise from the sympathetic ganglia and from chromaffin cells of the adrenal medulla are referred to as *catecholamine-secreting paragangliomas* and *pheochromocytomas*, respectively. The distinction between paraganglioma and pheochromocytoma is an important one because of implications for associated neoplasms, risk for malignancy, and genetic testing. The term *paraganglioma*, introduced in 1908, is defined as an extra-adrenal chromaffin tumor arising in a paraganglion.

Etiology
Catecholamine-secreting tumors are rare, with an annual incidence of 2–8 cases per million people. Paragangliomas occur with equal frequency in men and women, primarily in the third, fourth, and fifth decades. These tumors are rare in children, and when discovered, they may be multifocal and associated with a hereditary syndrome. A "rule of 10" has been quoted for describing the characteristics of catecholamine-secreting tumors: 10% are extra-adrenal; 10% occur in children; 10% are multiple or bilateral; 10% recur after surgical removal; 10% are malignant; 10% are familial; and 10% of benign, sporadic adrenal pheochromocytomas are found as adrenal incidentalomas. None of these rules is precisely 10%. For example, recent studies have suggested that up to 30% of catecholamine-secreting tumors are familial. Because of the increased use of computed imaging and familial testing, paraganglioma is diagnosed in up to 50% of patients before any symptoms develop.

Signs and symptoms
When symptoms are present, they are due to the pharmacologic effects of excess concentrations of circulating catecholamines. The resulting hypertension may be sustained (in approximately half of patients) or paroxysmal (in approximately a one-third of patients). The remaining patients have normal blood pressure. Episodic symptoms may occur in spells, or paroxysms, that can be extremely variable in presentation, but typically include forceful heartbeat, pallor, tremor, headache, and diaphoresis. Spells may be either spontaneous or precipitated by postural change, anxiety, medications (e.g. metoclopramide, anesthetic agents), exercise, or maneuvers that increase intra-abdominal pressure (e.g. change in position, lifting, defecation, exercise, colonoscopy, pregnancy, trauma). Spells may occur multiple times daily or as infrequently as once monthly. The typical duration of a catecholamine-secreting tumor-related spell is 15–20 minutes, but it may be much shorter or last several hours.

Diagnosis

Laboratory findings
The diagnosis must be confirmed biochemically by the presence of increased concentrations of fractionated catecholamines and fractionated metanephrines in the blood or a 24-hour urine collection. Localization studies should not be initiated until biochemical studies have confirmed the diagnosis of a catecholamine-secreting tumor.

Paragangliomas occur where there is chromaffin tissue: along the para-aortic sympathetic chain (Fig. 3.31), within the organs of Zuckerkandl (at the origin of the inferior mesenteric artery), in the wall of the urinary bladder (Fig. 3.32), and along the sympathetic chain in the neck or mediastinum. During early postnatal life, the extra-adrenal sympathetic paraganglionic tissues are prominent; then they degenerate, leaving residual foci associated with the vagus nerves, carotid vessels, aortic arch, pulmonary vessels, and mesenteric arteries. Unusual locations for paragangliomas include the intra-atrial cardiac septum, spermatic cord, vagina, scrotum, and sacrococcygeal region. Paragangliomas in the skull base and neck region (Fig. 3.33) (e.g. carotid body tumors, glomus tumors, chemodectomas) usually arise from parasympathetic tissue and typically do not hypersecrete catecholamines and metanephrines, whereas paragangliomas in the mediastinum, abdomen, and pelvis usually arise from sympathetic chromaffin tissue and typically do hypersecrete catecholamines and metanephrines.

Imaging tests
Iodine-123 metaiodobenzylguanidine scintigraphy should be obtained in all patients with paragangliomas to determine if there is more than one paraganglioma and whether there are sites of metastatic disease (Fig. 3.34). Positron emission tomography (PET) scanning with ^{18}F-fluorodeoxyglucose (FDG) is very effective in identifying sites of metastatic paraganglioma (Fig. 3.35).

Treatment
The treatment of choice for paraganglioma is complete surgical resection. For those patients with catecholamine-secreting paragangliomas, careful preoperative pharmacologic preparation with α- and β-adrenergic blockade is crucial for successful treatment. Most paragangliomas are benign and can be totally excised.

Illustrations (Figs 3.31–3.35)

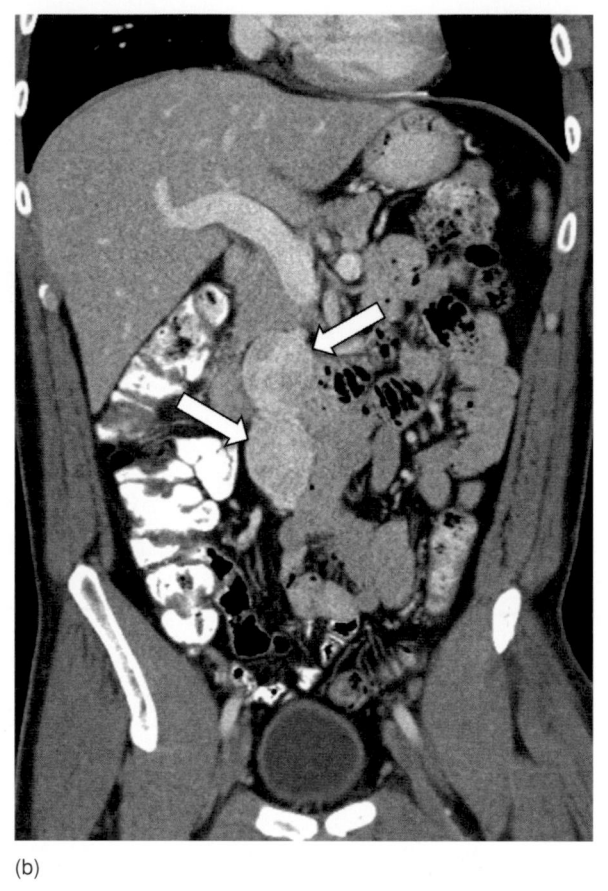

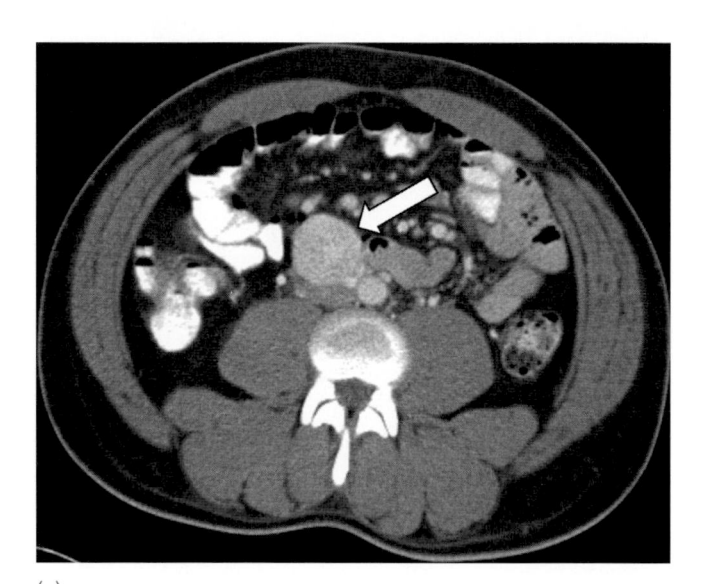

(a)
(b)

Figure 3.31 Computed tomography (CT) shows a 4.4 × 3.8 × 8.7 cm dumbbell-shaped right para-aortic paraglanglioma (arrows). (a) Axial view; (b) coronal view.

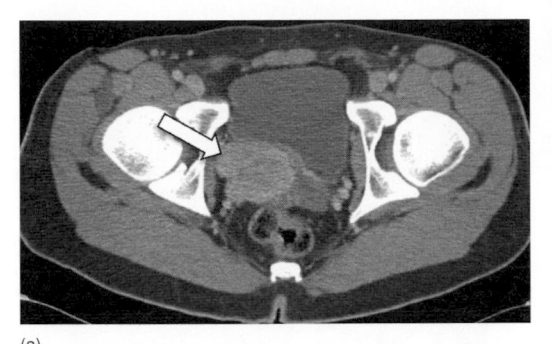

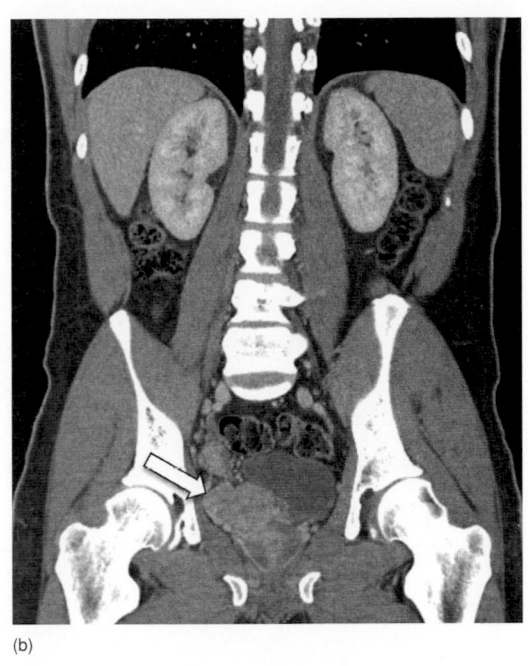

(a)

(b)

Figure 3.32 Computed tomography (CT) shows a 4.4 × 5.4 × 5.8 cm irregularly shaped paraganglioma involving the wall of the urinary bladder. (a) Axial view; (b) coronal view.

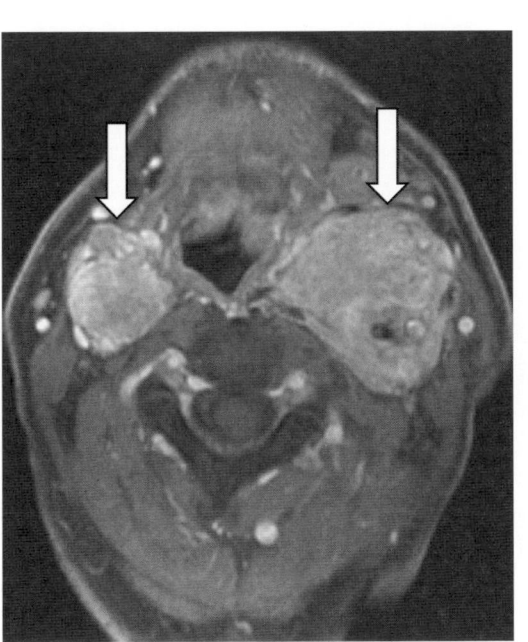

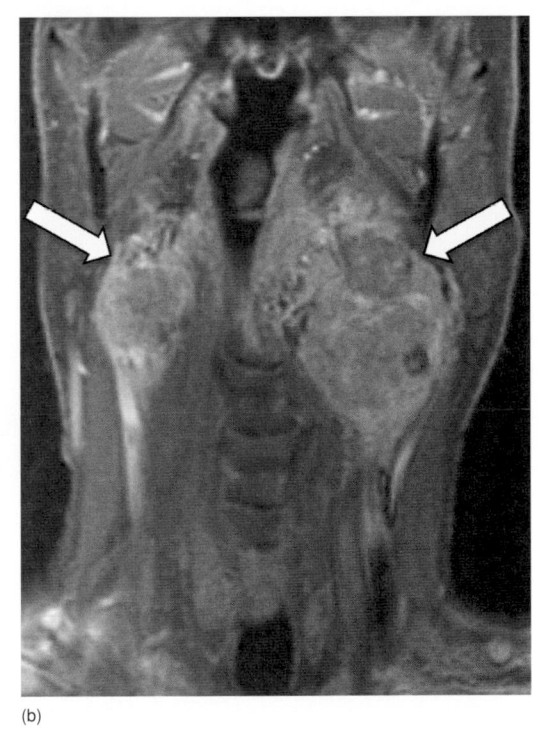

(a)

(b)

Figure 3.33 Neck magnetic resonance imaging (MRI) shows large bilateral carotid body tumors. The right carotid body tumor measures 2.5 × 3.3 × 4.8 cm and splays the internal and external carotid arteries. The left carotid body tumor measures 5.1 × 5.2 × 8.0 cm and encases the left internal carotid artery. (a) Axial view; (b) coronal view.

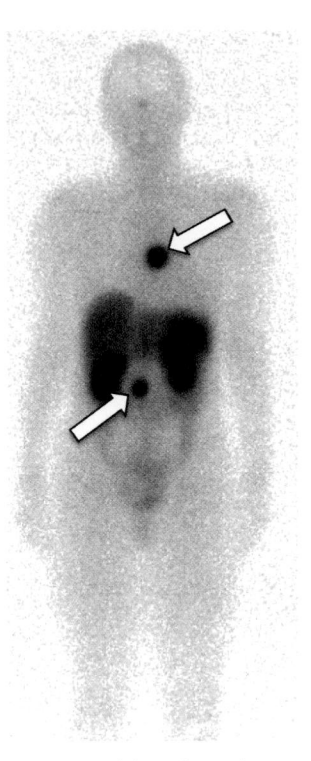

Figure 3.34 Iodine-123 metaiodobenzylguanidine scintigraphy showing two paragangliomas – one pericardiac (upper arrow) and one abdominal periaortic (lower arrow). Normal uptake is seen in the liver, spleen, and kidneys.

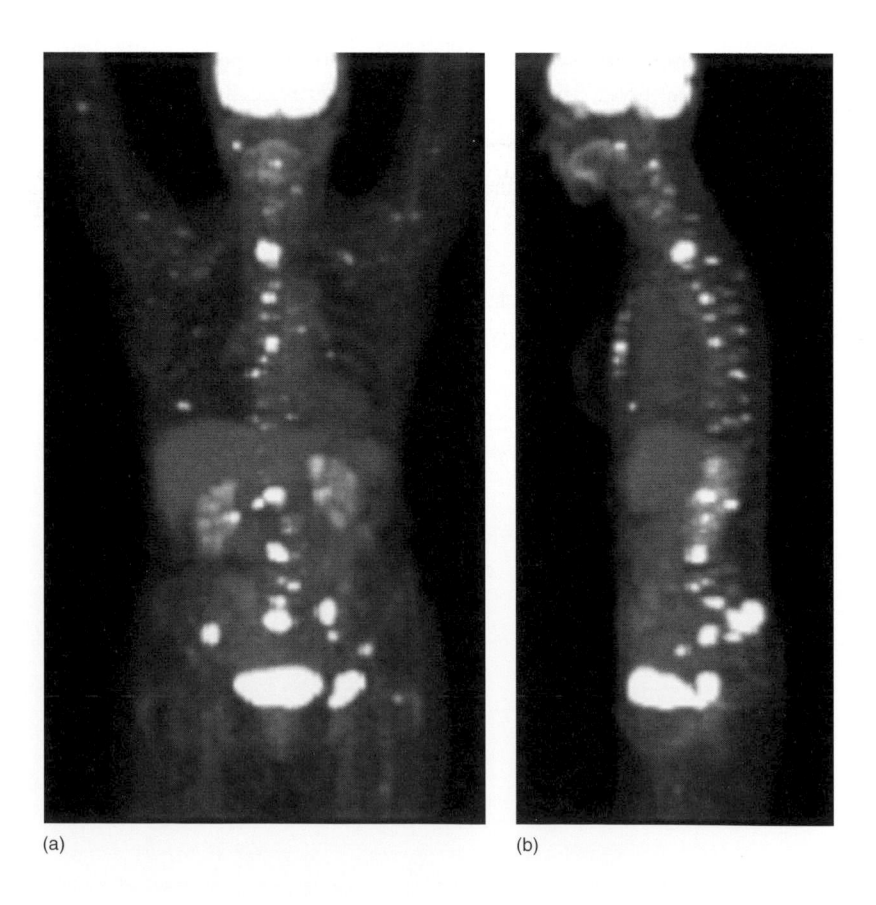

Figure 3.35 Positron emission tomography (PET) scanning with ^{18}F-fluorodeoxyglucose (FDG) images showing diffuse osseous metastases in a patient with metastatic paraganglioma. (a) Coronal image; (b) sagittal image.

(a)

(b)

Adrenal infarction

Definition
Adrenal infarction results from either hemorrhage (an acute event where there is interruption of the contiguous vascular supply to one or both adrenal glands) or adrenal vein thrombosis. The hemorrhage grossly expands the adrenal capsule and usually results in failure of adrenal gland function.

Etiology
The major risk factors for adrenal hemorrhage or infarction are anticoagulant therapy, coagulopathy, or blunt abdominal trauma. Intra-adrenal bleeding may occur in severe septicemia – especially in children with *Pseudomonas aeruginosa* septicemia. Fulminating meningococcal septicemia may result in hemorrhagic destruction of both adrenal glands and is known as the Waterhouse–Friderichsen syndrome, most often occurring in children and young adults. These patients present with extensive purpura, meningitis, prostration, and shock. Regardless of the etiology, if acute adrenal failure is not recognized, diagnosed, and treated, it can progress to shock, coma, and death.

Signs and symptoms
Adrenal hemorrhage should be considered in the setting of circulatory collapse and known underlying infection, trauma, anticoagulant therapy (e.g. heparin or warfarin), or coagulopathy (e.g. antiphospholipid syndrome). Adrenal hemorrhage may be associated with upper back, flank, abdominal pain, fever, anorexia, nausea and vomiting, and confusion.

Diagnosis

Laboratory findings
Laboratory findings consistent with adrenal hemorrhage include a sudden fall in hemoglobin and hematocrit, hyperkalemia, hyponatremia, and volume contraction. Acute adrenal failure associated with adrenal infarction should be treated before laboratory confirmation (high serum corticotropin concentration and inappropriately low serum cortisol) becomes available.

Imaging tests
Computed adrenal imaging should be obtained in those patients with localizing symptoms (e.g. pain in the flanks, upper back, or abdomen). Computed tomography (CT) in this setting shows enlarged mixed density adrenal glands that do not enhance with contrast administration (Fig. 3.36a). With time the hemorrhagic adrenal glands shrink and become atrophic (Fig. 3.36b). Occasionally the hemorrhagic adrenal may not involute and it develops an eggshell calcification pattern (Fig. 3.37).

Treatment
Acute adrenal failure or adrenal crisis is an endocrine emergency and fatal if untreated. Empiric treatment for possible adrenal failure should be considered in all severely ill patients with shock that is refractory to volume expansion and pressor agents.

The therapeutic approach to acute adrenal insufficiency should include:
• Hydrocortisone sodium succinate at a dose of 100 mg administered intravenously as a bolus.
• Rapid intravascular volume repletion with dextrose in isotonic saline (approx. 2–4 L over the first 4 h) depending on the degree of dehydration, presence of other cardiovascular or renal disorders, and the clinical response.
• Diagnostic assessments for the precipitating cause (e.g. infection).
• Frequent monitoring of serum electrolytes, acid–base balance, blood glucose level, and renal function.
The dosage of hydrocortisone sodium succinate is continued at 100 mg intravenously every 6–8 hours until remission of the underlying illness; the dosage may then be decreased by 50% per day until maintenance dosages are achieved.

Illustrations (Figs 3.36 & 3.37)

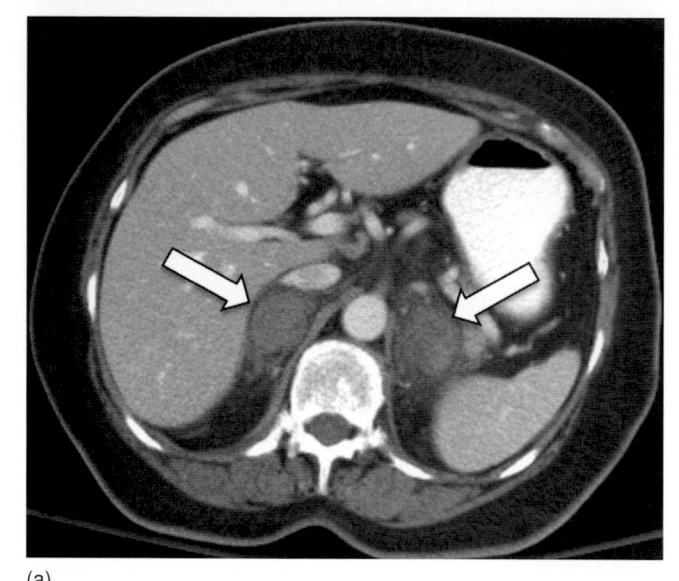

(a)

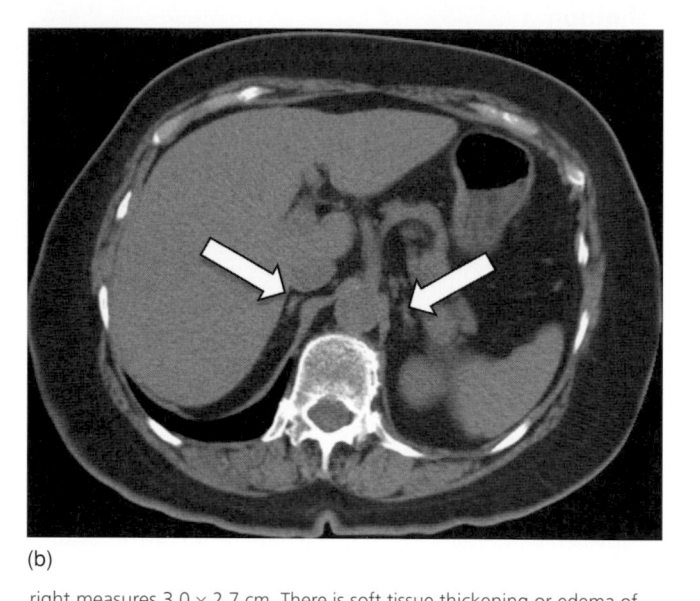

(b)

Figure 3.36 Computed tomography (CT) (axial views) images from a 68-year-old woman who recently started warfarin therapy. (a) CT obtained when the patient presented with bilateral flank pain and signs and symptoms of acute adrenal failure. Bilateral heterogeneous adrenal masses are seen (arrows); the left adrenal mass measures 3.2 × 2.6 cm and the right measures 3.0 × 2.7 cm. There is soft tissue thickening or edema of the adjacent mesenteric fat. After contrast administration, there is minimal enhancement. (b) This CT image was obtained 3 years following the adrenal hemorrhage and atrophic adrenal glands are seen (arrows). The patient had permanent primary adrenal insufficiency.

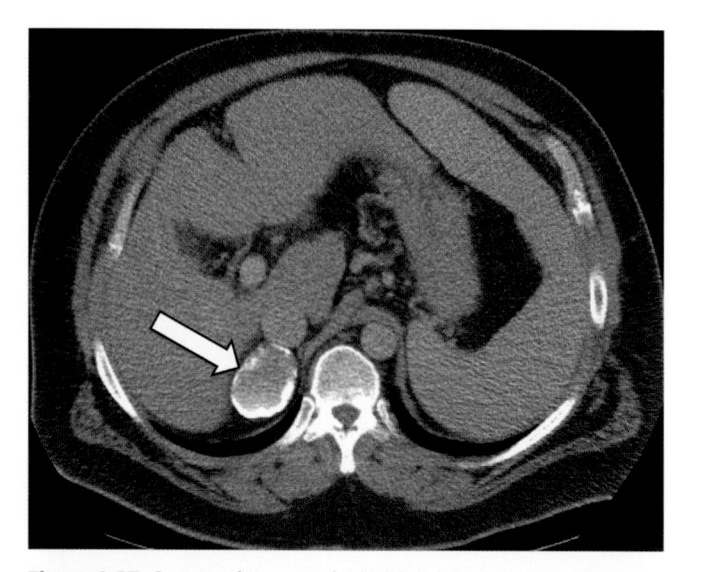

Figure 3.37 Computed tomography (CT) (axial view) image from a patient with distant history of right adrenal hemorrhage. Note the residual right adrenal mass (arrow) and eggshell calcification.

Tumors metastatic to the adrenal glands

Definition
Metastatic disease to the adrenal glands is common. Although the reason for its frequency is not clear, it likely relates to the high concentrations of glucocorticoids and the rich sinusoidal blood supply.

Etiology
At autopsy, adrenal metastases are found in 50% of patients with disseminated breast or lung cancer, in 30% of patients with melanoma, and in 15% of patients with colon or stomach cancer. When present, adrenal metastases are bilateral in approximately half of the cases (Fig. 3.38). However, clinically evident adrenal metastases or adrenal insufficiency is seen in only 4% of patients with tumors metastatic to the adrenal glands because most of the adrenal cortex of both adrenal glands must be destroyed before hypofunction becomes symptomatic. The most common organ locations for the primary malignancy (in order of frequency) are: lung, stomach, kidney, breast, colon, skin (melanoma), and pancreas. Adrenal metastases from primary tumors of the esophagus, liver, and bile ducts are more common in individuals of Asian ancestry.

Signs and symptoms
Prior to the advent of computed abdominal imaging the most common clinical presentation of metastatic disease to the adrenal glands was an insidious onset of signs and symptoms related to primary adrenal insufficiency (e.g. fatigue, myalgias, nausea, anorexia, orthostatic hypotension, hyper-pigmentation) or flank pain. However, with the widespread use of computed imaging and positron emission tomography (PET) in staging malignancies, asymptomatic metastases to the adrenal glands are becoming more commonly detected during life. In approximately 70% of cases, the adrenal metastasis is discovered concurrently with the primary malignancy – in the remaining patients, the adrenal metastases are typically found over a median duration of 7–30 months after the detection of the primary tumor.

Diagnosis
Accurate identification of the type of metastatic lesion usually relies on image-guided fine needle aspiration biopsy (Fig. 3.39b). The possibility of an incidentally discovered adrenal pheochromocytoma should be excluded with biochemical tests before proceeding with any biopsy procedure. Most of these patients have metastatic disease to sites in addition to the adrenal glands.

Treatment
Metastatic disease to the adrenal glands is a poor prognostic sign – the 1-year mortality is 80%. However, patients with adrenal metastases that are removed surgically have better survival rates than patients who do not have surgery. Percutaneous needlescopic adrenal ablative therapy has been used for the management of small (e.g. < 5 cm in largest lesional diameter) adrenal masses. Needlescopic ablation offers an effective minimally morbid intervention for patients who are poor surgical candidates. Ablative techniques include radiofrequency ablation, cryoablation, and chemical ablation. Most of these procedures can be performed under percutaneous radiographic guidance in the outpatient setting.

Illustrations (Figs 3.38 & 3.39)

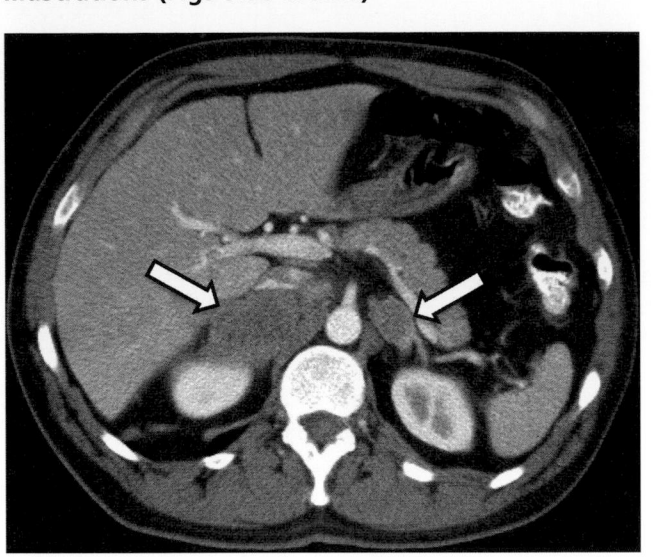

Figure 3.38 Computed tomography (CT) (axial view) image shows bilateral heterogeneous adrenal masses (arrows) with indistinct margins, which proved to be due to metastatic breast cancer.

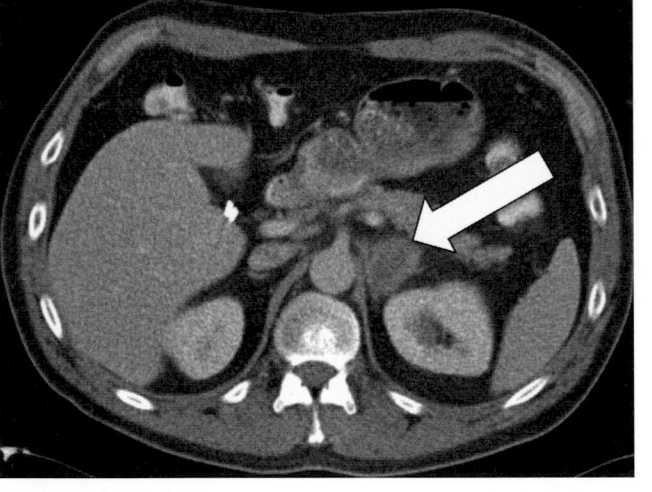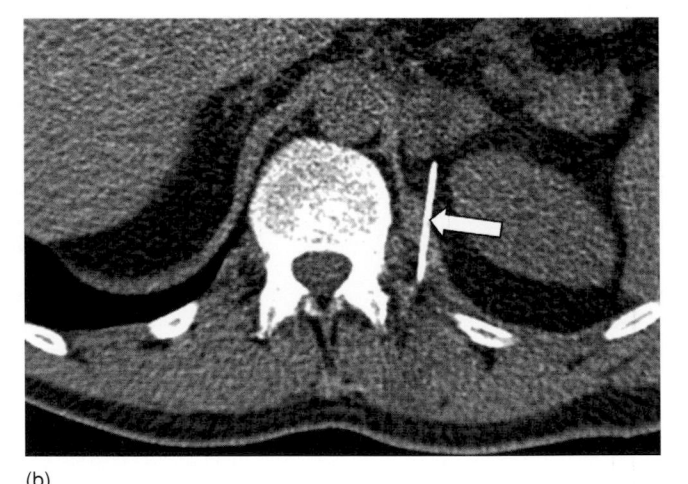

(a)   (b)

Figure 3.39 (a) Computed tomography (CT) (axial view) image showing a 3.3 cm inhomogeneous and irregularly shaped left adrenal mass (large arrow). (b) Fine needle aspiration biopsy (small arrow points to the needle) shows findings consistent with metastatic nonsmall cell lung cancer.

4   Pancreas

Diabetes

Diabetes and cardiovascular disease

Definition and pathogenesis
The most important long-term effects of diabetes mellitus manifest principally in the cardiovascular system in the form of accelerated atherosclerosis and hyaline arteriosclerosis (diabetic macroangiopathy).

People with diabetes are two to four times more likely to develop cardiovascular disease (CVD) than people without diabetes, making it the most common complication of diabetes.

Etiology
Smoking, high cholesterol, high blood pressure, stress from social inequality and oppressive work environments, poor diet, and abdominal fat all increase the likelihood of CVD events in people living with diabetes and impaired glucose tolerance.

Signs and symptoms

Symptoms
Patients with diabetes and CVD are often asymptomatic, especially women. The following are common symptoms:
• Any complaint of chest discomfort (from mid-abdomen to jaw) on exertion. Description of chest discomfort may vary depending on age, gender, education, ethnicity, and duration of diabetes
• Any limitation in walking or decreased exercise tolerance
• Snoring or sleep disturbance
• Increasing fatigue in people middle-aged or older
• Erectile dysfunction in younger men

Examination and testing
Tests of cognition, such as the Mini-Mental Exam, should be part of the intake exam for patients with diabetes and CVD who are at great risk of cognitive decline over time.

During a physical examination, the following signs may found:
• Blood pressure > 135/80, resting heart rate > 80 bpm, respiratory rate > 15
• Corneal arcus
• Poor dentition / periodontal disease
• Stiff blood vessels
• Increased pulse pressure (> 50 mmHg)
• Carotid bruit or murmur of aortic stenosis
• A loud S4 or any S3 gallop
• Signs of neuropathy
• Decreased ankle or knee jerks
• Decreased pedal pulses
• Ulcerations or severe calluses on the feet

Screening
Screening should include:
• *Clinical suspicion:* Those at highest risk of future cardiovascular events are those with previous history of heart failure or stroke.
• *History:* Family history of early onset CVD (< 55 years in men, < 65 years in women) is an important risk factor. Drawing a family pedigree for diabetes and heart disease is important during initial assessment.
• *Laboratory findings*: Measure non-fasting total cholesterol and high-density lipoprotein (HDL) cholesterol and their ratio. A ratio of > 3 : 1 is associated with progression of carotid intimal thickness. High-sensitivity C-reactive protein (HSCRP) testing may be helpful in people with intermediate CVD risk.
• *Imaging tests:* Electrocardiogram (ECG), stress testing

Imaging in Endocrinology, First Edition. Paolo Pozzilli, Andrea Lenzi, Bart L Clarke and William F Young Jr.
© 2014 John Wiley & Sons, Ltd. Published 2014 by John Wiley & Sons, Ltd.

Diagnosis

Clinical presentation

The most important clinical manifestations of diabetic vascular disease can be divided into three groups:

• *Coronary heart disease*: Angina (including silent ischemia), heart attack (including silent heart attack), sudden death, heart failure, fainting attacks

• *Cerebrovascular disease*: Stroke, transient ischemic attack, dementia

• *Peripheral vascular disease*: Gangrene, intermittent claudication, foot ulcers

Imaging tests

The following imaging tests are useful for diagnosis (Figs 4.1–4.5):

• Echocardiography for left ventricular hypertrophy, left ventricle size, and function.

• Carotid ultrasound for intimal thickness (Fig. 4.1).

• Coronary computed tomography (CT) can be a useful imaging test to establish coronary risk for those at intermediate risk (this includes all people with diabetes above age 45) (Fig. 4.5a). Coronary artery calcium (CAC) scores directly measure coronary artery disease burden.

• Coronary angiography (Fig. 4.3 & Fig. 4.5b)

Treatment

Optimize risk factors:

• *Smoking cessation*

• *Blood pressure* < 130/85 (although there is limited data on the efficacy for lower blood pressure in elderly patients who may become orthostatic)

• *Lipids*: Ratio of total cholesterol to HDL cholesterol < 3 : 1, low-density lipoprotein (LDL) < 100 mg/dL (target for people with known CVD is probably < 70 mg/dL)

• *Triglycerides* < 150 mg/dL (for people with known disease, target probably < 100 mg/dL)

• *A1C* < 7.0 (benefits for reducing risk of CVD below this level are uncertain)

• *Weight loss*

• *Lifestyle modification* (diet and exercise)

• *Antiaggregant therapy*: Indicated in anyone with a history of CVD and in people with diabetes who have > 10% risk of CVD over the next 10 years

• *Revascularization*: Percutaneous transluminal coronary angioplasty or bypass surgery are two possible options

Illustrations (Figs 4.1–4.5)

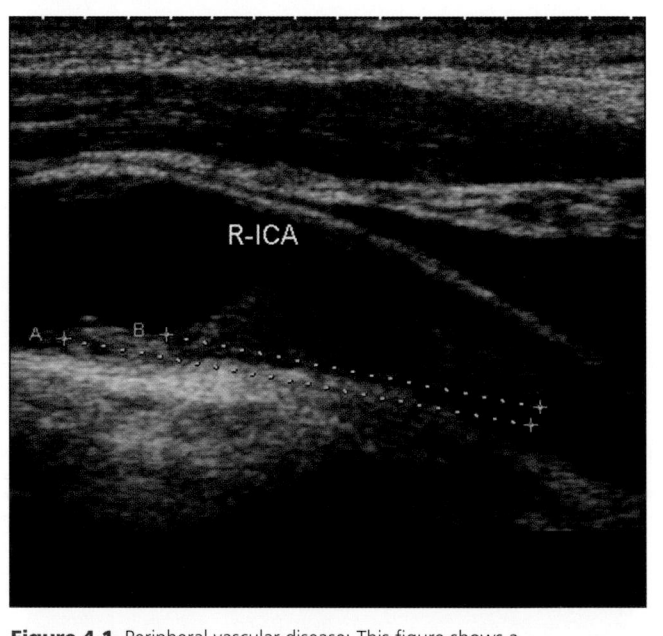

Figure 4.1 Peripheral vascular disease: This figure shows a hyperechogenic plaque in the bulb of the right internal carotid artery (R-ICA) determining a high-grade stenosis.

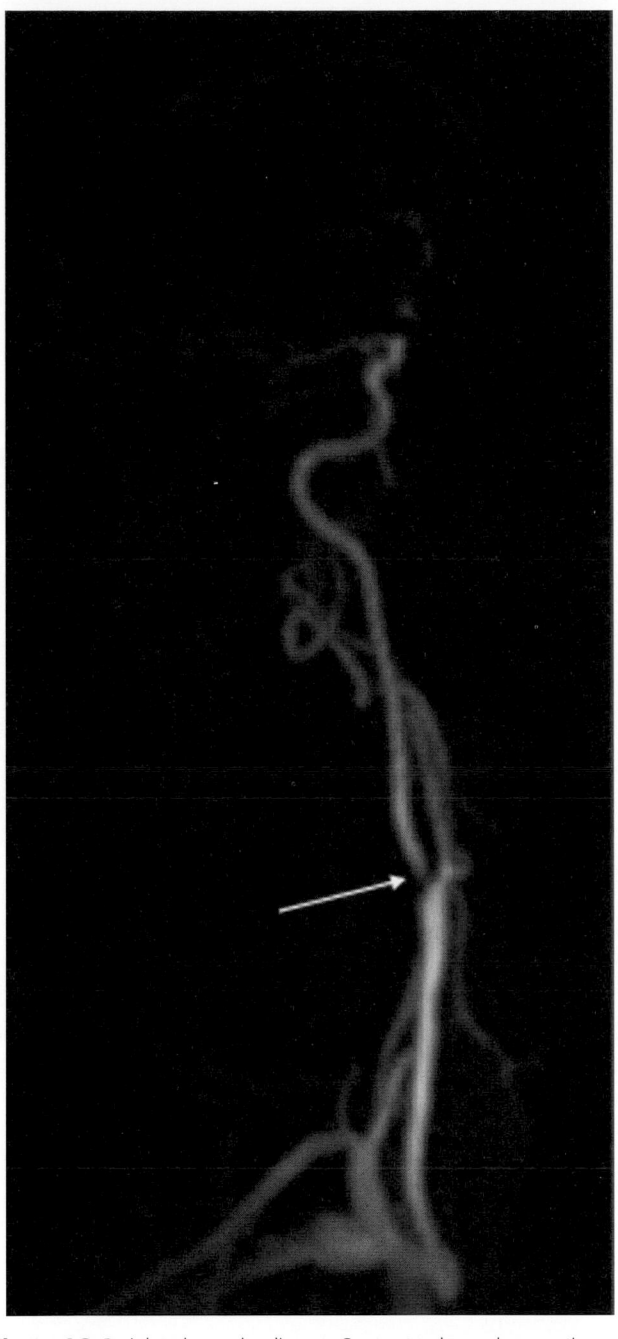

Figure 4.2 Peripheral vascular disease: Contrast-enhanced magnetic resonance (MR) angiogram with mixed integer programming (MIP) reconstruction shows a severe stenosis of the right internal carotid artery (white arrow).

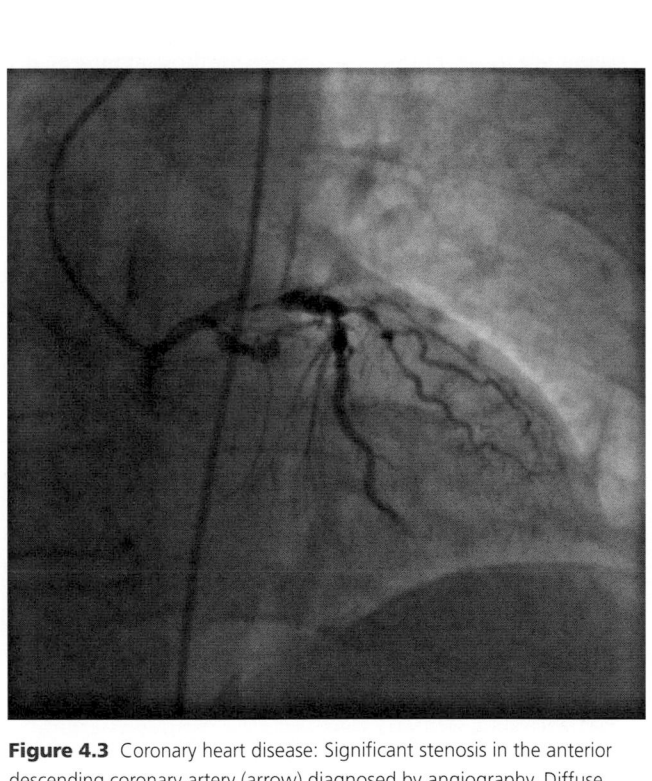

Figure 4.3 Coronary heart disease: Significant stenosis in the anterior descending coronary artery (arrow) diagnosed by angiography. Diffuse stenosis are also visible in the other coronary segment.

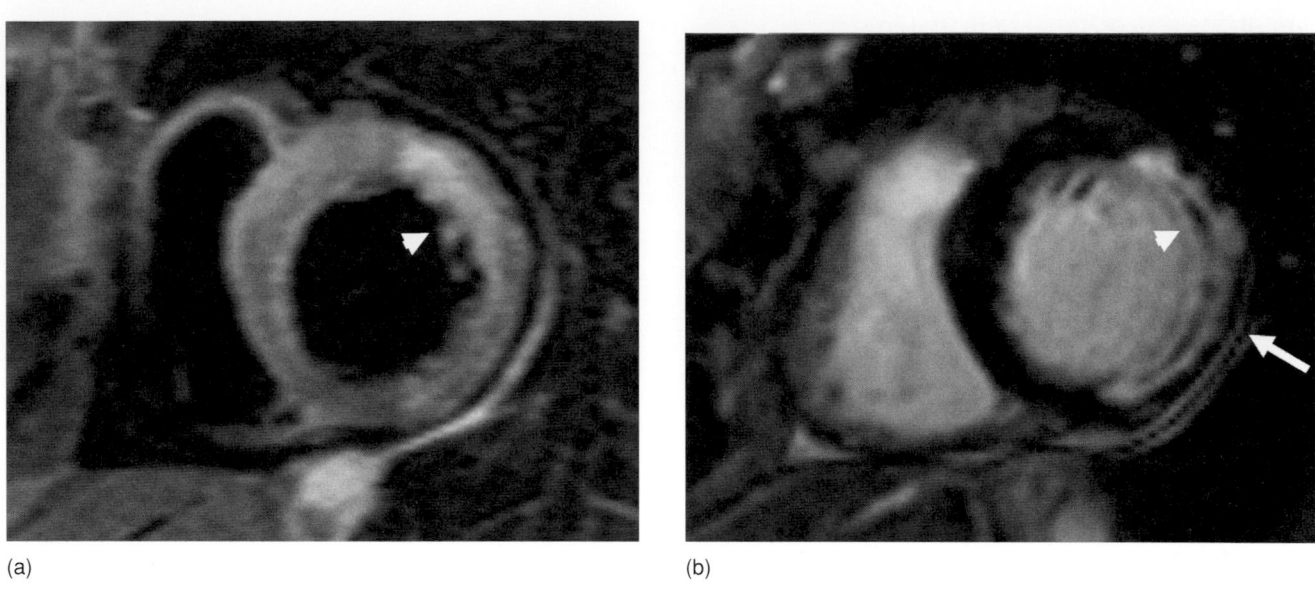

(a)   (b)

Figure 4.4 Acute myocardial infarction: (a) Subendocardial hyperintensity in the lateral wall (arrowhead) suggestive for myocardial edema. (b) Post-contrast late phase shows transmural late enhancement (arrow) of the lateral wall indicative of myocardial infarction. The subendocardial hypointense line (arrowhead) reveals a "no-reflow" phenomenon suggestive for microvascular obstruction.

Figure 4.5 Significant stenosis in the right coronary artery distal segment (arrow) diagnosed with coronary computed tomography (CT) (a) and confirmed by angiography (b). Diffuse atherosclerotic disease is also visible in the proximal coronary segment (a: arrowhead).

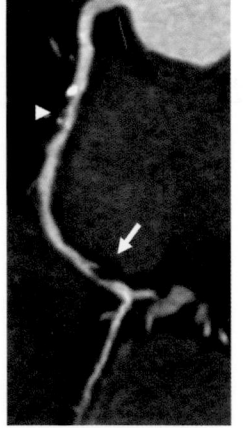

(a)

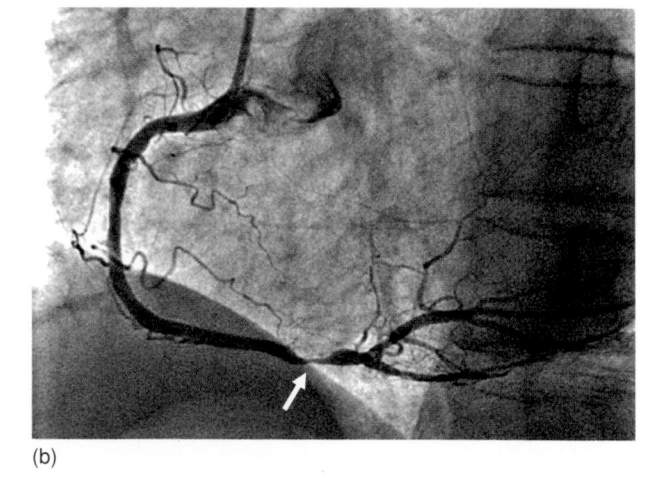

(b)

Skin diseases associated with diabetes

Definition
Skin diseases associated with diabetes can be divided into two main categories:
• *Diabetic dermopathy*, also known as shin spots or pigmented pretibial patches, is a skin condition usually found on the lower legs of people with diabetes.
• *Collagen disorders* such as necrobiosis lipoidica.

Etiology
Diabetic dermopathy is thought to result from changes in the small blood vessels that supply the skin and from minor leakage of blood products from these vessels into the skin.

Necrobiosis lipoidica is a disorder of collagen degeneration with a granulomatous response, thickening of blood vessel walls, and fat deposition. The exact cause of necrobiosis lipoidica is unknown, but the leading theory has focused on diabetic microangiopathy.

Signs and symptoms

Diabetic dermopathy
Diabetic dermopathy appears as pink to red or tan to dark-brown patches, which are found most frequently on the lower legs. The patches are slightly scaly and are usually round or oval. Long-standing patches may become faintly indented. They don't typically itch, burn, or sting (Fig. 4.6).

Possible locations are shins (the pretibial area), thighs, sides of feet, and forearms. Up to 50% of diabetics have shin spots and these are even more common in people with long-standing or poorly controlled diabetes.

Necrobiosis lipoidica
Patients usually present with asymptomatic shiny patches that slowly enlarge over months to years. The patches are initially red-brown and progress to yellow, depressed atrophic plaques. Ulcerations can occur typically after trauma and are occasionally associated with pain.

Classic skin lesions begin as 1–3 mm well-circumscribed papules or nodules that expand with an active border to become waxy, atrophic, round plaques centrally. Initially, these plaques are red-brown in color but progressively become more yellow and atrophic (Fig. 4.7).

Most cases of necrobiosis lipoidica occur on the pretibial area. The lesions of necrobiosis lipoidica are typically multiple and bilateral. In 75% of cases the lesions become painless because of cutaneous nerve damage, or in 25% of cases they can be extremely painful.

Diagnosis
Diagnosis is made through signs and symptoms (see above). There are no particular laboratory or imaging tests for making a diagnosis.

Treatment
The skin lesions of diabetic dermopathy often improve over time. Keeping the skin moisturized and trying to avoid any injury to the legs should help prevent the development of some lesions. Diabetic dermopathy is harmless and does not require any treatment.

Necrobiosis lipoidica can respond to topical or locally injected steroids.

Illustrations (Figs 4.6 & 4.7)

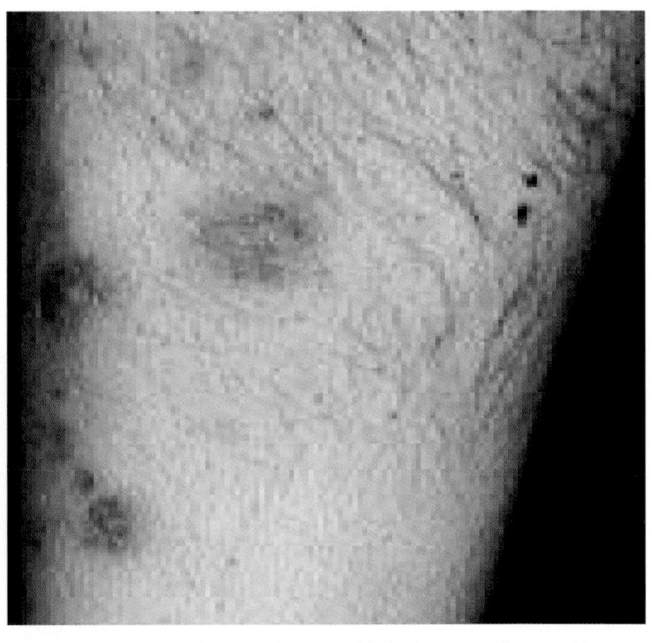

Figure 4.6 Diabetic dermopathy: Round light brown, scaly, atrophic patches on the skin of the lower leg.

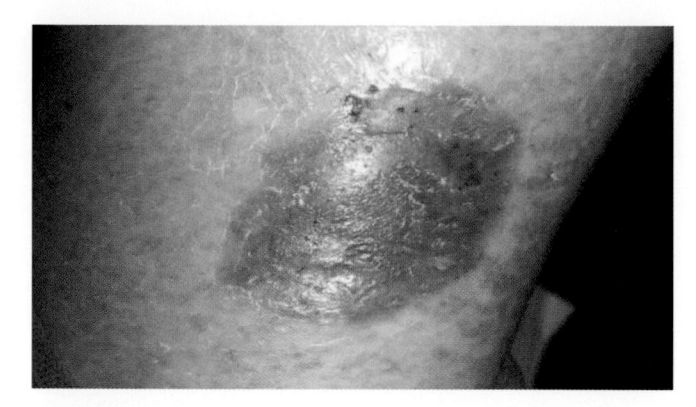

Figure 4.7 Necrobiosis lipoidica: Well-demarcated, atrophic, fibrotic yellowish-reddish-brown plaques with overlying telangiectasias.

Diabetic foot

Definition

The diabetic foot is defined by the World Health Organization as the foot of a diabetic patient that has the potential risk of pathologic consequences, including infection, ulceration, and/or destruction of deep tissues associated with neurologic abnormalities, various degrees of peripheral vascular disease, and/or metabolic complications of diabetes in the lower limb (WHO, *Adv Exp Med Biol* 2012;771:123–38). Ten to fifteen percent of diabetic patients develop foot ulcers at some point in their lives and foot-related problems are responsible for up to 50% of diabetes-related hospital admissions.

Pathophysiology and etiology

The pathophysiology of diabetic foot is divided into two categories:

• Damage to the nervous system
• Damage to blood vessels

Damage to the nervous system

People with long-standing or poorly controlled diabetes are at risk for peripheral neuropathy, which compromises the ability to feel the foot properly, and also impairs the normal sweat secretion and oil production that lubricates the skin. These factors together can lead to abnormal pressure on the skin, bones, and joints of the foot during walking and can lead to breakdown of the skin.

Damage to blood vessels

Wounds can be difficult to heal because of the poor blood flow, and so bacterial infection of the skin, connective tissues, muscles, and bones may then occur. These infections can also develop into gangrene because the antibiotics cannot get to the site of the infection easily. Many histopathologic studies show prolonged inflammatory phase in diabetic wounds, which causes delay in the formation of mature granulation tissue and a parallel reduction in wound tensile strength.

The combination of mechanical and vascular factors resulting from diabetic peripheral neuropathy may become Charchot osteoarthropathy (see below).

Signs and symptoms

History and physical examination should include the patient's vital signs (temperature, pulse, blood pressure, and respiratory rate), examination of the sensation in the feet and legs, an examination of the circulation in the feet and legs, and a thorough examination of any problem areas.

Vascular foot

The vascular foot has evidence of peripheral arterial disease signs such as absence of foot pulses, decrease in skin temperature, thin skin, lack of skin hair, and bluish skin color. However, these signs are neither sensitive nor specific enough to be helpful to an individual patient. The absence of pedal pulses, the presence of femoral bruits, or the prolongation of venous filling should prompt referral for more detailed evaluation. An ankle–brachial index (ABI) < 0.9 is very declarative of a vascular problem. Ischemic ulcers often occur on the great toe, medial and lateral surfaces of the forefoot, or on the heel.

Neuropathic foot

The foot needs evaluating for the presence of peripheral neuropathy, signs such as difficulty or absent capability to feel vibration, temperature, pressure sensation (monofilament), and superficial pain (pinprick) (Figs 4.8–4.12).

Deformation

The presence of a hammer toe can favor the formation of ulcers localized on metatarsal head of plantar side. Neuropathic ulcers often occur under the metatarsal heads, at the tips of the toes, or between the toes.

Charchot osteoarthropathy

Charchot osteoarthropathy is a chronic and progressive disease of bone and joints, defined by painful or relatively painless bone and joint destruction in limbs that have lost sensory innervation. It is characterized by pathologic fractures, joint dislocation, loss of plantar arches, overriding toes, and deformity. A common feature is bone reabsorption. The neuroarthropathy (Figs 4.13 & 4.14) is bilateral in about 20% of cases. The arthropathy is relatively painless. Although pain is often felt, the severity is less than might be expected from the clinical and radiologic appearance of the affected joint.

Diagnosis

Clinical stages
A widely used classification of diabetic foot ulcers is that proposed by Wagner:
• *Grade 0*: No ulcer in a high-risk foot (Fig. 4.8 & 4.9)
• *Grade 1*: Superficial ulcer involving the full skin thickness but not underlying tissues (Fig. 4.10)
• *Grade 2*: Deep ulcer, penetrating down to ligaments and muscle, but no bone involvement or abscess formation (Fig. 4.11)
• *Grade 3*: Deep ulcer with cellulitis or abscess formation, often with osteomyelitis (Fig 4.12)
• *Grade 4*: Localized gangrene (Fig. 4.15)
• *Grade 5*: Extensive gangrene involving the whole foot (Fig. 4.16 and see Fig. 4.22)

Laboratory findings
The following laboratory tests should be considered:
• Complete blood cell count in order to evaluate the potential infection
• Erythrocyte sedimentation rate (ESR)
• Polymerase chain reaction (PCR)

Imaging and diagnostic tests
The following imaging and diagnostic tests may be needed (Figs 4.17–4.19):
• Ankle–brachial index (ABI)
• Ultrasound
• X-ray
• Angiogram
• Contrast-enhanced magnetic resonance imaging (MRI)
• Contrast-enhanced Tc scan

Treatment
Treatment of the diabetic foot consists of the following points:
• Wearing sturdy, comfortable shoes whenever feasible to protect the feet.
• Regular exercise to improve bone and joint health in the feet and legs, improve circulation to the legs, and to also help to stabilize blood sugar levels.
• Good diabetes control
• Antibiotics
• Hyperbaric oxygen therapy
• Arterial revascularization (Figs 4.21 & 4.22)
• Amputation

Illustrations (Figs 4.8–4.22)

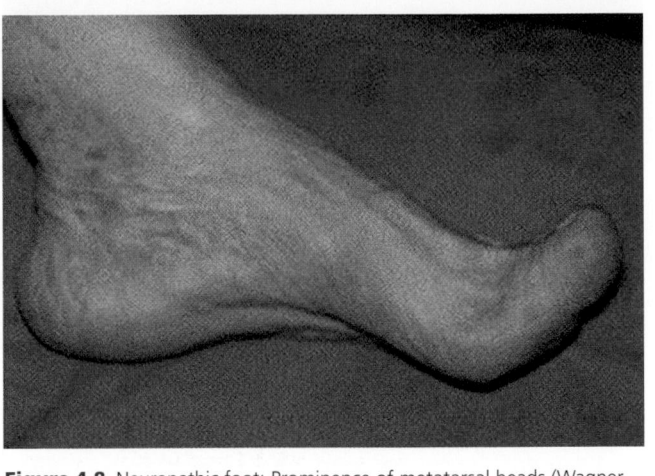

Figure 4.8 Neuropathic foot: Prominence of metatarsal heads (Wagner grade 0).

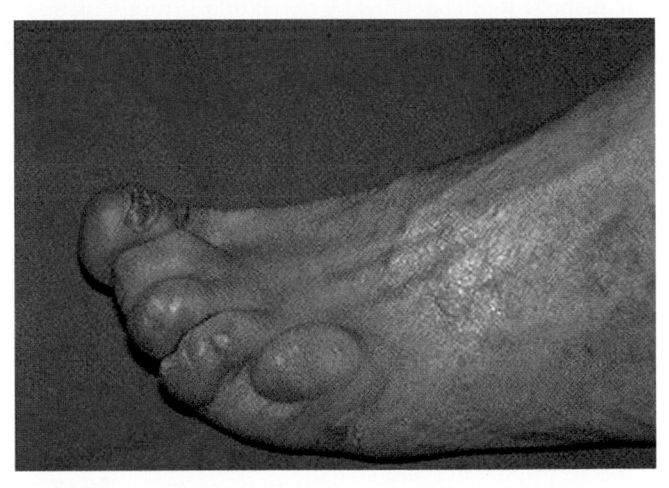

Figure 4.9 Neuropathic foot: Clawing toes and dilated foot veins indicating autonomic dysfunction (Wagner grade 0).

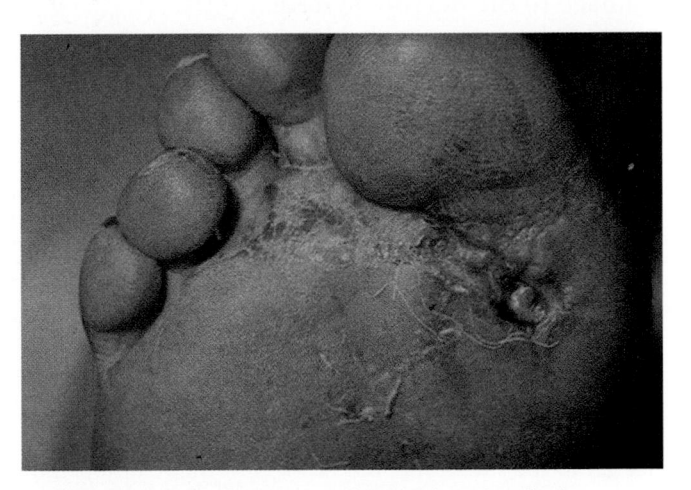

Figure 4.10 Neuropathic foot: Superficial skin breach under the metatarsal head (Wagner grade 1).

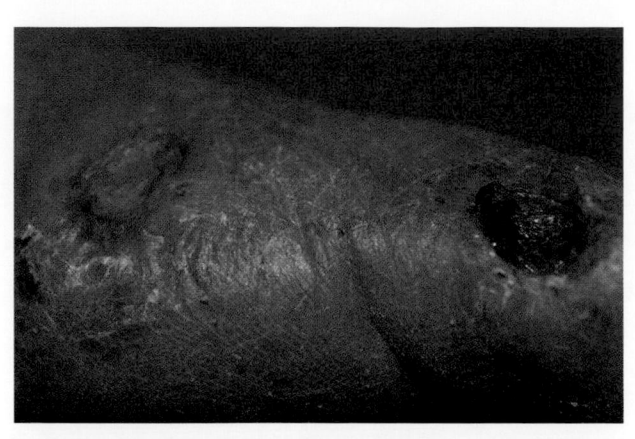

Figure 4.11 Neuropathic foot: Deep, punched-out ulcer on the lateral aspect of the foot with surrounding cellulitis (Wagner grade 2).

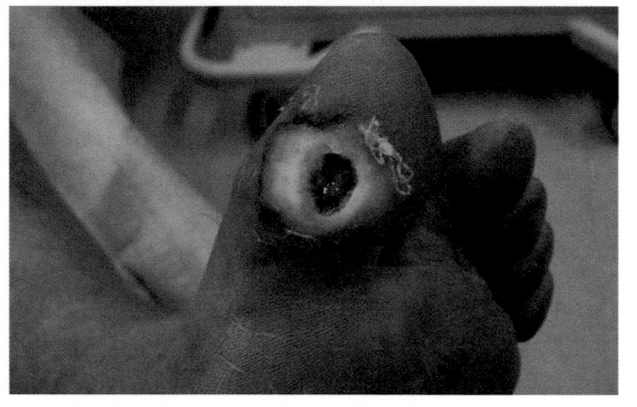

Figure 4.12 Neuropathic foot: Deep ulcer with abscess formation and bone involvement (Wagner grade 3).

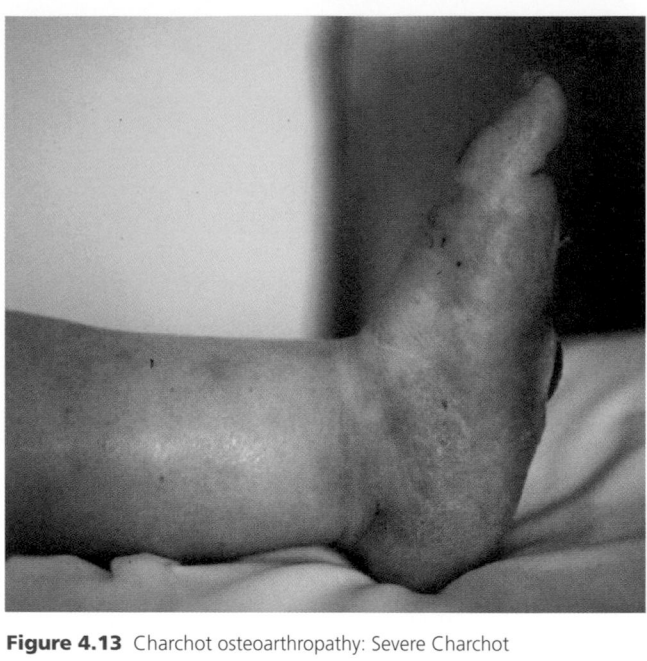

Figure 4.13 Charchot osteoarthropathy: Severe Charchot osteoarthropathy characterized by unilateral swelling, erythema, dry and flaking skin, collapse of the joints, and bone destruction of cuboid, navicular, and ankle bone.

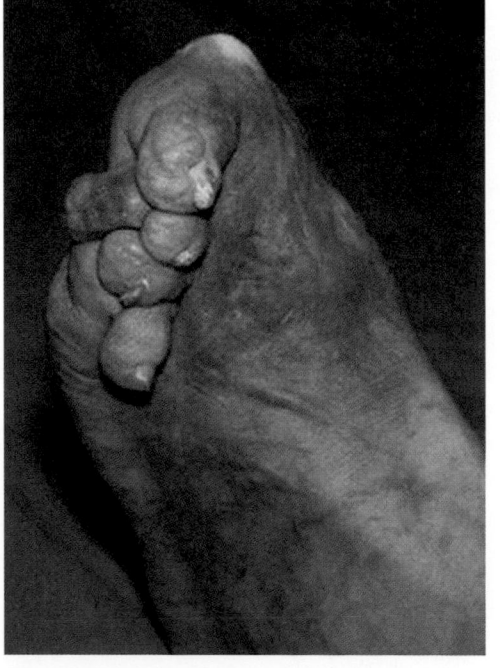

(a)

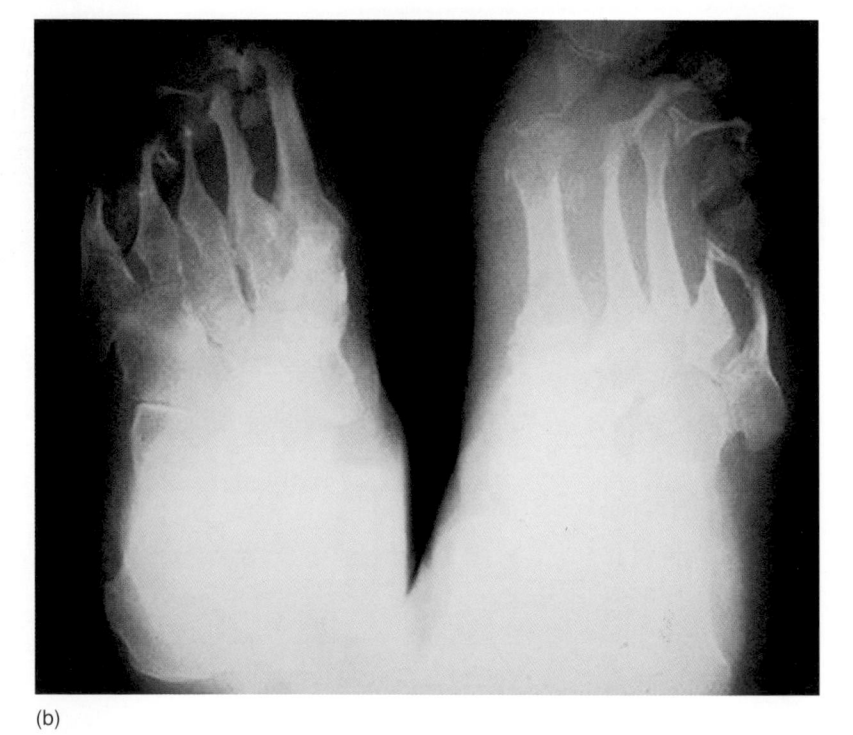

(b)

Figure 4.14 Charchot osteoarthropathy: Dilated foot veins indicated autonomic dysfunction and abnormal shape of the foot, such as a rocker bottom appearance with superimposition of the toes and general deformity.

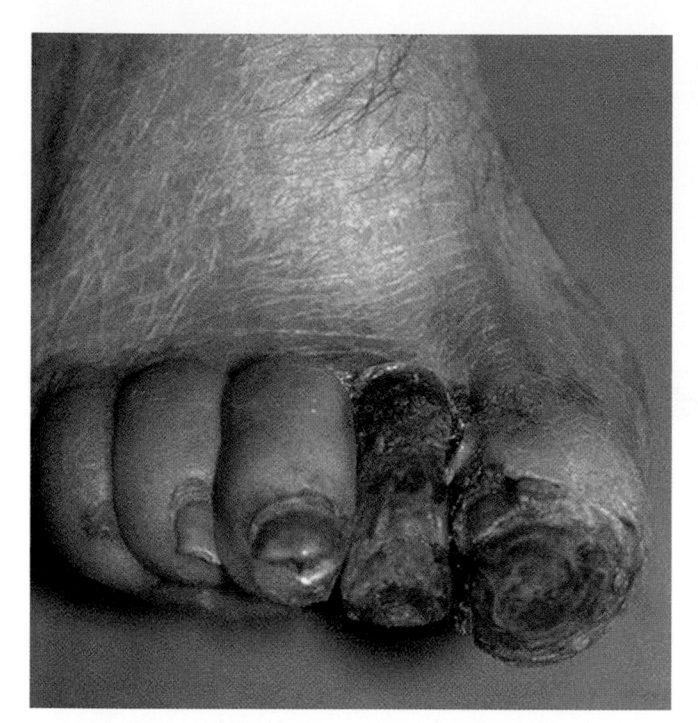

Figure 4.15 Vasculopathic foot: Localized toe gangrene with dry and flaking skin (Wagner grade 4).

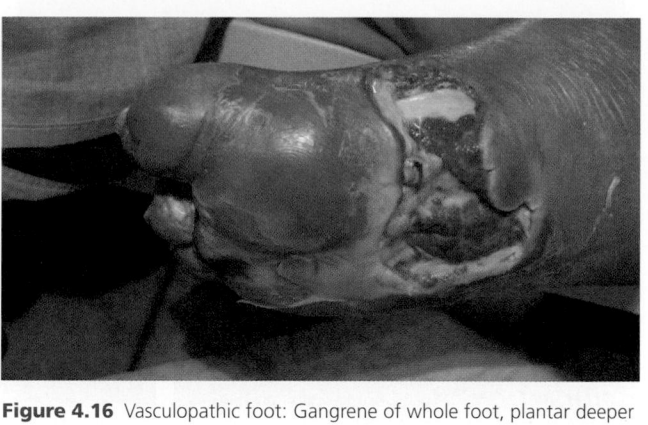

Figure 4.16 Vasculopathic foot: Gangrene of whole foot, plantar deeper ulcer with abscess formation and bone involvement. Erythema, purulent discharge and crepitation indicate the presence of a gas-forming organism.

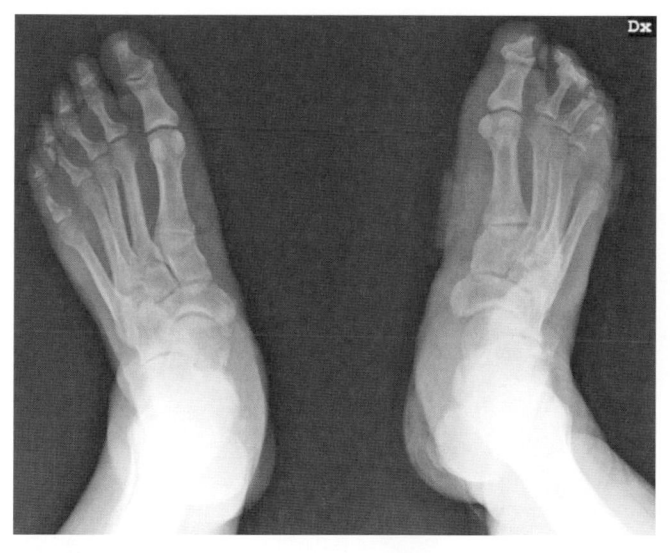

Figure 4.17 Vasculopathic foot: Bone involvement (osteomyelitis) of the distal phalange of right great toe (red arrow).

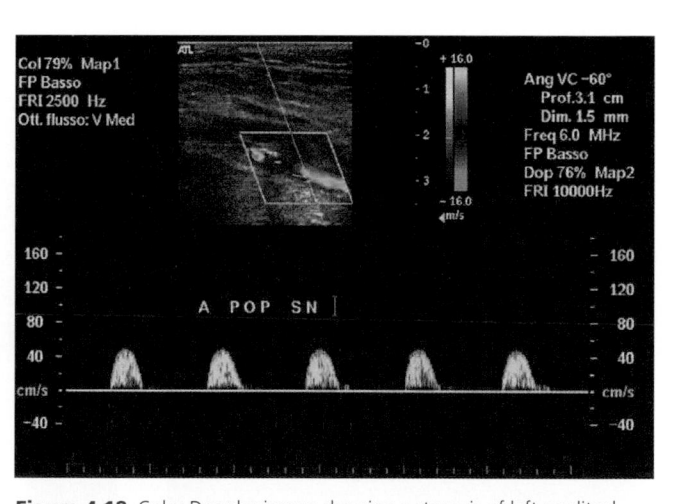

Figure 4.18 Color Doppler image showing a stenosis of left popliteal artery. There is low peak systolic velocity (< 50 cm/s) and absent diastolic forward flow.

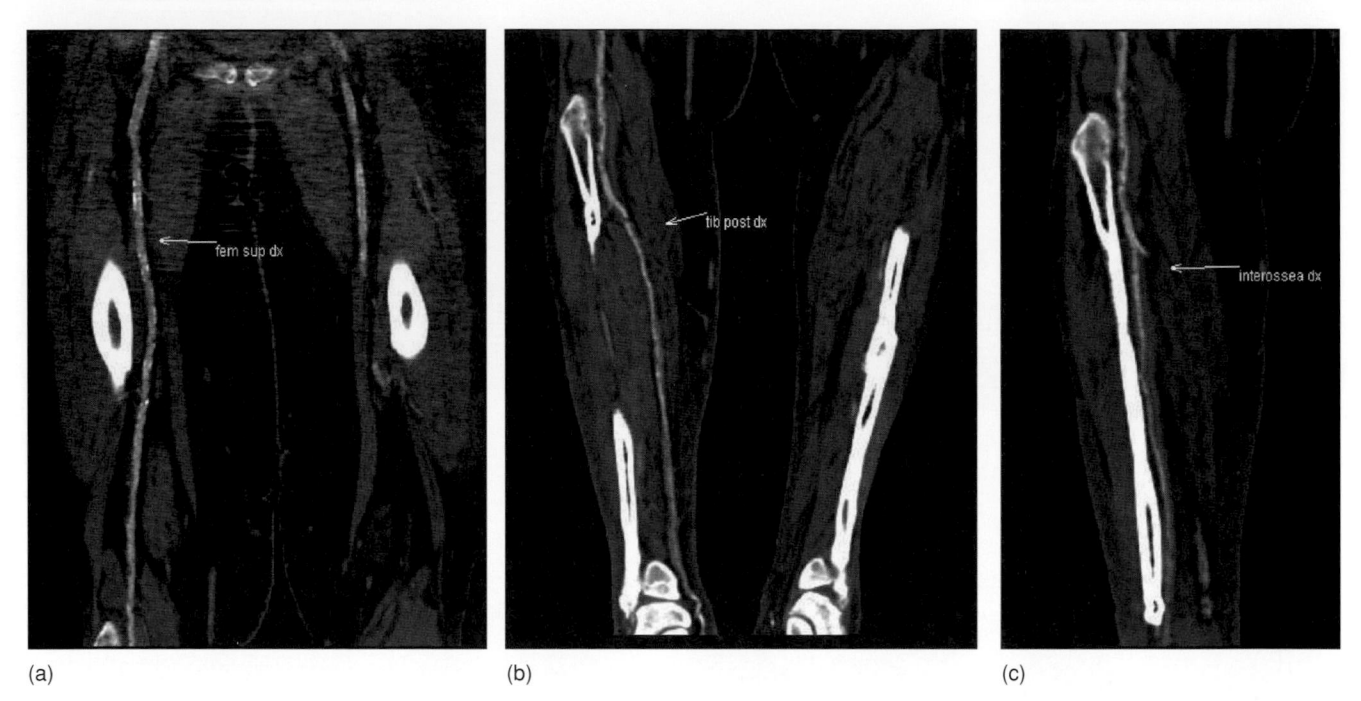

(a)   (b)   (c)

Figure 4.19 Computed tomography (CT) angiogram shows multiple stenosis of right femoral artery (a); occlusion of proximal part of right posterior tibial (b); and interosseous artery (c).

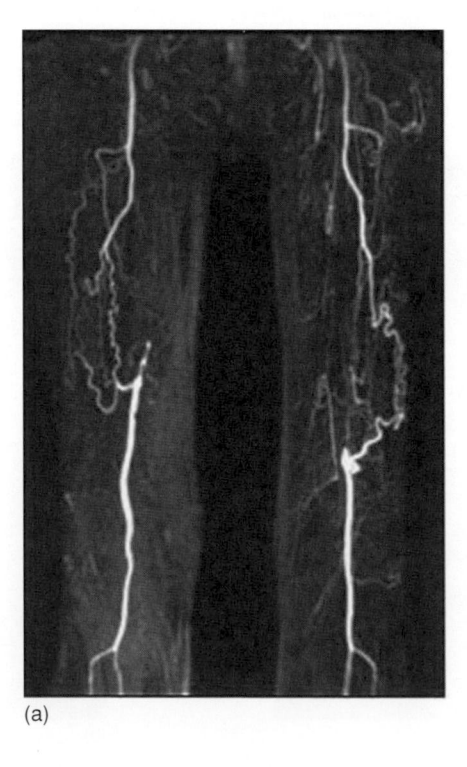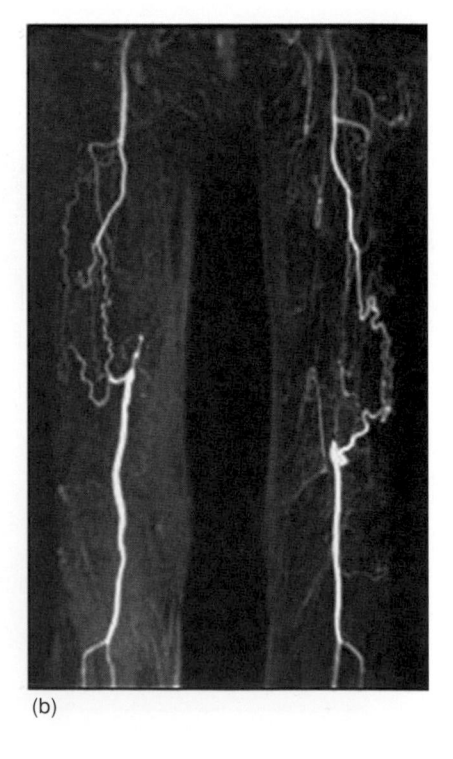

Figure 4.20 Axial T-1-weighted magnetic resonance images (a & b) demonstrate bilateral occlusion of superficial femoral artery.

(a)   (b)

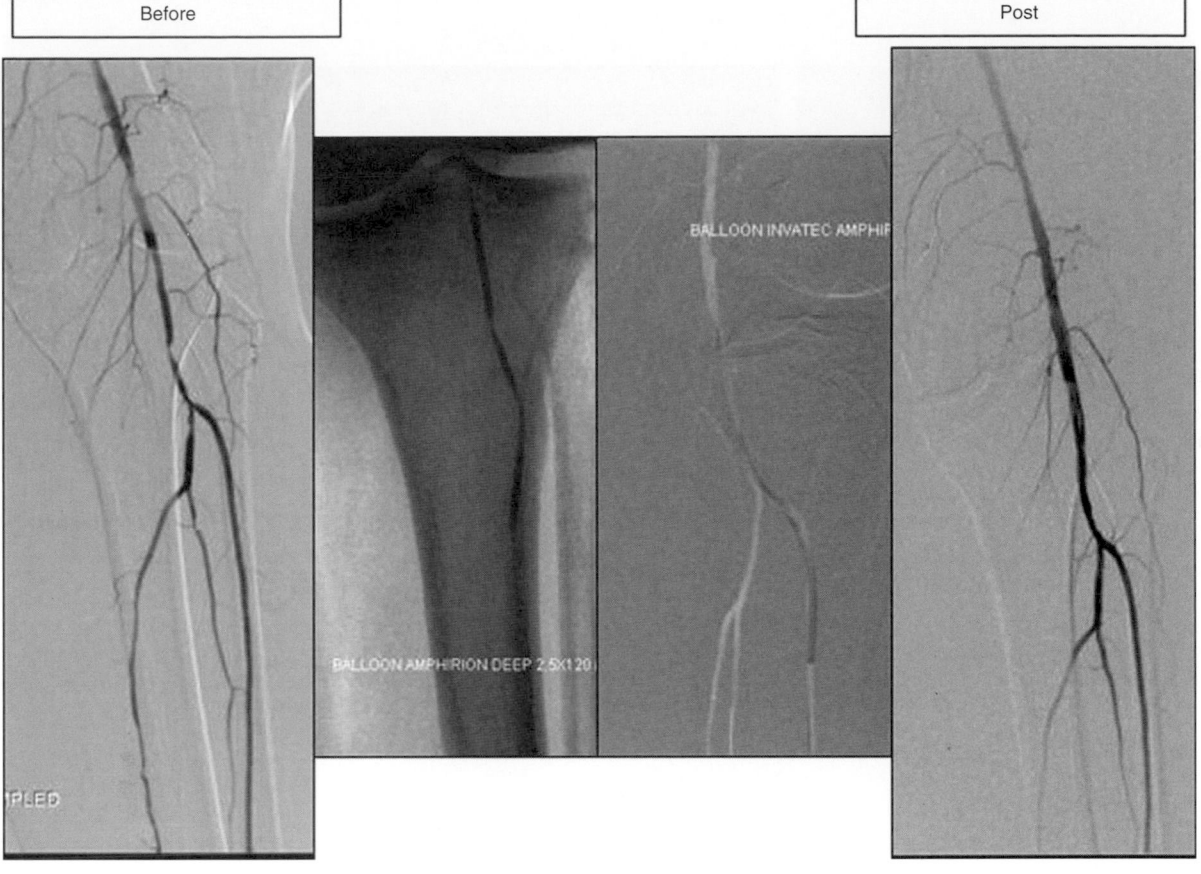

Before

Post

Figure 4.21 Arteriogram shows high-grade focal lesions of right femoral artery and occlusion of proximal part of right posterior tibial artery before angioplasty. Arteriogram obtained after angioplasty demonstrates good treatment results.

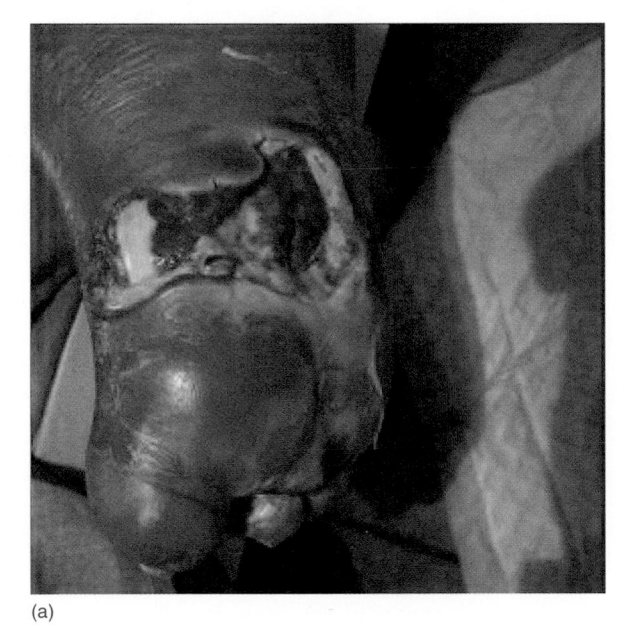

(a)

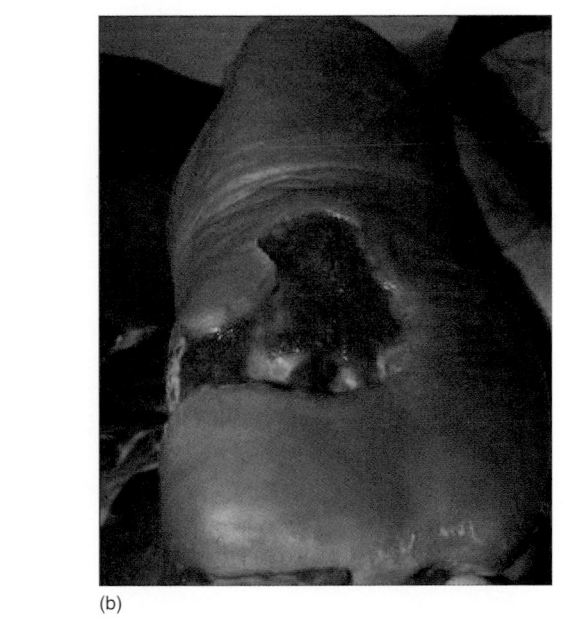

(b)

Figure 4.22 Gangrene of whole foot (a), plantar deeper ulcer with erythema, crepitation, abscess formation, and bone involvement (Wagner grade 5) before percutaneous angioplasty. After treatment (b): Wagner grade 3.

Diabetic neuropathy

Definition

Disorders of peripheral nerves are among the most frequent neurologic complications of diabetes. It can affect multiple sensory and motor nerves in distal parts of the limbs (diabetic polyneuropathy) or affect one nerve at a time (diabetic mononeuropathy). It can also primarily affect the autonomic nerves and cause diabetic autonomic neuropathy.

Etiology

The proximate cause of diabetic neuropathy is a length-dependent "dying back" axonopathy, primarily involving the distal portions of the longest myelinated and unmyelinated sensory axons, with relative sparing of motor axons. Morphologic abnormalities of the vaso nervorum are present early in the course of the disease and parallel the severity of the nerve fiber loss.

Evidence is accumulating to suggest that metabolic and ischemic factors interact with nerve repair mechanisms to cause diabetic polyneuropathy.

Diabetic neuropathy is classified into distinct clinical syndromes. The most frequently encountered neuropathies are described below.

Distal symmetric polyneuropathy

Peripheral neuropathy, also called sensor–motor neuropathy, is nerve damage in the arms and legs. Feet and legs are likely to be affected before hands and arms. The patient may experience unusual sensations (paresthesias), numbness, and pain in their hands and feet. In addition, there may be weakness of the muscles in the feet and hands.

Autonomic neuropathy

Autonomic neuropathy can affect any organ of the body, from the gastrointestinal system to the skin, and its appearance portends a marked increase in the mortality risk of diabetic patients. The patients may experience persistent nausea, vomiting, diarrhea, constipation, incontinence, sweating abnormalities, or sexual dysfunction.

The diagnosis of diabetic autonomic neuropathy is one of exclusion, and many other causes of autonomic dysfunction should first be ruled out (cancer, drug use, alcohol use, HIV exposure, *Trypanosoma cruzi*, and amyloidosis).

Individual cranial and peripheral nerve involvement

Individual cranial and peripheral nerve involvement causes focal mononeuropathies, especially affecting the oculomotor nerve (cranial nerve III) and the median nerve.

Thoracic and lumbar nerve root disease

Thoracic and lumbar nerve root disease causes polyradiculopathies

Asymmetric involvement of multiple peripheral nerves

Asymmetric involvement of multiple peripheral nerves results in a mononeuropathy multiplex.

Diagnosis

Along with the signs and symptoms (above), no particular laboratory tests are needed but the following imaging tests may be useful (Figs 4.23 & 4.24):
• Electroneurography
• Electromyography
• Ultrasound

In addition, quantitative sensory testing and/or nerve or skin biopsy may be needed.

Treatment

Treatment of diabetic neuropathy is as follows:
• The most important treatment of diabetic neuropathy is its prevention by optimal glucose control.
• Duloxetine and pregabalin are the only drugs formally approved by the European Medicines Agency and by the US Food and Drug Administration for the treatment of painful diabetic polyneuropathy.
• Alpha lipoic acid is an antioxidant used to improve the underlying pathophysiology of neuropathy and to reduce pain.
• Transcutaneous electrical nerve stimulation is a possible treatment for patients who continue to have pain despite combination drug therapy.

Illustrations (Figs 4.23 & 4.24)

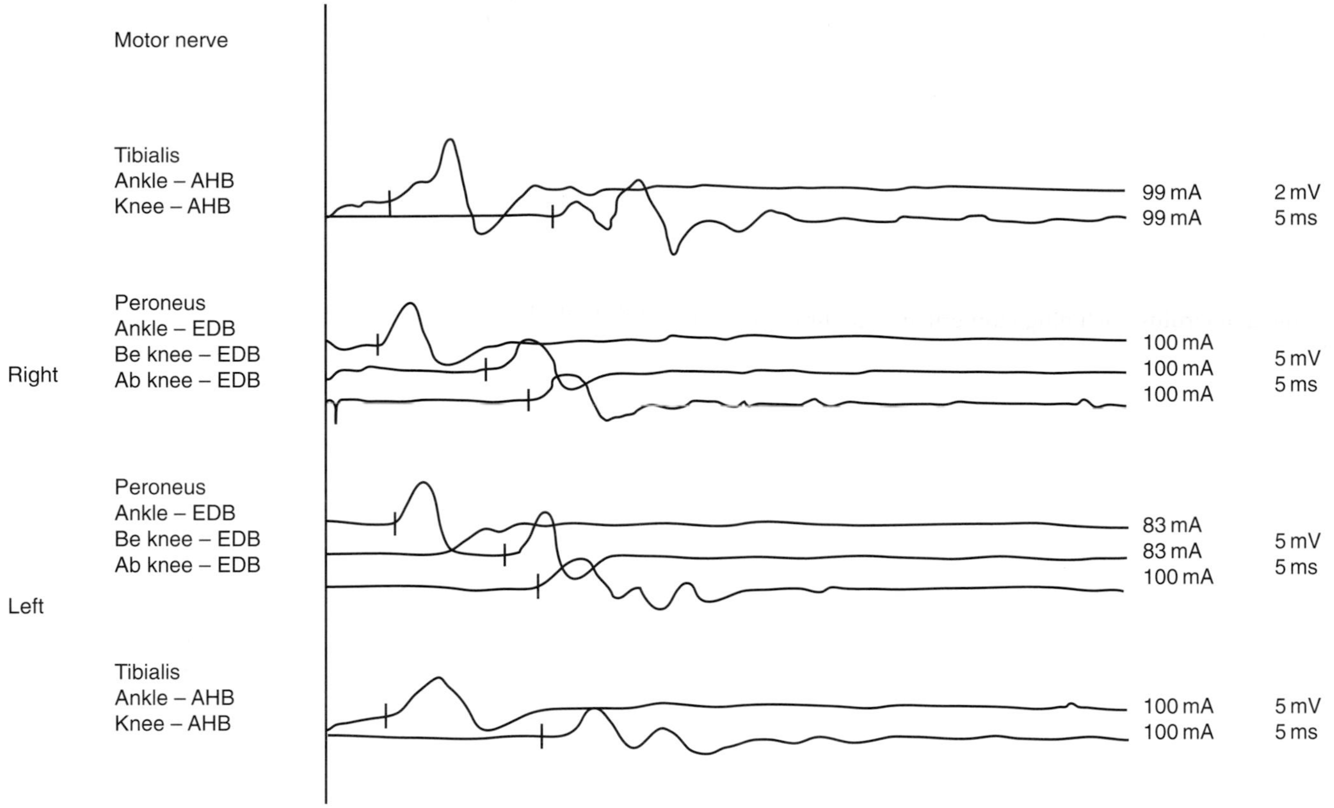

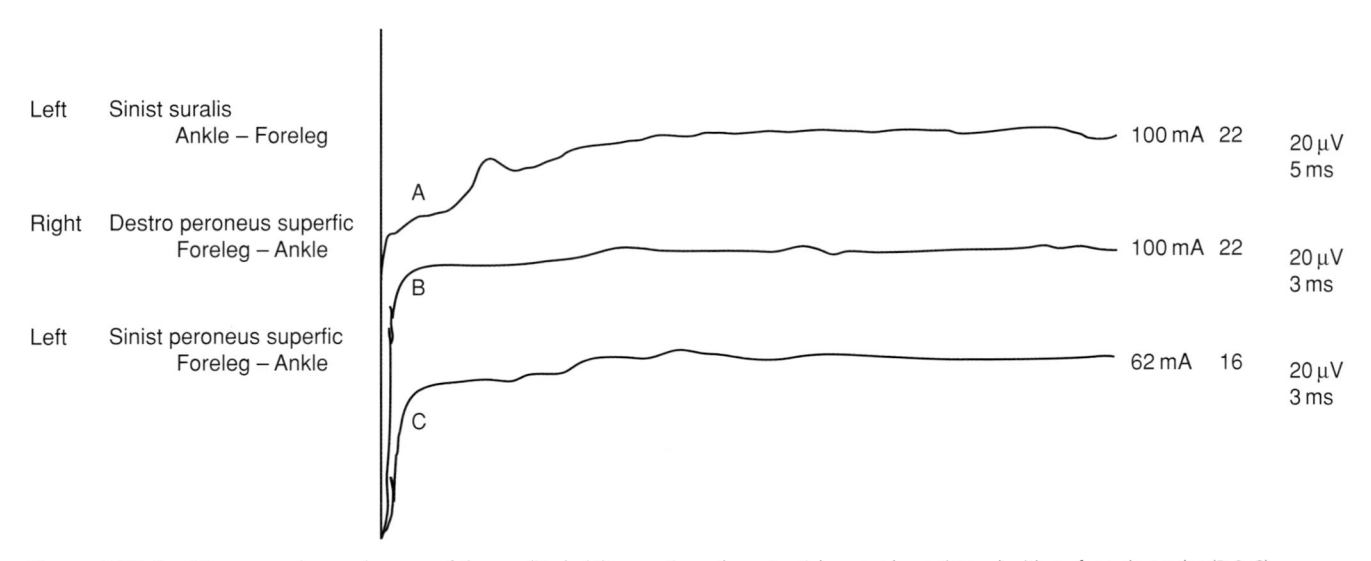

Motor nerve

Tibialis
Ankle – AHB
Knee – AHB

Right

Peroneus
Ankle – EDB
Be knee – EDB
Ab knee – EDB

Left

Peroneus
Ankle – EDB
Be knee – EDB
Ab knee – EDB

Tibialis
Ankle – AHB
Knee – AHB

99 mA · 2 mV
99 mA · 5 ms

100 mA · 5 mV
100 mA · 5 ms
100 mA

83 mA · 5 mV
83 mA · 5 ms
100 mA

100 mA · 5 mV
100 mA · 5 ms

Figure 4.23 Electroneurography: Distal symmetric polyneuropathy. Motor nerves show a decrease of amplitude and the spreading of the potential in time; generally, potential velocity is conserved or slightly decreased.

Left — Sinist suralis
Ankle – Foreleg

Right — Destro peroneus superfic
Foreleg – Ankle

Left — Sinist peroneus superfic
Foreleg – Ankle

A

B

C

100 mA 22 · 20 μV · 5 ms

100 mA 22 · 20 μV · 3 ms

62 mA 16 · 20 μV · 3 ms

Figure 4.24 Sensitive nerves show a decrease of the amplitude (A); sometimes the potential cannot be registered with surface electrodes (B & C). Generally potential velocity is conserved or slightly decreased.

Diabetic nephropathy

Definition

Diabetic nephropathy is a progressive kidney disease caused by the angiopathy of capillaries in the kidney glomeruli. It is characterized by nephrotic syndrome and diffuse glomerulosclerosis. It is due to longstanding diabetes mellitus and is a prime indication for dialysis in many Western countries.

Etiology

Diabetic nephropathy has several distinct phases of development. Functional changes occur in the nephron at the level of the glomerulus, including glomerular hyperfiltration and hyperperfusion, before the onset of any measurable clinical changes. Subsequently, thickening of the glomerular basement membrane, glomerular hypertrophy, and mesangial expansion take place.

Multiple mechanisms contribute to the development and outcomes of diabetic nephropathy, such as an interaction between hyperglycemia-induced metabolic and hemodynamic changes and genetic predisposition, which sets the stage for kidney injury.

Signs and symptoms

Throughout its early course, diabetic nephropathy has no symptoms. Symptoms develop in the late stages and may be a result of excretion of high amounts of protein in the urine or due to renal failure. The symptoms are:
- Edema
- Foamy appearance or excessive frothing of the urine (caused by the proteinura)
- Unintentional weight gain (from fluid accumulation)
- Anorexia
- Nausea and vomiting
- Malaise
- Fatigue
- Headache
- Frequent hiccups
- Generalized itching

Diagnosis

In the screening and diagnosis of diabetic nephropathy, the first step is to measure albumin in a spot urine sample. In addition, serum creatinine and blood urea nitrogen (BUN) may be increased (as kidney damage progresses). A kidney biopsy confirms the diagnosis, although it is not always necessary if the case is straightforward with a documented progression of proteinuria over time and the presence of diabetic retinopathy (Figs 4.25–4.28).

Clinical stages

Diabetic nephropathy has been didactically categorized into stages based on the values of urinary albumin excretion (UAE): microalbuminuria and macroalbuminuria. The cutoff values adopted by the American Diabetes Association (timed, 24-h, and spot urine collection) for the diagnosis of micro- and macroalbuminuria, as well as the main clinical features of each stage, are depicted in Table 4.1.

Laboratory findings

Glomerular filtration rate (GFR) is the best parameter of overall kidney function and should be measured or estimated in micro- and macroalbuminuric diabetic patients

Imaging tests

Imaging of the kidneys, usually by ultrasonography, should be performed in patients with symptoms of urinary tract obstruction, infection, or kidney stones, or with a family history of polycystic kidney disease.

Table 4.1 The cutoff values adopted by the American Diabetes Association (timed, 24-h, and spot urine collection) for the diagnosis of micro- and macroalbuminuria, as well as the main clinical features of each stage

Stages	Albuminuria cutoff values	Clinical characteristics
Microalbuminuria	20–199 µg/min 30–299 mg/24 h 30–299 mg/g	Abnormal nocturnal decrease of blood pressure and increased blood pressure levels Increased triglycerides, total and LDL cholesterol, and saturated fatty acids Increased frequency of metabolic syndrome components Endothelial dysfunction Association with diabetic retinopathy, amputation, and cardiovascular disease Increased cardiovascular mortality Stable GFR
Macroalbuminuria	≥ 200 µg/min ≥ 300 mg/24 h > 300 mg/g	Hypertension Increased triglycerides and total and LDL cholesterol Asymptomatic myocardial ischemia Progressive GFR decline

GFR, glomerular filtration rate; LDL, low-density lipoprotein.
Courtesy of TODAY Study Group. (2013) Rapid rise in hypertension and nephropathy in youth with type 2 diabetes: the TODAY clinical trail. *Diabetes Care* **36**(6):1735–41.

Table 4.2 Strategies and goals for reno- and cardioprotection in patients with diabetic nephropathy

	Goal	
Intervention	**Microalbuminuric patients**	**Macroalbuminuric patients**
ACE inhibitor and/or ARB, and low-protein diet (0.6–0.8 g/kg/wt per day)	Reduction of albuminuria or reversion to normoalbuminuria	Proteinuria as low as possible or < 0.5 g/24 h; and GFR mL/min/1.73 m² per year
	GFR stabilization	
Antihypertensive agents	Blood pressure < 130/80 or 125/75 mmHg	
Strict glycemic control	A1c < 7%	
Statins	LDL < 2.6 mmol/L (< 100 mg/dL)	
Acetyl salicylic acid	Thrombosis prevention	
Smoking cessation	Prevention of atherosclerosis progression	

ACE, angiotensin-converting enzyme; ARB, angiotensin-receptor blocker; GFR, glomerular filtration rate; LDL, low-density lipoprotein.
Courtesy of TODAY Study Group. (2013) Rapid rise in hypertension and nephropathy in youth with type 2 diabetes: the TODAY clinical trail. *Diabetes Care* **36**(6):1735–41.

Prevention and treatment

The basis for the prevention and treatment of diabetic nephropathy is the treatment of its known risk factors: hypertension, hyperglycemia, smoking, and dyslipidemia. These are also risk factors for cardiovascular disease and should be vigorously treated.

Strategies and goals for reno- and cardioprotection in patients with diabetic nephropathy are described in Table 4.2.

Illustrations (Figs 4.25–4.28)

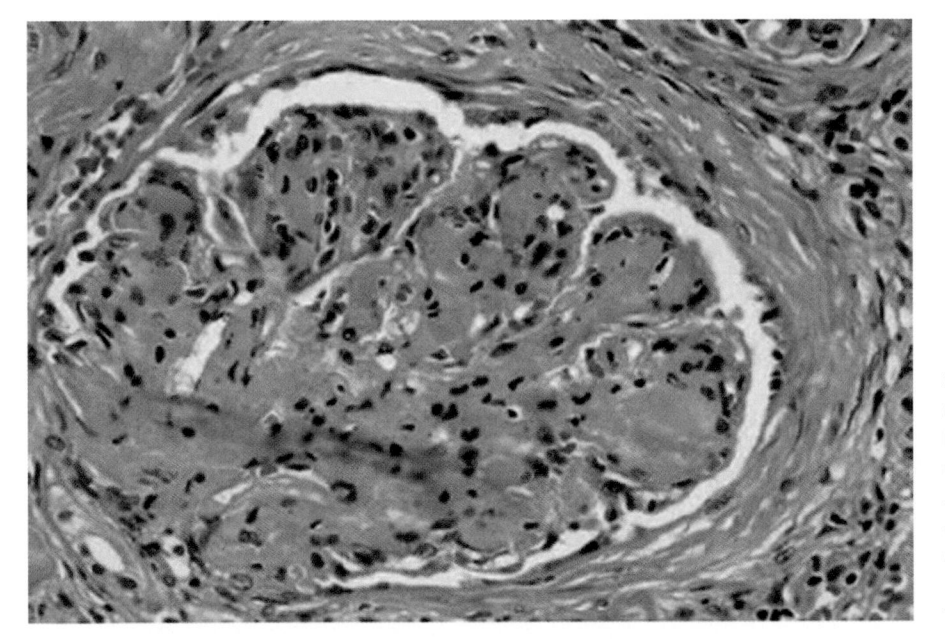

Figure 4.25 Histopathological image of diabetic nephropathy. Glomerulosclerosis: Mesangial nodules are located in the periphery of the glomerulus. The nodules contain lipids and fibrin. The nodules expand obliterating the glomerulus. The renal parenchyma invariably develops ischemia leading to tubular atrophy, interstitial fibrosis, and decreased renal size and function.

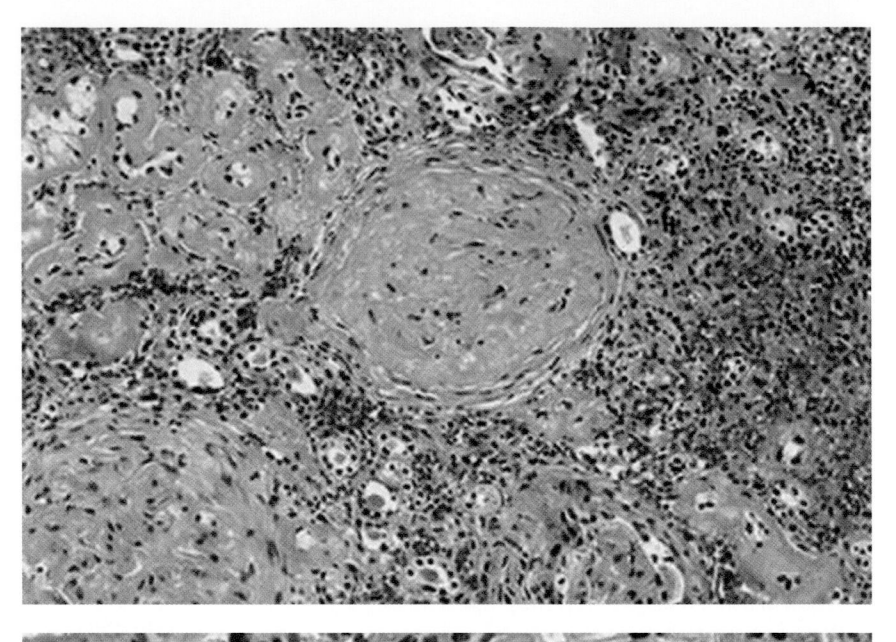

Figure 4.26 Histopathological image of diabetic nephropathy. The glomerulus in the center of the microphotograph is completely sclerotic.

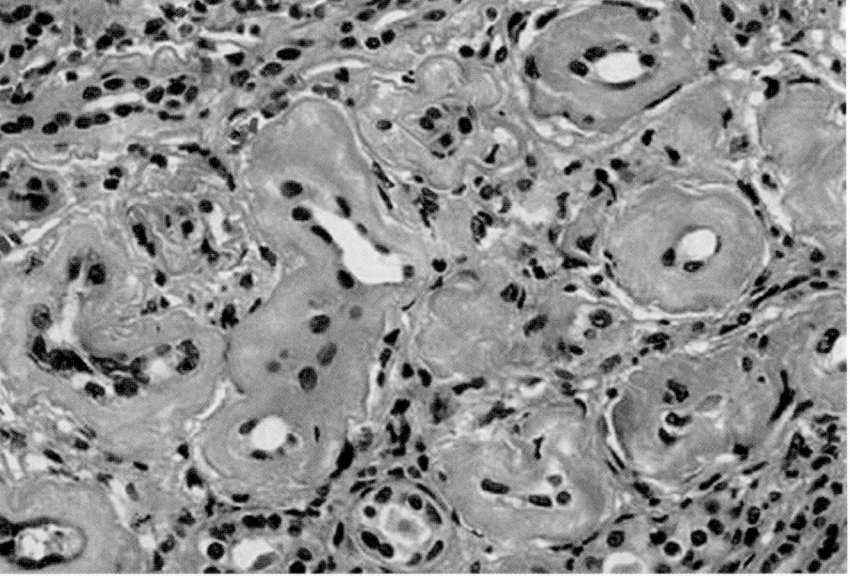

Figure 4.27 Histopathological image of diabetic nephropathy. Renal tubules. The basement membrane of the tubules are markedly thickened leading to tubular atrophy and dysfunction.

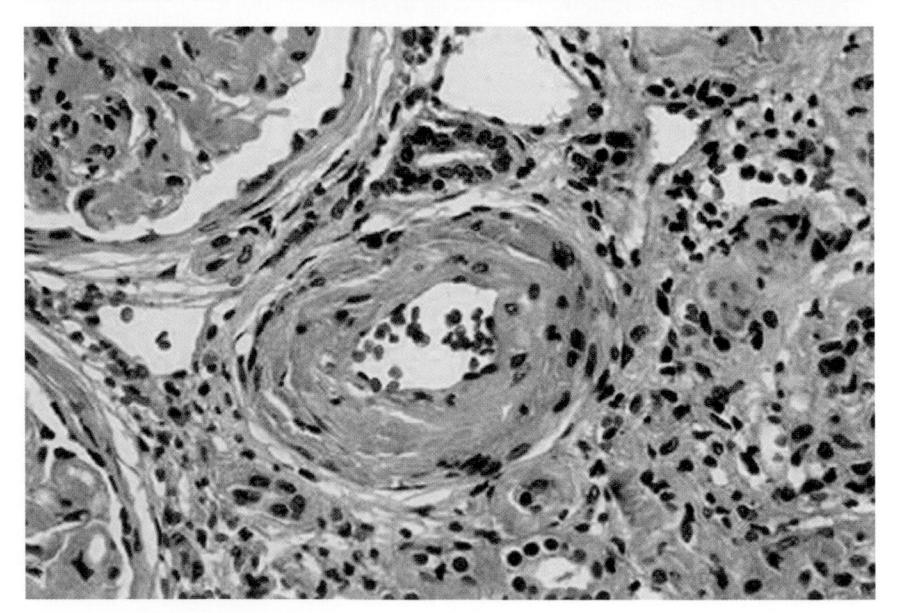

Figure 4.28 Histopathological image of diabetic nephropathy. Renal hyaline arteriolosclerosis. The arteriole in the center of the microphotograph is severely thickened, which is characteristic of hyaline arteriolosclerosis.

Diabetic retinopathy

Definition
Diabetic retinopathy is a complication of diabetes that results from damage to the blood vessels of the retina.

Etiology
Chronic hyperglycemia, hypertension, and hyperlipidemia contribute to the pathogenesis of diabetic retinopathy. Hyperglycemia damages retinal vasculature in several ways and progression is generally related to the severity and duration of hyperglycemia. The exact mechanism by which raised glucose levels lead to vascular disruption seen in retinopathy is poorly defined. Among these pathways, increased activity of protein kinase C (PKC) and glycation of key proteins that lead to formation of advanced glycation end (AGE) products are more important than polyol accumulation or oxidative stress.

Signs and symptoms
It is possible to have diabetic retinopathy and not know it. In fact, it is uncommon to have symptoms in the early stages.

As the condition progresses, diabetic retinopathy symptoms may include:
• Spots or dark strings floating in your vision (floaters)
• Blurred vision
• Fluctuating vision
• Dark or empty areas in your vision
• Poor night vision
• Impaired color vision
• Vision loss
Diabetic retinopathy usually affects both eyes.

Diagnosis
Diabetic retinopathy is best diagnosed with fundus oculi exam (Figs 4.29–4.31). Another imaging diagnostic test is optical coherence tomography (OCT) (Fig. 4.32). The clinical stages for diabetic retinopathy are as listed below.

Background retinopathy
Microaneurysms are outpouchings of capillaries and are among the first clinically detectable signs (Figs 4.29, 4.33 & 4.34). They appear as tiny red dots, commonly temporal to the macula. Hard exudates are the result of precipitation of lipoproteins and other circulating proteins through abnormally leaky retinal vessels. They appear as yellow lipid deposits with a waxy or shiny appearance and may form a circinate pattern around foci of leaking capillaries.

Maculopathy
Maculopathy is a disease of macula and can accompany any stage, including background retinopathy (Fig. 4.31). It is characterized by macular edema and ischemic maculopathy. Macular edema is due to extravasation of plasma proteins due to damage of the blood–retinal barrier. Clinically significant macular edema is defined as any one of the following:

• Retinal edema within 500 μm (one third of a disc diameter) of the fovea
• Hard exudates within 500 μm of the fovea if associated with adjacent retinal thickening
• Retinal edema that is one disc diameter (1500 μm) or larger, any part of which is within one disc diameter of the fovea

Preproliferative retinopathy
This stage is characterized by worsening retinal ischemia, which may lead to formation of new vessels (neovascularization) (Figs 4.35 & 4.36). It is characterized by the presence of one of the following:
• Multiple large dark blot hemorrhages
• Multiple (> 5) cotton wool spots appearing as dead white patches with vague margins and representing microinfarcts in the nerve fiber layer
• Venous beading, looping, and duplication
• Intraretinal microvascular abnormalities (IRMA)

Proliferative retinopathy
This stage is characterized by new vessel formation which appears as arcade of abnormal structures commonly arising on the optic disc (new vessel disc or NVD) or elsewhere on the retina (new vessel elsewhere or NVE) (Figs 4.30, 4.37 & 4.38). Fibrous tissue and hemorrhages may also accompany. Abnormal new vasculature may threaten vision due to complications such as retinal detachment, hemorrhage, and glaucoma. NVD carries a worse prognosis than NVE, and if left untreated often leads to vitreous hemorrhage and increases chances of blindness.

Advanced eye disease
This stage represents advanced retinal damage that leads to blindness in the absence of intervention. This stage is characterized by vitreous hemorrhage, progressive fibrovascular proliferation, retinal detachment, rubeosis iridis, and neovascular glaucoma, which may lead to a painful blind eye.

Laboratory and imaging tests
Along with the above signs and symptoms, no particular laboratory tests are needed but fluorescein angiography and optical coherence tomography may be useful imaging tests.

Treatment
Treatment for diabetic retinopathy depends on the stage of this condition:
• For early diabetic retinopathy, no treatment is necessary
• For advanced diabetic retinopathy, proliferative diabetic retinopathy needs prompt surgical treatment. Options may include focal laser treatment, scatter laser treatment, or vitrectomy

Illustrations (Figs 4.29–4.38)

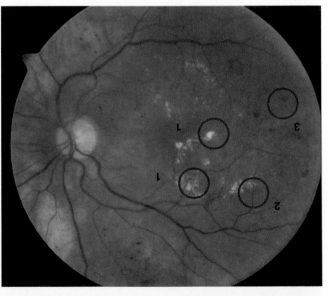

Figure 4.29 Fundus oculi exam: Background retinopathy. There are: white patches hard exudates (1); microaneurysms (2); hemorrhages "dot-blot," and flame shaped (3).

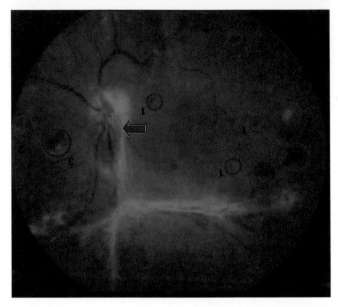

Figure 4.30 Fundus oculi exam: Proliferative diabetic retinopathy. It is possible to see neovessels around the optic disc. There are also superficial microhemorrhages (1); cotton whole spots (2); deep retinal hemorrhages (3); new vessel formation (arrow).

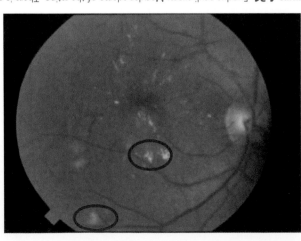

Figure 4.31 Fundus oculi exam: Macular edema of the retina. There is a ring of hard lipid exudates superior to the center of the macula, which is the dark circular zone near the center of the picture. Lipid rings often surround a zone of retinal thickening (edema). Hard exudates (1); cotton-wool spots (2).

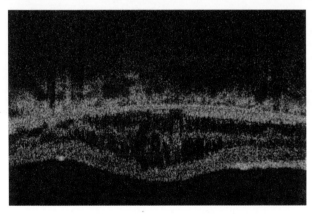

Figure 4.32 Diabetic retinopathy: Optical coherence tomography (OCT) shows a cross section of the central retina with marked fluid accumulation and cystoid formation leading to severe vision loss.

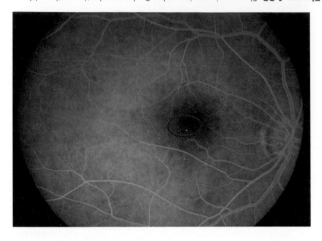

Figure 4.33 Fluorescein angiography: Background retinopathy with no lesions other than microaneurysms.

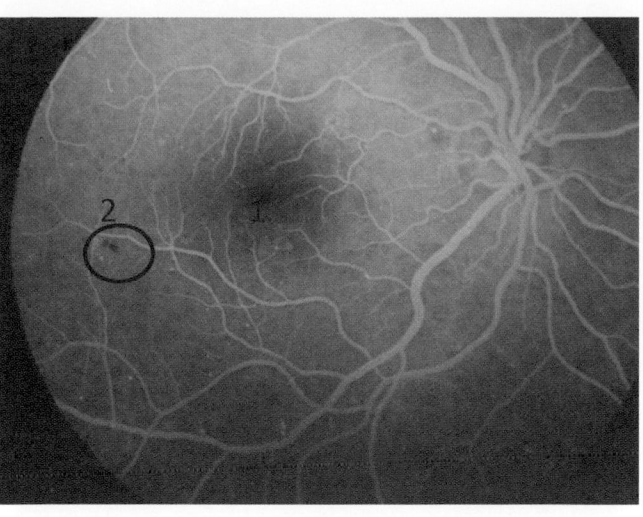

Figure 4.34 Fluorescein angiography: Mild nonproliferative diabetic retinopathy with microaneurysms (1) and dot blot hemorrhages (2).

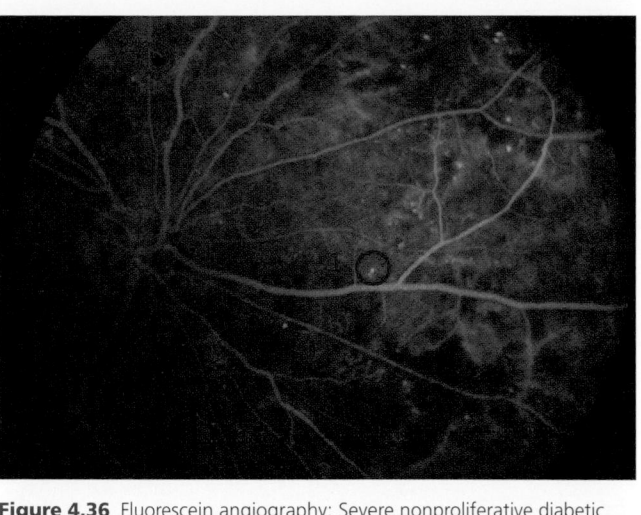

Figure 4.36 Fluorescein angiography: Severe nonproliferative diabetic retinopathy with microaneurysms (1), dot blot hemorrhages (2), and areas of ischemia.

Figure 4.37 Fluorescein angiography: Proliferative diabetic retinopathy with areas of ischemic retina, spots of laser photocoagulation (1), and leakage of fluorescein from the neovascular frond (2).

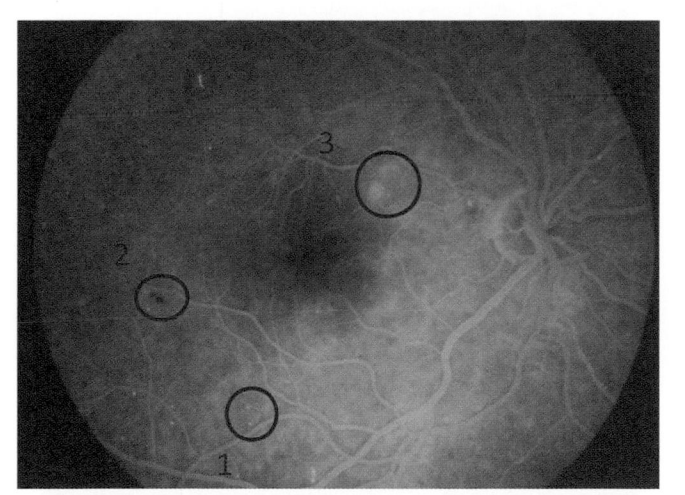

Figure 4.35 Fluorescein angiography: Mild nonproliferative diabetic retinopathy with microaneurysms (1), dot blot hemorrhages (2), and mild leakage (3) during the late phases of the angiogram.

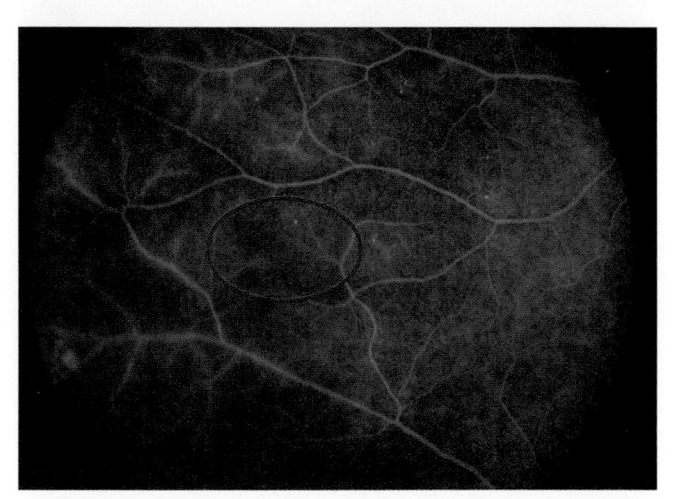

Figure 4.38 Fluorescein angiography: Area of ischemic retina with severe capillaropathy (drop-out spaces).

Insulinoma

Definition

Insulinoma is a tumor of the pancreas that is derived from beta cells and secretes insulin.

Etiology

Over 99% of insulinomas originate in the pancreas, with rare cases from ectopic pancreatic tissue. About 5% of cases are associated with tumors of the parathyroid glands and the pituitary (multiple endocrine neoplasia type 1) and are more likely to be multiple and malignant.

Signs and symptoms

Patients with insulinomas usually develop neuroglycopenic symptoms. These include recurrent headache, lethargy, diplopia, and blurred vision, particularly with exercise or fasting. Severe hypoglycemia may result in seizures, coma, and permanent neurological damage. Symptoms resulting from the catecholaminergic response to hypoglycemia (i.e. tremulousness, palpitations, tachycardia, sweating, hunger, anxiety, and nausea) are not as common. Sudden weight gain (the patient can become massively obese) is sometimes seen.

Diagnosis

The diagnosis of insulinoma is suspected in a patient with symptomatic fasting hypoglycemia. The conditions of Whipple's triad need to be met for the diagnosis of "true hypoglycemia" to be made. These conditions are:

- Symptoms and signs of hypoglycemia
- Concomitant plasma glucose level of ≤ 45 mg/dL (2.5 mmol/L)
- Reversibility of symptoms with administration of glucose

Laboratory findings

A 72-hour fast, usually supervised in a hospital setting, may be done to see if insulin levels fail to suppress, which is a strong indicator of the presence of an insulin-secreting tumor.

Imaging and other diagnostic tests

The following tests may help with diagnosis:

- Ultrasound (low sensitivity)
- Computed tomography (CT) (low sensitivity) (Figs 4.39 & 4.40)
- Magnetic resonance imaging (MRI) (low sensitivity)
- Endoscopic ultrasound (high sensitivity) (Figs 4.41 & 4.42)
- Angiography with percutaneous transhepatic pancreatic vein catheterization to sample the blood for insulin levels may be required.

Treatment

The definitive management is surgical removal of insulinoma.

Medication such as somatostatin and diazoxide can be used to block the release of insulin for patients who are not candidates.

Illustrations (Figs 4.39–4.42)

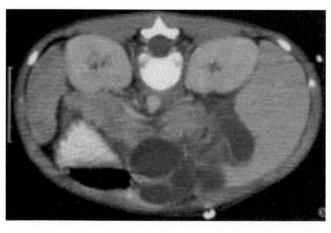

Figure 4.39 Computed tomography (CT) scan of the abdomen in a child with traumatic pancreatitis. The fluid collection adjacent to the pancreas will become a pseudocyst. Note that the pancreas is lacerated, nearly cut in half, by the force of the abdominal trauma. Also, note the typical location of this injury in relation to the vertebral column.

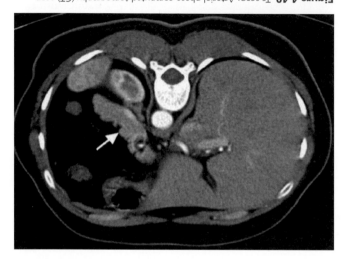

Figure 4.40 Tc scan: Arterial phase computed tomography (CT) scan. This lesion (white arrow) remains isoattenuating to the surrounding pancreatic parenchyma.

Acute pancreatitis

Definition

Acute pancreatitis is inflammation of the pancreas that occurs suddenly and usually resolves in a few days with treatment. However, acute pancreatitis can be a life-threatening illness with severe complications.

Etiology

While alcohol exposure and biliary tract disease do determine most cases, pancreatitis has numerous etiologies: 10–30% of cases have an unknown etiology, although studies have suggested that up to 70% of cases of idiopathic pancreatitis are secondary to biliary microlithiasis.

Causes of acute pancreatitis include:
• Biliary tract disease (approx. 40%)
• Alcohol (approx. 35%)
• Post-endoscopic retrograde cholangiopancreatography (ERCP) (approx. 4%)
• Drugs (approx. 2%)
• Infection (< 1%)
• Trauma (approx. 1.5%)
• Hereditary pancreatitis (< 1%)
• Hypercalcemia (< 1%)
• Developmental abnormalities of the pancreas (< 1%)
• Hypertriglyceridemia (< 1%)
• Tumor (< 1%)
• Toxins (< 1%)
• Postoperative (< 1%)
• Vascular abnormalities (< 1%)

Signs and symptoms

Acute pancreatitis usually begins with gradual or sudden pain in the upper abdomen that sometimes extends through the back. The pain may be mild at first and feel worse after eating, but it is often severe and it may become constant and last for several days.

Other symptoms may include:
• Swollen and tender abdomen
• Nausea and vomiting
• Fever
• Rapid pulse

Severe acute pancreatitis may cause dehydration and low blood pressure.

Diagnosis

Clinical features (abdominal pain and vomiting) together with elevation of plasma concentrations of pancreatic enzymes are the cornerstones of diagnosis.

Laboratory findings

Initial investigations (acute phase):
• Pancreatic enzymes in plasma
• Liver function tests
Followup (recovery phase):
• Fasting plasma lipids
• Fasting plasma calcium
• Viral antibody titers
Further investigations (usually appropriate for recurrent idiopathic acute pancreatitis):
• Autoimmune markers
• Pancreatic function tests to exclude chronic pancreatitis

Imaging tests

Initial investigations (acute phase):
• Ultrasound of gallbladder
Followup (recovery phase):
• Repeat biliary ultrasound

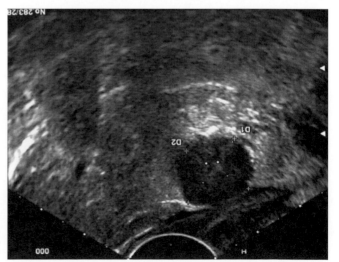

Figure 4.41 Pancreatic endoscopic ultrasound. Insulinoma – hypoechoic nodule with sharp margins in the isthmus of the pancreas.

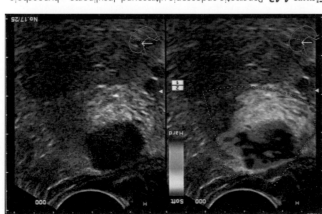

Figure 4.42 Pancreatic endoscopic ultrasound. Insulinoma – hypoechoic nodule with moderate consistency at elastosonographic examination.

- Magnetic resonance cholangiopancreatography (MRCP)
- Computed tomography (CT) (helical or multislice with pancreas protocol) (Figs 4.43 & 4.44)

Further investigations (usually appropriate for recurrent idiopathic acute pancreatitis):

- Further ultrasound
- Endoscopic ultrasound
- ERCP – bile for crystals and pancreatic cytology (Fig. 4.45)
- ERCP – bile and pancreatic cytology
- Sphincter of Oddi manometry

Treatment

It is necessary remove the cause of pancreatitis.

The medical management of mild acute pancreatitis is based on early oxygen supplementation and intravenous fluid hydration with analgesics that could be provided for pain relief.

For patients with severe acute pancreatitis the aims of medical care are to provide aggressive supportive care, to decrease inflammation, to limit infection or superinfection, and to identify and treat complications as appropriate using fluids, enteral nutrition, antibiotics, ERCP (if necessary), or surgical intervention.

Illustrations (Figs 4.43–4.45)

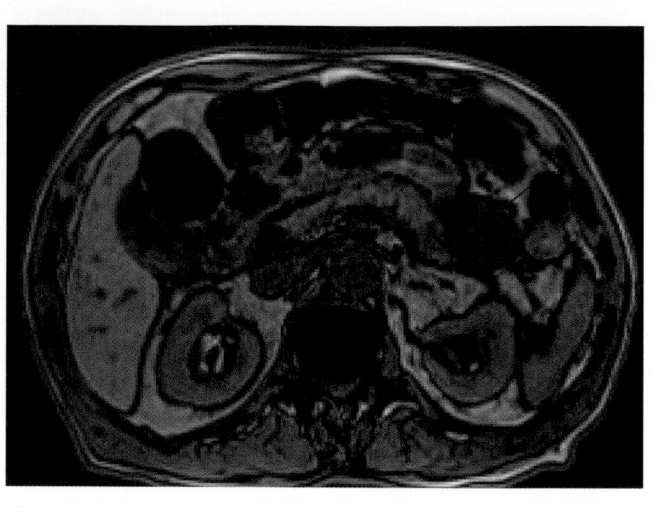

Figure 4.44 A T-1-weighted axial image of the same patient obtained in the subacute phase. The pseudocyst is still present (red arrow) and the pancreatic parenchyma is atrophic with irregular borders.

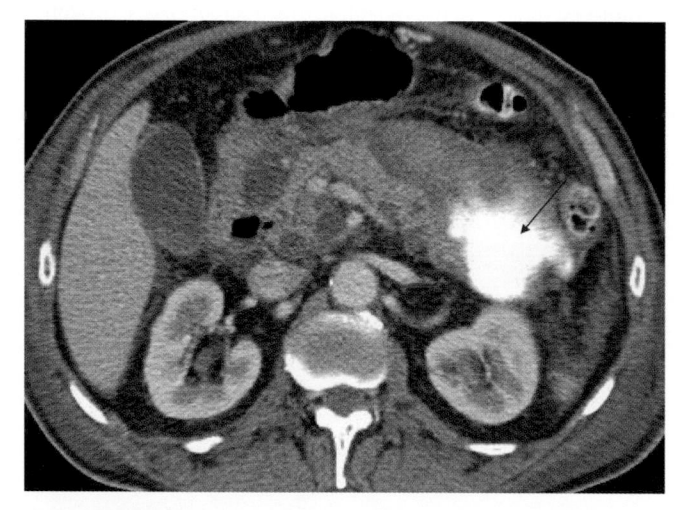

Figure 4.43 A computed tomography (CT) scan obtained in the axial plane showing a massive acute pancreatitis. There is no residual gland and the pancreatic lodge is replaced by necrotic tissue. Notice the f-contrast medium filling a huge pseudocysts (red arrow), which was drained.

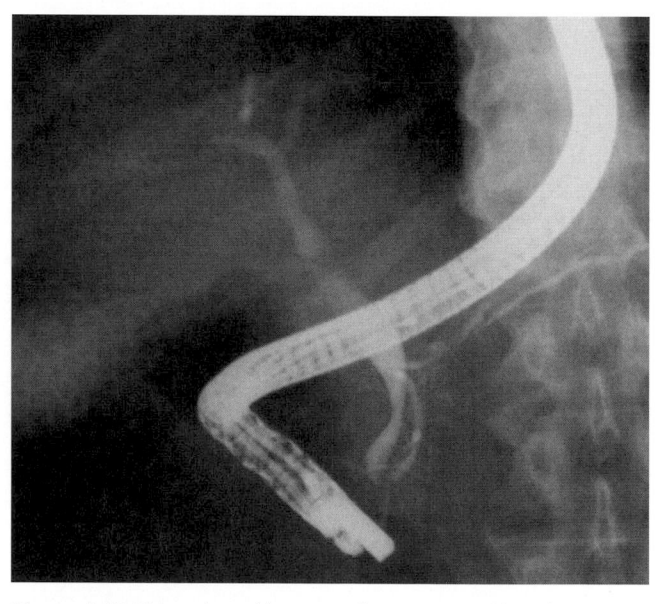

Figure 4.45 This patient with acute gallstone pancreatitis underwent endoscopic retrograde cholangiopancreatography (ERCP). The cholangiogram shows no stones in the common bile duct and multiple small stones in the gallbladder. The pancreatogram shows narrowing of the pancreatic duct in the area of the genu, the result of extrinsic compression of the ductal system by inflammatory changes in the pancreas.

Chronic pancreatitis

Definition
Chronic pancreatitis is a progressive and destructive necroinflammatory disorder of the pancreas characterized by irreversible fibrosis of the gland with eventual failure of exocrine and endocrine functions.

Etiology
Causes of chronic pancreatitis are shown in Table 4.3.

Signs and symptoms
Typical symptoms include:
• Pain radiating to the back
• Malabsorption, malnutrition, and pancreatic endocrine insufficiency
• The classic disease triad – pancreatic calcification, diabetes mellitus, and clinically significant malabsorption – but this emerges only in advanced disease
In most cases, physical examination does not help establish a diagnosis of chronic pancreatitis.

Diagnosis
There is no consensus on the diagnostic criteria for chronic pancreatitis. Diagnostic tests for chronic pancreatitis include fecal elastase measurement (to prove pancreatic insufficiency) and imaging.

A biopsy may be required to resolve diagnostic uncertainty.

Laboratory findings
Although there is no single test that is diagnostic for early chronic pancreatitis, the following laboratory testing may help in the diagnosis:
• Trypsin
• Amylase and lipase

• Test for genetic mutations in cationic trypsinogen and *CFTR*
• Fecal tests
• Pancreatic function tests

Imaging tests
Transabdominal ultrasound, computed tomography (CT), and magnetic resonance imaging (MRI) can all assist in the diagnosis and management of chronic pancreatitis (Figs 4.46–4.48). All of these studies may show calcifications, ductal dilation, pancreatic enlargement, and fluid collections (i.e. pseudocysts) adjacent to the gland.

Although endoscopic retrograde cholangiopancreatography (ERCP) is used as a reference standard (see Fig. 4.47b), a contrast-enhanced CT scan of the abdomen is the initial imaging modality of choice because it is reasonably sensitive and specific at a relatively low cost (Fig. 4.46).

Treatment
The aims of treatment are to minimize pain of chronic pancreatitis, alleviate symptoms and sequelae of pancreatic exocrine insufficiency, improve quality of life, and reduce complications, with minimal adverse effects of treatment.

Avoiding alcohol consumption may be beneficial in people with alcoholic chronic pancreatitis (where there is usually prolonged exposure to large amounts of alcohol) by preventing further injury to the pancreas and other organs (such as the liver, heart, and nervous system).

Treatment may include pancreatic enzyme replacement.

Illustrations (Figs 4.46–4.48)

Table 4.3 Causes of chronic pancreatitis

	Frequency (%)
Common	
Alcoholic	65–80
Idiopathic	15–30
Uncommon	
Autoimmune	3–5
Obstructive	3–5
Rare	
Hereditary	< 1
Hypertriglyceridemia	< 1
Hyperparathyroidism	< 1

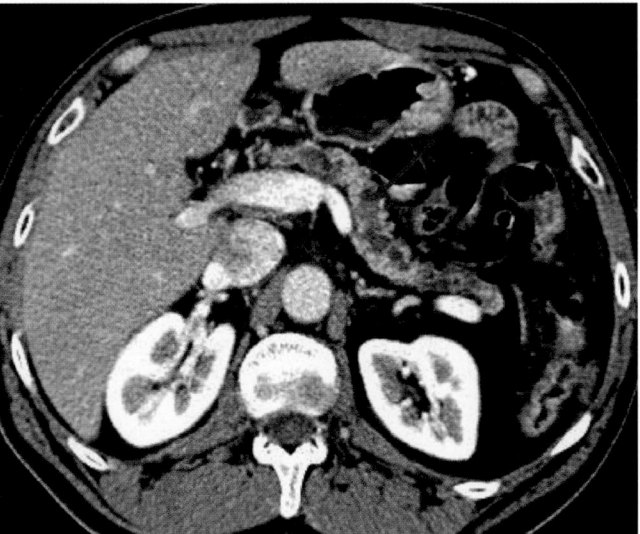

Figure 4.46 A computed tomography (CT) scan of a 63-year-old man with chronic pancreatitis. Notice the dilation of the primary and secondary pancreatic ducts. Note also the luminal foci of isodense material (red arrow), consistent with litiasic spots.

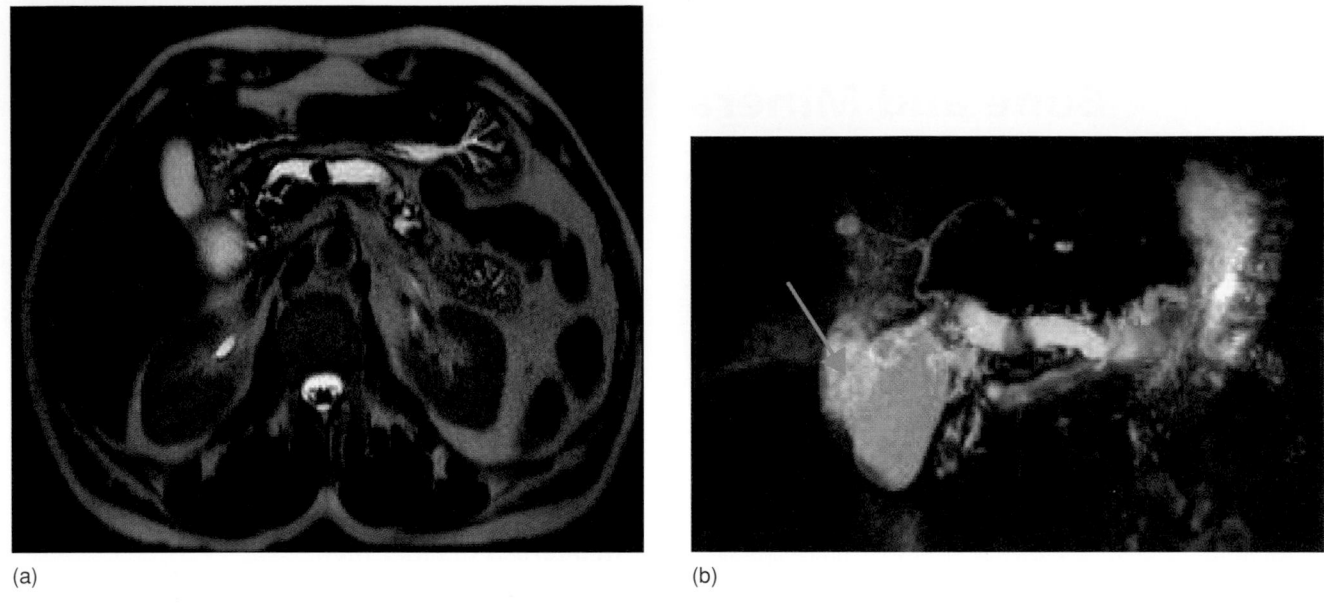

(a)   (b)

Figure 4.47 A T-2-weighted image obtained in the axial plane showing an intraluminal spot of low intensity within the Wirsung duct (red arrow), consistent with a litiasic spot (a). A T-2-weighted image of the same patient obtained in the coronal plane and reformatted with a mixed integer programming (MIP) algorithm (b) showing the same finding within the Wirsung duct lumen. Moreover, a huge pseudocyst is visible within the pancreatic head (green arrow).

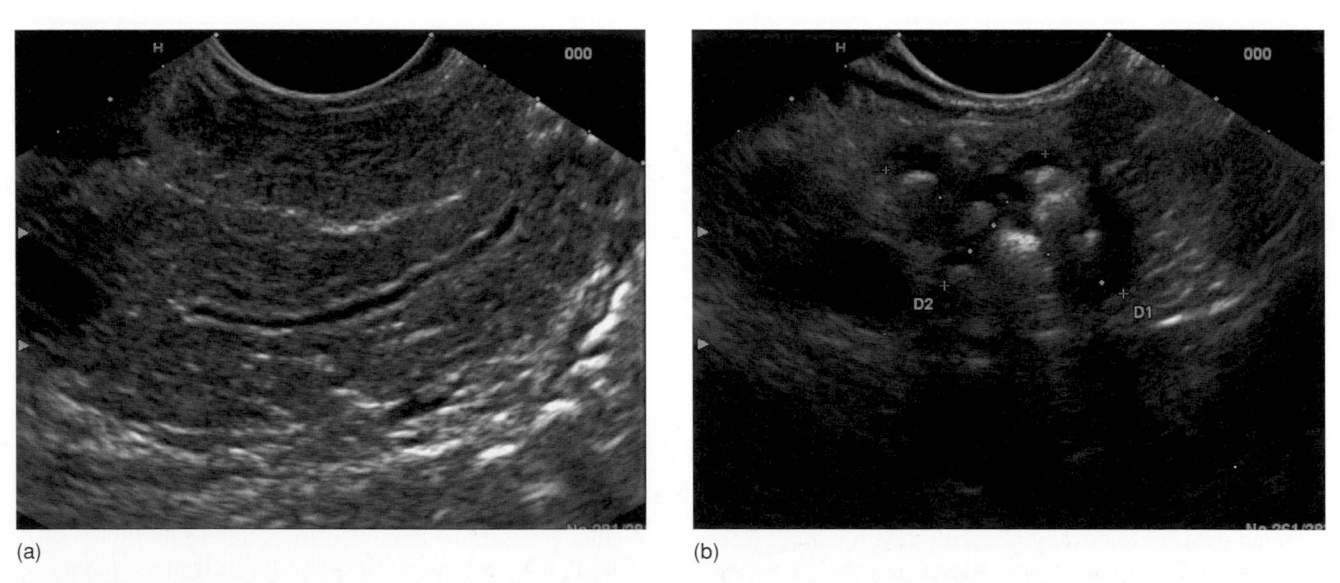

(a)   (b)

Figure 4.48 Endoscopic ultrasound (EUS) images (a & b) show features consistent with the diagnosis of chronic pancreatitis. (a) Hyperechoic spots and lines in the parenchyma of the pancreas. (b) Major pancreatic duct lithiasis with increased echogenicity of the wall of the duct.

5 Bone and Mineral Metabolism

Osteoporosis

Definition

Osteoporosis is characterized by decreased bone strength associated with increased risk of fracture.

Etiology

Postmenopausal osteoporosis

Postmenopausal osteoporosis results from physiologic changes associated with normal aging. Bone loss during normal aging is primarily associated with gonadal sex steroid deficiency in both women and men. Mechanisms by which gonadal sex steroid deficiency cause bone loss include increased receptor activator of nuclear factor kappa B ligand (RANKL) and decreased osteoprotegerin (OPG), resulting in an increased RANKL/OPG ratio that increases osteoclast recruitment and activation, and decreases osteoclast apoptosis. Estrogen deficiency upregulates cytokines that stimulate bone resorption, such as interleukin (IL)-1, IL-6, tumor necrosis factor (TNF)-α, macrophage colony-stimulating factor (M-CSF), and prostaglandins. Estrogen deficiency also decreases production of transforming growth factor (TGF)-β by osteoblast precursor cells, thereby reducing osteoclast apoptosis. Estrogen deficiency directly decreases apoptosis of osteoclast precursor cells, and increases osteoclast precursor differentiation by stimulating RANKL/M-CSF-induced activator protein (AP)-1-dependent transcription by increasing c-jun activity. C-jun activity is increased by upregulating c-jun transcription and increasing phosphorylation. Estrogen deficiency also stimulates activity of mature osteoclasts by direct receptor-mediated mechanisms. It is likely that the major direct effect of estrogen deficiency is mediated by alteration in the ratio of RANKL to OPG in the bone microenvironment, thereby leading to increased osteoclast activity and bone resorption. However, the multiple other changes induced by estrogen deficiency also likely play a significant role in causation of early postmenopausal bone loss.

Osteoporosis in older men

Osteoporosis in older men also appears to be due primarily to gonadal sex steroid deficiency. Estrogen deficiency appears to have a greater effect on causation of bone loss in men than testosterone deficiency.

Other age-related factors

Age-related bone loss is due to multiple factors other than gonadal sex steroid deficiency, including vitamin D deficiency, secondary hyperparathyroidism, decreased bone formation, decreased adrenal secretion of weak androgens such as DHEA-S, increased leptin secretion, increased intestinal serotonin secretion, relative tissue hypoxia and increased generation of reactive oxygen species, and decreased physical activity and muscle mass. Genetic influences explain between 50 and 85% of the variability in measurement of bone density. Genetic inheritance impacts peak bone mass and the rate of postmenopausal bone loss. Numerous sporadic factors also contribute to age-related bone loss, including glucocorticoid therapy, malabsorption, anorexia nervosa, idiopathic hypercalciuria, or behavioral factors such as excess alcohol intake, cigarette smoking, high-caffeine or high-sodium diet, or physical inactivity. Age-related bone loss occurs independently of gonadal sex steroid deficiency-related bone loss.

Premenopausal low bone density

Premenopausal low bone density is due to multiple factors that affect bone mass acquisition during growth and development. Multiple disorders that affect growth and development limit acquisition of peak bone density in the late 20s or early 30s, and increase rate of bone loss after peak bone density is achieved.

Imaging in Endocrinology, First Edition. Paolo Pozzilli, Andrea Lenzi, Bart L Clarke and William F Young Jr.
© 2014 John Wiley & Sons, Ltd. Published 2014 by John Wiley & Sons, Ltd.

Signs and symptoms

Low trauma or atraumatic fractures are the classical hallmark of osteoporosis. These fractures are typically defined as occurring with falls from standing height or less, or with minimal or no trauma. However, traumatic fractures may also be due to osteoporosis. Bone pain is commonly present after fracture, but patients may have X-ray evidence of vertebral fractures without associated pain. Asymptomatic fractures have the same significance as symptomatic fractures in the diagnosis of osteoporosis, and increased risk of future fractures. Patients with multiple vertebral fractures typically lose height, and may develop kyphosis, depending on the location of the vertebral fractures (Fig. 5.1).

Diagnosis

Diagnosis of osteoporosis is based on clinical evidence of fractures, X-ray evidence of asymptomatic fractures, or bone density test results when fractures are not present. The World Health Organization defines osteoporosis in postmenopausal women and older men based on bone mineral density T-scores less than –2.5. The International Society of Clinical Densitometry defines low bone density in women or men less than 50 years old based on bone mineral density Z-scores of less than –2.0.

Imaging tests

When classical low trauma or atraumatic clinical fractures of the hip, lumbar spine, or wrist are not evident, bone density assessment by dual energy X-ray absorptiometry (DXA) is the current gold standard for diagnosing osteoporosis. Other imaging modalities are occasionally used, including calcaneal ultrasound or quantitative CT scanning. X-rays or DXA vertebral morphometry of the lumbar spine in asymptomatic patients may detect unsuspected vertebral fractures (Fig. 5.2).

Laboratory findings

Laboratory testing reveals clinically unrecognized secondary causes of bone loss in as many as 40% of women with postmenopausal osteoporosis, and in as many as 50% of older men with osteoporosis. Younger adults with low bone density, with or without fractures, also frequently have unrecognized secondary causes of bone loss. Frequently detected secondary causes of bone loss with biochemical testing include vitamin D deficiency, primary hyperparathyroidism, hypogonadism, and hypercalciuria. Less common secondary causes of low bone density or osteoporosis include endogenous hypercortisolism, mastocytosis, or osteogenesis imperfecta.

Treatment

Treatment of osteoporosis depends on the underlying causes of osteoporosis or low bone density.

In postmenopausal women or older men with gonadal sex steroid deficiency, hormone therapy may be appropriate, if not contraindicated for other reasons. However, oral bisphosphonates such as alendronate, risedronate, or ibandronate, or intravenous zoledronic acid, ibandronate, or pamidronate are usually efficacious and well-tolerated regardless of age or co-morbid conditions. Raloxifene may be helpful in some women with postmenopausal osteoporosis, especially when breast cancer prevention is a concern. Salmon calcitonin may be useful in patients not able to tolerate other medications. Teriparatide (recombinant human parathyroid hormone 1–34) is approved for use in patients with severe osteoporosis, those with multiple fractures, or those not able to tolerate other osteoporosis medications. Denosumab is a monoclonal antibody to RANKL that potently suppresses bone loss, but does not have long-term suppressive effects on bone turnover.

Complications of long-term use of oral or intravenous bisphosphonates may include osteonecrosis of the jaw (Figs 5.3 & 5.4) or atypical subtrochanteric fractures. Vertebroplasty may be used to treat painful vertebral fractures in some cases (Fig. 5.5).

Illustrations (Figs 5.1–5.5)

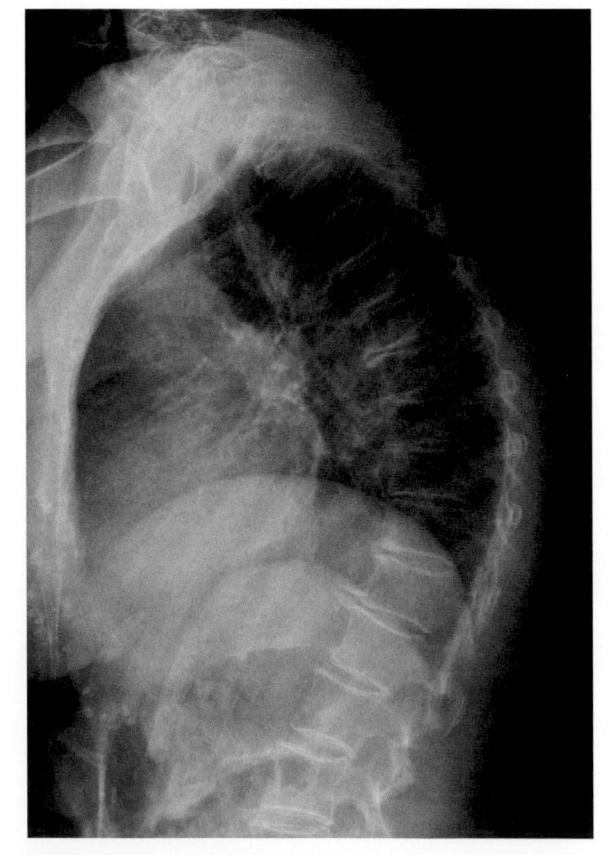

Figure 5.1 Moderate kyphosis due to postmenopausal osteoporosis. Courtesy of Dr. Bart L. Clarke.

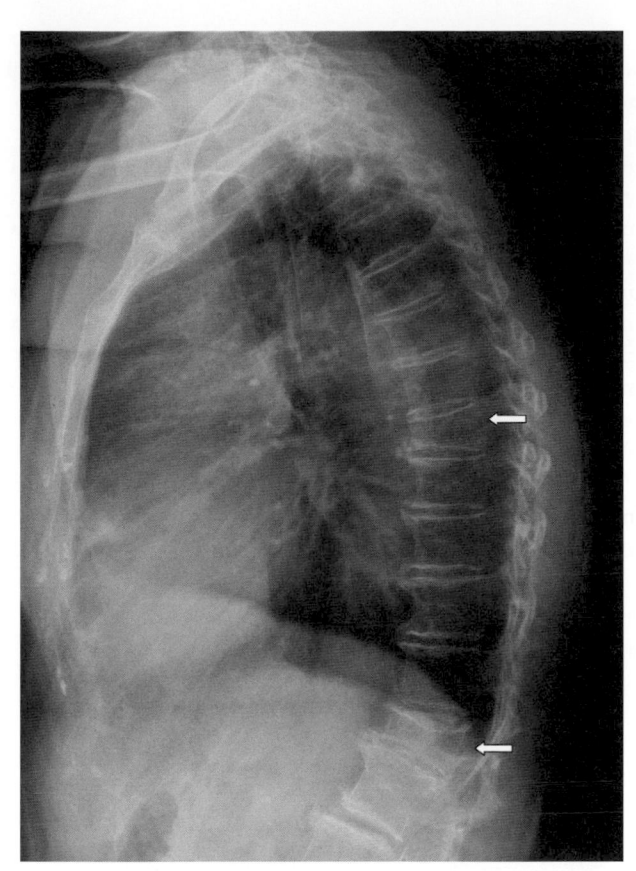

Figure 5.2 Asymptomatic mid-thoracic and lumbar vertebral fractures (arrows). Courtesy of Dr. Bart L. Clarke.

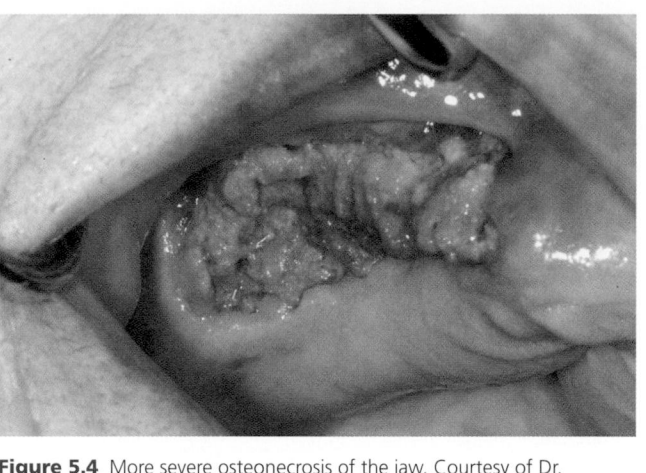

Figure 5.4 More severe osteonecrosis of the jaw. Courtesy of Dr. Christopher F. Viozzi.

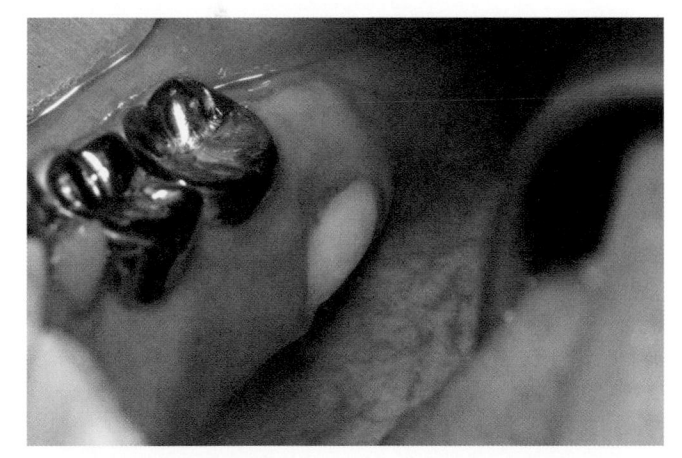

Figure 5.3 Mild osteonecrosis of the jaw. Courtesy of Dr. Christopher F. Viozzi.

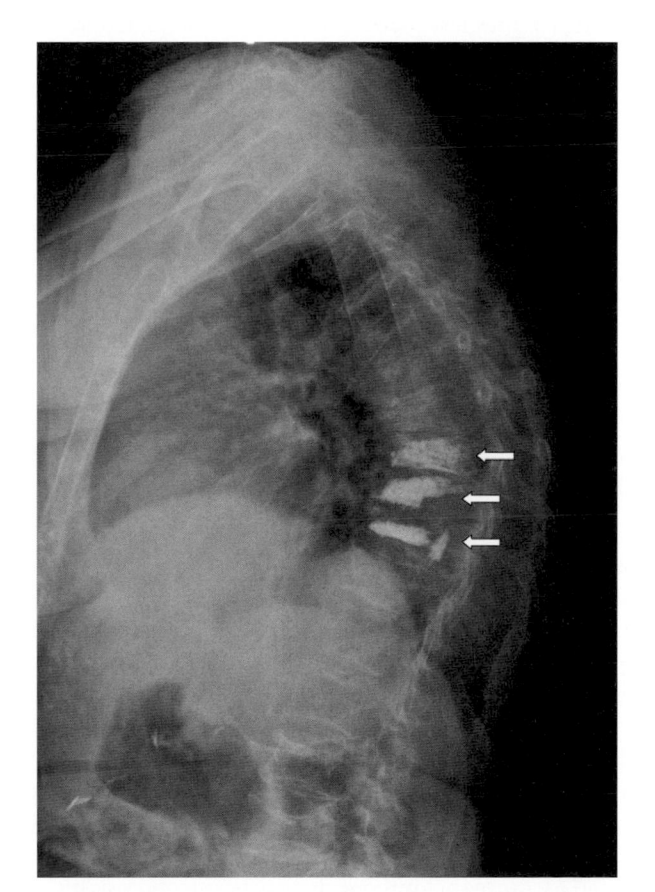

Figure 5.5 Vertebroplasty after thoracic vertebral compression fractures. Courtesy of Dr. Bart L. Clarke

Primary hyperparathyroidism

Definition

Primary hyperparathyroidism is characterized by hypercalcemia associated with excessive or inappropriate parathyroid hormone (PTH) secretion.

Etiology

Primary hyperparathyroidism results from increased or inappropriate PTH secretion, typically associated with hypercalcemia. Solitary parathyroid adenomas cause primary hyperparathyroidism 80–85% of the time, whereas four-gland hyperplasia is found in 15–20% of cases, and parathyroid cancer in < 0.5% of cases. As with other endocrine tumors, pathologic diagnosis of parathyroid carcinoma is difficult and is usually based on examination of local tissue, presence of vascular invasion, or detection of metastatic disease. Most single adenomas are due to sporadic disease, whereas four-gland hyperplasia may be associated with a familial disorder, most commonly MEN type I or IIA. Excessive secretion of PTH by an adenoma results from loss of feedback control of PTH secretion by extracellular calcium at the cellular level, causing an increased set-point, whereas excessive secretion of PTH by hyperplastic cells is due to an increased number of cells with a normal calcium set-point.

The cause of sporadic primary hyperparathyroidism is not well understood. Previous exposure to neck irradiation contributes in a minority of cases, typically 20–30 years after such exposure. More commonly, adenomas represent clonal expansion of a single or several abnormal cells, attributable to a genetic abnormality that results in either stimulation of cell proliferation or loss of inhibition of cell proliferation. A small number of adenomas have been reported with a *PRAD1* (cyclin D1) proto-oncogene rearrangement, in which the *PRAD1* gene is inserted close to enhancer elements of the *PTH* gene; consequently, parathyroid cell division is provoked whenever PTH secretion is stimulated. PRAD1 protein expression is increased in about 20% of parathyroid adenomas. Up to 17% of parathyroid adenomas have been reported with a mutation in the *MEN1* (menin) gene, a tumor suppressor gene. Loss of heterozygosity analysis of parathyroid adenomas has shown several other potential sites for parathyroid oncogenes on chromosomes 16p and 19, and loss of tumor suppressor genes on chromosomes 1p, 1q, 6q, 13q, and other sites. Several recent studies have shown mutations in the calcium-sensing receptor (CaSR) in parathyroid adenomas.

Eucalcemic hyperparathyroidism, in which serum calcium is normal but PTH is increased, has recently been described. This condition requires that serum 25-hydroxyvitamin D and 24-hour urine calcium levels be normal, in order to rule out other causes of physiological hyperparathyroidism. Eucalcemic hyperparathyroidism is thought to be an early stage of evolving primary hyperparathyroidism, with increased complications compared to asymptomatic primary hyperparathyroidism.

Signs and symptoms

Most patients with primary hyperparathyroidism have asymptomatic mild hypercalcemia, typically with serum calcium levels < 1.0 mg/dL above the upper end of the normal range. More severe cases have classical bone features, including osteitis fibrosa cystica (Fig. 5.6), characterized by distal phalangeal subperiosteal bone resorption (Fig. 5.7), distal clavicular resorption (Fig. 5.8), "salt and pepper" skull (Fig. 5.9), bone cysts (Fig. 5.10), and brown tumors of long bones (Fig. 5.11), or osteoporosis, predominantly at cortical sites such as the distal third of the radius. Fractures may be increased. Bone disease is currently diagnosed in < 5% of patients with primary hyperparathyroidism. Renal disease, including nephrocalcinosis (Fig. 5.12), calcium-containing nephrolithiasis (Fig. 5.13), or renal insufficiency, may be found in up to 20% of patients. Hypercalciuria is reported in up to 30% of patients.

Patients with primary hyperparathyroidism often report fatigue or weakness with subtle cognitive impairment. Associations with peptic ulcer disease and pancreatitis are probably not causally related, unless associated with MEN syndromes. Mild hypertension, coronary artery and cardiac valvular calcifications, and septal and left ventricular hypertrophy may be present in patients with more symptomatic hyperparathyroidism.

Other classical abnormalities of primary hyperparathyroidism, such as gout or pseudogout, anemia, band keratopathy (Fig. 5.14), or loosened teeth due to lamina densa resorption (Fig. 5.15), are rarely seen today. On initial assessment, occasional patients may have severe hypercalcemia, as a form of acute primary hyperparathyroidism or parathyroid crisis.

Diagnosis

Patients with primary hyperparathyroidism most often have high-normal or mildly increased serum total calcium and ionized calcium values. Most patients diagnosed today have asymptomatic primary hyperparathyroidism without symptoms or recognized complications. Rare patients may have eucalcemic primary hyperparathyroidism, in which serum calcium is normal but PTH levels are increased.

Imaging tests

Preoperative localization of parathyroid adenomas before initial neck exploration may be unnecessary because of extremely high cure rates (95–98%) with standard neck exploration. Patient or physician interest in minimally invasive parathyroidectomy requires use of parathyroid imaging studies, including ultrasonography, ^{99m}Tc-thallium or ^{99m}Tc-sestamibi-^{123}I subtraction scanning (Fig. 5.16), computed

tomography (CT), or magnetic resonance imaging (MRI) of the neck, before the initial operation. ^{99m}Tc-sestamibi subtraction scanning is capable of detecting as many as 90% of parathyroid adenomas before surgery. False-negative and false-positive imaging results, however, are relatively common.

Laboratory findings

Other than increased serum calcium and PTH levels, serum phosphorus is usually low normal or mildly decreased, with normal or mildly increased levels of serum total or bone alkaline phosphatase, and normal serum creatinine. Intact PTH is mildly increased or inappropriately high-normal for the level of serum calcium. Patients treated with thiazide-type diuretics or lithium may have increased serum calcium and PTH levels without primary hyperparathyroidism.

Markers of bone turnover such as bone alkaline phosphatase or beta-CTx-telopeptide may be increased without obvious bone disease, possibly due to increased IL-6 or tumor necrosis factor-α. PTH renal tubular effects may cause mildly increased serum chloride and decreased bicarbonate levels. Serum 1,25-dihydroxyvitamin D levels are usually high-normal or mildly increased, and serum 25-hydroxyvitamin D levels are typically low-normal. Studies show that 24-hour urinary calcium excretion is increased in 25–30% of patients with primary hyperparathyroidism.

Treatment

Patients with single adenomas should undergo resection of the tumor by minimally invasive surgery, or alternatively, by full neck exploration with identification of the remaining normal glands. Patients with four-gland hyperplasia should undergo removal of 3.5 glands, with one-half gland left in place, or alternatively, removal of all 4 parathyroid glands followed by autotransplantation of part of one gland in forearm or neck muscle.

In patients cured of their primary hyperparathyroidism, serum calcium promptly normalizes, often after a brief period of asymptomatic mild hypocalcemia. "Hungry bones" syndrome, with rapid skeletal calcium and phosphorus uptake postoperatively, may develop in patients with bone disease. Usually, intravenously and orally administered calcium and vitamin D supplementation is necessary to prevent symptomatic hypocalcemia. Potential complications of parathyroid surgery include hypocalcemia from chronic hypoparathyroidism, or recurrent laryngeal nerve damage. In most patients, bone density improves rapidly postoperatively, when measured at the lumbar spine and radius.

Reoperation for persistent or recurrent primary hyperparathyroidism is technically difficult. Most surgeons require preoperative imaging to localize a parathyroid tumor before a repeat operation. Invasive arteriography and selective venous sampling may be helpful if available, although these are expensive and time-consuming. Reconfirmation of the diagnosis is helpful before a second operation, primarily to rule out unsuspected familial benign hypercalcemia (FBH). Intraoperative ^{99m}Tc-sestamibi scanning with a handheld gamma counter, coupled with rapid intraoperative PTH assay, may be useful in difficult cases.

Medical options are limited for patients with symptomatic hypercalcemia who are unable to tolerate a surgical procedure. Patients should maintain hydration and remain physically active, and use of thiazides or lithium should be avoided. Daily calcium intake of 800–1000 mg/day is advised to minimize bone loss and avoid aggravation of hypercalcemia or hypercalciuria. Daily calcium intake of < 600 mg/day will cause physiologic hyperparathyroidism. Oral or intravenous phosphate should be avoided because this may precipitate ectopic calcification.

Estrogen replacement therapy may help normalize serum calcium levels and prevent bone loss in postmenopausal women, although PTH and phosphate levels do not change. Orally administered bisphosphonates may be beneficial, but etidronate and clodronate have not shown long-term benefit. Alendronate, risedronate, raloxifene, and salmon calcitonin administered by nasal spray or injection have not been extensively investigated for this indication, although alendronate or raloxifene have been reported to decrease serum calcium levels. The CaSR agonist (calcimimetic) cinacalcet HCl has been shown to decrease serum calcium and maintain normal levels of serum calcium for as long as 5 years without affecting bone mineral density, and to improve serum calcium levels in patients with intractable primary hyperparathyroidism. Patients with identifiable tumors on ultrasound studies who do not desire, or are not candidates for, surgical treatment may benefit from alcohol ablation of their tumor under ultrasound guidance, usually requiring several initial treatments over 1 month or so, but hyperparathyroidism may recur later. Asymptomatic patients with primary hyperparathyroidism who do not have parathyroidectomy tend to do well, although as many as one-quarter of these patients develop progression of disease, defined as development of at least one new indication for surgery, over 15 years of follow-up, and younger patients < 50 years old tend to have a higher incidence of progressive disease.

Illustrations (Figs 5.6–5.16)

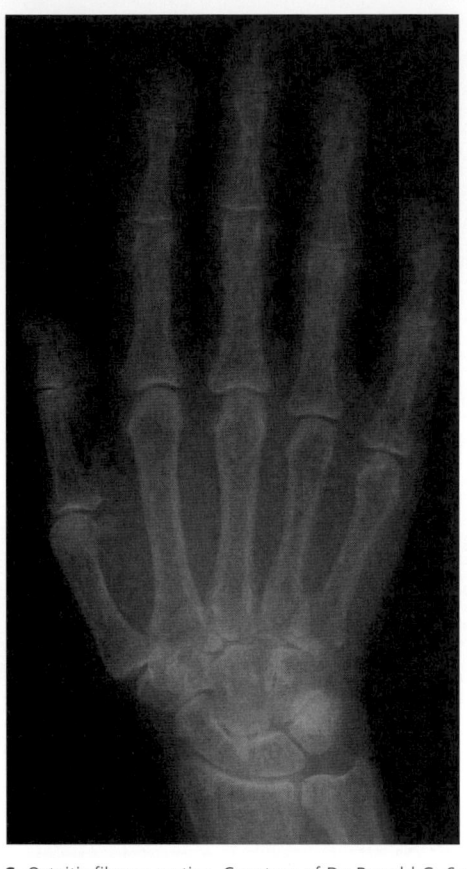

Figure 5.6 Osteitis fibrosa cystica. Courtesy of Dr. Ronald G. Swee.

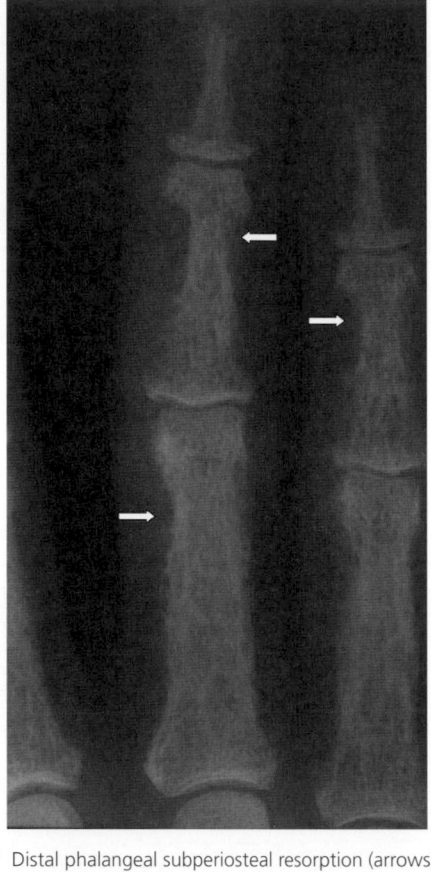

Figure 5.7 Distal phalangeal subperiosteal resorption (arrows). Courtesy of Dr. Ronald G. Swee.

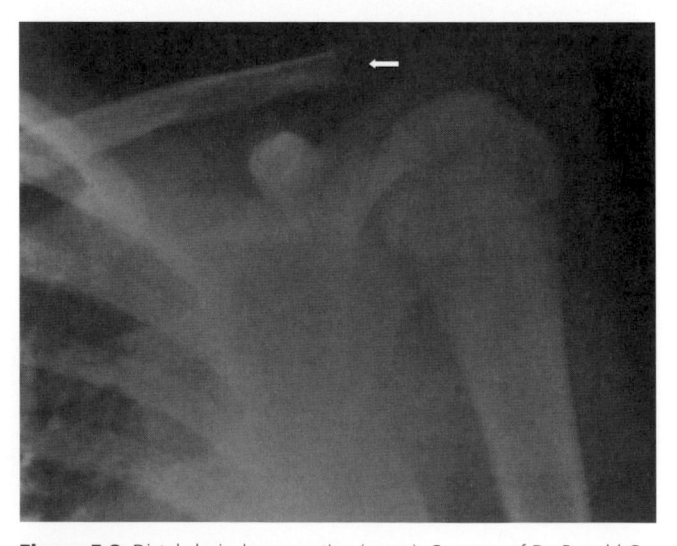

Figure 5.8 Distal clavicular resorption (arrow). Courtesy of Dr. Ronald G. Swee.

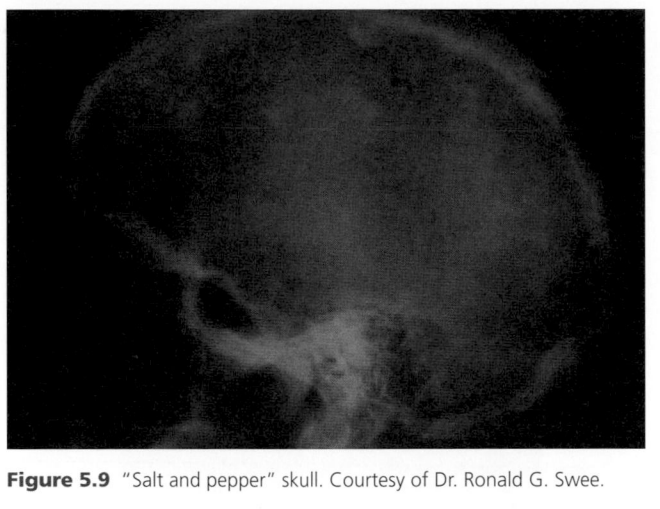

Figure 5.9 "Salt and pepper" skull. Courtesy of Dr. Ronald G. Swee.

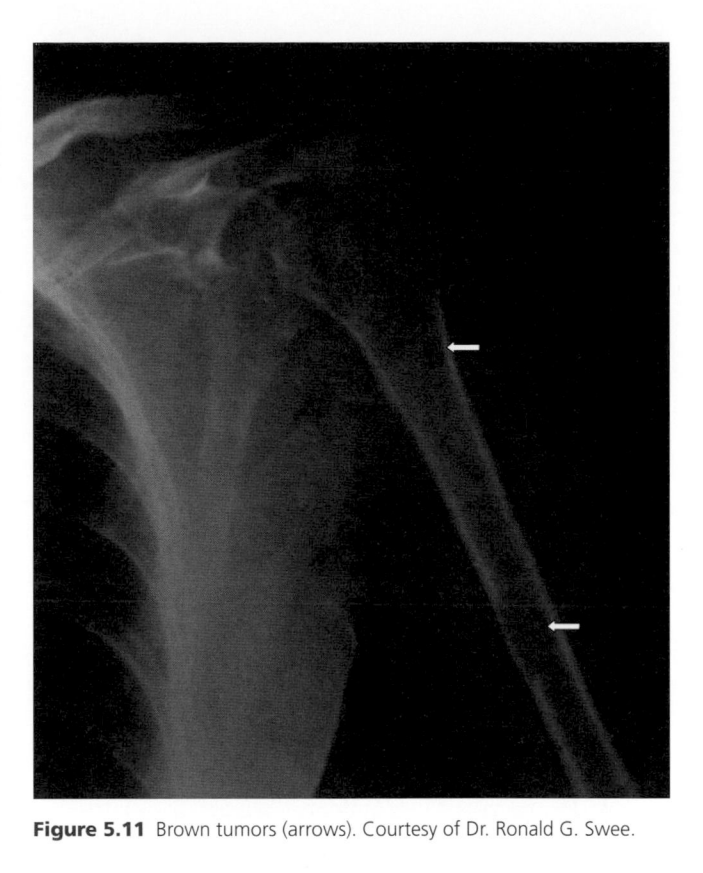

Figure 5.11 Brown tumors (arrows). Courtesy of Dr. Ronald G. Swee.

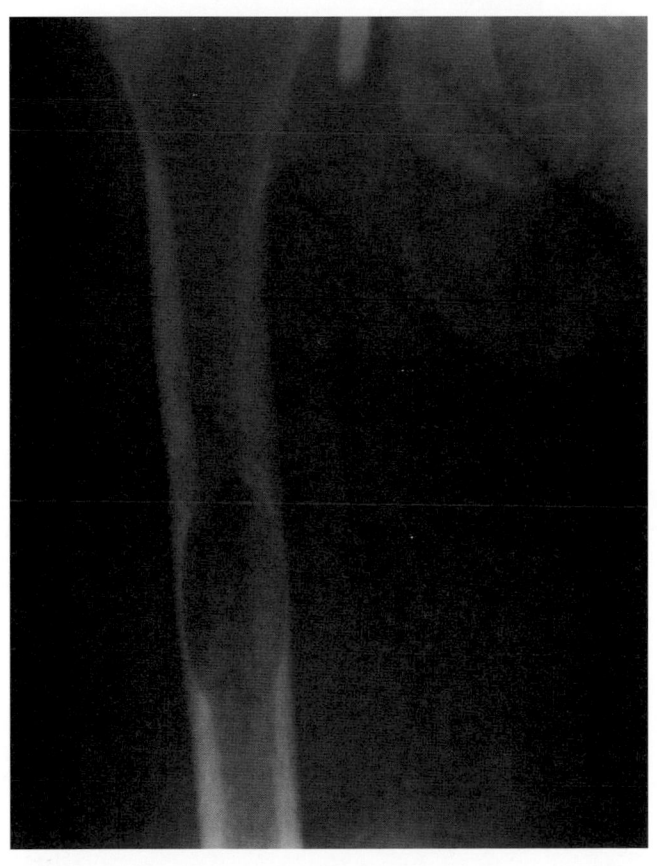

Figure 5.10 Bone cyst. Courtesy of Dr. Ronald G. Swee.

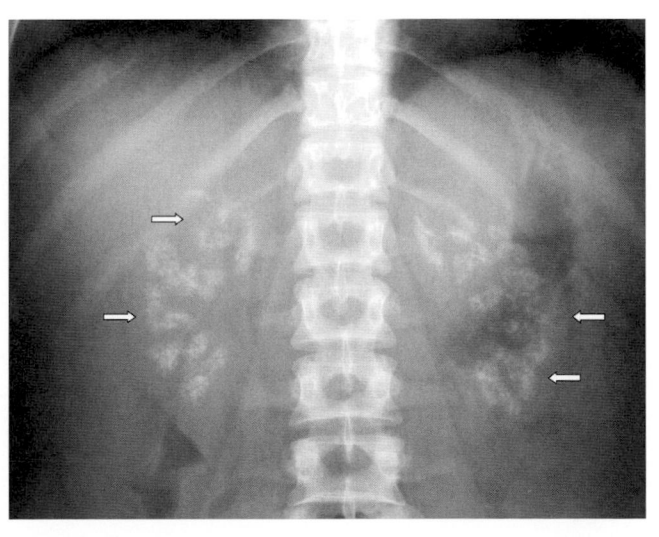

Figure 5.12 Nephrocalcinosis (arrows). Courtesy of Dr. Terri J. Vrtiska.

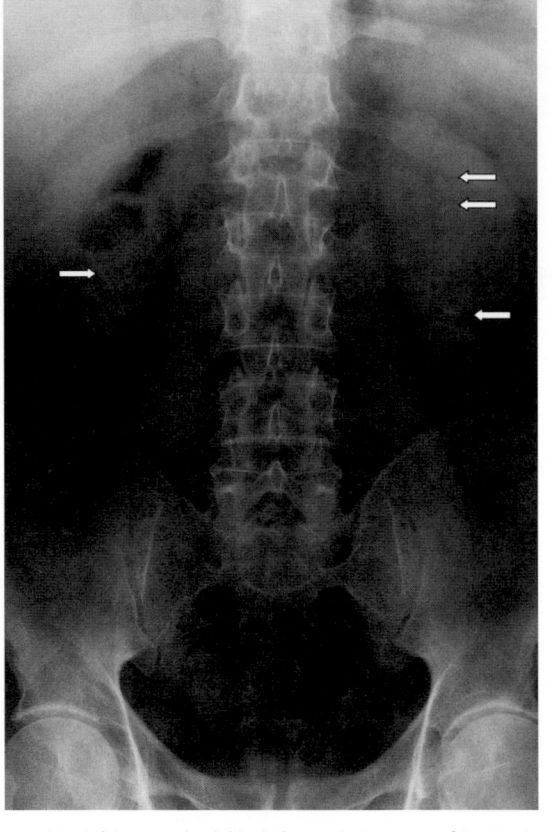

Figure 5.13 Calcium nephrolithiasis (arrows). Courtesy of Dr. Terri J. Vrtiska.

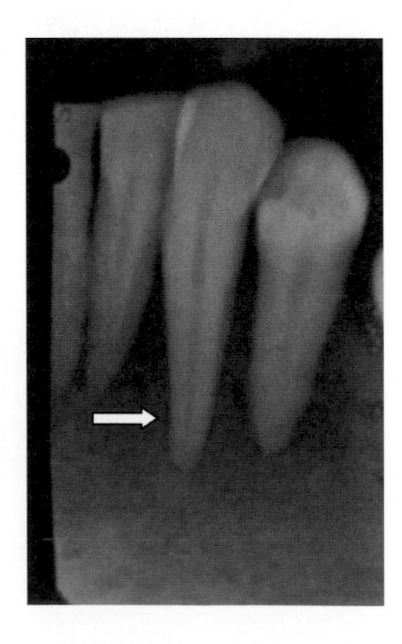

Figure 5.14 Band keratopathy. Courtesy of Dr. James A. Garrity.

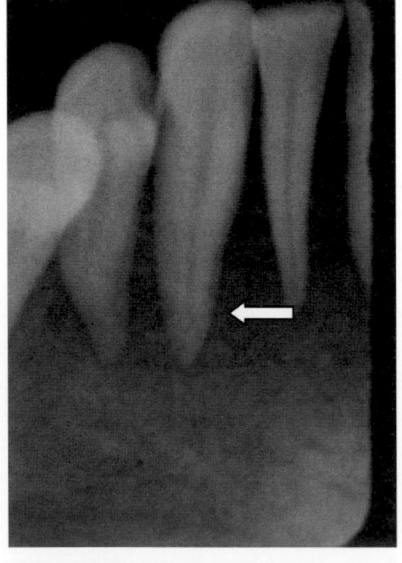 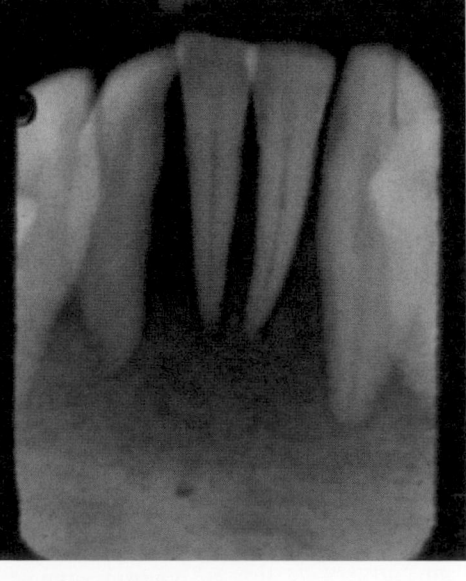 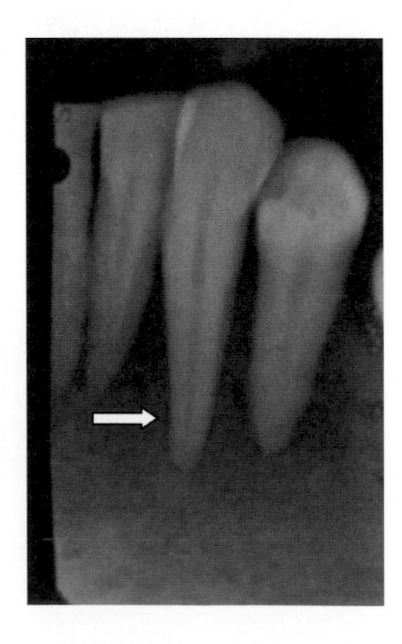

Figure 5.15 Lamina densa resorption (arrows). Courtesy of Dr. Ronald G. Swee.

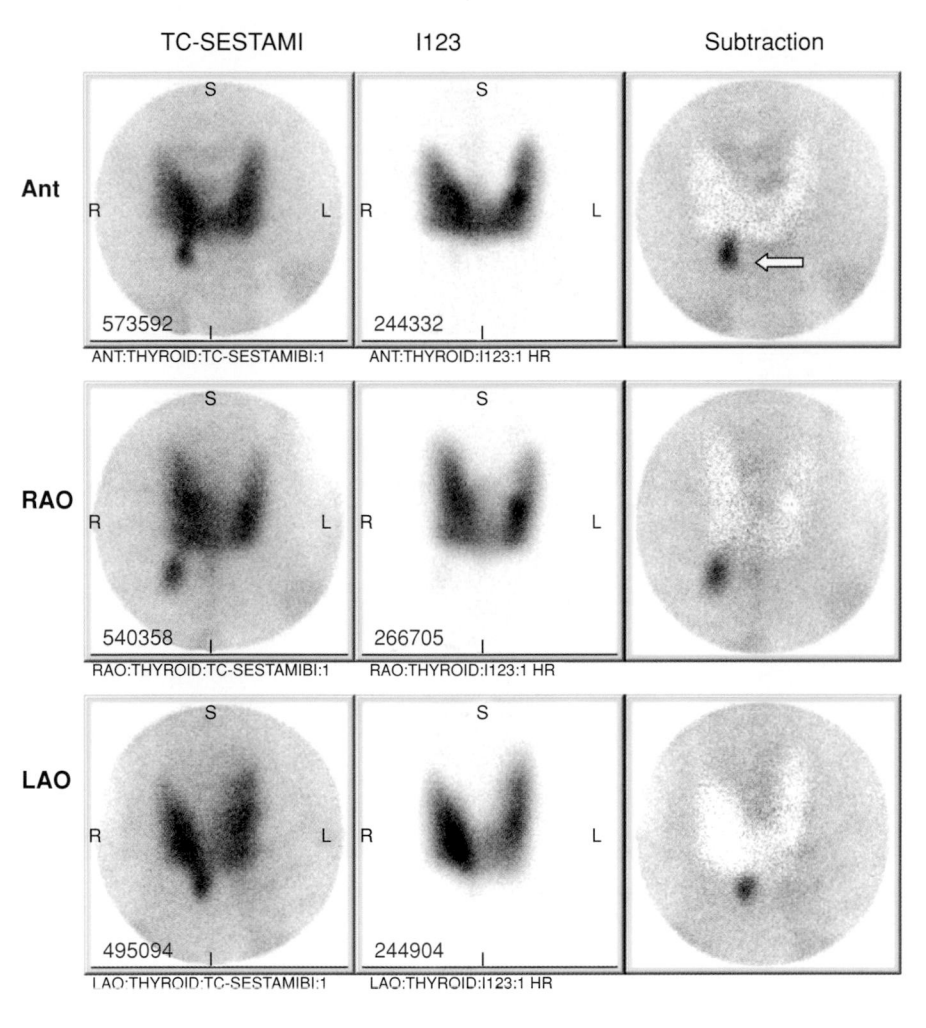

Figure 5.16 Classical parathyroid adenoma.

Hypoparathyroidism

Definition
Hypoparathyroidism is characterized by hypocalcemia associated with increased hyperphosphatemia and decreased parathyroid hormone (PTH) secretion.

Etiology
Hypoparathyroidism results from decreased PTH secretion, almost always associated with hypocalcemia. Patients with hypoparathyroidism typically present with subacute onset of tingling paresthesias, cramps, or tetany, but may also manifest with seizures, bronchospasm, laryngospasm, or cardiac rhythm disturbances. Hypoparathyroidism occurs in both acquired and inherited forms.

Postsurgical hypoparathyroidism
The most common acquired cause of hypoparathyroidism in adults is postsurgical hypoparathyroidism. Surgery on the thyroid or parathyroid glands, or adjacent neck structures, or neck dissection surgery for malignancy, may lead to acute

or chronic hypoparathyroidism. Postsurgical hypoparathyroidism is usually due to inadvertent removal of, or damage to, the parathyroid glands and/or their blood supply. While transient hypoparathyroidism after neck surgery is relatively common, chronic partial hypoparathyroidism is less common, and chronic complete hypoparathyroidism relatively rare. Diagnosis of chronic hypoparathyroidism requires that hypoparathyroidism persist for at least 6 months after surgery. Most patients with postsurgical hypoparathyroidism recover parathyroid gland function within several weeks to months after surgery.

Autoimmune hypoparathyroidism
After postsurgical hypoparathyroidism, autoimmune hypoparathyroidism is thought to be the next most common form of hypoparathyroidism in adults. Autoimmune hypoparathyroidism may be isolated, or part of an autoimmune polyglandular syndrome. Autoimmune polyglandular syndrome type I (APS-1) is caused by autosomal recessive mutations in the autoimmune regulator gene (*AIRE*) on chromosome 21q22.3.

Other acquired causes

Other less common acquired causes of hypoparathyroidism include excessive accumulation of iron in the parathyroid glands due to thalassemia or hemochromatosis. Excessive accumulation of copper in Wilson's disease is estimated to have a prevalence of 1 : 50 000 to 1 : 100 000. Acquired hypoparathyroidism has been reported to occur very rarely after iodine-131 therapy, and relatively rarely with metastatic infiltration of the parathyroid glands. Magnesium deficiency, due to proton pump inhibitor therapy, or magnesium excess, due to tocolytic therapy during labor, may cause hypoparathyroidism infrequently.

Inherited disorders

Inherited disorders are a relatively rare cause of hypoparathyroidism. DiGeorge (velocardiofacial) syndrome is estimated to occur in about 1 : 2000 to 1 : 3000 live births, and is due to *TBX1* and other gene mutations located on chromosome 22q11.2. Autosomal dominant familial hypocalcemia caused by activating mutations in the calcium-sensing receptor (CaSR) on chromosome 3q13 may be among the more common causes of inherited isolated hypoparathyroidism, but a prevalence estimate has not yet been established. Familial isolated hypoparathyroidism due to autosomal recessive or dominant mutations in the *pre-proPTH* gene on chromosome 11p15, or parathyroid gland dysgenesis due to mutations in various transcription factors regulating parathyroid gland development such as *GCMB* (glial cells missing B) or *GCM2* (glial cells missing 2), *GATA3*, or sry-box 3 (*SOX3*), are thought to be very rare. Autosomal dominant hypoparathyroidism associated with deafness and renal anomalies is due to mutations in the *GATA3* gene on chromosome 10p14-10-pter. Hypoparathyroidism has also very rarely been associated with X-linked recessive mutations on Xq26-27, leading to effects on SOX3 transcription. The syndrome of autosomal recessive hypoparathyroidism, growth and mental retardation, and dysmorphism due to mutations in the *TBCE* gene on chromosome 1q42-q43 is thought to be a very rare cause of hypoparathyroidism. Hypoparathyroidism with metabolic disturbances and congenital anomalies is associated with rare maternal mitochondrial gene defects.

Signs and symptoms

Symptomatic hypocalcemia most often presents with tingling paresthesias, especially in the distal fingers, toes, and perioral and nasal area. Neuromuscular irritability may be demonstrated by facial muscle twitching in response to tapping the facial nerve just anterior to the ear (Chvostek's sign), or by carpal spasm after inflating a blood pressure cuff 20 mmHg above the systolic blood pressure for 3 minutes (Trousseau's sign). Muscle cramps are frequently seen, but their significance may be overlooked. Tetany, laryngospasm, and bronchospasm may occur with severe or acute hypocalcemia. Seizures may occur with either acute or chronic hypocalcemia. Other central nervous system signs may include irritability, personality change, or impaired intellectual function. The presence and severity of signs and symptoms reflect the degree of hypocalcemia, and/or the acuteness of the decline in serum calcium.

Diagnosis

Patients with hypoparathyroidism typically have decreased serum total calcium, ionized calcium, and parathyroid hormone values. Most patients diagnosed today have symptomatic hypoparathyroidism with tingling paresthesias or muscle cramps, unless they are found to have mild or relatively asymptomatic transient hypoparathyroidism while being monitored after surgery. Occasional patients have low-normal serum calcium or ionized calcium, with inappropriately low parathyroid hormone levels, due to an early or very mild form of the disease.

Imaging tests

Imaging studies are not typically used in the diagnosis or management of hypoparathyroidism. Patients treated for hypoparathyroidism with calcium and vitamin D supplementation over many years frequently develop basal ganglia or other soft tissue calcification (Figs 5.17 & 5.18), cataracts, nephrocalcinosis, or calcium-containing kidney stones, which may be detected on computed tomography (CT) scans of the head, or kidney X-rays or CT scans. Skeletal X-rays may show increased bone mineralization (Fig. 5.19). Parathyroid imaging studies, including ultrasonography, ^{99m}Tc-thallium or ^{99m}Tc-sestamibi-^{123}I subtraction scanning, CT or magnetic resonance imaging (MRI) of the neck, are not helpful in localizing hypofunctioning parathyroid glands.

Laboratory findings

Other than decreased serum calcium and PTH levels, serum phosphorus is usually upper-normal or increased. Serum total alkaline phosphatase and creatinine are usually normal. Serum magnesium levels may be decreased or increased, and thereby limit PTH secretion. Markers of bone turnover, such as bone alkaline phosphatase or beta-CTx-telopeptide may be low-normal or mildly decreased with normal or mildly increased bone density. Lack of PTH renal tubular effects may cause mildly decreased serum chloride or increased bicarbonate levels. Serum 1,25-dihydroxyvitamin D levels are usually low-normal or mildly increased, and serum 25-hydroxyvitamin D levels are typically low-normal. Most patients with hypoparathyroidism have low-normal or decreased 24-hour urinary calcium, and upper-normal or mildly increased 24-hour urinary phosphorus excretion before diagnosis. Patients treated with calcium and calcitriol supplementation often have significant hypercalciuria.

Treatment

Symptomatic or severe acute hypocalcemia due to hypoparathyroidism typically requires parenteral calcium therapy. Intravenous calcium gluconate is the preferred preparation. An infusion of 10 ampules of calcium gluconate, containing 90 mg elemental calcium/10 mL ampule, in 1 L D5W allows titration of the infusion rate to achieve a serum calcium level in the range of 8.0–8.5 mg/dL. To prevent recurrence of hypocalcemia after stopping the infusion, oral therapy with calcium supplementation of 1000–2000 mg elemental calcium each day, and calcitriol (1,25-dihydroxyvitamin D3) 0.5–1.0 μg each day, are started as soon as the patient is able to tolerate oral intake. In many cases patients require daily calcium supplementation in the range of 3000–5000 mg elemental calcium, and daily calcitriol supplementation of 0.5–1.0 μg, to maintain serum calcium close to the normal range.

Forms of vitamin D other than calcitriol may be less expensive and equally effective, but if hypercalcemia develops due to vitamin D toxicity, their long half-life results in persistent hypercalcemia lasting for weeks or months, rather than days. Hypercalciuria is frequently seen in patients with chronic hypoparathyroidism, but this may be limited with use of thiazide-type diuretics. Twice daily injections of PTH 1-34, or once daily injections of PTH 1-84, have been demonstrated in short-term trials to normalize serum and urine calcium and phosphate levels in hypoparathyroid patients, but these therapies remain investigational. Successful parathyroid allograft transplants in the setting of renal transplantation have been reported in a few individuals. Stem cell therapy is under investigation.

Illustrations (Figs 5.17–5.19)

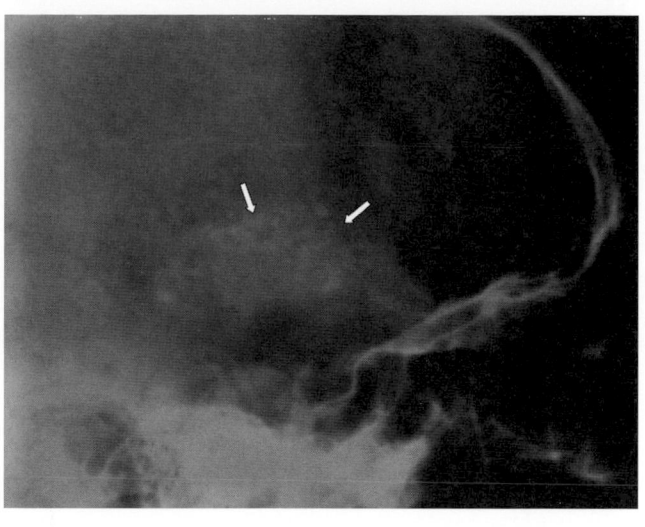

Figure 5.18 Basal ganglia calcification (arrows) seen on lateral skull view. Courtesy of Dr. Ronald G. Swee.

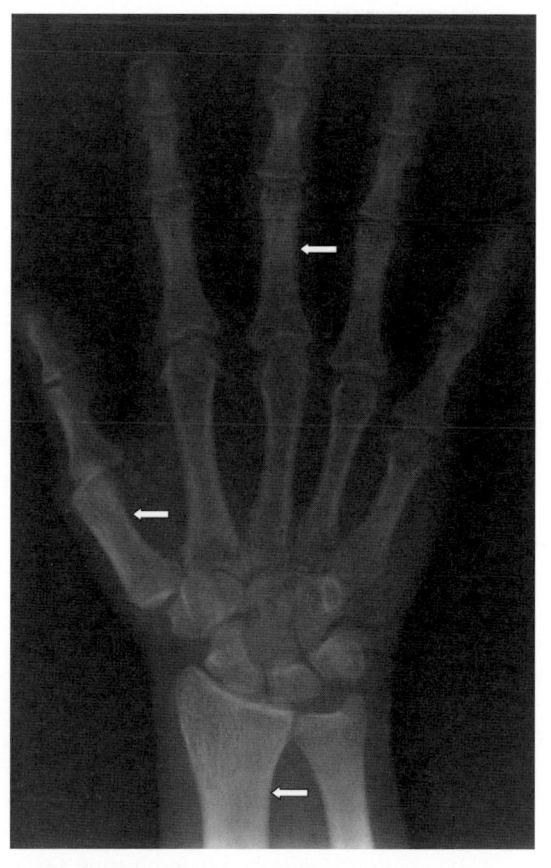

Figure 5.19 Increased skeletal mineralization (arrows) in hypoparathyroidism. Courtesy of Dr. Ronald G. Swee.

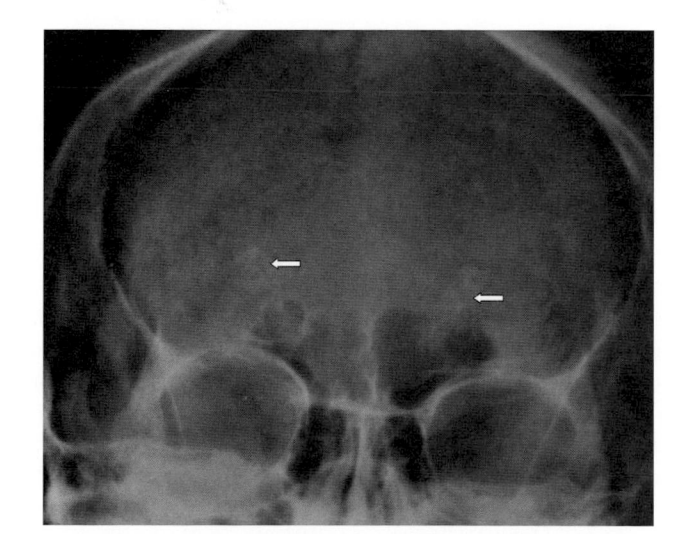

Figure 5.17 Basal ganglia calcification (arrows) seen on AP skull view. Courtesy of Dr. Ronald G. Swee.

Pseudohypoparathyroidism

Definition

Pseudohypoparathyroidism is characterized by hypocalcemia associated with excessive or inappropriate parathyroid hormone (PTH) secretion.

Etiology

Classical hypoparathyroidism is characterized by hypocalcemia, hyperphosphatemia, and decreased PTH levels. Pseudohypoparathyroidism, a group of disorders of tissue resistance to PTH, is characterized by hypocalcemia, hyperphosphatemia, and upper-normal or increased PTH levels. Patients with pseudohypoparathyroidism are not born with hypocalcemia, but develop hypocalcemia during early childhood.

Normal subjects infused with PTH during an Ellsworth–Howard test transiently increase their urinary cyclic adenosine monophosphate (cAMP) excretion, whereas patients with pseudohypoparathyroidism type 1a do not. The PTH1 receptor (PTH1R) is a member of the seven-transmembrane G-protein-coupled receptor family. Binding of PTH to PTH1R causes a conformational change in the receptor, allowing the receptor to bind to G_s protein. The guanosine diphosphate (GDP) bound to G_s is replaced by guanosine triphosphate (GTP), and the subunits of G_s dissociate. $G\alpha_s$ subunit binds to adenylate cyclase, stimulating synthesis of cAMP. In pseudohypoparathyroidism type 1a, $G\alpha_s$ expression or activity is reduced by about 50%, thereby disrupting the PTH signaling cascade. In this situation, both PTH and PTHR1 function normally, but target tissues are unable to respond normally. Patients with pseudohypoparathyroidism type 1a may also have resistance to other hormones, such as thyroid stimulating hormone (TSH), which also rely on this G-protein-coupled receptor signal transduction mechanism.

Patients with pseudohypoparathyroidism type 1a have a constellation of developmental and somatic defects called Albright's hereditary osteodystrophy (AHO). This constellation includes short stature, rounded facies, obesity, brachydactyly, and subcutaneous ossifications. Individuals who manifest AHO but do not have PTH resistance are classified as having pseudopseudohypoparathyroidism. Patients with pseudohypoparathyroidism type 1a or pseudopseudohypoparathyroidism both have approximately 50% decreases in $G\alpha_s$ activity. Analysis of pedigrees of patients with these disorders has shown that genomic imprinting of the $G\alpha_s$ gene (GNAS1) explains the differences in phenotype. Maternal transmission of $G\alpha_s$ deficiency leads to pseudohypoparathyroidism type 1a, whereas paternal transmission leads to pseudopseudohypoparathyroidism. The mechanism of imprinting is complex, and does not yet fully explain all manifestations of these disorders.

Other forms of pseudohypoparathyroidism are molecularly and clinically distinct from pseudohypoparathyroidism type 1a. Individuals with pseudohypoparathyroidism type 1b lack phenotypic features of AHO, have normal $G\alpha_s$ function, and are resistant only to PTH. This condition appears to be due to an imprinting defect of GNAS1 and selective deficiency of $G\alpha_s$ limited to the proximal renal tubule. A few individuals have been described with pseudohypoparathyroidism type 1c, which is characterized by normal G-protein function and resistance to multiple hormones. Pseudohypoparathyroidism type 2 is a heterogeneous disorder, with PTH resistance characterized by normal urinary cAMP response but decreased phosphaturic response to PTH. The genetic and molecular bases for the pseudohypoparathyroidism types 1c and 2 are not yet known.

The gold standard for diagnosis of pseudohypoparathyroidism is demonstration of end-organ resistance to PTH by provocative testing, but this is rarely performed today due to lack of available PTH. A positive family history, or the same biochemical or physical findings in other family members, tends to confirm the diagnosis.

Signs and symptoms

Most patients with pseudohypoparathyroidism have asymptomatic or mildly symptomatic hypocalcemia, hyperphosphatemia, and increased PTH levels. There is a moderate degree of heterogeneity in the degree of hypocalcemia among patients with pseudohypoparathyroidism. Patients with pseudohypoparathyroidism type 1a or pseudopseudohypoparathyroidism have features of AHO, whereas patients with pseudohypoparathyroidism type 1b, 1c, or 2 do not have these features.

Diagnosis

Diagnosis is usually based on biochemical findings, sometimes buttressed by physical exam findings. Patients with pseudohypoparathyroidism typically have low-normal or mildly decreased serum total calcium and ionized calcium values, with hyperphosphatemia and increased PTH levels.

Imaging tests

Imaging studies are not often useful in diagnosing pseudohypoparathyroidism. Classical phenotypic physical features of AHO and/or biochemical findings of pseudohypoparathyroidism are sufficient for clinical diagnosis of this group of disorders. Shortened fourth and/or fifth metacarpals or metatarsals may be seen on hand or foot X-rays in patients with pseudohypoparathyroidism type 1a with AHO, but are not seen in patients with pseudohypoparathyroidism type 1b (Fig. 5.20). However, these findings are not pathognomic of this group of disorders. Individuals with shortened fourth or fifth metacarpals have dimples where their knuckles should be when clenching their fists (Fig. 5.21).

Laboratory findings

Patients with pseudohypoparathyroidism have low-normal or decreased serum calcium, increased serum phosphorus,

and increased serum PTH levels. Serum total alkaline phosphatase is usually low-normal or normal, and serum creatinine is normal. Markers of bone turnover such as bone alkaline phosphatase or beta-CTx-telopeptide are usually normal or mildly decreased, without obvious bone disease. Resistance to PTH renal tubular effects may cause mildly decreased serum chloride and increased bicarbonate levels. Serum 1,25-dihydroxyvitamin D levels are usually low-normal or normal, and serum 25-hydroxyvitamin D levels are typically low-normal. Pseudohypoparathyroidism is associated with normal or mildly decreased 24-hour urinary calcium excretion.

Treatment

Patients with pseudohypoparathyroidism are treated with calcium and calcitriol (1,25-dihydroxyvitamin D3) supplementation as needed to maintain normal serum calcium levels. Supplement doses required to treat this group of disorders are usually less than those required to treat hypoparathyroidism.

Illustrations (Figs 5.20 & 5.21)

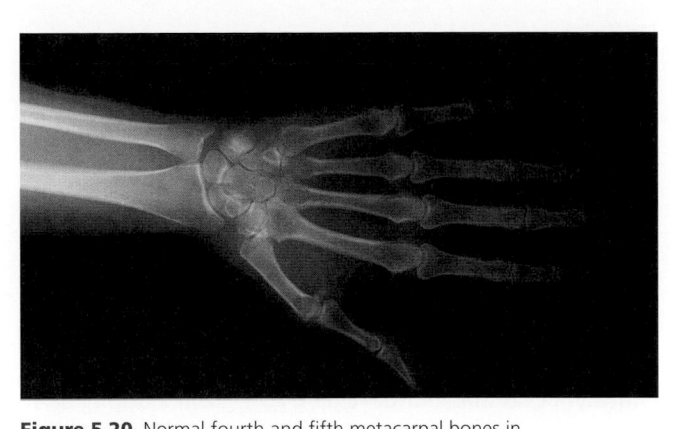

Figure 5.20 Normal fourth and fifth metacarpal bones in pseudohypoparathyroidism type 1b. Courtesy of Dr. Ronald G. Swee.

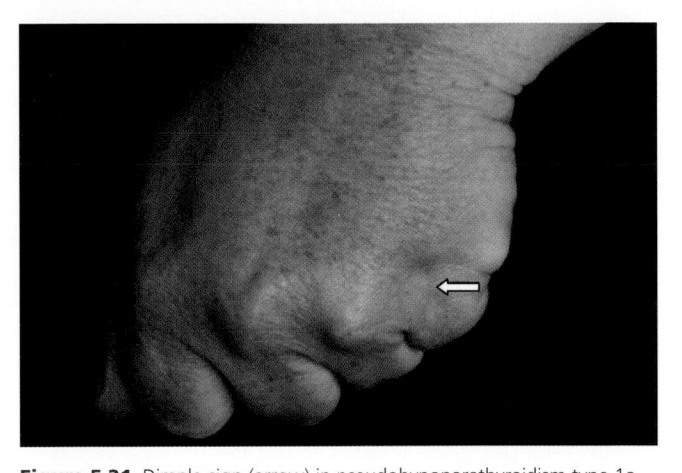

Figure 5.21 Dimple sign (arrow) in pseudohypoparathyroidism type 1a, with shortened fifth metacarpal.

Paget's disease of bone

Definition

Paget's disease is a focal progressive disorder of increased bone remodeling, characterized by mixed lytic and sclerotic bone lesions.

Etiology

Osteoclasts in pagetic bone are markedly increased in size and number, and may contain up to as many as 100 nuclei, in comparison with the usual 5–10 nuclei in a normal osteoclast. Because bone resorption and formation are coupled in Paget's disease, increased bone resorption results in a secondary increase in bone formation, and up to 10-fold increased bone turnover. Bone that is remodeled by pagetic osteoclasts and osteoblasts becomes enlarged and structurally weakened. Pain, skeletal deformity, and fractures may develop as a consequence of these changes.

Monostotic Paget's disease involves only one bone, but more commonly this disorder involves multiple skeletal sites (polyostotic), and is asymmetric in skeletal distribution. The most common sites of involvement are the pelvis, lumbar spine, and femur. At least one of these sites is involved in more than 75% of patients. Other sites that are commonly affected are the skull, tibia, scapula, sternum, and humerus.

Pagetic bone is remodeled at an accelerated rate. During remodeling, bone collagen is deposited in a random, disorganized fashion that produces woven bone, rather than normal lamellar bone. Woven bone is less strong than lamellar bone, and this contributes to the fractures and deformity that develop in patients with Paget's disease.

Pagetic bone is characterized by increased osteoclasts and osteoblasts, increased osteoid surface, thickness, and volume, bone marrow fibrosis, and increased vascular spaces within the marrow. Trabeculae are thickened and irregular, with increased trabecular bone volume, and cortical bone is thickened because of increased periosteal bone formation. In early Paget's disease, bone resorption predominates, and lytic lesions are frequently seen. As the disease progresses, increased bone formation results in a mixed lytic and sclerotic picture. In late Paget's disease, bony sclerosis is the predominant finding.

Several mutations have been described that predispose patients to Paget's disease. Susceptibility loci for Paget's disease have been identified on chromosomes 18, 5, 6, 2, and 10. Mutations in the *Sequestasome 1* gene (*SQSTM1*) on chromosome 5q35, important in nuclear factor-κB (RANK) ligand (RANKL)-induced osteoclastogenesis, have been reported in both familial and sporadic Paget's disease. *Sequestasome 1* is thought to be most important gene associated with classical late-onset Paget's disease, and is estimated to account for 20–50% of familial, and 5–20% of

sporadic, cases of Paget's disease. Chromosome 18 contains the RANK gene, which is directly involved in osteoclast formation and activation. Mutations in RANK (*TNFRSF11A* gene) have been identified as a cause of familial expansile osteolysis (FEO), expansile skeletal hyperphosphatasia (ESH), and early-onset familial Paget's disease. Inactivating mutations of osteoprotegerin (OPG) (*TNFRSF11B* gene), an endogenous inhibitor of osteoclastic bone resorption secreted by osteoblasts and a decoy receptor for RANKL, have been found in patients with juvenile Paget's disease. Polymorphisms in the *TNFRSF11B* gene are also associated with sporadic Paget's disease. Finally, mutations in the valosin-containing protein (VCP) gene, which is involved in RANK signaling, have been reported to cause inclusion body myopathy with Paget's disease of bone and frontotemporal dementia (IBMPFD).

Ultrastructural studies have identified nuclear inclusions resembling paramyxovirus nucleocapsids in osteoclasts from pagetic lesions in patients with Paget's disease. Molecular and immunologic studies have shown that nuclear inclusions in pagetic osteoclasts may cross-react with antibodies to nucleocapsids from measles virus, respiratory syncytial virus, or canine distemper virus. Transfection of measles virus nucleocapsid gene into normal osteoclast precursors has resulted in osteoclasts that resemble pagetic osteoclasts. Specific viruses have not been isolated from patients with Paget's disease, and the role of viruses in development of Paget's disease is the subject of ongoing research.

Signs and symptoms

Most patients with Paget's disease of bone are asymptomatic at diagnosis. However, pain is the most common clinical manifestation, followed by bone deformities. Potential causes of pain include pagetic bone pain, stress fracture or complete fracture, secondary arthritis, neurologic compression syndromes, or sarcomatous transformation. Patients with Paget's disease may have a significantly reduced quality of life due to decreased ability to function physically. Survival is not reduced in Paget's disease.

Pagetic bone pain is often present at rest and aggravated by weight-bearing activity when the spine or lower extremities are involved. Patients with skull involvement frequently complain of a band-like discomfort or headache. In areas where bone is close to the skin surface, increased vascularity may increase skin temperature.

Secondary arthritis is common in Paget's disease, and most commonly found in the hip, knee, and ankle joints. In patients with pain involving the spine, hip, or knee, determining whether the pain is pagetic in origin or due to secondary arthritis may be difficult. Injection of a local anesthetic agent is a useful diagnostic test in these patients. As many as 11% of Paget's patients may require a hip or knee replacement.

Diagnosis

Diagnosis is usually based on classic X-ray findings, increased serum total or bone alkaline phosphatase, and sometimes by physical exam findings. X-ray findings include bony enlargement, cortical thickening, thickened trabecular markings, osteolysis, or loss of the cortical-medullary junction (Fig. 5.22). Early stages of Paget's disease are characterized by bone lysis, leading to the classic "blade of grass" lesion in long bones (Fig. 5.23), and osteoporosis circumscripta in the skull (Fig. 5.24). Late changes in the skull may have a "cotton wool" appearance (Fig. 5.25). Individually, none of these findings are specific for Paget's disease, but in combination, they are diagnostic in almost all cases. Paget's disease usually has an insidious onset, and occurs later in life. The disease seldom develops before the age of 40. Both men and women are affected, with a slight male preponderance.

Imaging tests

Imaging studies are critical in diagnosing Paget's disease. Plain X-rays (Fig. 5.26) or computed tomography (CT) scans are relatively specific for Paget's disease, especially when findings are noted incidentally. A bone scan is useful in defining the extent of disease in patients who are found to have Paget's disease (Fig. 5.27), and in assessing causes for an unexplained increase in serum bone alkaline phosphatase. Areas of unexplained increased uptake on a bone scan should be imaged by X-ray to clarify the diagnosis.

Identification of new foci of Paget's disease is extremely rare after the initial discovery of Paget's disease. Radiographs should be considered if new symptoms develop, when symptoms become more severe, or if a fracture is suspected. X-rays are also useful for monitoring lytic lesions in weight-bearing bones. X-rays, CT or magnetic resonance imaging (MRI), or bone biopsy, are useful in assessing patients for sarcomatous transformation of Paget's disease (Fig. 5.28).

Laboratory findings

Patients with Paget's disease often have increased serum bone alkaline phosphatase, but not always. Patients with quiescent Paget's disease may have normal serum bone alkaline phosphatase levels. Other markers of bone formation, such as P1NP or osteocalcin are often increased dramatically, as are markers of bone resorption, such as serum CTx-telopeptide or urinary NTx-telopeptide or deoxypyridinoline. Paget's disease is most often associated with normal serum calcium, unless an adult patient is immobilized, in which case hypercalcemia may be present. Serum phosphorus, creatinine, and parathyroid hormone (PTH) levels are usually normal. Serum 25-hydroxyvitamin D is usually normal or low-normal. Serum 1,25-dihydroxyvitamin D is usually normal or upper-normal, depending on serum creatinine and PTH levels. 24-hour urinary calcium may be increased with active Paget's disease, but is otherwise usually normal.

Treatment

Paget's disease typically responds quickly to intravenous zoledronic acid, with reduction in symptoms and serum alkaline phosphatase within several weeks to months. Approved oral bisphosphonate therapies such as alendronate, risedronate, or tiludronate, or intravenous pamidronate, also reduce symptoms and serum alkaline phosphatase, albeit more slowly, often over months. Rapidity of response to bisphosphonates may correlate with time to relapse, with more rapid response leading to a more prolonged decrease in bone turnover. Salmon or human calcitonin by daily subcutaneous injection has also been approved for treatment of Paget's disease, but calcitonin is less potent than any of the bisphosphonates. Occasional patients refractory to therapy with one agent may benefit from combination therapy.

Surgical treatment is reserved for specific indications in Paget's disease. These include secondary arthritis that fails to improve with medical therapy, progressive skeletal deformities that impair mobility, spinal stenosis, unstable fractures, or fractures with delayed union.

Illustrations (Figs 5.22–5.28)

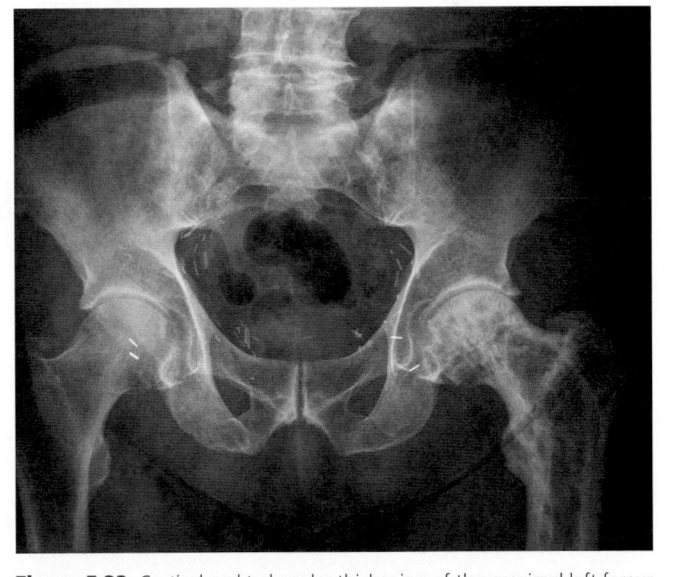

Figure 5.22 Cortical and trabecular thickening of the proximal left femur due to Paget's disease of bone. Courtesy of Dr. Bart L. Clarke.

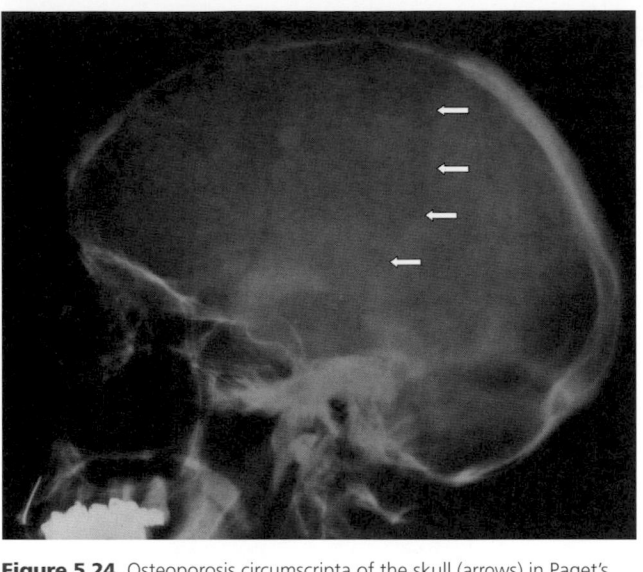

Figure 5.24 Osteoporosis circumscripta of the skull (arrows) in Paget's disease of bone. Courtesy of Dr. Ronald G. Swee.

Figure 5.23 "Blade of grass" lesion (arrows) in mid-femoral shaft. Courtesy of Dr. Ronald G. Swee.

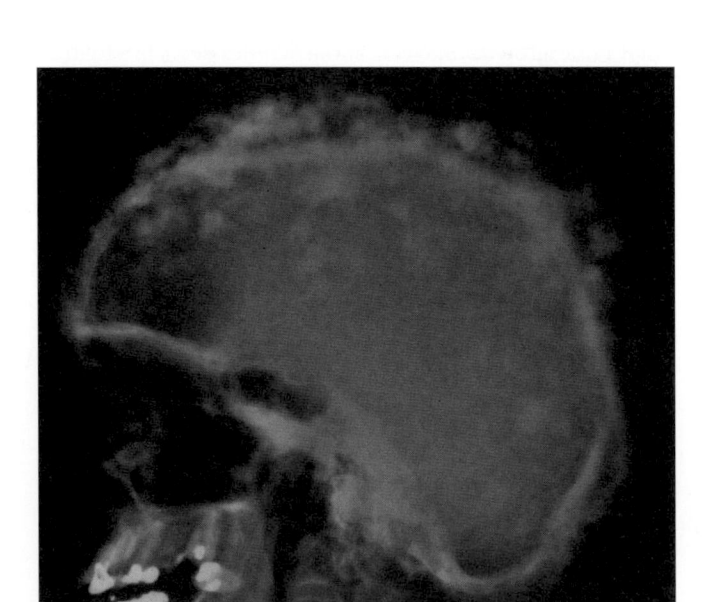

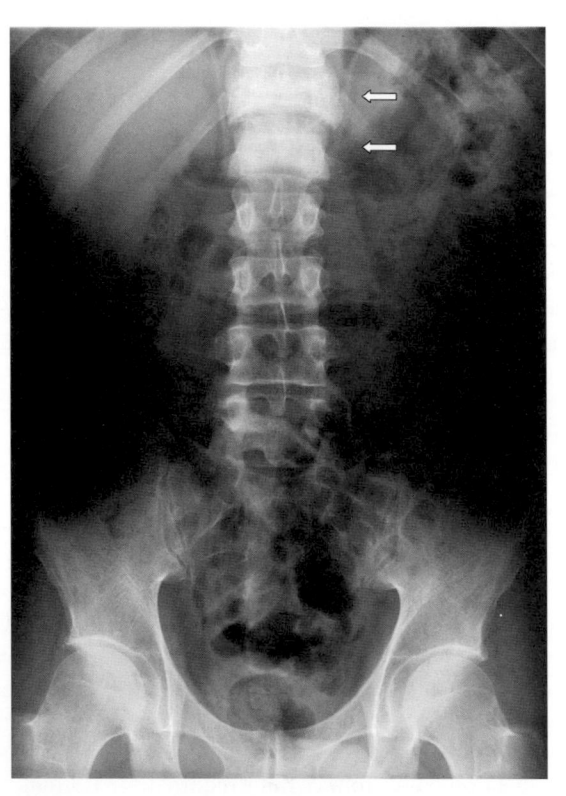

Figure 5.25 Cotton-wool patches over the skull in advanced Paget's disease of bone. Courtesy of Dr. Ronald G. Swee.

Figure 5.26 Incidental finding of increased vertebral body sclerosis and thickening (arrows) in Paget's disease of bone. Courtesy of Dr. Bart L. Clarke.

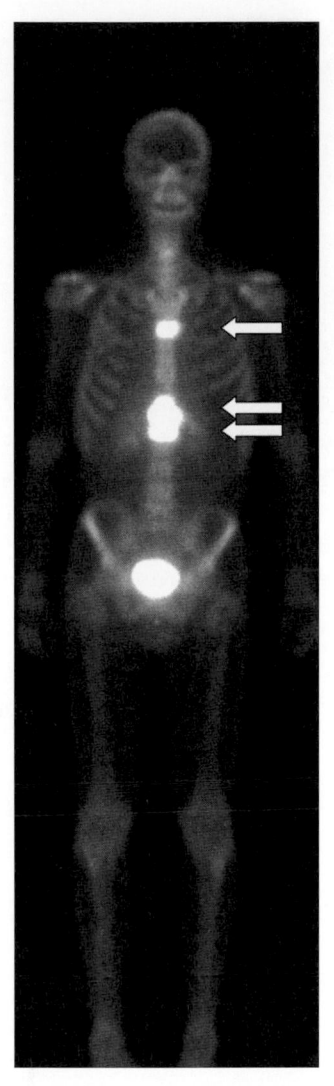

Figure 5.27 Increased uptake in multiple vertebral bodies on ^{99}Tc bone scan (arrows) in Paget's disease of bone. Courtesy of Dr. Bart L. Clarke.

Osteomalacia

Definition

Osteomalacia is a disorder characterized by defective mineralization of osteoid matrix at sites of bone turnover or periosteal or endosteal apposition in the mature skeleton in adults. The major abnormalities seen on bone biopsy are excessive amounts of inadequately mineralized osteoid, and prolonged mineralization lag time. In most cases, inadequately mineralized osteoid is due to lower circulating calcium-phosphate product than required for normal mineralization. Osteomalacia is a general term describing similar histopathologic and radiologic changes seen in a large group of diverse disorders.

Rickets is due to failure or delay in mineralization of endochondral new bone formation at the growth plates in children. This causes disorganized cartilage development, with

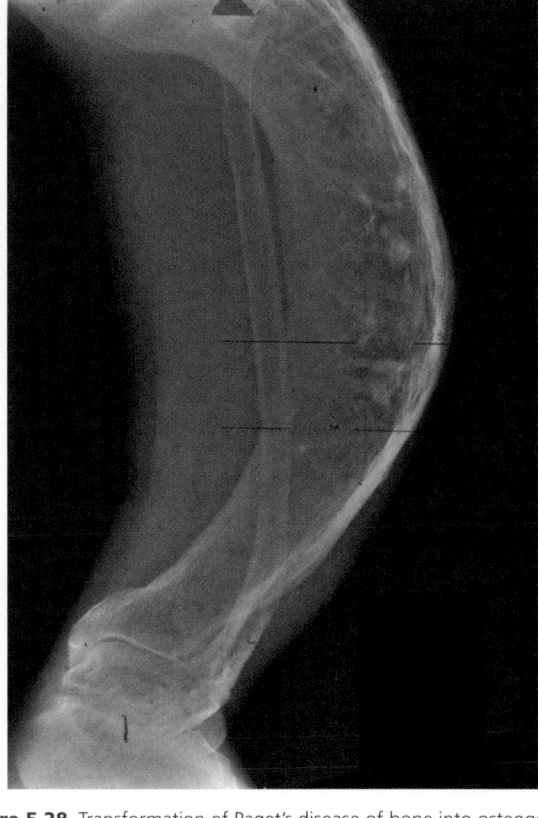

Figure 5.28 Transformation of Paget's disease of bone into osteogenic sarcoma. Courtesy of Dr. Robert D. Tiegs and Dr. Frank H. Sim.

widening of the ends of long bones, and slowing of longitudinal bone growth. Skeletal abnormalities seen in children with rickets, or adults who had rickets in childhood, include short stature and bowing of the legs.

Etiology

Osteomalacia results from multiple diverse causes. Abnormalities in vitamin D metabolism may be due to vitamin D deficiency, resulting from nutritional deficiency, lack of adequate sunlight exposure, or intestinal malabsorption after partial or total gastrectomy, small bowel disease, or pancreatic insufficiency. Defective skin production of vitamin D3 may play a role in chronic kidney disease or normal aging. Defective liver 25-hydroxylation of vitamin D plays a role in primary biliary cirrhosis, biliary atresia, or biliary fistula. Defective renal 1α-hydroxylation of 25-hydroxyvitamin D may cause osteomalacia in patients with hypoparathyroidism, pseudohypoparathyroidism, chronic kidney disease, autosomal recessive pseudovitamin D deficiency rickets (previously known as vitamin D-dependent rickets type I), hypophosphatemic osteomalacia, tumor-induced (oncogenic) osteomalacia, or age-related osteomalacia. Hereditary vitamin D-resistant rickets (previously known as vitamin D-dependent rickets type II) is associated with defective target organ response to 1,25-dihydroxyvitamin D because of

vitamin D receptor mutations, in association with alopecia totalis in some kindreds, and occasionally chronic anticonvulsant therapy. Renal loss of vitamin D-binding protein may contribute to osteomalacia in patients with nephrotic syndrome.

Vitamin D deficiency

Vitamin D deficiency in healthy adults is more prevalent than previously thought in many countries. Recent reports suggest that in most cases serum 25-hydroxyvitamin D levels are mildly decreased (in the 15–25 ng/dL range), but not sufficiently decreased to cause osteomalacia, which requires serum 25-hydroxyvitamin D levels < 10 ng/mL. While not sufficiently decreased to cause osteomalacia, suboptimal vitamin D levels have been linked to bone loss and osteoporosis, as well as prostate, breast, and colon cancer, type 1 diabetes mellitus, hypertension, cardiovascular disease, psoriasis, multiple sclerosis, osteoarthritis, periodontal disease, depression, schizophrenia, and other disorders.

Phosphate deficiency

Phosphate deficiency may occur in patients with diminished oral intake, resulting in hypophosphatemic neonatal rickets, or in patients ingesting excess aluminum hydroxide antacid, which blocks intestinal phosphate absorption. Cadmium, ifosfamide, tenofovir, efavirenz, and saccharated ferric oxide or iron polymaltose may impair renal phosphate reabsorption. Impaired renal tubular reabsorption of phosphate occurs in several disorders. Primary renal tubular defects are seen in X-linked hypophosphatemic osteomalacia, adult-onset hypophosphatemic osteomalacia, sporadic acquired hypophosphatemic osteomalacia, and Fanconi syndromes.

Genetic mutations

X-linked hypophosphatemic vitamin D-resistant rickets is due to mutations in the *PHEX* gene (Phosphate-regulating gene with Homologies to Endopeptidases on the X chromosome) located on Xp22.1-22.2. These mutations result in decreased production of the endopeptidase PHEX, which normally cleaves and inactivates circulating fibroblast growth factor-23 (FGF-23). Increased circulating FGF-23 levels cause decreased sodium-dependent phosphate transporter 2A (NaPi-2A) activity at the renal tubular brush border membrane, resulting in increased urinary phosphate wasting. Autosomal dominant hypophosphatemic rickets is due to mutations in the *FGF-23* gene, which result in resistance of FGF-23 protein to enzymatic cleavage. This leads to elevated circulating FGF-23 levels, which cause decreased NaPi-2A activity, leading to increased urinary phosphate wasting. Hereditary hypophosphatemic rickets with hypercalciuria is due to biallelic mutations in the *SLC34A3* gene, causing abnormalities in the sodium-phosphate cotransporter type IIc (NaPi-IIc).

Tumor-induced osteomalacia

Secondary renal tubular defects may be seen in primary and secondary hyperparathyroidism, renal tubular acidosis, and tumor-induced osteomalacia. In tumor-induced osteomalacia, tumors of mesenchymal origin oversecrete FGF-23, which leads to decreased NaPi-2A activity and increased urinary phosphate wasting. Other mesenchymal tumors causing tumor-induced osteomalacia may oversecrete other "phosphatonins," which are products that cause renal tubular phosphate wasting in a manner similar to FGF-23, including secreted frizzled related protein 4 (sFRP4), matrix extracellular phosphoglycoprotein (MEPE), FGF-7, or FGF-2. Patients with tumor-induced osteomalacia typically have low-normal or decreased serum 1,25-dihydroxyvitamin D levels in spite of hypophosphatemia because the phosphatonin suppresses renal 1α-hydroxylase activity. However, not all patients with mesenchymal tumors of this type secrete phosphatonins.

Calcium deficiency

Calcium deficiency may occur in children in certain developing countries with very low dietary calcium intakes, but this is not a common cause of osteomalacia in adults. Excessive use of sunscreens, avoidance of sunlight, or high-dose cholestyramine may cause low vitamin D levels, leading to hypocalcemia. Phenobarbital, phenytoin, or carbemazepine may also cause low vitamin D levels due to increased liver metabolism, resulting in hypocalcemia.

Mineralization defects

Mineralization defects may be due to deficiency of tissue-nonspecific alkaline phosphatase enzyme in hypophosphatasia, circulating inhibitor(s) of calcification in chronic kidney disease or hypophosphatasia (due to increased pyrophosphate), or therapy with certain drugs or ions such as high-dose bisphosphonates, fluoride, or aluminum intoxication. Mineralization defects may also occur in patients with abnormal bone collagen or matrix, as seen in chronic kidney disease, osteogenesis imperfecta, or fibrogenesis imperfecta ossium.

Rapid bone formation

Patients with rapid bone formation rates may develop osteomalacia, such as after surgical cure of primary hyperparathyroidism with pre-existing osteitis fibrosa cystica, or in osteopetrosis. Patients treated with parenteral alimentation without adequate vitamin or mineral supplementation may develop osteomalacia.

Signs and symptoms

Most patients with recognized osteomalacia have diffuse bone pain or proximal muscle weakness at diagnosis. However, patients with mild osteomalacia may be relatively asymptomatic.

Skeletal pain associated with osteomalacia is typically dull and aching, and worsens with weight-bearing or physical activity. Pain is most often present in the lower back, hips, and at fracture sites, and most often distant from joints. Patients often have tenderness to palpation of the bones and muscles between the joints.

Patients with long-standing or severe osteomalacia may develop significant muscle weakness. Muscle weakness may be severe, with muscle wasting, and usually involves the proximal muscles of the lower extremities, resulting in a waddling gait. Muscle weakness due to osteomalacia is thought to be due to multiple causes, and may be due to myopathic changes, usually associated with neurogenic atrophy or type II muscle fiber atrophy. Muscle weakness in many cases may be due to prolonged hypophosphatemia or the effect of prolonged secondary hyperparathyroidism on muscles.

Fractures most commonly occur in the ribs, vertebrae, and long bones and may lead to deformities, depending on their location.

Diagnosis

Diagnosis of osteomalacia is usually suspected based on classical physical symptoms, increased serum total or bone alkaline phosphatase, and classical imaging findings. The only way to confirm osteomalacia, however, is by tetracycline-labeled iliac crest bone biopsy. Iliac crest biopsy shows increased unmineralized osteoid width, surface, and volume (Fig. 5.29), and prolonged mineralization lag time. Fluoroscopic microscopic examination of a tetracycline-labeled bone biopsy from a patient with osteomalacia shows smudging of the label (Fig. 5.30).

Imaging tests

Radiographic findings associated with osteomalacia include decreased skeletal bone density, often characterized as osteopenia, but this is nonspecific. Trabecular coarsening may be due to loss of secondary trabeculae or inadequate mineralization of osteoid. In advanced disease, vertebral bodies may soften and endplates become concave, producing "codfish" vertebrae (Fig. 5.31), with enlarged and biconvex intervertebral disks.

Changes of rickets are best seen at the distal radius and ulna, or the tibial and femoral growth plates around the knee (Fig. 5.32). Classical changes of rickets include widening of the growth plate with fraying, cupping, and splaying of the metaphyses and underdevelopment of the epiphyses. At the wrist, the earliest change of rickets is loss of the clear demarcation between the growth plate and the metaphysis, with loss of the provisional zone of calcification.

Looser's zones (pseudofractures) are narrow radiolucent lines that transect and lie at right angles or obliquely to the cortical margins of bones (Figs 5.34 & 5.35). These are often bilateral and symmetric, and they may be commonly found at the axillary margins of the scapulae, lower ribs, superior and inferior pubic rami, inner margins and neck of proximal femurs, and posterior margins of proximal ulnae. Milkman's syndrome is characterized by multiple, bilateral, symmetric pseudofractures. Pseudofractures are thought to be due to stress fractures inadequately repaired by unmineralized osteoid, or possibly due to mechanical erosion of bone caused by arterial pulsations at the site of the pseudofracture.

Skeletal deformities occur at sites of rapid skeletal growth in childhood rickets. Skeletal changes vary with age because the rate of bone growth varies with age. The types of changes seen indicate the age of onset of rickets in a child. The skull is prominently affected in neonates, with craniotabes (softening of the cranium) associated with parietal flattening, frontal bossing, and widened sutures of the skull. Arms and ribs seem to be predominantly affected in childhood onset of rickets, with widening of the forearms at the wrists, thickening of the costochondral junctions ("rachitic rosary"), and indentation of the lower ribs at the site of attachment to the diaphragm (Harrison's groove). Classical bowing of the lower extremity long bones and deformities of pelvic bones typically begins with weight bearing.

Areal bone densitometry typically shows reduced bone density in adults with osteomalacia. Bone scans show an increased uptake of technetium-99 pyrophosphate in long bones, wrists, calvaria, and mandible, as well as the sternum ("tie sternum"). Pseudofractures typically appear as hot spots on the scan. Venous sampling and nuclear imaging of various types (octreotide scan, Sestamibi scan, or positron emission tomography [PET] scan) or MRI scans may be used to try to localize tumors causing tumor-induced osteomalacia.

Laboratory findings

Patients with osteomalacia most often have normal serum calcium or hypocalcemia, hypophosphatemia, and increased serum alkaline phosphatase, but some patients with mild osteomalacia do not have these findings. Measurement of serum parathyroid hormone (PTH), 25-hydroxyvitamin D, or 1,25-dihydroxyvitamin D levels is often helpful in establishing the cause of increased serum alkaline phosphatase. Serum PTH levels are often increased in osteomalacia, and serum 25-hydroxyvitamin D levels decreased to < 10 ng/mL (optimal, 30–80 ng/mL). Serum 1,25-dihydroxyvitamin D levels may be decreased, normal, or increased. Serum fibroblast growth factor-23 levels are typically increased in oncogenic osteomalacia or other hypophosphatemic disorders. Twenty-four hour urine calcium, phosphorus and creatinine will establish hypocalciuria or hyperphosphaturia.

Treatment

Treatment of osteomalacia includes correcting hypocalcemia, hypophosphatemia, and vitamin D deficiency, correcting skeletal deformities if present, and preventing hypercalcemia and hyperphosphatemia during treatment.

Calcium replacement is typically given as calcium carbonate 1000–2000 mg each day for the duration of disease. Phosphate replacement is typically given as potassium neutral phosphate 2–3 g each day for the duration of disease. A high sodium load in sodium neutral phosphate preparations may increase urinary calcium loss. Some patients require treatment for several months, whereas others need life-long therapy.

Vitamin D replacement may be given in different ways, including vitamin D2 (ergocalciferol) or vitamin D3 (cholecalciferol) 50 000–100 000 units 2–3 times each week, 25-hydroxyvitamin D3 (calcifediol 50 μg capsules) 50–100 μg each day, or 1,25-dihydroxyvitamin D3 0.25–1.0 μg twice a day. In some countries, a single oral or intramuscular dose of vitamin D 600 000 units is available. Ultraviolet irradiation of the skin (e.g. in tanning beds) may be effective in some settings. In patients with pseudovitamin D deficiency rickets, therapy with 1,25-dihydroxyvitamin D3 is effective, whereas most patients with hereditary vitamin D-resistant rickets typically respond to high-dose vitamin D or 1,25-dihydroxyvitamin D3 with calcium infusions.

Once effective therapy is started, symptoms of osteomalacia, including bone pain and proximal muscle weakness, typically improve within 4–6 weeks. Complete resolution of symptoms may take as long as six months. Increased serum alkaline phosphatase levels typically normalize over 3–6 months, but may take as long 6–9 months in some cases.

Orthopedic surgery may be required in patients with marked bowing of the legs. Osteotomies may be necessary to straighten bones deformed by osteomalacia.

Illustrations (Figs 5.29–5.35)

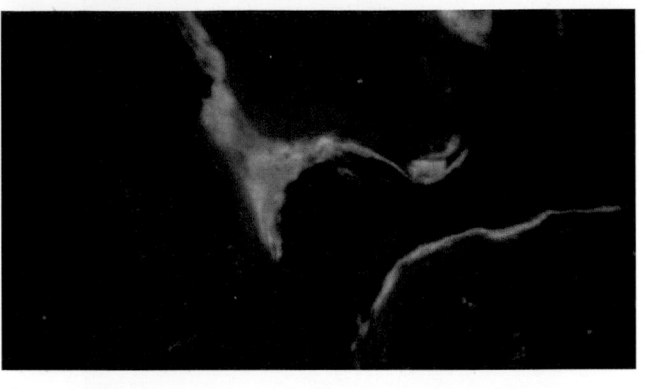

Figure 5.30 Iliac crest bone biopsy showing smudging of fluorescent green tetracycline label using fluorescence microscopy. Courtesy of Dr. Lorraine A. Fitzpatrick.

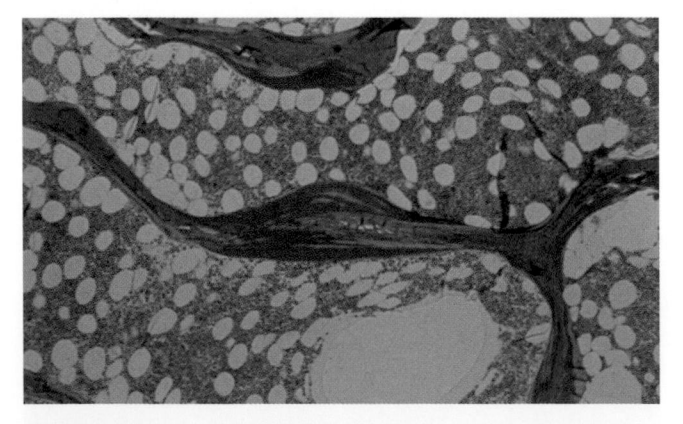

Figure 5.29 Iliac crest bone biopsy showing increased unmineralized osteoid width, surface, and volume (in red) using Goldner–Masson–Trichrome stain. Courtesy of Dr. Lorraine A. Fitzpatrick.

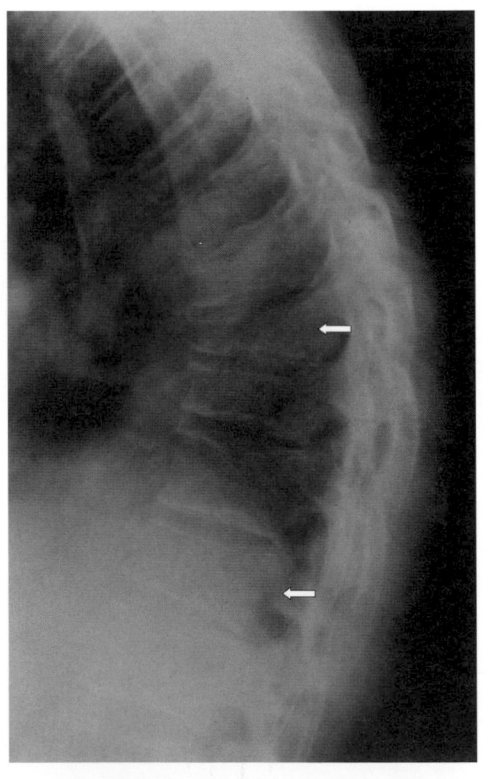

Figure 5.31 Enlarged and biconvex intervertebral disks resulting in biconcave "codfish" vertebrae (arrows). Courtesy of Dr. Ronald G. Swee.

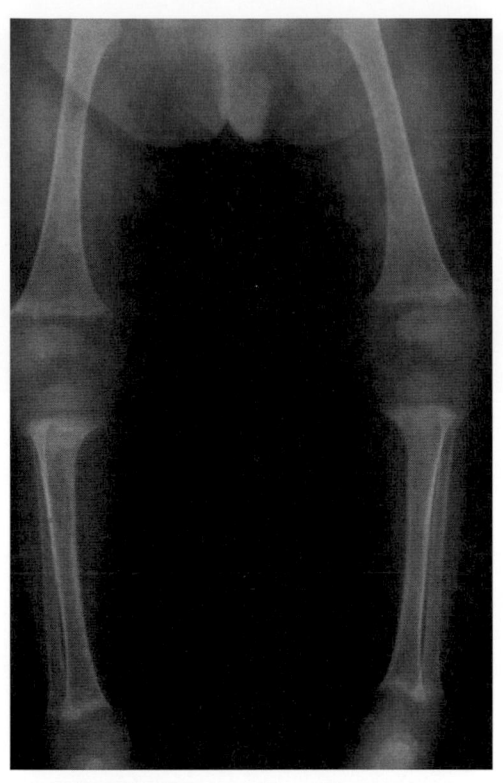

Figure 5.32 Widening and fraying of the epiphyses in a child with rickets. Courtesy of Dr. Ronald G. Swee.

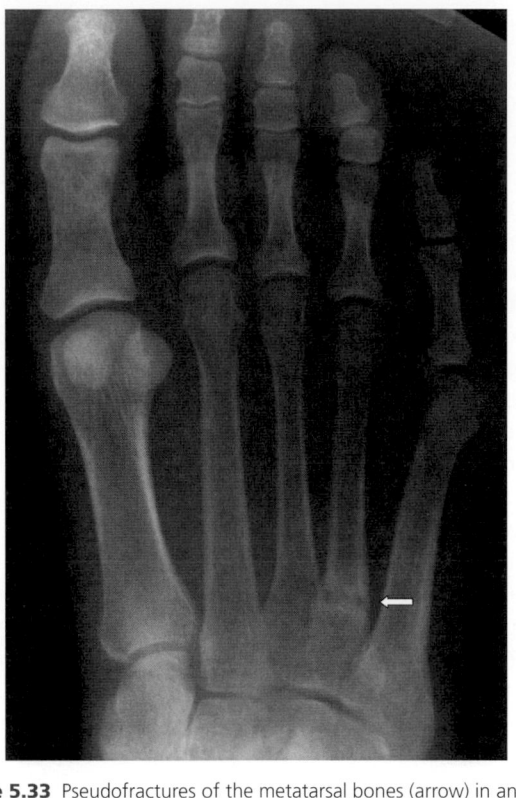

Figure 5.33 Pseudofractures of the metatarsal bones (arrow) in an adult with osteomalacia. Courtesy of Dr. Ronald G. Swee.

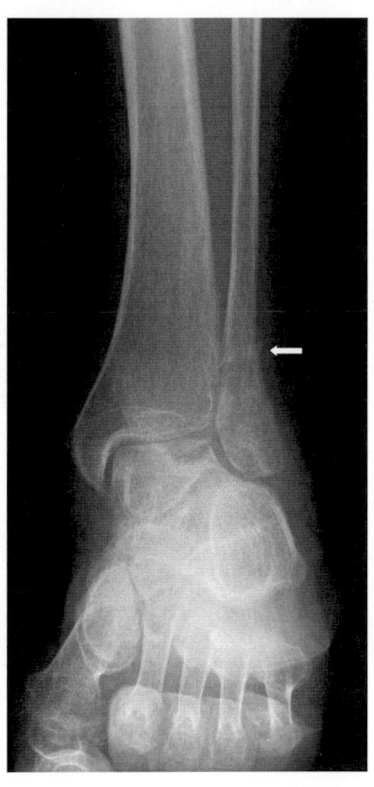

Figure 5.34 Pseudofracture of the distal fibula (arrow) in an adult with osteomalacia. Courtesy of Dr. Lorraine A. Fitzpatrick.

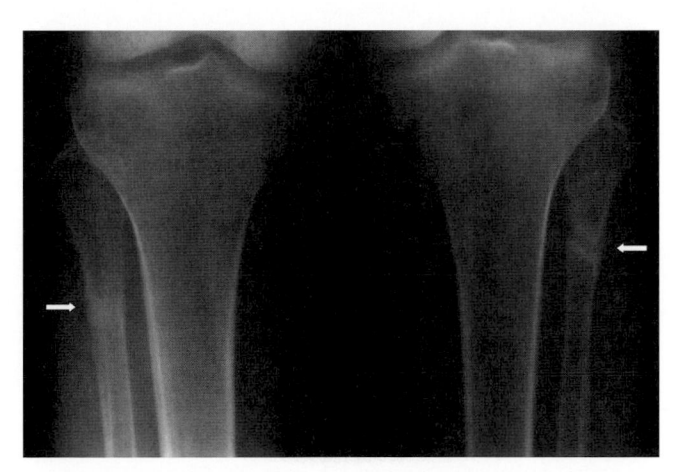

Figure 5.35 Pseudofractures of the proximal fibulae (arrows) in an adult with osteomalacia. Courtesy of Dr. Lorraine A. Fitzpatrick.

Chronic kidney disease

Definition

Chronic kidney disease (CKD) is associated with a spectrum of metabolic bone disease, ranging from high-turnover osteitis fibrosa cystica in earlier stages to low-turnover adynamic bone disease in later stages. Metabolic bone disease associated with CKD is heterogeneous, with variation at each stage of CKD.

Etiology

Chronic kidney disease affects between 5 and 10% of the general world population, and about 20 million patients in the United States. Prevalence of CKD generally increases with age, and incorporation of estimated glomerular filtration rate (GFR) in laboratory reports has raised awareness of significant renal dysfunction in many older patients with normal or only mildly increased serum creatinine. As renal function declines over time, mineral homeostasis progressively deteriorates, with alterations in normal serum and tissue concentrations of calcium and phosphorus, and changes in circulating levels of serum parathyroid hormone (PTH), 1,25-dihydroxyvitamin D and other vitamin D metabolites, fibroblast growth factor-23 (FGF-23), and growth hormone (GH). The ability of the kidneys to appropriately excrete phosphorus gradually diminishes, leading eventually to hyperphosphatemia, elevated serum PTH, decreased serum 1,25-dihydroxyvitamin D, and increased serum FGF-23. Recent studies have shown that serum FGF-23 rises earlier than serum phosphorus in early stage CKD. Conversion of serum 25-hydroxyvitamin D to 1,25-dihydroxyvitamin D by renal 1α-hydroxylase gradually becomes impaired, leading to reduced intestinal calcium absorption and further increased PTH secretion. The kidneys fail to respond adequately to serum PTH, which normally promotes urinary phosphate excretion and calcium reabsorption, and fail to respond to serum FGF-23, which normally stimulates urinary phosphate excretion. In addition, vitamin D receptor (VDR) production is downregulated at the tissue level. Parathyroid hormone skeletal resistance gradually develops for multiple reasons. Therapy of CKD–metabolic bone disease focuses on correcting the recognized biochemical and hormonal abnormalities in an effort to limit their consequences.

Chronic kidney disease is categorized into stages 1–5, based on the estimated or measured glomerular filtration rate:
- *Stage 1*: Kidney damage with normal or increased GFR of ≥ 90 mL/min/1.73 m^2.
- *Stage 2*: Kidney damage with mildly decreased GFR of 60–89 mL/min/1.73 m^2.
- *Stage 3*: Moderately decreased GFR of 30–59 mL/min/1.73 m^2.
- *Stage 4:* Severely decreased GFR of 15–29 mL/min/1.73 m^2.
- *Stage 5*: Kidney failure with GFR < 15 mL/min/1.73 m^2 or on renal replacement therapy (either hemodialysis or peritoneal dialysis).

Patients with chronic kidney disease who have already had a renal transplant are described as having CKD stages 1–5T, and those with stage 5 CKD on hemodialysis or peritoneal dialysis are described as having CKD stage 5D.

The mineral and endocrine functions disrupted in CKD are critically important in the regulation of initial bone formation during skeletal growth and development, adaptation of the skeleton to biomechanical stresses (bone modeling), and also bone structure and function during adulthood (bone remodeling). As a result, bone abnormalities are found almost universally in patients with CKD stage 5D, and in the majority of patients with CKD stages 3–5. More recently, there has been increasing recognition that extraskeletal calcification or mineralization likely also results from the deranged mineral and bone metabolism of CKD, particularly increased serum phosphorus, or from the therapies used to correct these abnormalities.

Observational cohort studies have demonstrated associations between disorders of mineral metabolism and fractures, cardiovascular disease, and mortality in patients with CKD. These studies have broadened the focus of CKD-related mineral and bone disorders to include cardiovascular disease, which is the leading cause of death in patients at all stages of CKD. Abnormal mineral metabolism, bone metabolism, and extra-skeletal (including vascular and cardiac) calcification are closely interrelated, and all are believed to contribute to the morbidity and mortality of patients with CKD.

Signs and symptoms

Most patients with CKD are relatively asymptomatic at diagnosis. However, bone pain may occur, especially with high turnover osteitis fibrosis cystica or osteomalacia. Patients experience symptoms most often dominated by their stage of chronic renal disease. Bone fractures may occur, as may bone deformities. Potential causes of bone pain include stress fracture or complete fracture, or joint pain due to secondary arthritis. Survival is reduced in CKD, mainly due to cardiovascular complications.

Diagnosis

The traditional definition of renal osteodystrophy does not accurately describe the more diverse clinical spectrum of chronic kidney disease–mineral and bone disorder (CKD–MBD), which has been more recently recognized as a result of analysis of serum minerals, hormones, and biomarkers, noninvasive imaging studies, and bone abnormalities. The absence of a generally accepted definition or diagnosis of renal osteodystrophy has prompted the international kidney organizations Kidney Disease: Improving Global

Outcomes (KDIGO) and Kidney Disease Outcomes Quality Initiative (K/DOQI) to re-evaluate the definition, evaluation, and classification of renal osteodystrophy. It is currently recommended that the term *CKD–MBD* be used to describe the broader clinical syndrome, including mineral, bone, and calcific cardiovascular abnormalities, which develops as a complication of CKD. It is also recommended that the term *renal osteodystrophy* be restricted to the description of the bone pathology associated with CKD. The evaluation and definitive diagnosis of renal osteodystrophy requires a bone biopsy, using an expanded classification system developed at a recent consensus conference, based on parameters of bone turnover, mineralization, and volume (TMV).

The KDIGO definition of CKD–MBD incorporates elements of abnormal mineral metabolism, altered bone structure and composition, and extraskeletal calcification. In general, in adult patients CKD–MBD applies only to those with GFR of < 60 mL/min/1.73 m^2, as this is the level of GFR below which abnormalities in calcium, phosphorus, PTH, and vitamin D metabolism become detectable, and are most likely attributable to kidney dysfunction. In pediatric patients the level of GFR at which CKD–MBD abnormalities may become detectable is as high as < 89 mL/min/1.73 m^2. In kidney transplant recipients, there may be residual CKD–MBD which persists in the post-transplant period, even with higher GFR.

Bone disease and vascular calcification are both multifactorial processes, and disturbances in mineral metabolism due to CKD may not be the primary underlying etiology for either process. Increased bone fragility observed with normal aging or postmenopausal osteoporosis, and atherosclerotic disease with calcification, may develop independently of CKD, and can be present in patients with CKD who have normal or only slightly reduced kidney function, and can co-exist with CKD–MBD after its onset. This is important, as CKD may alter the diagnosis, treatment, and prognosis of osteoporosis and atherosclerosis. Thus, bone disease and vascular calcification of CKD–MBD are discrete entities that are not exclusive to the CKD population. The evidence for a link between mineral disturbances and vascular calcification in CKD is not yet fully established, and the pathogenesis of the latter is likely to be multifactorial.

In patients with CKD Stages 3–5D a bone biopsy should be considered in the evaluation of unexplained bone fractures, bone pain, hypercalcemia, hypophosphatemia, or to rule out aluminum toxicity.

Imaging tests

Imaging studies are not often used to diagnose CKD–MBD, but may be helpful in classifying the type of bone disease present. Plain X-rays may be helpful in assessing bone pain due to high turnover osteitis fibrosa cystica (Figs 5.36–5.38), fractures, or stress fractures. Patients with later stage CKD often have osteopenia on X-ray. X-rays of patients with osteomalacia or adynamic bone disease appear to show osteopenia, often without other characteristic findings. Bone scans may be useful in detecting increased skeletal turnover due to hyperparathyroidism, or stress fractures. Focal areas of unexplained increased uptake on bone scans should be imaged by X-ray or computed tomography (CT) to clarify the diagnosis. Bone density testing is more difficult to interpret in the setting of CKD, and is less predictive of fracture risk than in postmenopausal osteoporosis.

Iliac crest bone biopsies may be used to classify the type of renal osteodystrophy present in patients with CKD. Patients with early stage CKD tend to have high turnover hyperparathyroidism, characterized by very active osteoclast bone resorption (Fig. 5.39), and those with late stage CKD have low turnover or adynamic bone disease, characterized by very low osteoblast and osteoclast numbers, and very low bone formation (Fig. 5.40).

Laboratory findings

Given the relatively early development of metabolic abnormalities related to CKD–MBD, assessment for biochemical abnormalities is recommended starting in patients with CKD stage 3. Parameters that should be checked include serum calcium, phosphorus, and PTH. Patients typically have low or normal serum calcium, upper-normal or increased serum phosphorus, and increased PTH levels. Serum alkaline phosphatase may be increased, especially with hyperparathyroid bone disease or after fracture or stress fracture. Serum 25-hydroxyvitamin D is usually low-normal or mildly decreased unless patients are taking supplemental vitamin D. Serum 1,25-dihydroxyvitamin D is usually decreased, especially in later stages of CKD, due to decreased renal 1α-hydroxylase activity. The frequency of monitoring for laboratory abnormalities should be based on the presence and magnitude of the abnormalities, as well as the rate of progression of CKD. For patients on treatment for osteoporosis or other mineral and bone disorders, monitoring frequency should be individualized to assess for efficacy and adverse effects.

Treatment

Patients with CKD–MBD stages 3–5D frequently have increased serum phosphorus levels. Therapy is typically directed toward lowering serum phosphorus into, or closer to, the normal range. Methods to lower serum phosphorus include reduction of phosphorus in the diet, use of pharmacological phosphate binding agents, and increased duration or frequency of dialysis in CKD stage 5D.

Due to changes in PTH assays in recent years, it has become more difficult to establish an optimal range for serum PTH in patients with CKD stage 5D. It has been recommended that the target for circulating intact PTH should be between two and nine times the upper limits of normal for the assay used. Treatment options for lowering increased serum PTH include calcitriol, vitamin D analogs (paricalcitol,

doxercalciferol, others), and calcimimetics (cinacalcet). The choice of pharmacologic agent should be influenced by a patient's serum calcium and phosphorus levels. In patients with serum PTH less than two times the upper limit of normal for the assay used, calcitriol, vitamin D analogs and/or calcimimetics should be withheld, reduced, or withdrawn to prevent over-suppression of PTH secretion. Circulating PTH, calcium, and phosphorus should be monitored more frequently during treatment with any PTH-altering treatment. There are no specific indications for parathyroidectomy, but surgery should be considered when severe hyperparathyroidism is resistant to medical pharmacologic therapy.

Calcium supplementation has been shown to increase risk of myocardial infarction and death in patients with renal failure, particularly in those on hemodialysis. However, calcium supplementation lowers parathyroid hormone secretion in CKD stages 3–4. Clinical trials have not yet distinguished a threshold of renal function at which calcium supplementation may be harmful.

Vitamin D supplementation in patients with chronic kidney disease increases intestinal absorption of phosphorus, which may accelerate vascular disease, but vitamin D deficiency has been shown to increase mortality in chronic kidney disease stage 5D. Treatment of patients with chronic kidney disease with vitamin D analogues has been shown to reduce proteinuria, suppress the renin–angiotensin–aldosterone system, and cause anti-inflammatory and immunomodulatory effects that may protect the kidney. Current guidelines focus on use of vitamin D receptor activating agents mainly to suppress hyperparathyroidism.

Patients with CKD stages 1–2 with osteoporosis and/or high risk of fracture as identified by World Health Organization (WHO) bone density criteria should be managed as patients in the general population. Patients with CKD stage 3 with osteoporosis and/or high risk of fracture, as identified by WHO criteria, who are postmenopausal, but have normal serum PTH, vitamin D, and alkaline phosphatase levels, should be treated with drugs that have been evaluated for fracture prevention in the CKD stage 3 population. Because there are insufficient data on safety and efficacy in patients with CKD stages 3–5D and biochemical abnormalities of CKD–MBD to routinely recommend use of fracture-preventing drugs in patients with low bone mineral density and/or increased fracture risk as identified by WHO criteria, caution should be used in these patients. Bisphosphonates are cleared by the kidneys without further metabolism, and are not approved for use in patients with CKD worse than stage 3 with GFR < 30 mL/min because they have not been investigated in this setting, except for zoledronic acid in patients with multiple myeloma. Zoledronic acid infusion is approved for patients with multiple myeloma at a dose of 4 mg for GFR > 60 mL/min, 3.5 mg for GFR of 50–60 mL/min, 3.3 mg for GFR of 40–49 mL/min, and 3.0 mg for GFR of 30–39 mL/min.

Illustrations (Figs 5.36–5.40)

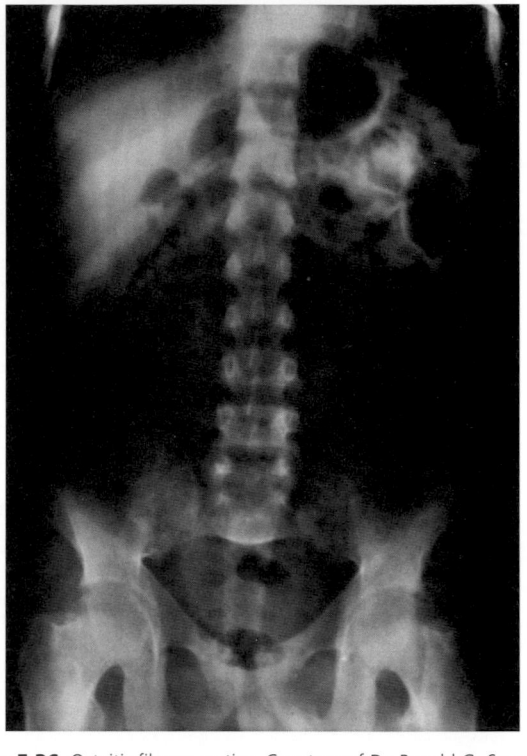

Figure 5.36 Osteitis fibrosa cystica. Courtesy of Dr. Ronald G. Swee.

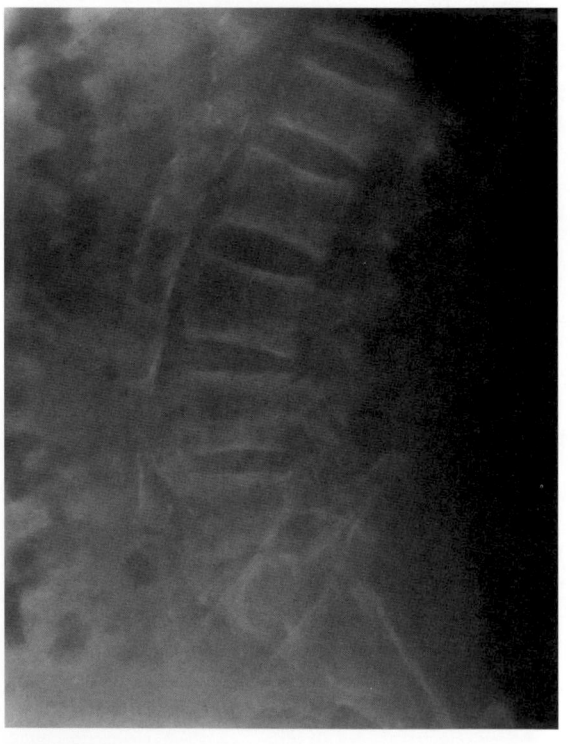

Figure 5.37 Rugger-jersey spine with hyperparathyroid bone disease in chronic kidney disease. Courtesy of Dr. Ronald G. Swee.

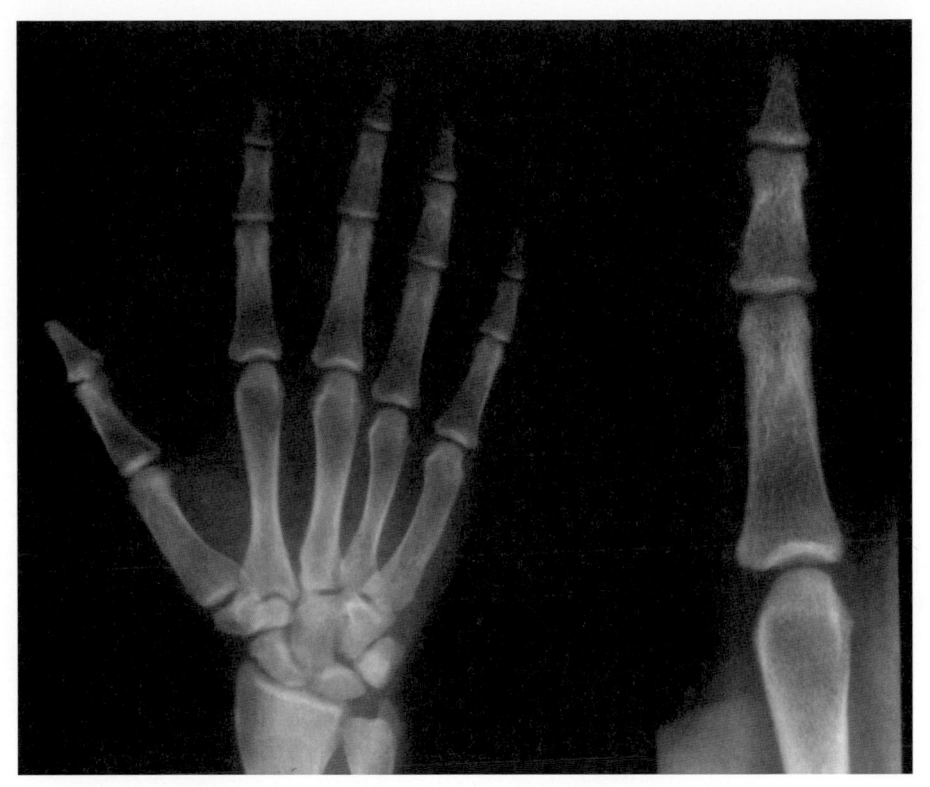

Figure 5.38 Hyperparathyroid bone disease in chronic kidney disease. Courtesy of Dr. Ronald G. Swee.

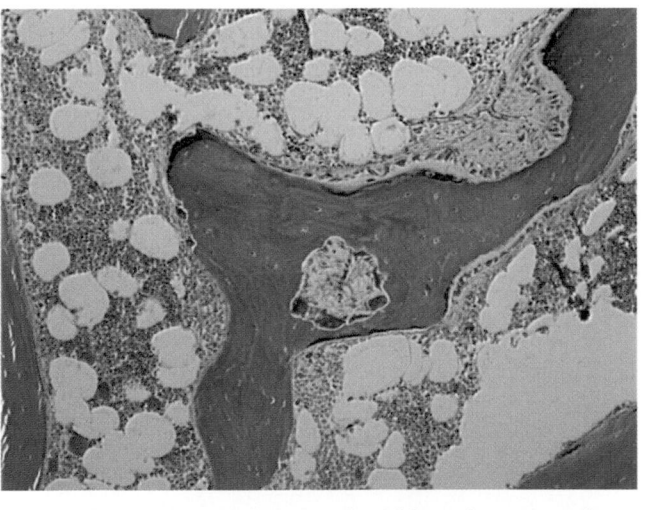

Figure 5.39 High-turnover (hyperparathyroid) bone disease. Note the increased osteoclast bone resorption and increased osteoblast bone formation, as well as bone marrow fibrosis. Courtesy of Glenda L. Evans.

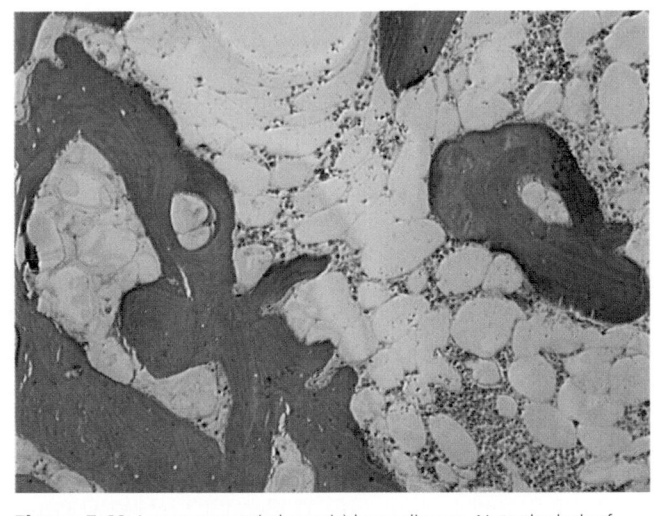

Figure 5.40 Low-turnover (adynamic) bone disease. Note the lack of bone turnover on trabecular surfaces, with markedly decreased osteoclasts and osteoblasts. Courtesy of Glenda L. Evans.

Fibrous dysplasia

Definition

Fibrous dysplasia is an uncommon skeletal disorder characterized by fibrous skeletal lesions affecting single or multiple bones, occasionally associated with extraskeletal lesions or dysfunction, most commonly skin hyperpigmentation or hyperfunctioning endocrinopathies, known as McCune–Albright syndrome.

Etiology

Fibrous dysplasia is caused by dominant gain-of-function (activating) missense mutations of the *GNAS* gene, which encodes the α-subunit of the stimulatory G-protein $G_s\alpha$. Mutations in this disorder occur post-zygotically, and therefore are never inherited. Affected individuals with the mutation are somatic mosaics, with some of their non-gonadal cells normal, and other nongonadal cells containing the constitutively activated $G_s\alpha$ protein.

Arginine-201 in the stimulatory G-protein Gsalpha is most commonly replaced by histidine or cysteine, and rarely other amino acids, although mutations at Q227 have also recently been reported. The two most common mutations at arginine-201 occur early in development, and result from methylation and deamination of cytosines within the CpG dinucleotide in the arginine-201 codon, most likely during de novo methylation of cells in the inner cell mass of the trophoblast. Because inner cell mass cells are multipotent, mutations in these cells may be passed on to cells in all three germ layers, which likely explains why severe forms of the disease may affect multiple tissues and organs. The size and variability of the clone arising from the single, original mutated cell is thought to explain the distribution and frequency of mutated cells in postnatal life, and the subsequent extent and severity of the disease. Because of the activating mutation, catalysis of guanosine triphosphate (GTP) to guanosine diphosphate (GDP) by $G_s\alpha$ is decreased. This leads to constitutive activation of adenylate cyclase, with increased cyclic adenosine monophosphate (cAMP) generated within affected cells thought to mediate pathological effects.

In bone, mutations frequently affect cells of the osteogenic lineage, with adverse effects on both osteoprogenitor cells and more mature osteoblasts. $G_s\alpha$ is not imprinted, and is normally biallelically expressed in bone, but asymmetric expression of the $G_s\alpha$ alleles in osteoprogenitor cells is thought to explain the distribution and severity of skeletal lesions.

Local expansion of affected osteoprogenitor cells results in marrow space accumulation, displacement of hematopoietic cells, and marrow fibrosis. Mutated cells are functionally and morphologically abnormal, and deposit abnormal matrix. Trabecular bone is abnormally shaped, with abnormal collagen fibril orientation and biochemical composition, leading to severe undermineralization and abnormal compliance.

Increased serum fibroblast growth factor (FGF)-23 produced by highly activated mutant osteoblastic cells in fibrous dysplasia lesions may result in renal tubular phosphate loss commonly associated with fibrous dysplasia. Histological patterns in bone are usually different in different affected bones, and unusual patterns may be seen in craniofacial bones. However, Sharpey fibers and retracted osteoblasts are seen at virtually all affected skeletal sites.

The rate of bone remodeling in skeletal lesions is stimulated by gonadal sex steroid secretion, and may worsen with puberty or postmenopausal hormone therapy. Fibrous dysplasia lesions are highly vascular, and may bleed spontaneously or with minor trauma, leading to development of posthemorrhagic cysts.

Signs and symptoms

Fibrous dysplasia ranges in expression from incidentally discovered asymptomatic monostotic bone abnormalities to more severe, extensive, polyostotic disease. In occasional patients, the entire skeleton may be affected. Patients with polyostotic disease often, but not always, have affected limb bones on the same side.

Patients with fibrous dysplasia and extraskeletal lesions or dysfunction, including skin hyperpigmentation (café-au-lait spots) (Figs 5.41 & 5.42) and hyperfunctioning endocrinopathies, such as precocious puberty, hyperthyroidism, increased growth hormone secretion, and Cushing syndrome, have McCune–Albright syndrome. Fibrous dysplasia frequently is associated with renal tubular phosphate loss due to increased serum FGF-23 levels in polyostotic disease. Myxomas of skeletal muscle (Mazabraud syndrome) or dysfunction of the heart, liver, pancreas, or other organs may be seen in McCune–Albright syndrome.

The skeletal distribution of fibrous dysplasia is usually apparent at an early age. About 90% of craniofacial lesions are evident by age 5 years, and roughly 75% of other skeletal lesions are recognized by age 15 years. Effects of $G_s\alpha$ mutations in osteoprogenitor cells and osteoblasts are most clinically evident during rapid growth associated with onset of puberty. Fractures associated with fibrous dysplasia are most common during rapid skeletal growth.

Pain, fracture, and bone deformity are the most common presenting features in adolescents or adults. Infants are rarely affected, but most often have a severe form of disease. Children less commonly complain of pain. Adult pain is

common in affected ribs, long bones, and craniofacial bones, and usually less severe in vertebral or pelvic lesions. Pathological fractures or stress fractures may occur in affected limb bones, with deformity in limb bones due to fracture malunion, expansion and abnormal compliance of bone lesions, and hemorrhagic cyst formation. Craniofacial bone deformities are typically due only to overgrowth of affected bone(s).

Fibrous dysplasia skeletal lesions rarely undergo malignant transformation, but the risk of this may be increased by high-dose external beam radiation therapy. Sarcomatous transformation is often associated with rapid lesion expansion, disruption of the cortex, and increase in pain. Osteogenic sarcoma is the most common malignancy seen in fibrous dysplasia, but other tumors may also develop. Malignancies tend to be aggressive, and surgery is the current primary treatment, with chemotherapy or radiation offering little improvement in prognosis.

Diagnosis

Diagnosis is usually based on classic physical, X-ray, and histopathological findings. Mutation analysis may help distinguish between fibrous dysplasia and other fibro-osseous skeletal lesions such as osteofibrous dysplasia, ossifying fibromas of the jaw, multiple nonossifying fibromas, skeletal angiomatosis, and Ollier's disease.

Imaging tests

The extent of skeletal disease is best assessed by total body bone scan (Fig. 5.43) and/or skeletal surveys. The most commonly affected bones are the proximal femoral metaphysis and skull base (Fig. 5.44). On X-ray, femoral lesions in younger individuals most often are expansile, deforming, medullary abnormalities with cortical thinning and ground glass appearance (Fig. 5.45). As individuals age, femoral lesions become more sclerotic and heterogeneous, and may develop aneurysmal bone cysts. Sclerosis may imply relatively quiescent disease.

Lesions in the skull base and facial bones may cause skull or facial asymmetry in childhood, sometimes with greater bony prominence on one side or area of the skull (Fig. 5.46). Skull lesions may progress in adulthood, especially when associated with growth hormone oversecretion, sometimes causing cranial neuropathies due to compression. Craniofacial bone involvement may lead to bleeding, herniation through cranial foramina or vascular passages, or posthemorrhagic cysts. Blindness may result from optic nerve compression. Craniofacial lesions in children often have a ground glass appearance, but in adults are more sclerotic, and may be similar to pagetic lesions.

Fibrous dysplasia lesions in the spine, ribs, and pelvis may be difficult to detect on X-ray, but are easily detected on bone scan or computed tomography (CT) scan (Fig. 5.47). Bone scanning is the most sensitive technique to detect fibrous dysplasia at present. Fibrous dysplasia in the spine may cause progressive scoliosis into adulthood requiring surgery.

Laboratory findings

Serum total or bone alkaline phosphatase, and other markers of bone turnover, are usually increased in fibrous dysplasia. Serum phosphorus may be decreased if renal tubular loss of phosphorus due to increased serum FGF-23 levels is present. Patients with hypophosphatemia and growth hormone oversecretion tend to have a worsened prognosis.

Treatment

Fibrous dysplasia of the proximal femur, with fracture or impending fracture, is usually treated with intramedullary nailing to prevent deformity or limb length discrepancy. Craniofacial fibrous dysplasia should generally be treated with surgery only when hearing or vision loss are present, and prophylactic optic nerve decompression is not recommended. Bisphosphonates are often recommended to reduce bone pain, decrease markers of bone turnover, and improve skeletal X-ray appearance. A recent open-label clinical trial with bisphosphonates showed reduction in bone pain, but no improvement on X-rays or histologically. Placebo-controlled trials are underway to establish the role of bisphosphonates in treatment of fibrous dysplasia.

Illustrations (Figs 5.41–5.47)

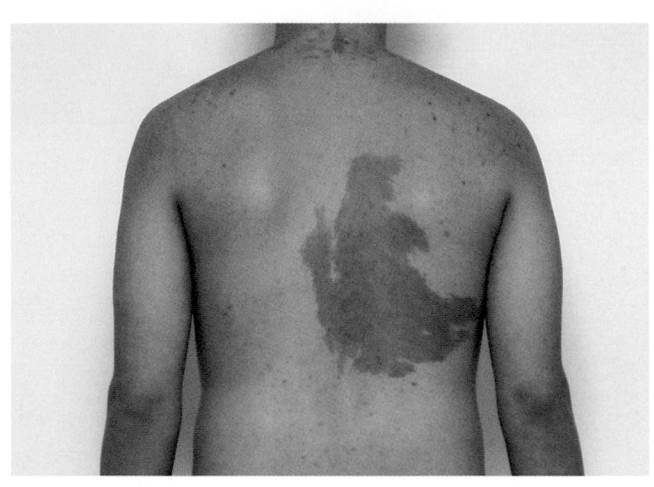

Figure 5.41 Café-au-lait spot. Courtesy of Dr. Peter J. Tebben.

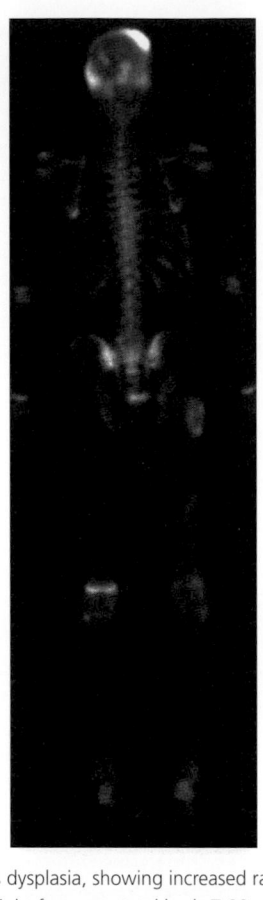

Figure 5.43 Fibrous dysplasia, showing increased radiotracer uptake in skull, mandible, and right femur on total body Tc99-sestamibi bone scan. Courtesy of Dr. Peter J. Tebben.

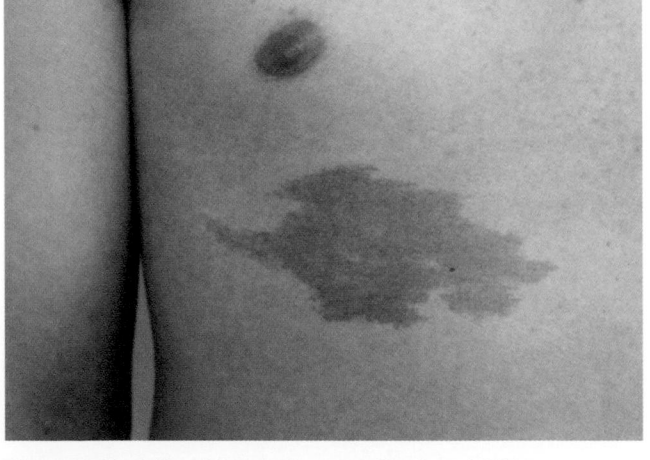

Figure 5.42 Café-au-lait spot. Courtesy of Dr. Peter J. Tebben.

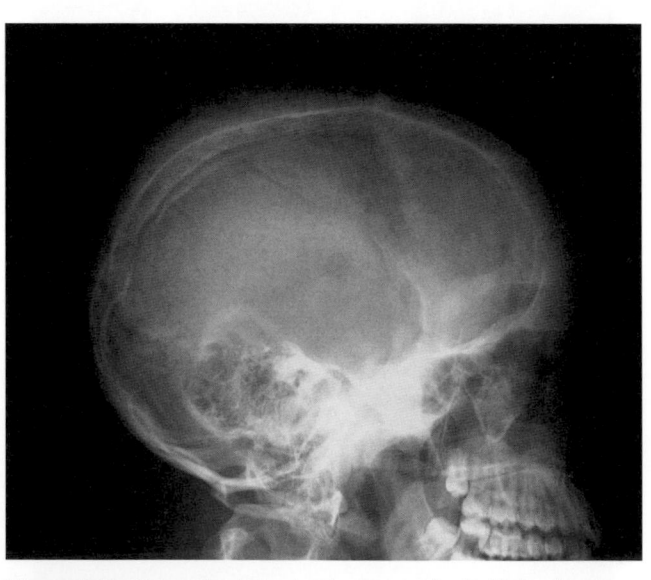

Figure 5.44 Fibrous dysplasia, showing increased mixed lytic-sclerotic appearance of skull base. Courtesy of Dr. Peter J. Tebben.

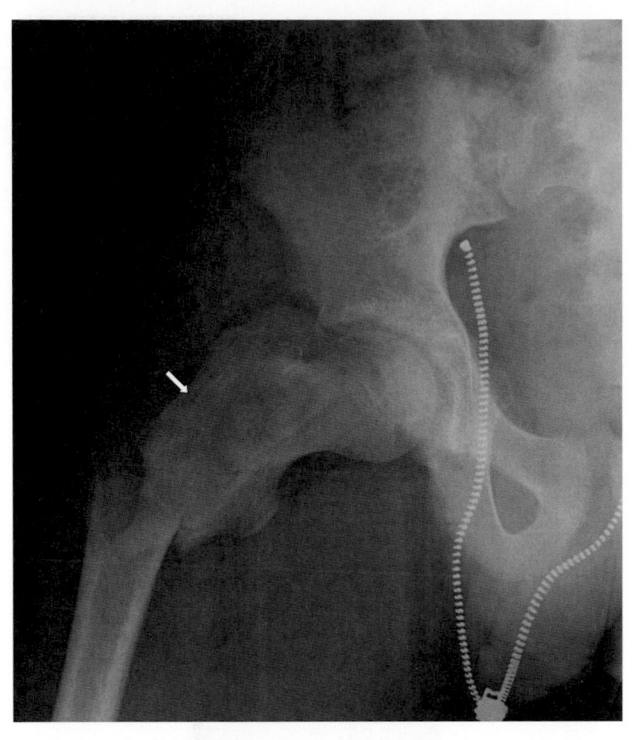

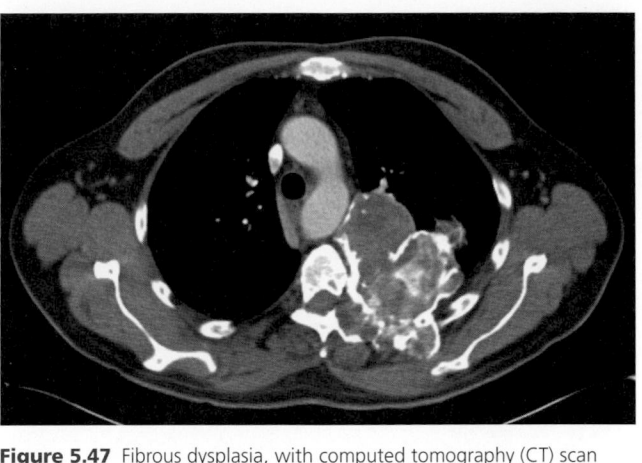

Figure 5.47 Fibrous dysplasia, with computed tomography (CT) scan showing vertebral and pelvic involvement. Courtesy of Dr. Naveen S. Murthy.

Figure 5.45 Fibrous dysplasia, showing expansile, deforming, medullary proximal femur involvement (arrow) in young patient. Courtesy of Dr. Peter J. Tebben.

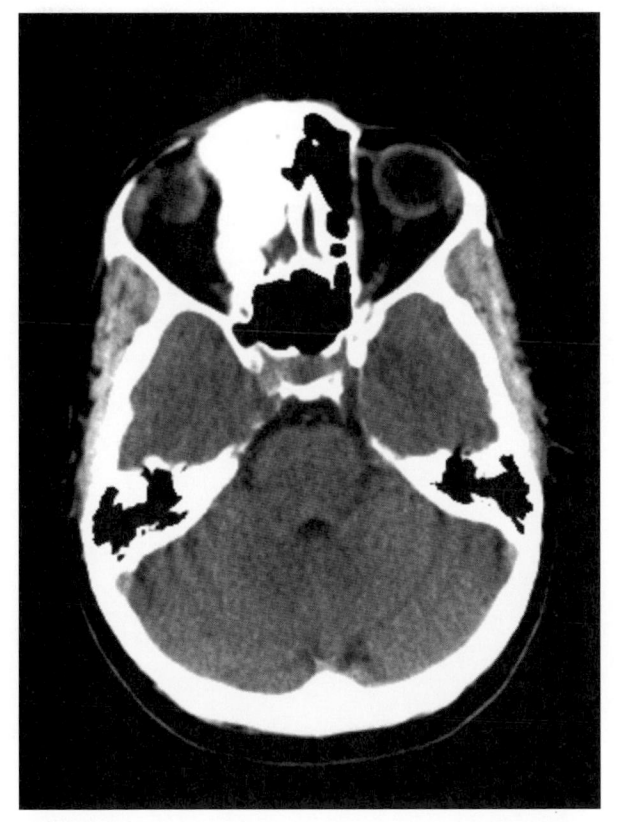

Figure 5.46 Fibrous dysplasia, with computed tomography (CT) scan showing involvement of nasal and facial bones. Courtesy of Dr. Peter J. Tebben.

Selected sclerosing bone disorders

Definition

This family of disorders is characterized by decreased bone resorption or increased bone formation, resulting in trabecular and cortical bone thickening, and increased bone density. Disorders may be due to many inherited osteochondrodysplasias, as well as a variety of dietary, metabolic, endocrine, hematologic, infectious, or neoplastic conditions.

Metabolic bone disorders associated with sclerosis include carbonic anhydrase type 2 deficiency, fluorosis, heavy metal poisoning, hepatitis C-associated osteosclerosis, hypervitaminosis A and D, hyper-, hypo-, and pseudohypoparathyroidism, hypophosphatemic osteomalacia, activating mutations of LRP5 (high bone mass phenotype), milk-alkali syndrome, and X-linked hypophosphatemia.

Other disorders associated with sclerosis include axial osteomalacia, diffuse idiopathic skeletal hyperostosis (DISH), Erdheim–Chester disease, fibrogenesis imperfecta ossium, hypertrophic osteoarthropathy, ionizing radiation, leukemia, lymphomas, mastocytosis, multiple myeloma, myelofibrosis, osteomyelitis, osteonecrosis, Paget's disease, sarcoidosis, sickle cell disease, skeletal metastases, and tuberous sclerosis.

Osteopetrosis

Etiology

Osteopetrosis has many potential complex causes. Mutations affecting the stem cell for osteoclastogenesis or its microenvironment, mononuclear precursor cell, or mature heterokaryon could lead to decreased bone resorption. An osteoblast mutation has been reported that stimulates new bone formation. Resistance of bone matrix to resorption would cause the same phenotype. Defective lysosomes may cause osteopetrosis accompanied by neuronal storage disease, associated with accumulation of ceroid lipofuscin. Virus-like inclusion bodies in osteoclasts have been reported in a few mild cases of osteopetrosis. Abnormal PTH, interleukin (IL)-2 or superoxide production might cause the same presentation. Leukocyte function may be reduced in infantile osteopetrosis. Impaired skeletal resorption causes skeletal fragility because collagen fibers do not interconnect osteons, and woven bone remodels poorly to compact bone.

Mutations in three genes that regulate acidification by osteoclasts cause osteopetrosis in the majority of affected patients. Haploinsufficiency for chloride channel 7 activity caused by inactivating mutations in *CLCN7* causes Albers–Schönberg disease. Autosomal recessive infantile osteopetrosis is most often due to mutations in *TCIRG1* (*ATP6I*) that encodes the α3 subunit of the vacuolar proton pump. Autosomal recessive malignant or intermediate osteopetrosis may also be due to *CLCN7* mutations. Inactivation of *CAII* leads to carbonic anhydrase II deficiency. Loss of function of the *GL* (grey-lethal) gene that encodes osteopetrosis-associated transmembrane protein 1 (*OSMT1*) causes severe osteopetrosis. Inactivation of a key modulator of NF-κB causes X-linked osteopetrosis, lymphedema, anhydrotic ectodermal dysplasia, and immunodeficiency (OL-EDA-ID) in boys. Inactivation of the *RANKL* gene causes a rare form of osteopetrosis with decreased osteoclast number, which does not respond to bone marrow transplantation. Osteopetrosis may also be due to *RANK* inactivation.

Signs and symptoms

This disorder, also called "marble bone disease" or Albers–Schönberg disease, was first recognized in 1904. It typically presents as an autosomal dominant adult benign form with relatively few symptoms, or an autosomal recessive infantile aggressive form that is fatal in childhood if not treated. A rarer intermediate childhood form has been reported, of uncertain impact on survival. Osteopetrosis with renal tubular acidosis and cerebral calcification is due to CAII deficiency. Malignant osteopetrosis may occur in association with neuronal storage disease. Other forms of osteopetrosis have been labeled "lethal," "transient infantile," or "postinfectious." Drug-induced osteopetrosis was first reported in 2003 in an adolescent male receiving long-term high-dose pamidronate infusions.

Infantile osteopetrosis

Infantile osteopetrosis is usually diagnosed during the first year of life. Nasal stuffiness due to failure of paranasal sinuses to enlarge may be an early symptom, and cranial foramina fail to widen, so the optic, oculomotor, and facial nerves may become paralyzed. Hearing loss is common. Blindness may develop because of retinal degeneration or increased intracranial pressure. Hydrocephalus or central sleep apnea may occur. Tooth eruption is delayed, and children fail to thrive. The skeleton is denser than normal on X-ray, but bones are fragile and may fracture. Recurrent infections and spontaneous bruising or bleeding occur following myelophthisis with narrowing of the marrow cavities of long bones. Hypersplenism and hemolysis may worsen the anemia. Affected children have short stature, macrocephaly, frontal bossing, "adenoid" appearance, nystagmus, hepatosplenomegaly, and genu valgum. Untreated patients usually die during the first decade due to hemorrhage, severe anemia, pneumonia, or sepsis.

Intermediate osteopetrosis

Intermediate osteopetrosis causes short stature, cranial nerve deficits, ankylosed teeth that predispose to jaw osteomyelitis, recurrent fractures, and mild or moderate anemia.

Adult osteopetrosis

Adult osteopetrosis results in increased X-ray density of bones in childhood, with carriers apparently unaffected. The long bones are brittle and may fracture. Cranial nerve palsies may affect the facial, optic, or oculomotor nerves. Psychomotor delay, jaw osteomyelitis, carpal tunnel syndrome, slipped femoral capital epiphyses, and osteoarthritis may occur. Adult osteopetrosis type 1 has been reclassified as high bone mass phenotype due to activating mutations of LRP5, and adult osteopetrosis type 2 is now called Albers–Schönberg disease.

Osteopetrosis associated with neuronal storage disease

Osteopetrosis associated with neuronal storage disease presents with a severe skeletal phenotype with epilepsy and neurodegenerative disease. Lethal osteopetrosis is evident in utero and usually causes stillbirth. Transient infantile osteopetrosis completely resolves during the first few months of life for unclear reasons.

Diagnosis

This disorder is most often diagnosed based on the constellation of physical exam and radiological findings, with supportive biochemical and histological evidence. Genetic testing may help confirm the diagnosis.

Imaging tests

Skeletal surveys show diffuse symmetrically increased bone density, with thickening of both trabecular and cortical bone (Figs 5.48 & 5.49). Growth, modeling, and remodeling are all affected in the more severe forms. Alternating sclerotic and radiolucent bands may develop in the iliac wings and long bone metaphyses. Metaphases may flare and take on a club or "Erlenmeyer flask" shape. The distal phalanges of the hands may be eroded, similar to what is seen in pycnodysostosis. Pathological fractures of long bones are relatively common. Rachitic-like changes in growth plates may occur because of hypocalcemia with resultant secondary hyperparathyroidism. The skull is typically thickened and dense, especially at the base, with paranasal and mastoid sinuses underpneumatized. Lateral spine X-rays may show vertebrae with a "bone-in-bone" (endobone) appearance (Fig. 5.50). Albers–Schönberg disease is associated with a thickened skull base and "rugger-jersey" appearance of the vertebrae (Fig. 5.51). Radiological studies may detect malignant osteopetrosis late in pregnancy, but ultrasound studies have not been helpful.

Bone scans may detect fractures, stress fractures, or osteomyelitis. Magnetic resonance imaging (MRI) scans are useful after bone marrow transplantation in severe forms because they can detect medullary space enlargement after successful bone marrow engraftment.

Laboratory findings

Hypocalcemia may develop due to decreased bone resorption in infantile osteopetrosis as the infant transitions to dependence on intestinal calcium absorption. Secondary hyperparathyroidism and increased serum 1,25-dihydroxyvitamin D are usually present in this situation. These findings may be present in milder form in Albers–Schönberg disease. Serum acid phosphatase and creatine kinase BB-isoenzyme levels are usually increased due to overproduction by abnormal osteoclasts.

Because osteopetrosis is always associated with failure of osteoclast-mediated bone resorption, primary spongiosa (calcified cartilage deposited during endochondral bone formation) persists, and is regarded as a histological hallmark of this disorder. These remnants of primary spongiosa are described as "islands" or "bars" of calcified cartilage within trabecular bone. Osteoclast number may be increased, normal, or rarely decreased. Abundant osteoclasts are present in infantile osteopetrosis, with numerous nuclei and absent ruffled borders or clear zones associated with bone resorption. Marrow fibrosis is often present and crowding out the hematopoietic cells. Adult osteopetrosis is associated with increased osteoid and either reduced osteoclast numbers, again lacking ruffled borders, or increased large osteoclasts. Immature woven bone is common. Rounded osteoclasts with increased nuclei are seen detached from bone surfaces in bisphosphonate-associated osteopetrosis.

Treatment

Therapy depends on the underlying cause of the disorder. Mutation analysis is currently recommended to classify the osteoclast defect responsible for osteopetrosis within a given family. Some patients with infantile osteopetrosis respond well to HLA-matched bone marrow transplantation. Bone marrow transplantation does not work well when the causal mutation does not involve the osteoclast, such as in RANKL inactivating mutations. Hypercalcemia may occur with onset of osteoclast function after transplantation. Stem cell transplantation frequently is associated with severe acute pulmonary hypertension. Those with narrowed medullary cavities may be less likely to engraft. Bone marrow transplantation from HLA-nonidentical donors is not well-studied, and administration of progenitor cells in blood from HLA-haploidentical parents works for some patients.

Calcium-deficient diets may help reverse some of the changes in milder forms of osteopetrosis, but calcium supplementation is required in more severe cases with hypocalcemia. High-dose calcitriol supplementation may stimulate underactive osteoclasts in infantile osteopetrosis, usually given while calcium intake is restricted to prevent hypercalcemia and absorptive hypercalciuria. Resistance to this treatment may occur, however. Recombinant human interferon γ-1b has been used to treat malignant osteopetrosis, based on the observation that white blood cells in this

condition have reduced superoxide production. High-dose glucocorticoid therapy usually stabilizes pancytopenia and hepatosplenomegaly. Prednisone and a low-calcium, high-phosphate diet has been considered an alternative to bone marrow transplantation.

Hyperbaric oxygen may be useful in treatment of jaw osteomyelitis. Surgical decompression may help spare optic, oculomotor, and facial nerve function. Joint replacement is difficult but may be beneficial.

Illustrations (Figs 5.48–5.51)

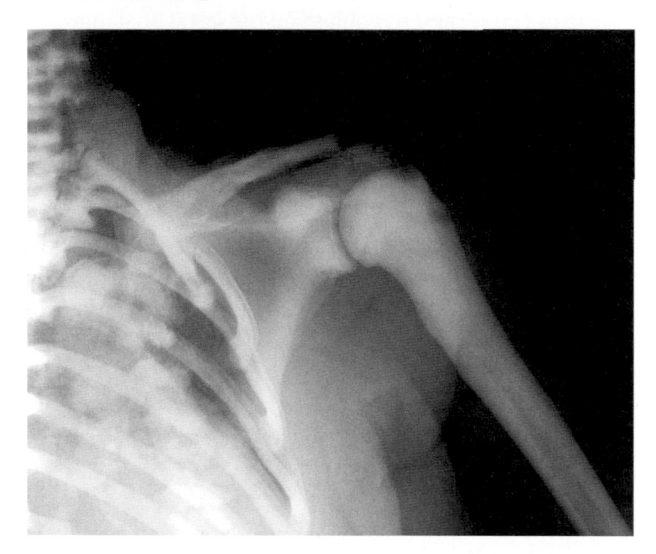

Figure 5.48 Osteopetrosis, with thickening of both cortical and trabecular bone in the shoulder. Courtesy of Dr. Naveen S. Murthy.

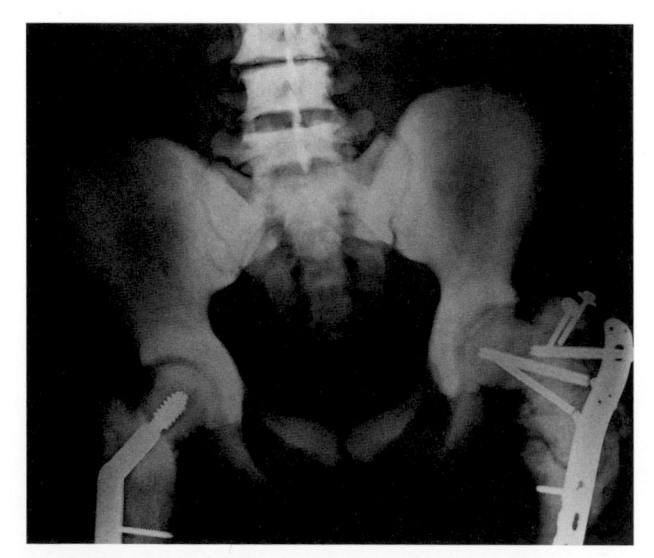

Figure 5.49 Osteopetrosis, with thickening of both cortical and trabecular bone in the lumbar spine, pelvis, and femurs. Courtesy of Dr. Naveen S. Murthy.

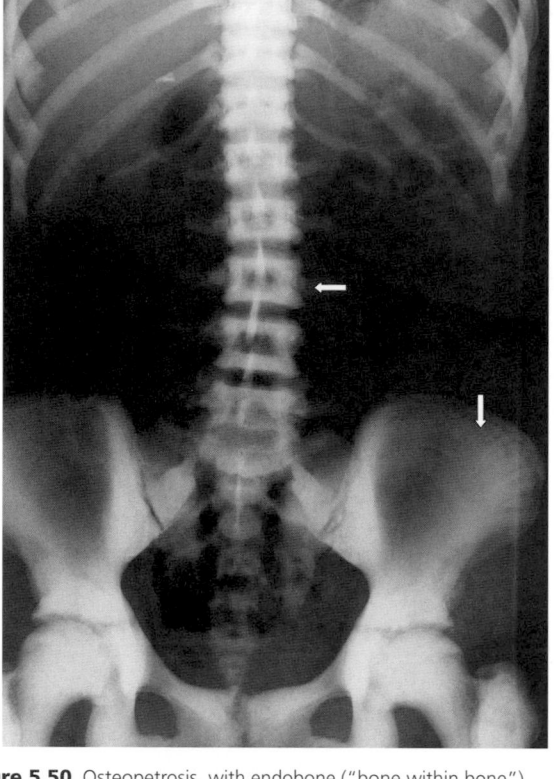

Figure 5.50 Osteopetrosis, with endobone ("bone within bone") appearance in lumbar and thoracic spine and pelvis (arrows). Courtesy of Dr. Naveen S. Murthy.

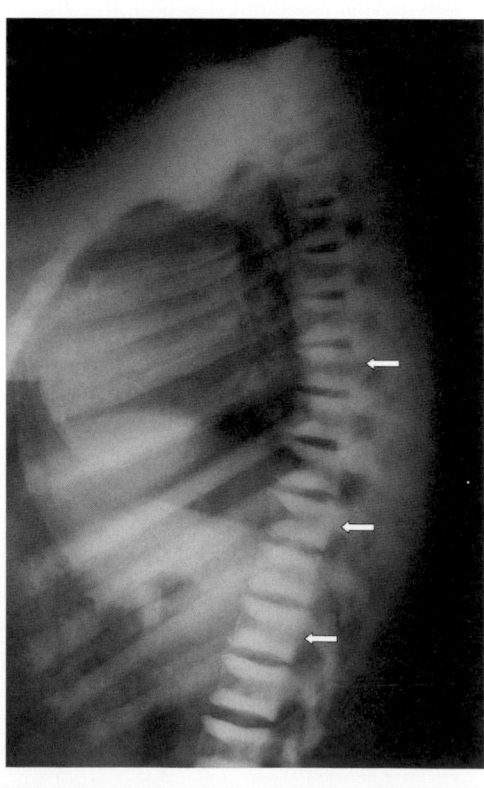

Figure 5.51 Osteopetrosis, with "rugger jersey" appearance of thoracic and lumbar spine (arrows). Courtesy of Dr. Naveen S. Murthy.

Pycnodysostosis

Etiology

This rare autosomal recessive disorder is due to loss of function mutations in the cathepsin K gene. Cathepsin K is a lysosomal cysteine protease normally expressed in high concentration in osteoclasts that is primarily responsible for collagen degradation during bone resorption. Deficiency of this enzyme results in high bone density with decreased bone quality. About 30% of cases are associated with parental consanguinity.

Signs and symptoms

Affected individuals are usually diagnosed in infancy or early childhood because of disproportionate short stature, relatively large skull, fronto-occipital prominence, small facies and chin, obtuse mandibular angle, high-arched palate, dental malocclusion with retained deciduous teeth, proptosis, and a beaked and pointed nose. Sclerae may be bluish. The anterior fontanelle and other cranial sutures often remain open. Fingers tend to be short and clubbed due to acro-osteolysis or terminal phalangeal aplasia, with the hands small and square. The thorax is narrow and pectus excavatum, kyphoscoliosis, or lumber lordosis may be present. Recurrent lower limb fractures in childhood or adulthood may cause genu valgum. Peak adult height may be < 152 cm. Mental retardation may affect up to 10% of cases. Recurrent upper respiratory infections and right heart failure may develop due to chronic upper airway obstruction due to micrognathia.

Diagnosis

This condition is diagnosed clinically based on classic phenotypic physical exam and X-ray features. Genetic testing is available.

Imaging tests

This condition resembles osteopetrosis, with uniform skeletal X-ray evidence of osteosclerosis in childhood, and increased osteosclerosis in adulthood (Figs 5.52 & 5.53). Recurrent fractures are typical. The calvarium, orbital ridges, and skull base are osteosclerotic (Fig. 5.54). The marked modeling defects of osteosclerosis do not occur, although the long bones typically have narrow medullary canals. Delayed closure of cranial sutures and fontanelles (especially the anterior fontanelle), obtuse mandibular angle, wormian bones, gracile clavicles with hypoplastic ends, partial absence of the hyoid bone, and hypoplasia of the distal phalanges and ribs are hallmarks of the condition. Endobones and skeletal striations are not present, as in osteopetrosis.

Laboratory findings

Serum calcium, phosphorus, and alkaline phosphatase are typically normal. Anemia is not present, as in osteosclerosis. Degradation of bone collagen appears defective on electron microscopy. Inclusion bodies have been reported in chondrocytes, and virus-like inclusion bodies have been reported in osteoclasts from brothers. Decreased growth hormone secretion and low insulin-like growth factor (IGF)-1 levels have been reported in five of six affected children in one family.

Treatment

There is no established medical therapy for this condition. Bone marrow transplantation has not been reported. Long bone fractures are typically transverse, and heal at normal rates, but may be associated with delayed union or significant callus formation. Internal fixation of long bones or tooth extraction are challenging because of skeletal hardness. Jaw fracture may occur. Mandibular osteomyelitis may require antibiotics and surgery.

Selected sclerosing bone disorders

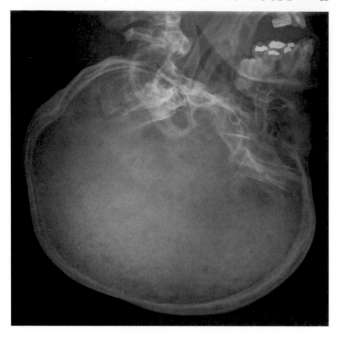

Figure 5.54 Pycnodysostosis, with osteosclerosis of the skull. Courtesy of Dr. Bart L. Clarke.

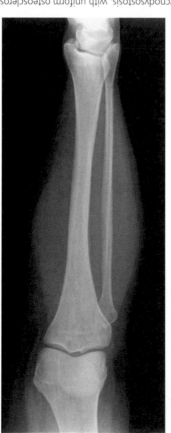

Figure 5.53 Pycnodysostosis, with uniform osteosclerosis of distal femur, tibia, and fibula. Courtesy of Dr. Bart L. Clarke.

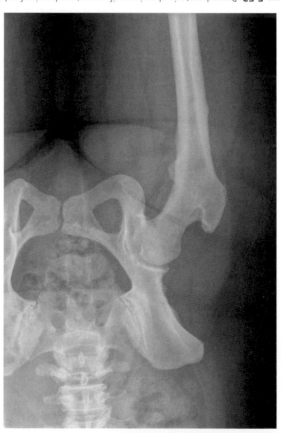

Figure 5.52 Pycnodysostosis, showing uniform osteosclerosis of pelvis and femur. Courtesy of Dr. Bart L. Clarke.

Melorheostosis

Etiology

This rare sporadic disorder is likely due to a segmentary embryonic defect, not yet defined. It occurs sporadically, even when it accompanies osteopoikilosis. Endosteal bone is thickened during growth and development, and periosteal new bone formation is common in adulthood. Affected bones are sclerotic with thickened, irregular lamellae, and marrow fibrosis is sometimes present. The collagen in scleroderma-like skin lesions is normal and not disorganized, as in true scleroderma.

Signs and symptoms

Melorheostosis is usually diagnosed in childhood. Monomelic involvement is typical, with bilateral disease usually asymmetrical. Cutaneous changes may overlie the skeletal lesions, including linear scleroderma-like patches or hypertrichosis. Fibromas, fibrolipomas, capillary hemangiomas, lymphangiectasia, and arterial aneurysms may occur. Soft tissue abnormalities are often noticed before the skeletal changes. Pain and stiffness are typical presenting features, usually associated with the degree of subperiosteal bone formation. Affected joints may develop contractures. Leg length discrepancy may occur after premature fusion of epiphyses. Bone lesions often progress more rapidly during childhood, and become less progressive in adulthood.

Diagnosis

Diagnosis is made through X-ray imaging and bone scans.

Imaging tests

X-rays classically show flowing hyperostosis, similar to wax dripping down a candle (Fig. 5.55). Dense hyperostosis that is irregular and eccentric on both periosteal and endosteal surfaces of single or multiple adjacent bones is typical (Fig. 5.56). Any bone may be affected, but the lower limb bones are most commonly affected. Bone may develop in soft tissues near skeletal lesions, typically near joints. Bone scanning shows increased uptake in active lesions due to hyperemia.

Laboratory findings

Serum calcium, phosphorus, alkaline phosphatase, and other markers of bone and mineral metabolism are normal.

Treatment

Surgical treatment of contractures is often difficult, with recurrent deformity common. No specific medical treatment is available.

Illustrations (Figs 5.55 & 5.56)

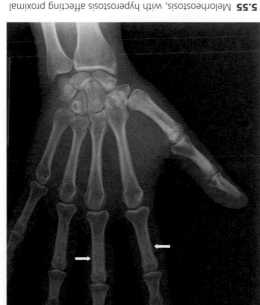

Figure 5.55 Melorheostosis, with hyperostosis affecting proximal phalanges (arrows). Courtesy of Dr. Peter J. Tebben.

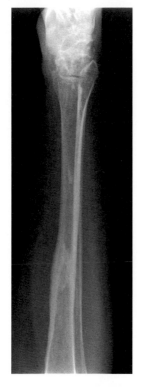

Figure 5.56 Melorheostosis, with hyperostosis involving the tibia. Courtesy of Dr. Peter J. Tebben.

Progressive diaphyseal dysplasia (Camurati–Engelmann disease)

Etiology

This disorder was first described by Cockayne in 1920. Camurati subsequently established that it was an inherited autosomal dominant disorder. Engelmann first reported cases with the severe form in 1929. The cause of progressive diaphyseal dysplasia was established in 2001 when mutations within the *TGFβ1* gene that encodes transforming growth factor (TGF)-β1 were first reported. These mutations prevent a latency-associated peptide from dissociating from TGF-β1, which keeps TGF-β1 constitutively active in the skeletal matrix, thereby continually stimulating osteoblast function.

Mild progressive diaphyseal dysplasia may reflect variable penetrance. Progressive diaphyseal dysplasia may worsen with succeeding generations, a phenomenon known as "anticipation." There does not appear to be a strong genotype–phenotype correlation, as there is heterogeneity of expression in different kindreds with the same mutation. Response of severe progressive diaphyseal dysplasia to glucocorticoid therapy suggests that it may be a systemic inflammatory connective tissue disorder.

Signs and symptoms

Clinical severity is quite variable, but all races are known to be affected. Hyperostosis gradually develops on the periosteal and endosteal surfaces of long bones, with the skull and axial skeleton also affected in severe cases. Carriers may have no detectable X-ray findings, but bone scans usually show diffusely increased uptake.

Patients typically present in childhood with limping or broad-based and waddling gait, leg pain, muscle atrophy, and decreased subcutaneous fat in the extremities, similar to patients with muscular dystrophy. More severely affected patients usually have a large head, prominent forehead, proptosis, and relatively thin extremities, with thickened, painful bones and decreased muscle development. Skull involvement may lead to cranial neuropathies or increased intracranial pressure. Puberty may be delayed.

Physical exam shows palpable widened and tender bones. Some patients develop hepatosplenomegaly, Raynaud's phenomenon, and other findings suggestive of vasculitis. The skeletal abnormalities usually progress with aging, although some patients experience spontaneous improvement in adulthood.

Diagnosis

Diagnosis is based on classic X-ray changes and physical exam findings. Genetic testing helps confirm the diagnosis.

Imaging tests

Skeletal surveys show hyperostosis affecting both periosteal and endosteal surfaces in the metaphyseal region of long bones, with thickening fairly symmetrical and progressive over time (Fig. 5.57). The epiphyses are spared. The diaphyses progressively widen and develop surface irregularities. The bones most commonly affected are the tibias and femurs, with radii, ulnae, humeri, scapulae, clavicles, pelvis, and occasionally, short tubular bones also affected. Age of onset, progression, and severity of skeletal changes are highly variable. In relatively mild disease in adolescents and young adults, skeletal findings may be limited to the legs.

X-rays, clinical findings, and bone scans are usually concordant. Bone scans typically show increased uptake in areas of active disease, but may be relatively unremarkable in patients with advanced but quiescent disease. Patients with early disease may have intense uptake on bone scans but relatively unremarkable X-ray findings.

Laboratory findings

Serum total or bone alkaline phosphatase and other markers of bone turnover are increased in some, but not all, patients. Severe active disease may be associated with mild hypocalcemia and marked hypocalciuria due to rapid skeletal mineral uptake. Serum calcium, phosphorus, creatinine, 25-hydroxyvitamin D, 1,25-dihydroxyvitamin D, and parathyroid hormone (PTH) are usually normal. Patients may have mild anemia, leukopenia, and an increased erythrocyte sedimentation rate.

Bone histomorphometry shows increased new bone formation along diaphyses, with endosteal surface woven bone undergoing centripetal maturation and incorporation into the cortex. Muscle and vascular abnormalities have been noted on electron microscopic studies.

Treatment

Because of the variable course of this disorder, spontaneous improvement or remission may occur during adolescence or adulthood. Glucocorticoid therapy in small doses given every other day may help bone pain and improve bone histology. Localized pain sometimes improves with resection of a "cortical window." Bisphosphonates may help pain symptoms after transient worsening of pain.

Hepatitis C-associated osteosclerosis

Etiology

This condition is associated with current hepatitis C viral infection in former intravenous drug abusers.

Signs and symptoms

Patients with this condition have severe, generalized hyperostosis and osteosclerosis throughout their skeleton, usually associated with pain in the forearms and legs when disease is initially active. Gradual, spontaneous remission over several years may occur in some cases.

Diagnosis

This disorder is diagnosed based on classic X-ray appearance, limb pain symptoms, and documentation of current hepatitis C viral infection.

Imaging tests

X-rays show diffuse periosteal, endosteal, and trabecular bone thickening throughout the skeleton, typically sparing the skull (Figs 5.58–5.60). Dual energy X-ray absorptiometry (DXA) bone density is usually increased two- to three-fold above age-matched controls. Spontaneous remission may lead to a return in increased DXA bone density toward normal.

Laboratory findings

Most biochemical parameters of bone and mineral metabolism are normal. The only reported abnormality is that serum insulin-like growth factor (IGF)-binding protein 2 and "big" IGF-2 are increased. Bone histomorphometry shows that remodeling of good quality excessive bone is accelerated during active disease.

Treatment

Bisphosphonates may slow down excessive bone remodeling and thereby improve bone pain symptoms.

Illustration (Fig. 5.57)

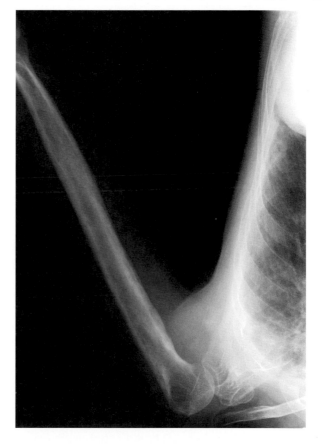

Figure 5.57 Progressive diaphyseal dysplasia (Camurati–Engelmann disease) with hyperostosis affecting the humerus.

Illustrations (Figs 5.58–5.60)

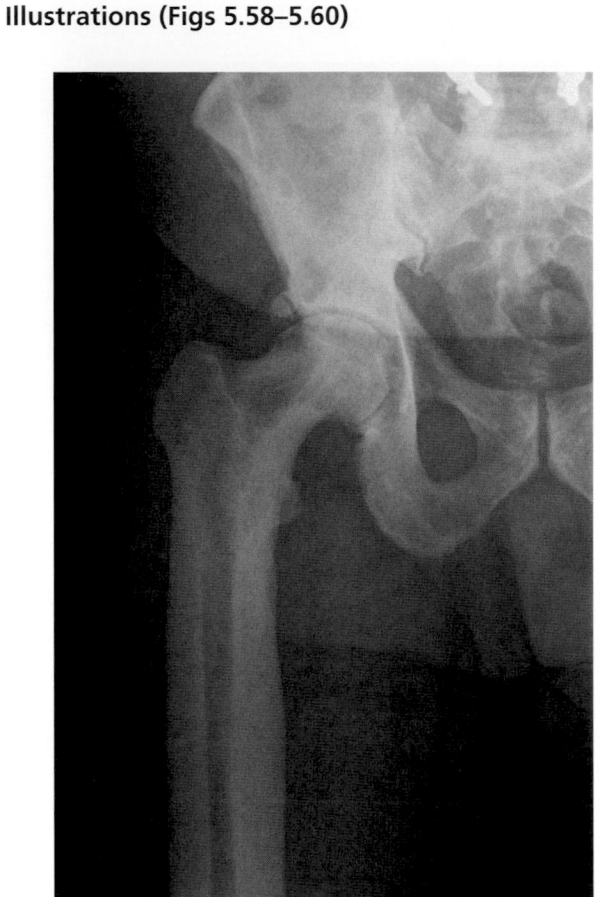

Figure 5.58 Hepatitis C-associated osteosclerosis, affecting the pelvis. Courtesy of Dr. Robert D. Tiegs.

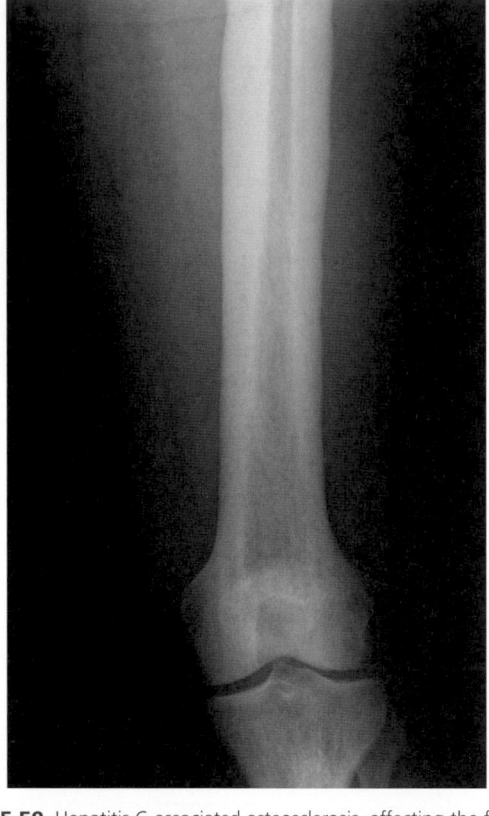

Figure 5.59 Hepatitis C-associated osteosclerosis, affecting the femur. Courtesy of Dr. Robert D. Tiegs.

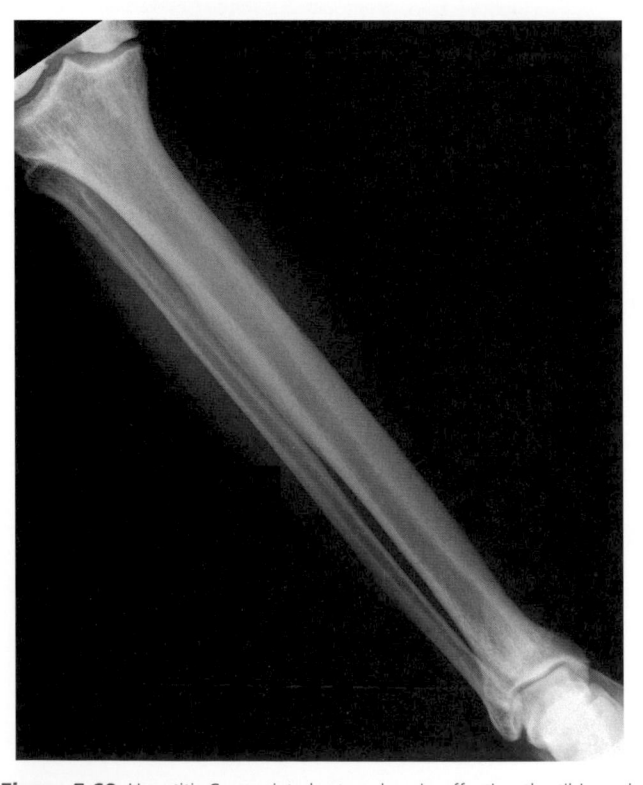

Figure 5.60 Hepatitis C-associated osteosclerosis, affecting the tibia and fibula. Courtesy of Dr. Robert D. Tiegs.

Familial high bone mass phenotype due to Lrp5 mutation

Etiology

This disorder is caused by autosomal dominant activating mutations in the first propeller domain of the *LRP5* gene that encodes the low-density lipoprotein receptor-related protein 5. These mutations result in constitutive stimulation of the canonical Wnt-signaling pathway in osteoblasts, thereby promoting osteoblastogenesis and increased osteoblast function, which results in diffusely increased bone density throughout the skeleton.

Signs and symptoms

Patients have high skeletal bone density, with good quality bone. They tend not to fracture despite trauma, and do not have bone pain. Some patients have torus palatinus, oropharyngeal exostoses, squaring of the mandible, or cranial neuropathies.

Diagnosis

This disorder is diagnosed clinically by classic X-ray findings of diffuse skeletal sclerosis, and moderately or markedly increased bone density. The diagnosis is confirmed by LRP5 mutation analysis.

Imaging tests

X-rays show uniformly dense bone throughout the skeleton (Figs 5.61 & 5.62). Dual energy X-ray absorptiometry (DXA) bone density testing shows bone density typically 2–3 or more standard deviations above age-matched controls.

Laboratory findings

Bone and mineral metabolism biochemical parameters are typically within the normal range. There is not a unique diagnostic biochemical test that has been reported.

Treatment

No treatment is usually necessary, since high bone density is protective against fracture, and skeletal pain is not a feature of this disorder. Glucocorticoid therapy could potentially improve compressive cranial or other neuropathies, but surgery is not typically required.

Illustrations (Figs 5.61 & 5.62)

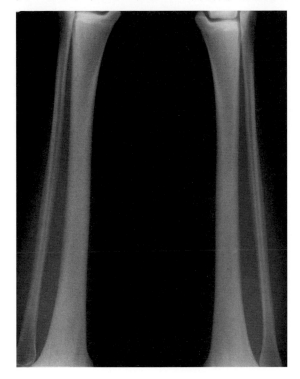

Figure 5.61 Familial high bone mass phenotype due to Lrp5 mutation, causing uniformly dense bone in the ribs and humerus. Courtesy of Dr. Ann E. Kearns.

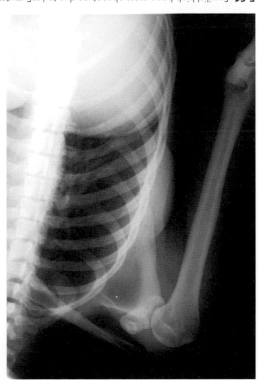

Figure 5.62 Familial high bone mass phenotype due to Lrp5 mutation, causing uniformly dense bone in the tibiae and fibulae. Courtesy of Dr. Ann E. Kearns.

Erdheim–Chester disease

Etiology

Erdheim–Chester disease is a rare form of systemic non-Langerhans' cell histiocytosis described initially by Erdheim and Chester in 1930. The cause of the disorder remains unknown. Affected tissues are typically infiltrated with xanthomatous histiocytes, Touton giant cells, lymphocytes, and plasma cells, with associated fibrosis. The clinical course depends on the severity and distribution of the disease. Some patients are asymptomatic or have only mild or limited symptoms, whereas others have a more aggressive form of the disease and deteriorate over 2–3 years.

Signs and symptoms

Symmetric bone pain in the extremities is the most common presenting symptom, most often affecting the lower extremities. However, about half of affected patients experience extraskeletal manifestations. These include effects on the central nervous system and pituitary gland, sometimes causing diabetes insipidus. The cardiovascular system and aorta may be affected, as may the lungs with interstitial lung disease. Retroperitoneal and perirenal infiltration may cause renal dysfunction. Osteosclerosis of the paranasal sinuses and exophthalmos have been reported. Skin lesions may be similar to subcutaneous fat necrosis.

Diagnosis

Diagnosis of this disorder is based on clinical history, radiological features, and pathologic findings that show infiltration of tissues with foamy histiocytes that are CD68$^+$ and CD1a$^-$.

Imaging tests

X-rays usually show sclerosis of the affected bones, typically with diffuse or patchy sclerosis symmetrically affecting the medullary cavities of the metaphyses of the long bones of the lower extremities, with relative epiphyseal sparing (Figs 5.63 & 5.64). Technetium-99 bone and positron emission tomography (PET) scans show increased uptake where the skeleton is involved, again typically symmetrically affecting the long bones of the extremities (Fig. 5.65). Computed tomography (CT) and magnetic resonance imaging (MRI) scans may further define the bone disease, but specific findings are not helpful in making a diagnosis.

Laboratory findings

Bone and mineral metabolism parameters are usually normal, except for serum total and bone alkaline phosphatase, which may be increased at the time of diagnosis, or when the disease flares. Increased erythrocyte sedimentation rate, C-reactive protein, or anemia may be present.

Treatment

Various treatments have been used for Erdheim–Chester disease in small numbers of patients, but none has been proven to be more effective than the others. Steroids, cytotoxic agents, interferon-α, the tyrosine kinase inhibitor imatinib mesylate, radiotherapy, and double autologous hematopoietic stem cell transplantation have each been tried. Bisphosphonates have been used with some success to treat bone pain in those with significant bone involvement.

Illustrations (Figs 5.63–5.65)

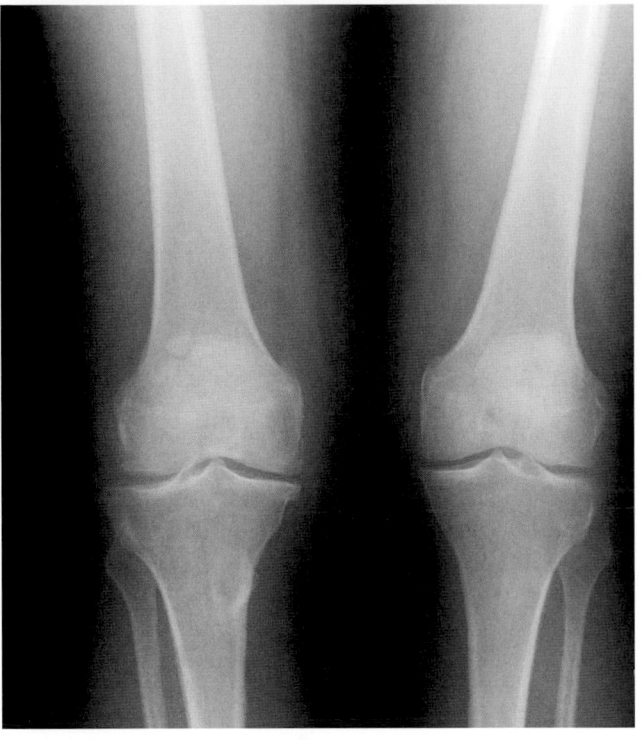

Figure 5.63 Erdheim–Chester disease, showing patchy sclerosis affecting the distal femurs and tibiae, with relative sparing of the epiphyses. Courtesy of Dr. Bart L. Clarke.

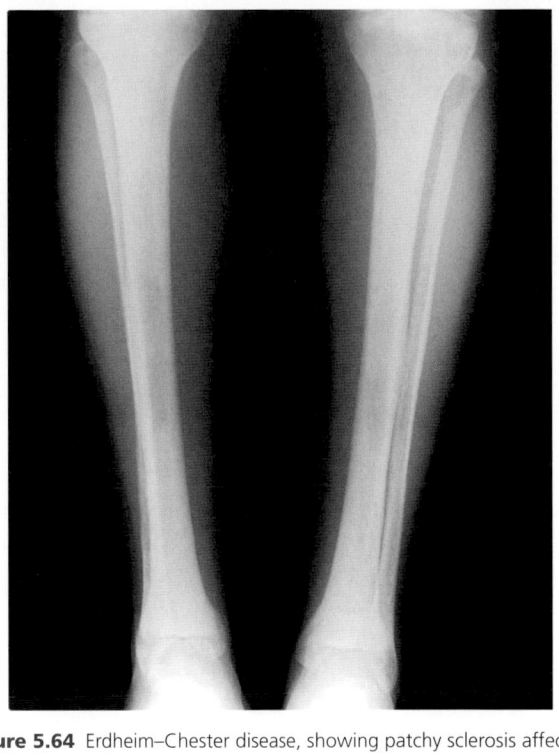

Figure 5.64 Erdheim–Chester disease, showing patchy sclerosis affecting the tibiae and fibulae, with relative sparing of the epiphyses. Courtesy of Dr. Bart L. Clarke.

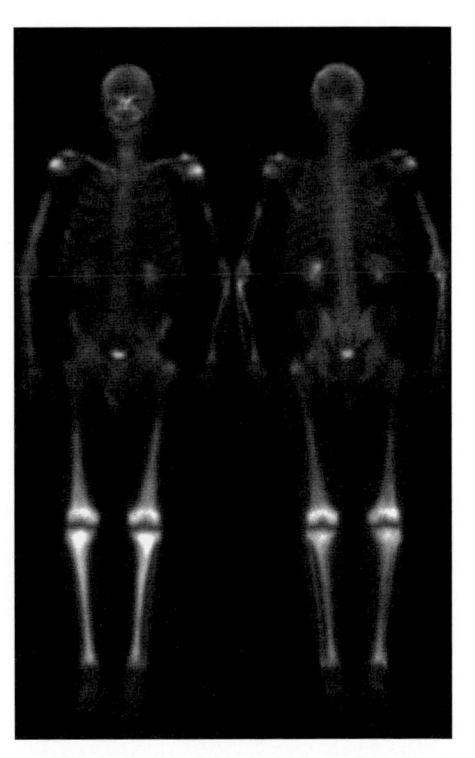

Figure 5.65 Erdheim–Chester disease, with bone scan showing distribution of symmetric osteosclerosis over the distal lower extremities. Courtesy of Dr. Bart L. Clarke.

Skeletal fluorosis

Etiology

Skeletal fluorosis occurs with excess exposure of the skeleton to fluoride, either by industrial, endemic (e.g. well water), dietary (e.g. high-fluoride content tea or dentifrice consumption), or supplemental intake of this mineral. High levels of fluoride in the skeleton may cause toxic effects on mineralization, impairment of normal bone resorption, and decreased strength per unit of bone. Sodium fluoride stimulates new bone formation by recruiting active, normally functioning osteoblasts independent of preceding bone resorption, similar to what is seen with aluminum. Fluoride also replaces the hydroxyl group in hydroxyapatite to form fluoroapatite, which has a more stable crystal structure than hydroxyapatite, which is therefore more resistant to osteoclast resorption.

Daily intake of sodium fluoride of < 30 mg/day produce no discernable effect on the skeleton, whereas intake of > 80 mg/day causes marked skeletal abnormalities, including woven, irregular bone matrix and irregularly distributed osteocytes in enlarged lacunae surrounded by haloes of low bone mineral density. Enhanced matrix deposition results in excess osteoid that is poorly mineralized, in some cases meeting criteria for generalized or focal osteomalacia. Osteomalacia often develops with increased fluoride intake without adequate calcium intake or supplementation, and this form of osteomalacia is not vitamin D dependent, nor does it respond to vitamin D therapy. Normal fluoride intake in the setting of renal dysfunction may also result in toxicity.

Signs and symptoms

Increased fluoride intake typically causes asymptomatic increased bone density. Excess fluoride intake may cause crippling bone and joint dysfunction, and marked bone pain.

Diagnosis

Fluorosis is characterized by increased bone density or sclerosis on X-ray or other imaging, associated with increased serum fluoride levels.

Imaging tests

X-rays show increased bone density and sclerosis throughout the skeleton (Figs 5.66 & 5.67). Bone scans usually show increased uptake throughout the skeleton, particularly in affected areas.

Laboratory findings

Most biochemical parameters of bone and mineral metabolism are normal, although increased serum total or bone alkaline phosphatase may occur. Normal serum fluoride levels in healthy adults aged 18–80 range from 0.5 to 2.3 μM.

Treatment

Patients with skeletal fluorosis are best treated by stopping all sources of fluoride intake. There is no evidence that chelation therapy reduces skeletal fluoride faster than conservative management. Low bone turnover will decrease clearance of skeletal fluoride, whereas high turnover will increase clearance.

Illustrations (Figs 5.66 & 5.67)

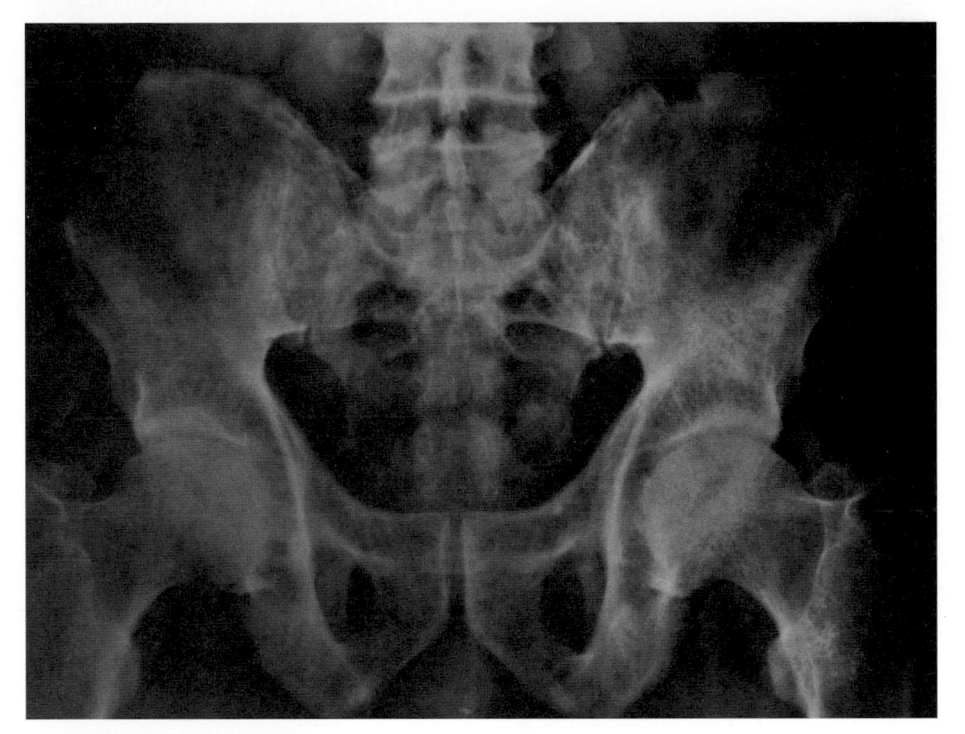

Figure 5.66 Skeletal fluorosis, showing patchy sclerosis affecting the pelvis. Courtesy of Dr. Ronald G. Swee.

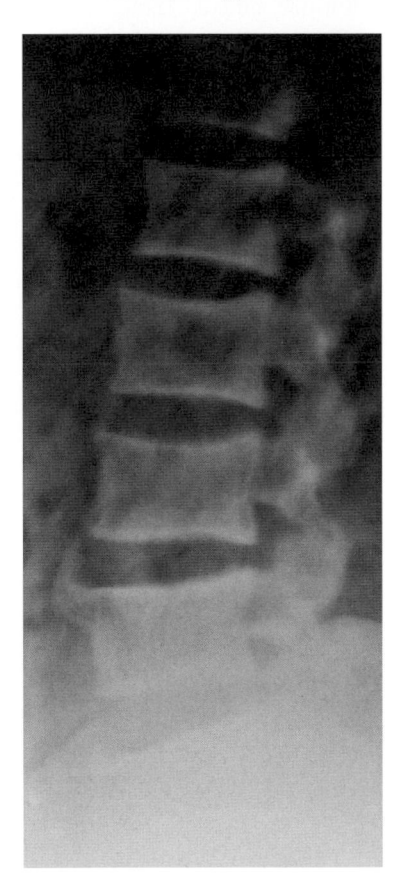

Figure 5.67 Skeletal fluorosis, showing patchy sclerosis affecting the lumbar spine. Courtesy of Dr. Ronald G. Swee.

Tumoral calcinosis

Definition
Tumoral calcinosis is a rare autosomal recessive metabolic bone disease characterized by progressive deposition of calcium phosphate crystals in soft tissues, especially around the joints.

Etiology
This disorder typically results in hyperphosphatemia due to increased renal tubular reabsorption of phosphate, but it may also occur without hyperphosphatemia. When hyperphosphatemia is present, the increased tissue calcium–phosphate product increases soft tissue deposition of calcium phophate crystals. Biallelic mutations in the *GALNT3* gene on chromosome 2q24-q31 were first identified to cause this disorder in Druze and black kindreds. The *GALNT3* gene is responsible for synthesis of a glycosyltransferase enzyme that initiates mucin-type O-glycosylation. This enzyme O-glycosylates a furin-like convertase recognition sequence in fibroblast growth factor (FGF)-23 that prevents proteolytic cleavage of the protein. In tumoral calcinosis, FGF-23 O-glycosylation does not occur, resulting in decreased secretion of intact FGF-23, which results in hyperphosphatemia and increased serum 1,25-dihydroxyvitamin D production by proximal renal tubular cells.

Families with normophosphatemic tumoral calcinosis do not have linkage to the *GALNT3* gene, but have been reported to have *FGF-23* gene mutations. These mutations result in secretion of incomplete FGF-23 protein from cells. It is not clear why these patients do not also have hyperphosphatemia.

A single 13-year-old girl with tumoral calcinosis has been reported to have a *KLOTHO* gene mutation associated with hyperphosphatemia, increased serum 1,25-dihydroxyvitamin D, hypercalcemia, and increased serum parathyroid hormone (PTH). She had increased serum intact FGF-23 and FGF-23 C-terminal fragments, but reduced FGF-23 bioactivity. KLOTHO protein is a cofactor required by FGF-23 for binding and signaling through its FGF receptors.

Signs and symptoms
Most patients with tumoral calcinosis present with calcium phosphate deposition causing masses in the soft tissues around their major joints. First lesions are reported to occur most often around the hips, elbows, shoulders, and scapulae, with onset from age 22 months to adulthood. Most patients are recognized with the disorder by their early 20s. Most case reports are from kindreds of African descent, with families usually demonstrating autosomal recessive or dominant inheritance.

The soft tissue masses reported around major joints are usually painless, and may grow as large as grapefruit. Because the soft tissue masses are extracapsular, they do not usually impair joint range of motion. However, the masses may cause sciatica or other neurological compression syndromes due to nerve compression, or erode through the skin and ooze chalky fluid, or become infected. Early lesions may be precipitated by local bleeding around major joints, followed by accumulation of foamy histiocytes, which become transformed into cystic cavities lined by osteoclast-like giant cells and histiocytes. Movement and friction caused by the location of the lesions seems to result in transformation of early lesions. Exuberant cellular proliferative changes are seen adjacent to cysts, consisting of ill-defined reactive-like perivascular solid cell nests mixed with mononuclear and iron-loaded macrophages, or well-defined fibrohistiocytic nodules of variable size included in dense collagenous stroma. Mature lesions are usually filled with chalky material in a viscous milky fluid.

Some patients develop findings suggestive of pseudoxanthoma elasticum, including skin changes, vascular calcification, and retinal angioid streaks. Patients may have dental hypoplasia, with short bulbous dental roots, and near-complete obliteration of dental pulp spaces by pulp stones.

Diagnosis

Diagnosis is usually based on classic X-ray findings, with increased serum phosphorus and 1,25-dihydroxyvitamin D levels, and family history.

Imaging tests

The earliest soft tissue lesions are usually located along bursae, and often distributed along para-articular regions along the extensor surfaces of major joints. The soft tissue lesions represent multiple globular collections of amorphous calcium phosphate separated by fibrous connective tissue (Fig. 5.68). Fluid levels may be seen within masses with cystic components. Inflammatory periostitis in the mid-diaphyseal region of long bones may be seen on routine X-rays, computed tomography (CT), or magnetic resonance imaging (MRI) scans. Vascular calcification may be seen on X-rays or CT scans. Bone scans show increased uptake in the skeletal areas affected by tumoral calcinosis (Fig. 5.69). Patients with chronic kidney disease may develop periarticular soft tissue masses due to calcium phosphate deposition that cannot be distinguished by X-ray from tumoral calcinosis.

Laboratory findings

Patients with tumoral calcinosis typically have increased serum phosphorus and 1,25-dihydroxyvitamin D levels. The tubular maximum for phosphate reabsorption in relation to glomerular filtration rate (TmPO$_4$/GFR) is increased, with normal renal function. Occasional patients have periarticular soft tissue masses but normal serum phosphorus. Serum calcium, alkaline phosphatase, and parathyroid hormone (PTH) are usually normal. Metabolic balance studies have shown increased calcium and phosphorus balance due to increased gastrointestinal absorption and decreased renal excretion.

Treatment

Surgical removal of calcified lesions is recommended if they cause pain, affect joint function, or for cosmetic reasons. Medical treatments have been variably successful. Aluminum hydroxide antacid, dietary phosphorus, and calcium restriction were reported to be helpful in a single case report. Calcitonin has been used to induce renal phosphate excretion. Acetazolamide and aluminum hydroxide in combination were used for 14 years to reduce the size of lesions. Oral alendronate was reported to reduce symptoms within 3 months in one patient. New therapies targeting FGF-23 may offer better opportunities to help these patients.

Illustrations (Figs 5.68 & 5.69)

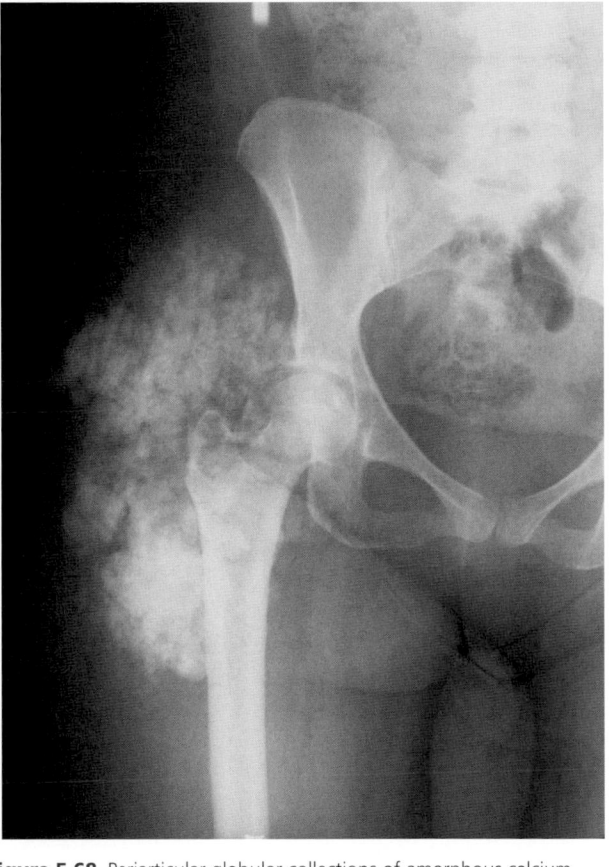

Figure 5.68 Periarticular globular collections of amorphous calcium phosphate in tumoral calcinosis. Courtesy of Dr. Naveen S. Murthy.

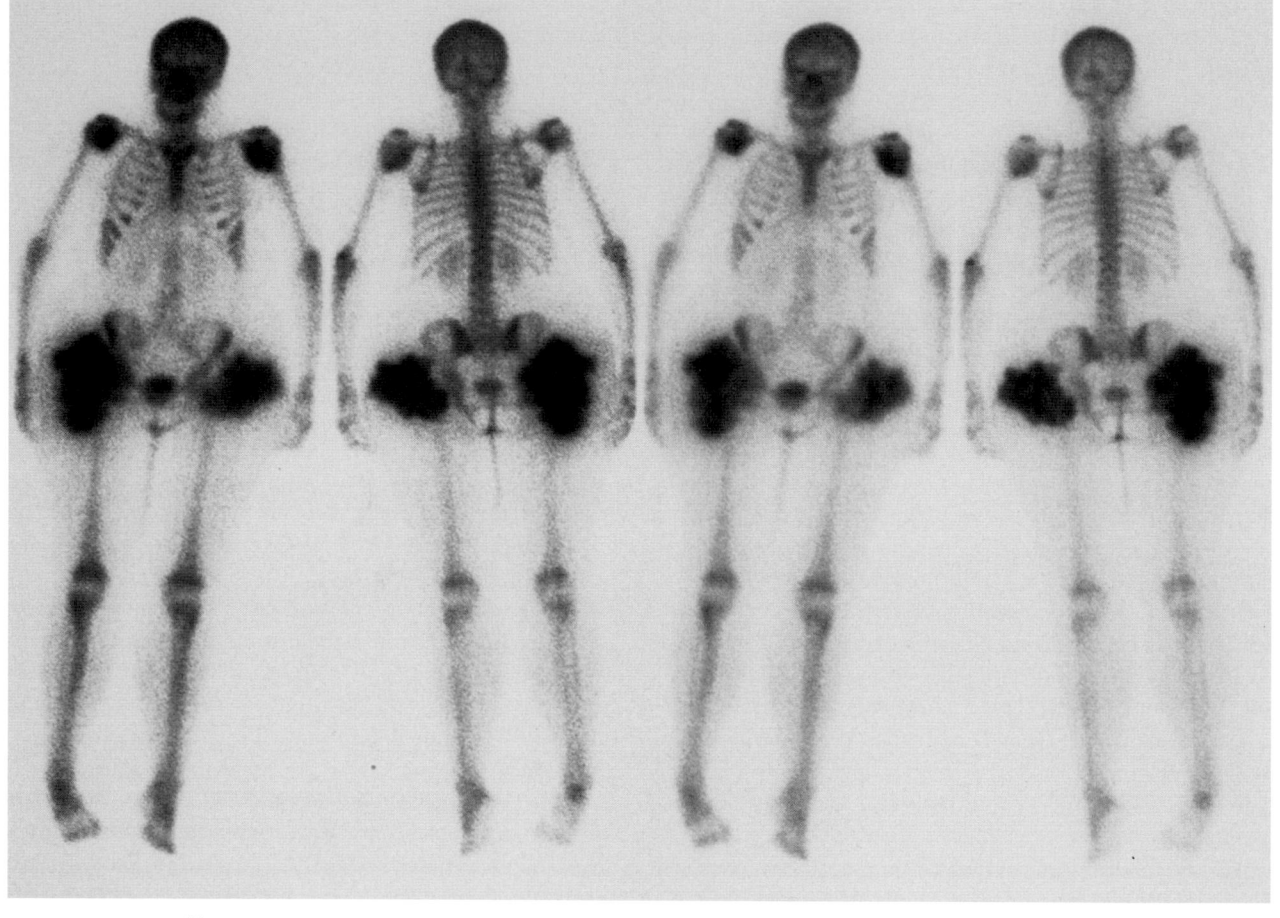

Figure 5.69 Increased ^{99}Tc bone scan uptake in tumoral calcinosis. Courtesy of Dr. Naveen S. Murthy.

Osteogenesis imperfecta

Definition

Osteogenesis imperfecta (OI) is a genetic disorder of connective tissue characterized by fragile bones and susceptibility to fracture, most frequently caused by mutations in type I collagen.

Etiology

Classical OI is due to autosomal dominant defects in type I collagen synthesis, which affects the bones, skin, and tendons. The Sillence classification proposed in 1979, based on clinical and radiographic criteria, categorized OI into four main types: mild (type I), lethal (II), progressive deforming (III), or moderate (IV). Type I OI is caused by decreased production of $\alpha 1$(I) collagen by at least 50%. Types II–IV are due to mutations in either of the two chains that form the type I collagen heterotrimer. Classic OI may occur in the children of unaffected parents due to parental mosaicism.

The four new types of OI (types V–VIII) are defined by different criteria than types I–IV, and most often are similar to type IV. Types V and VI are defined by histology and radiographic criteria, and are due to unknown mutations at present. Type VII was first described histologically and clinically, and is due to mutations in the *CRTAP* gene which produces cartilage-associated protein. Type VIII was first defined biochemically and molecularly as due to mutations in the *LEPRE1* gene. Types VII and VIII are transmitted by autosomal recessive inheritance, and overlap with the lethal and severe Sillence types II and III. Types VII and VIII are due to mutations in two members of the prolyl 3-hydroxylation complex, CRTAP and P3H1. This complex post-translationally 3-hydroxylates the $\alpha 1$(I)Pro986 residue in the endoplasmic reticulum. About 5% of cases of OI are not due to type I collagen or P3H1 hydroxylation complex mutations, and their etiology is currently not known.

Signs and symptoms

Osteogenesis imperfecta is known as brittle bone disease because affected individuals have increased risk of fracture with minor or no trauma. The range of clinical expression is extremely wide, ranging from lethality from multiple fractures in the perinatal period to presentation with early osteoporosis in adults. Individuals with osteogenesis imperfecta

may have varying combinations of short stature, defective tooth formation (dentinogenesis imperfecta), hearing loss, macrocephaly, bluish coloration of the sclerae, scoliosis, barrel chest, and increased joint flexibility or dislocation due to lax ligaments.

The eight types of OI vary significantly in their symptoms and timing of onset. Family history is usually negative for OI, as most individuals carry new mutations. The prenatal severe forms of types II, III, VII, or VIII are often difficult to distinguish from thanatophoric dysplasia, camptomelic dysplasia, or achondrogenesis type I. The neonatal form of types II or VIII present similarly to infantile hypophosphatasia, but infantile hypophosphatasia is associated with low serum alkaline phosphatase and bone spurs at the elbows and knees. Milder forms of OI diagnosed in childhood may be misdiagnosed as juvenile or idiopathic osteoporosis or child abuse. Because OI causes a generalized connective tissue defect, children with OI typically have characteristic facial features, including a flat midface, triangular facial shape, bluish sclerae, yellowish or opalescent teeth, relative macrocephaly, barrel chest or pectus excavatum, joint laxity, vertebral compression fractures, and growth deficiency in varying combinations. The autosomal recessive types VII and VIII overlap with types II and III in presentation, but have white sclerae.

Type I

Type I is the mildest form of the disorder, and may be diagnosed in adulthood as the cause of early osteoporosis. Fractures occur after birth, usually after children start to walk, stop at puberty, and then may recur in early to middle adulthood. Affected individuals usually have bluish sclerae (Fig. 5.70), often have easy bruising, may lose their hearing anywhere from late childhood to their third decade, and often have joint hyperextensibility. Growth deficiency and long bone deformity are generally mild. Dentinogenesis imperfecta is present in type A, and absent in type B.

Type II

Type II is usually lethal in the perinatal period due to respiratory infection, but affected individuals may survive for as long as 1 year or more. These children are typically born prematurely and are small for gestational age. The skeleton is extremely undermineralized, with in utero fractures, and the skull has open anterior and posterior fontanelles. Bones of affected infants are mostly woven bone, without Haversian canals or organized lamellae. The sclerae are usually blue-gray.

Type III

Type III is associated with severe bone dysplasia, but affected individuals usually survive childhood despite multiple fractures, which cause a progressive deforming phenotype. At birth the skeleton is similar to milder forms of type II.

These children have dozens or hundreds of fractures over their lifetime. Long bones deform from normal muscle tension and recurrent fractures. Growth deficiency is severe, with final height in the normal range for prepubertal children. Scoliosis is common, with metaphyseal flaring and "popcorn" formation at growth plates typical. Most require intensive physical rehabilitation and orthopedic care to walk with assistance in childhood; many depend on wheelchairs for mobility. Some individuals with this form have normal life expectancy, whereas others develop respiratory insufficiency and cor pulmonale by middle age, and some die in infancy or childhood from upper respiratory infection.

Type IV

Type IV is moderately severe, and usually diagnosed at birth or in early childhood. The sclerae are variably bluish. Affected children usually have several fractures each year and bowing of their long bones, but fractures decrease after puberty. Final height is reduced, often to the range of pubertal children, but many affected children respond to growth hormone. The skeleton is undermineralized with mild modeling abnormalities, and platybasia, vertebral compression fractures, and scoliosis are common. These individuals usually develop independent mobility and have normal life expectancy.

Types IV or III OI may overlap with Ehlers–Danlos syndrome, with joint laxity, hip dysplasia, or early progressive scoliosis. These individuals have a mutation in the N-terminal region of the type I collagen chains that interferes with collagen N-propeptide processing.

Type V

Type V is associated with radiographically dense bands of connective tissue adjacent to the growth plates of long bones, with hypertrophic calluses at the sites of fractures or surgical procedures, and calcification of the membrane between the radius and ulna, which leads to restricted wrist motion (Fig. 5.71). Their teeth are normal, and their sclerae are white. The microscopic appearance of their bony lamellae is described as mesh-like.

Type VI

Type VI is only diagnosable by bone biopsy, with bony lamellae having a "fish-scale"-like appearance on microscopy. Skeletal disease is moderate to severe, but their teeth and sclerae are normal. Serum alkaline phosphatase is mildly increased.

Type VII

Type VII was first identified in an isolated First Nations community in northern Quebec, Canada. Affected individuals have rhizomelia and moderate skeletal disease. Null mutations in the *CRTAP* gene are lethal, with rhizomelia, white sclerae, and a small-to-normal skull.

Type VIII

Type VIII has a similar phenotype to type VII. Null mutations in *LEPRE1* cause a phenotype similar to types II and III, but with white sclerae and extreme growth deficiency. A recurring *LEPRE1* mutation occurs in West Africans and North Americans of African descent, which is lethal in the homozygous form.

Diagnosis

Diagnosis is usually suspected based on classic X-ray and physical exam findings, with collagen biochemical studies or DNA sequencing of type I collagen, *CRTAP*, and *LEPRE1* used to help make the correct diagnosis.

Imaging tests

Skeletal surveys in patients with OI usually show diffuse osteopenia, with thin cortices and gracile appearance of the long bones and ribs (Fig. 5.72). In moderate and severe forms, bowing or bone modeling deformities are common, with metaphyseal flaring and "popcorn" appearance at the growth plates (Fig. 5.73). Vertebral endplate central compression is common in all forms, with moderate to severe forms often having compression fractures (Fig. 5.74). Scoliosis results from spinal ligamentous laxity and asymmetric vertebral compression fractures (Fig. 5.75). Wormian bones may be present in the skull (Fig. 5.76).

Platybasia occurs in types III and IV, and should be assessed serially with computed tomography (CT) scans for basilar impression and invagination. Bones of affected children with types VII and VIII are extremely underminer-alized, have a cylindrical shape, and may have cystic and disorganized bone structure. Surviving children with type VIII have flaring of the metaphyses, with gracile hands and shortened metacarpals.

Dual energy X-ray absorptiometry (DXA) bone density ranges from normal, in mild forms of OI, to very low, in severe forms of OI, with Z-scores generally correlating with severity of disease. Type I patients often have Z-scores in the −1.0 to −2.0 range, whereas children with type VIII may have Z-scores as low as in the −6.0 to −7.0 range.

Laboratory findings

Serum calcium, phosphorus, alkaline phosphatase, and creatinine are typically normal, although alkaline phosphatase may be increased after fractures or in type VI. Acid phosphatase is usually increased in type VIII or VII. Vitamin D levels are typically normal.

Bone histomorphometry usually shows defects in bone modeling and fewer but thickened trabeculae. Cortical width and trabecular bone volume are decreased in all forms of OI. Bone remodeling is increased, with increased osteoblast and osteoclast surfaces. Polarized light microscopy shows thinner and less smooth lamellae. Mineral apposition rate is normal. Hydroxyapatite crystal disorganization may contribute to bone structural weakness. Osteocytic lacunae are often larger than usual.

Skin biopsy and fibroblast culture allows biochemical type I collagen analysis. Type I OI results in 50% reduction in synthesis of structurally normal type I collagen due to inheritance of a null *COL1A1* allele. Cultured fibroblasts from individuals with type I OI show an increase in the COL3/COL1 protein ratio because they produce less than normal type I collagen. Patients with OI types II, III, and IV produce a mix of normal and abnormal type I collagen. The abnormal collagen produced in these forms has delayed helix folding and enzymatic overmodification that results in delayed electrophoretic migration. Biochemical testing is not able to detect abnormalities in the amino one-third of the α1(I) chain or amino one-half of the α2(I) chain. Collagen produced in types VII and VIII also has delayed helix folding and overmodification, indicating that the mutations in the P3H1 complex delay helical folding.

Mutation analysis by direct sequencing does not provide functional information, but is more sensitive at detecting mutations. Sequencing of DNA or transcript sequencing of cDNA are both available. These techniques may miss large deletions or rearrangements or low-percentage splice defects.

Genotype–phenotype modeling of the more than 800 type I collagen mutations currently recognized shows different roles for the two collagen α-chains. Roughly one-third of the α1(I) chain substitutions are lethal, especially those to residues with branched or charged side chains. Two exclusively lethal regions are associated with proposed major ligand-binding regions for the collagen monomer with integrins, matrix metalloproteinases, fibronectin, and cartilage oligomeric matrix protein. About one-fifth of the α2(I) chain substitutions are lethal, and these are clustered along eight regularly spaced regions along the chain that bind to proteoglycans.

Treatment

Physical rehabilitation exercises should be started early and continued consistently throughout life to optimize the physical abilities of OI patients. Necessary orthopedic procedures should be done by experienced orthopedic surgeons. Fractures should be reduced appropriately to prevent loss of function or ambulation. Osteotomies require fixation with intramedullary rods.

Complications of OI such as decreased pulmonary function, hearing loss, or basilar invagination, are best handled by programs offering coordinated specialized care. About half of children with type IV OI, and most children with type I OI, respond well to growth hormone treatment.

Bisphosphonates are useful for prevention of fractures and for increasing vertebral trabecular bone density over 1–2 years, with less definite effects on cortical long bones. Long-term use of intravenous pamidronate may result in

skeletal and reproductive risks, with defective bone remodeling and accumulation of bone microdamage, manifest as growth arrest lines in vertebrae (Fig. 5.77) or long bones. Delayed osteotomy healing may result with conventional doses. Most specialists recommend continuous treatment for a maximum of 2–3 years, with long-term follow-up afterwards.

Illustrations (Figs 5.70–5.77)

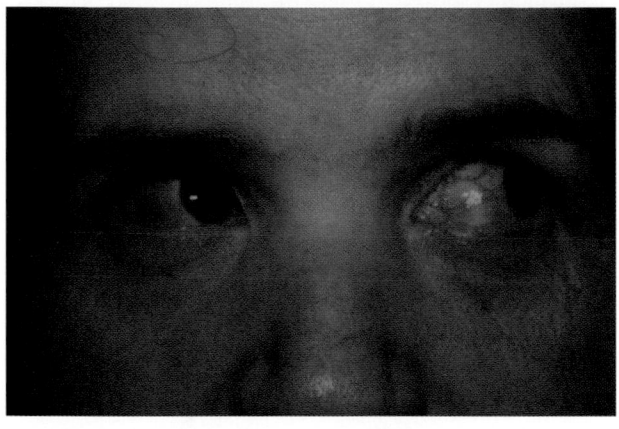

Figure 5.70 Blue sclerae in type I osteogenesis imperfecta. Courtesy of Dr. Bart L. Clarke.

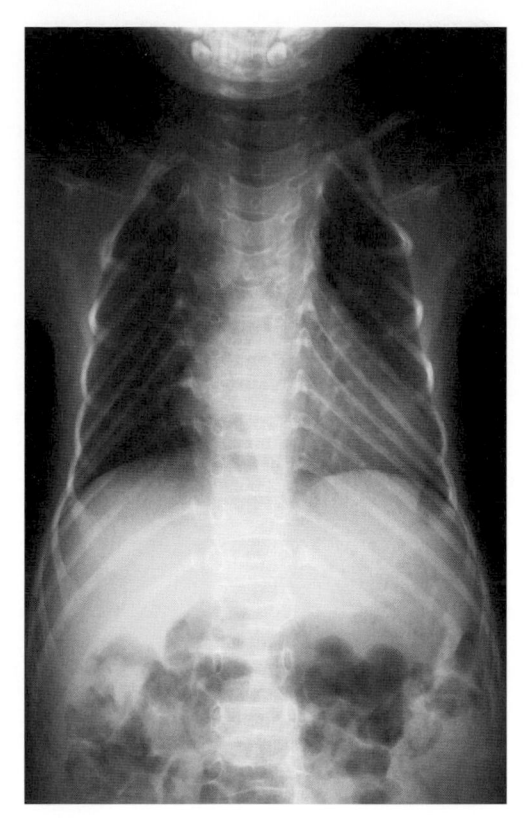

Figure 5.72 Gracile ribs in type I osteogenesis imperfecta. Courtesy of Dr. Peter J. Tebben.

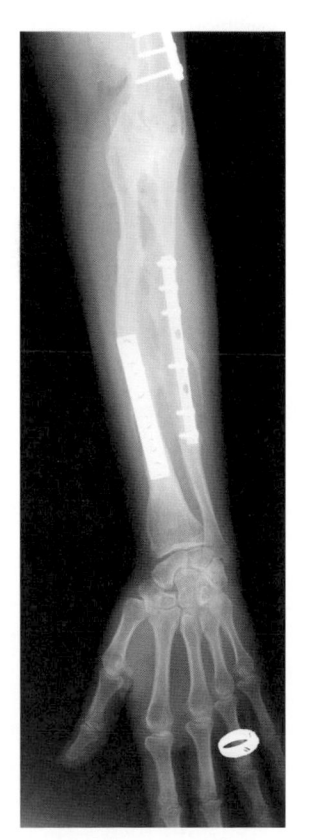

Figure 5.71 Restricted wrist motion in type V Osteogenesis imperfecta. Courtesy of Dr. Peter J. Tebben.

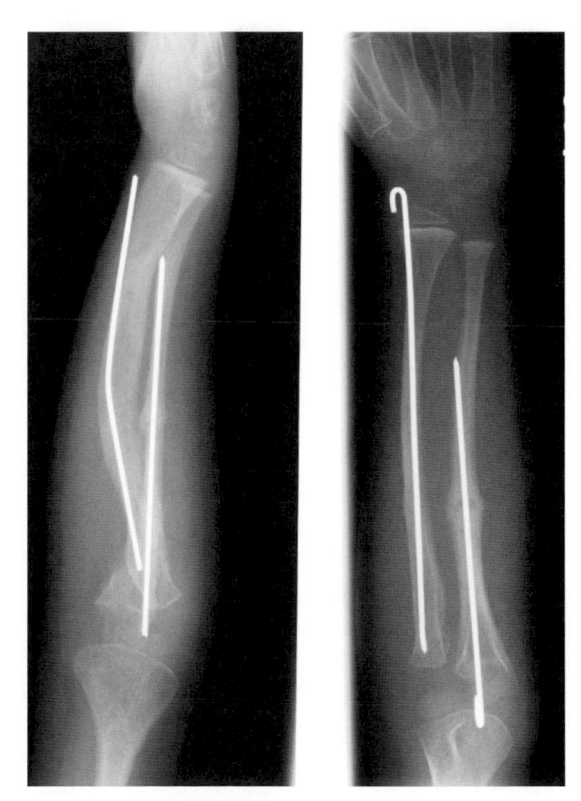

Figure 5.73 Bowing and metaphyseal flaring in type III osteogenesis imperfecta. Courtesy of Dr. Peter J. Tebben.

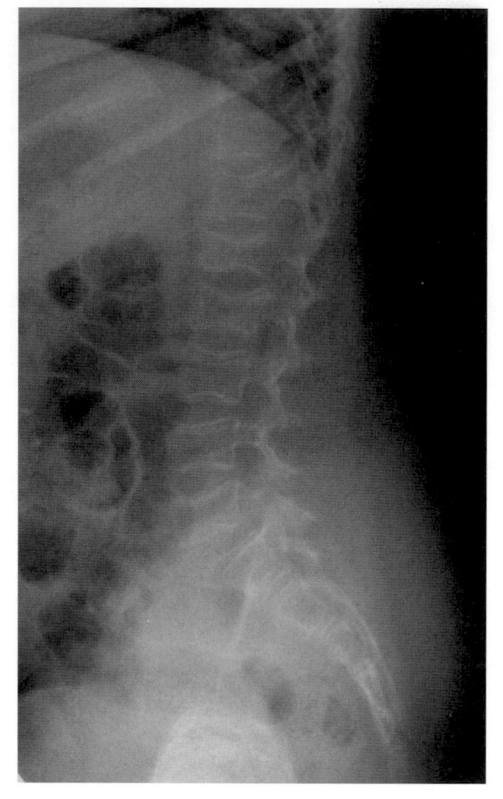

Figure 5.74 Vertebral compression fractures in type III Osteogenesis imperfecta. Courtesy of Dr. Peter J. Tebben.

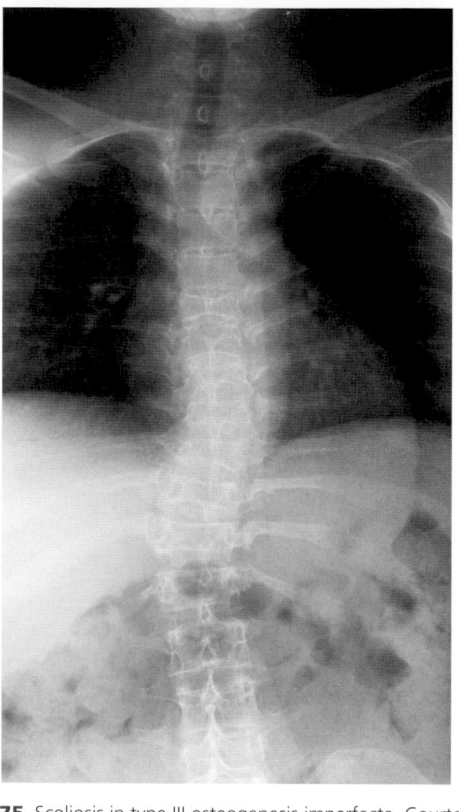

Figure 5.75 Scoliosis in type III osteogenesis imperfecta. Courtesy of Dr. Peter J. Tebben.

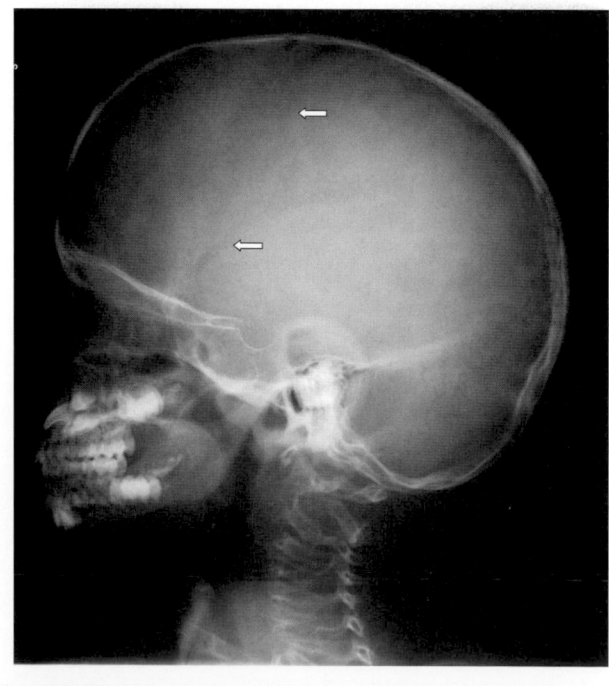

Figure 5.76 Skull wormian bones (arrows) in type III osteogenesis imperfecta. Courtesy of Dr. Peter J. Tebben.

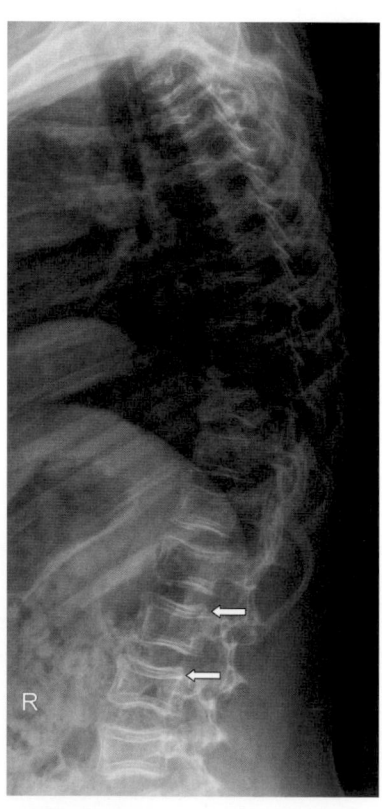

Figure 5.77 Growth arrest lines in vertebrae (arrows) in type III osteogenesis imperfecta. Courtesy of Dr. Peter J. Tebben.

Other skeletal disorders

Osteoporosis–pseudoglioma (OPPG) syndrome

Definition

Osteoporosis pseudoglioma syndrome is a genetic disorder characterized by childhood osteoporosis and congenital blindness.

Etiology

This rare autosomal recessive disorder characterized by childhood osteoporosis and congenital blindness is due to inactivating mutations in the low-density lipoprotein receptor-related protein 5 (*LRP5*) gene. *LRP5* is a membrane co-receptor in the canonical Wnt signaling pathway, and inactivating mutations in *LRP5* prevent binding of Wnt to LRP5, thereby resulting in pathway inactivation that leads to OPPG syndrome. Most homozygous and heterozygous mutations reported to cause OPPG occur in the second or third of its four beta-propeller domains, which are high affinity Wnt binding domains that are highly conserved. Inactivating *LRP5* mutations also cause about 20% of cases of the separate disorder familial exudative vitreoretinopathy (FEVR), which results in premature arrest in development of the retinal vasculature, which leads to retinal detachment and blindness in most. Many affected individuals have not had bone density assessment, but in those where it has been measured, low bone density or osteoporosis have been found, suggesting that OPPG and FEVR may be part of a single phenotypic spectrum.

Signs and symptoms

Affected homozygous or compound heterozygous individuals are typically diagnosed with childhood osteoporosis and ocular abnormalities leading to blindness. In most cases fractures develop after age 2 years. Blindness appears to result from persistence of the fetal ocular fibrovascular system and failure of retinal development. Short stature is common. Heterozygotes are reported to have low bone density but not eye pathology.

Diagnosis

Diagnosis is based on childhood medical history and physical exam findings, with low bone density or osteoporosis assessed by dual energy X-ray absorptiometry (DXA) measurement. Genetic testing confirms the diagnosis.

Imaging tests

X-rays show osteopenia throughout the skeleton, sometimes accompanied by fractures. Long bones may be gracile (Figs 5.78–5.81).

Laboratory findings

Serum calcium, phosphorus, and alkaline phosphatase, and urinary NTx-telopeptide have been reported to be normal. Urinary deoxypyridinoline has been reported to be mildly increased in one case. Serum 25-hydroxyvitamin D may be decreased due to lack of adequate intake or supplementation. Parathyroid hormone (PTH) is reported to be normal.

Treatment

Bisphosphonates have been reported to increase bone density in affected individuals.

Illustrations (Figs 5.78–5.81)

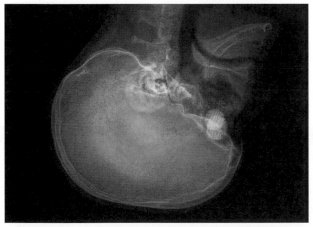

Figure 5.78 Osteoporosis–pseudoglioma syndrome. Courtesy of Dr. Peter J. Tebben.

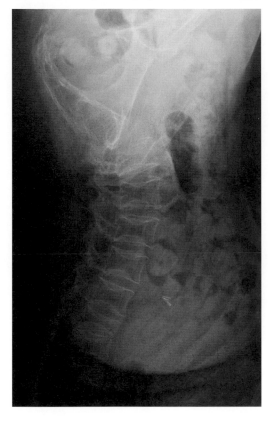

Figure 5.79 Osteoporosis–pseudoglioma syndrome. Courtesy of Dr. Peter J. Tebben.

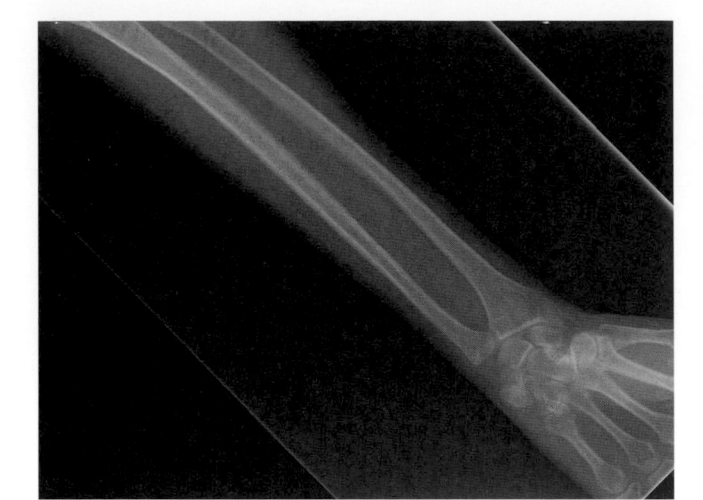

Figure 5.80 Osteoporosis–pseudoglioma syndrome. Courtesy of Dr. Peter J. Tebben.

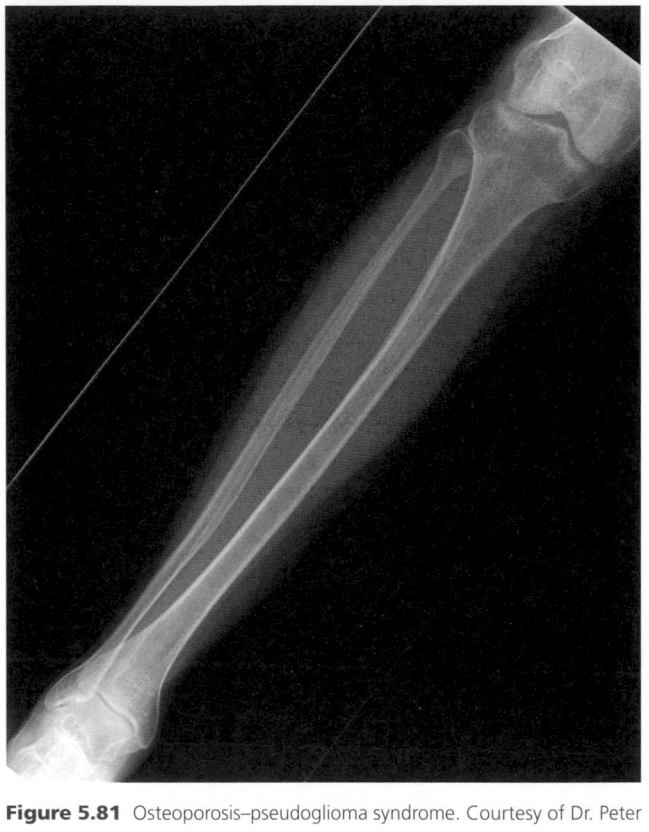

Figure 5.81 Osteoporosis–pseudoglioma syndrome. Courtesy of Dr. Peter J. Tebben.

Hajdu–Cheney syndrome (hereditary osteodysplasia with acro-osteolysis)

Definition

Hajdu–Cheney syndrome is characterized by severe osteoporosis, with associated distal phalangeal bone resorption in the hands and feet.

Etiology

Two groups recently reported that Hajdu–Cheney syndrome is due to mutations in the Notch 2 gene.

Signs and symptoms

Hajdu–Cheney syndrome is a rare autosomal dominant disorder characterized by progressive acro-osteolysis of the distal phalanges of the hands and feet, brachydactyly, Wormian bones or open sutures, platybasia, premature loss of dentition, micrognathia, midfacial flattening, coarse facies, coarse hair, dental anomalies, short stature, and severe osteoporosis. Renal cysts may occur more frequently than in the general population. Apparently sporadic cases may represent new mutations. Full expression of the syndrome is rarely seen in childhood, but clinical and X-ray abnormalities typically progress during adulthood. Acro-osteolysis first becomes apparent in late childhood or adolescence, and progresses slowly during long-term follow-up, with digital bone resorption not limited by joint spaces in the fingers and toes.

Diagnosis

The diagnosis is based on clinical history, physical examination, and classic radiological findings. Genetic testing is not yet available.

Imaging tests

X-rays show osteolysis in the distal phalanges of the fingers and toes (Fig. 5.82). Serial X-rays over time show progressive osteolysis proceeding distal to proximal within the affected digits. Dual energy X-ray absorptiometry (DXA) bone density testing shows osteoporosis in most affected adults.

Laboratory findings

Serum calcium, phosphorus, and alkaline phosphatase are normal in most patients. Biopsy of affected phalangeal osteolytic areas shows active bone resorption with increased numbers of mast cells, and replacement with fibrous and angiomatous tissue. Iliac crest biopsies and bone histomorphometry have shown high-turnover osteoporosis.

Treatment

Bisphosphonates have been used to decrease bone turnover and improve bone density. Integrated antiresorptive and anabolic therapy has been reported to prevent bone loss.

Illustration (Fig. 5.82)

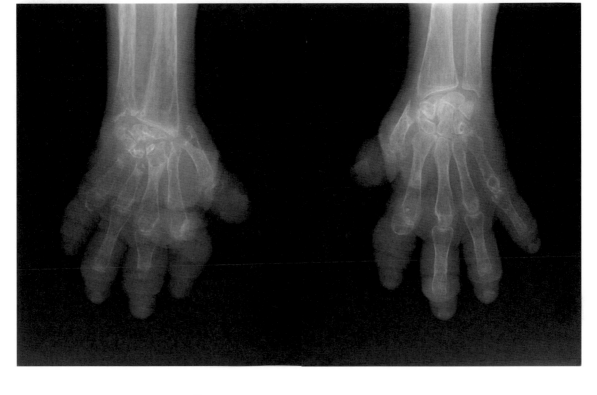

Figure 5.82 Hajdu–Cheney syndrome. Courtesy of Dr. Bart L. Clarke.

Hypophosphatasia

Definition
Hypophosphatasia is a form of osteomalacia that leads to low bone mineral density and fractures, characterized by a low serum alkaline phosphatase level.

Etiology
Hypophosphatasia is a rare heritable form of rickets or osteomalacia due to subnormal activity of the tissue non-specific isoenzyme of alkaline phosphatase. This enzyme is normally present in all tissues, but the disorder affects mostly the bones and dentition. Perinatal and infantile hypophosphatasia are inherited as autosomal recessive traits, with carrier parents or siblings often having low or low-normal serum alkaline phosphatase and mildly increased serum pyridoxal-5-phosphate. Childhood and adulthood hypophosphatasia and odontohypophosphatasia may be inherited as autosomal dominant or recessive traits.

Tissue nonspecific alkaline phosphatase functions as an ectoenzyme to dephosphorylate phosphorus-containing proteins and other compounds. Increased serum pyrophosphate levels due to lack of alkaline phosphatase activity causes inhibition of skeletal mineralization, leading to rickets or osteomalacia.

Signs and symptoms
The disorder presents with a wide range of severity. Four overlapping clinical forms have been described, depending on at what age the disorder is diagnosed. Odontohypophosphatasia is a milder form of the disorder that affects only the teeth. The younger the patient is at the time of diagnosis, the more severe the clinical course.

Perinatal hypophosphatasia
Perinatal hypophosphatasia is evident before birth with extreme skeletal undermineralization. At birth caput membranaceum and short, deformed limbs are present. Life expectancy is short due to respiratory difficulties, with prolonged survival rare. X-ray features are pathognomonic, with lack of skeletal mineralization of such severity that only the skull base may be seen, or that only the central calvarium is mineralized. The vertebral column may appear to be missing certain segments, and severe rachitic changes may be seen in the limbs.

Infantile hypophosphatasia
Infantile hypophosphatasia is diagnosed before 6 months of life. Poor feeding, inadequate weight gain, hypotonia, and widened fontanelles are characteristic, with rachitic deformities of the extremities. Vitamin B6-dependent seizures may occur. Hypercalcemia and hypercalciuria may be associated with recurrent nausea and vomiting, nephrocalcinosis, renal dysfunction. Functional craniosynostosis may occur. Flail chest may lead to pneumonia. Sometimes spontaneous improvement occurs, whereas progressive skeletal deterioration may also occur. Fifty percent of affected infants die in infancy. X-rays show typical but less striking findings compared to infantile hypophosphatasia, with abrupt transition from mineralized diaphyses to undermineralized metaphyses suggesting rapid metabolic deterioration. Progressive skeletal demineralization with fractures and thoracic deformity may result in demise of the infant.

Childhood hypophosphatasia
Childhood hypophosphatasia results in premature loss of deciduous teeth at < 5 years of age, without root resorption, from hypoplasia of dental cementum. Lower incisors are usually lost first, but all teeth may eventually be lost. Permanent teeth tend to be retained. Delayed walking with a waddling gait, short stature, and dolichocephaly are typical presenting features. Static myopathy may also occur for unclear reasons. Patients often improve at puberty, but skeletal symptoms often recur in middle age. X-rays show areas of lucency projecting from the epiphyses toward the metaphyses. Craniosynostosis may result in a "beaten copper" appearance of the skull.

Adult hypophosphatasia
Adult hypophosphatasia usually presents in middle age, often with recurrent, slowly healing metatarsal stress fractures. Pain in the thighs or hips may be due to femoral pseudofractures. Patients may report having had rickets or early tooth loss in childhood. Chondrocalcinosis from calcium pyrophosphate dihydrate deposition in cartilage may occur. X-rays usually show osteopenia, and may show chondrocalcinosis, metatarsal stress fractures, or proximal femoral pseudofractures.

Diagnosis
Diagnosis of hypophosphatasia is based on classic medical history, physical examination, and X-ray findings, with low serum alkaline phosphatase and increased serum pyridoxal-5-phosphate and urinary phosphoethanolamine. Oral pyridoxine supplementation causes marked increases in serum pyridoxal-5-phosphate in affected individuals and some carriers. Genetic testing for tissue non-specific alkaline phosphatase mutations is available to confirm the diagnosis.

Imaging tests
Hypophosphatasia is characterized by mild to severe undermineralization of the skeleton. X-rays in perinatal and infantile hypophosphatasia show severe osteopenia or apparent absence of bone, with rachitic changes, limb deformities, and fractures. In childhood hypophosphatasia, X-rays show osteopenia, as well as areas of lucency projecting from the

epiphyses toward the metaphyses (Fig. 5.83). If craniosynostosis is present, skull X-rays may show a "beaten copper" appearance. In the adult form, X-rays usually show osteopenia, metatarsal stress fractures, or proximal femoral pseudofractures, as typical for any form of osteomalacia (Fig. 5.84). Chondrocalcinosis may be present.

Laboratory findings

Unlike other forms or rickets or osteomalacia, serum calcium and phosphorus are typically normal, and serum total or bone alkaline phosphatase moderately or severely decreased. Hypercalcemia occurs frequently in perinatal and infantile hypophosphatasia due to inability of the skeleton to take up mineral adequately. Hyperphosphatemia occurs in about 50% of childhood and adult patients because of increased renal tubular reabsorption of phosphorus. Serum PTH and 1,25-dihydroxyvitamin D are usually decreased if hypercalcemia is present. Bone histomorphometry of undecalcified bone biopsies shows rickets or osteomalacia, without secondary hyperparathyroidism.

This disorder is characterized by increased serum pyridoxal-5-phosphate and pyrophosphate, and urinary phosphoethanolamine. Pyridoxal-5-phosphate is usually increased if vitamin B6 is not supplemented. Usually the lower the serum alkaline phosphatase, the higher the serum pyridoxal-5-phosphate, and the more severe the clinical presentation.

Treatment

No treatment for hypophosphatasia has yet been proven to benefit affected individuals. Bone marrow transplantation may be considered in severely affected individuals. Teriparatide (PTH 1-34) has been used to stimulate osteoblast synthesis of tissue non-specific alkaline phosphatase and heal fractures in a woman with adult hypophosphatasia. Clinical trials with enzyme replacement therapy using a bone-targeted recombinant form of tissue non-specific alkaline phosphatase are under way. Dietary phosphorus restriction and phosphate binders may be useful in decreasing serum pyrophosphate levels in patients with childhood hypophosphatasia who have hyperphosphatemia. Supplementation with calcium and vitamin D could potentially worsen hypercalcemia or hypercalciuria. Restriction of dietary calcium and use of calcitonin and/or glucocorticoid therapy may improve hypercalcemia in perinatal or infantile hypophosphatasia. Fractures may heal spontaneously, but healing may be delayed, including after osteotomy. Load-sharing intramedullary rods, rather than load-sparing plates, seem to work best after fractures or pseudofractures in adults. Expert dental care is necessary, and soft foods or dentures may be necessary, even in children.

Illustrations (Figs 5.83 & 5.84)

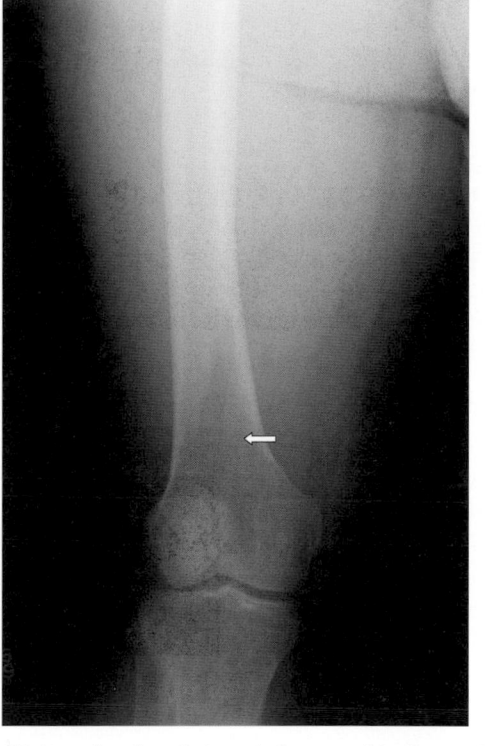

Figure 5.83 Hypophosphatasia (arrow). Courtesy of Dr. Naveen S. Murthy.

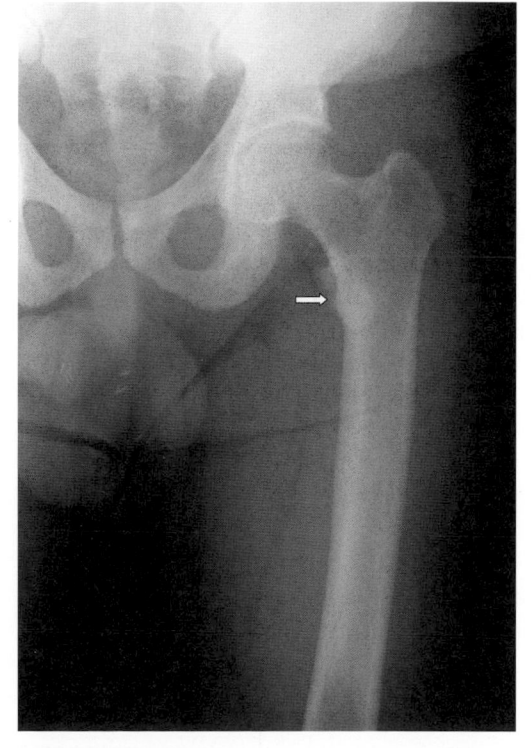

Figure 5.84 Proximal femur stress fracture in hypophosphatasia (arrow). Courtesy of Dr. Naveen S. Murthy.

6 Gonads

Male gonads

Testes

Definition

The testicle, or testis, is the male reproductive organ. Human males have two testicles, oval in shape, with an average volume of 18 ± 4 mL. They are located in the scrotum, outside the abdominal cavity (Fig. 6.1).

Function

Testes are covered with a fibrous capsule, called the tunica albuginea. This is itself covered with a double layer of serous peritoneum, the tunica vaginalis. The tunica albuginea is thicker on its dorsal surface, giving rise to the mediastinum. This is the point where blood vessels, lymphatic vessels, nerves, and ductus deferens, draining sperm from the epididymis, enter or leave the testes.

The tunica albuginea gives rise to around 250 fibrous trabeculae that migrate toward the center, dividing the testicular parenchyma into lobules. Each lobule contains from one to four seminiferous tubules, which make up 80–90% of the entire testicular volume. Spermatogenesis takes place in the seminiferous tubules. The seminiferous tubules converge in a canalicular system of convoluted ducts, giving rise to the epididymis. This is a long duct divided into three parts (head, body, tail). The ductus deferens are followed by the ejaculatory duct, both of which originate in the epididymis. All these structures secrete substances and allow sperm to pass, contributing to their development and metabolism.

The testicle has two important functions: spermatogenesis and steroidogenesis. Androgen and sperm production take place in two different testicular compartments: the first in the interstitial cell compartment (Leydig cell) and the second in the seminiferous tubule compartment (Sertoli cells and germinal epithelium).

Spermatogenesis

Spermatogenesis is the entire process of germ cell development within the seminiferous epithelium of the adult testis. It can be divided into four phases: (i) proliferation and differentiation of spermatogonia; (ii) meiotic division of spermatocytes (Fig. 6.2); (iii) transformation of haploid round spermatids arising from the second meiotic division into spermatozoa (spermiogenesis); and (iv) release of spermatozoa into the lumen of the seminiferous tubules (spermiation). A complete spermatogenesis cycle takes 74 ± 5 days.

Sertoli cells, stimulated by follicle-stimulating hormone (FSH) to secrete substances involved in spermatogenesis regulation, act as a mechanical and nutritional support for germ cells.

Hormone synthesis

Androgens are produced in the Leydig cells, in the interstitium adjacent to the seminiferous tubules. The interstitium also contains fibrocytes, blood vessels, lymph vessels, and leukocytes (especially macrophages, T lymphocytes, and mast cells). The main androgen produced by Leydig cells is testosterone, but they also produce growth factor, neuropeptides, and cytokines. Leydig cell function depends on luteinizing hormone (LH), produced by the pituitary gland.

Tests

Imaging tests

Scrotal ultrasound

Ultrasound is the main imaging technique for the scrotum. Each testis and epididymis should be examined separately and the anatomy recorded on longitudinal and transverse scans. Images should be acquired in both grayscale and Color Doppler modes (Fig. 6.3).

The development stage of the germ cell elements and tubular maturation determines the echotexture of the testicles. Prepubertal testes are typically of low echogenicity,

Imaging in Endocrinology, First Edition. Paolo Pozzilli, Andrea Lenzi, Bart L Clarke and William F Young Jr.
© 2014 John Wiley & Sons, Ltd. Published 2014 by John Wiley & Sons, Ltd.

which increases progressively to reach a medium echogenicity in postpubertal testicles. The normal adult testis has a homogeneous granular echotexture composed of uniformly distributed medium level echoes, resembling the echogenicity of the normal thyroid gland.

The vessels, rete testis, mediastinum, and testicular parenchyma should all have a homogeneous echotexture, even in prepuberty. Nonhomogeneity should be interpreted as a pathologic finding.

The echogenicity of the epididymis is comparable to that of the testis. The head of the epididymis is usually slightly more echogenic than the body or tail, probably because it contains more tubules and therefore has an increased number of interfaces. Blood flow can be detected using Color Flow Doppler or Power Doppler imaging.

Color Doppler is particularly useful in establishing a diagnosis of testicular torsion, scrotal trauma, testicular abscess, and varicocele. The evaluation of intratesticular vascularization, especially of benign and malignant lesions, is now gaining a major role in the differential diagnosis of small unsuspected nonpalpable lesions.

Scanning tomography and magnetic resonance imaging
These techniques may be useful in the diagnosis and staging of testicular tumors and in studying the undescended testis.

Laboratory findings
The following laboratory tests may be needed:
• Evaluation of the hypothalamic–pituitary–gonadal axis: LH, FSH, prolactin, testosterone, estradiol, and inhibin B.
• Evaluation of fertility by semen analysis.
• Genetic screening for men with genetic azoospermia or severe oligozoospermia. In all cases of ambiguous genitalia, perform karyotype and Y-microdeletion testing.
• Testicular biopsy in cases of azoospermia to examine the testicular parenchyma or spermatogenesis (Fig. 6.4).

Treatment
Specific treatment of testicular diseases are explained in the individual entries.

Illustrations (Figs 6.1–6.4)

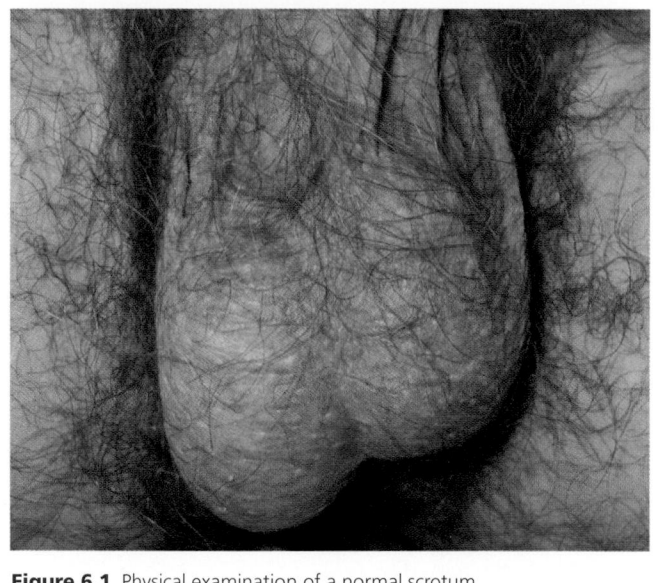

Figure 6.1 Physical examination of a normal scrotum.

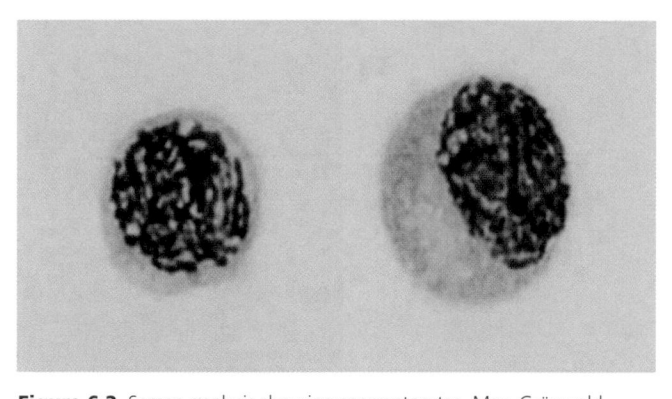

Figure 6.2 Semen analysis showing spermatocytes, May–Grünwald–Giemsa 1000 × . Courtesy of Gandini L, Lombardo F, Dondero F, & Lenzi A. (2004) *Atlante di Seminologia*. Carocci Editore, Rome, Italy.

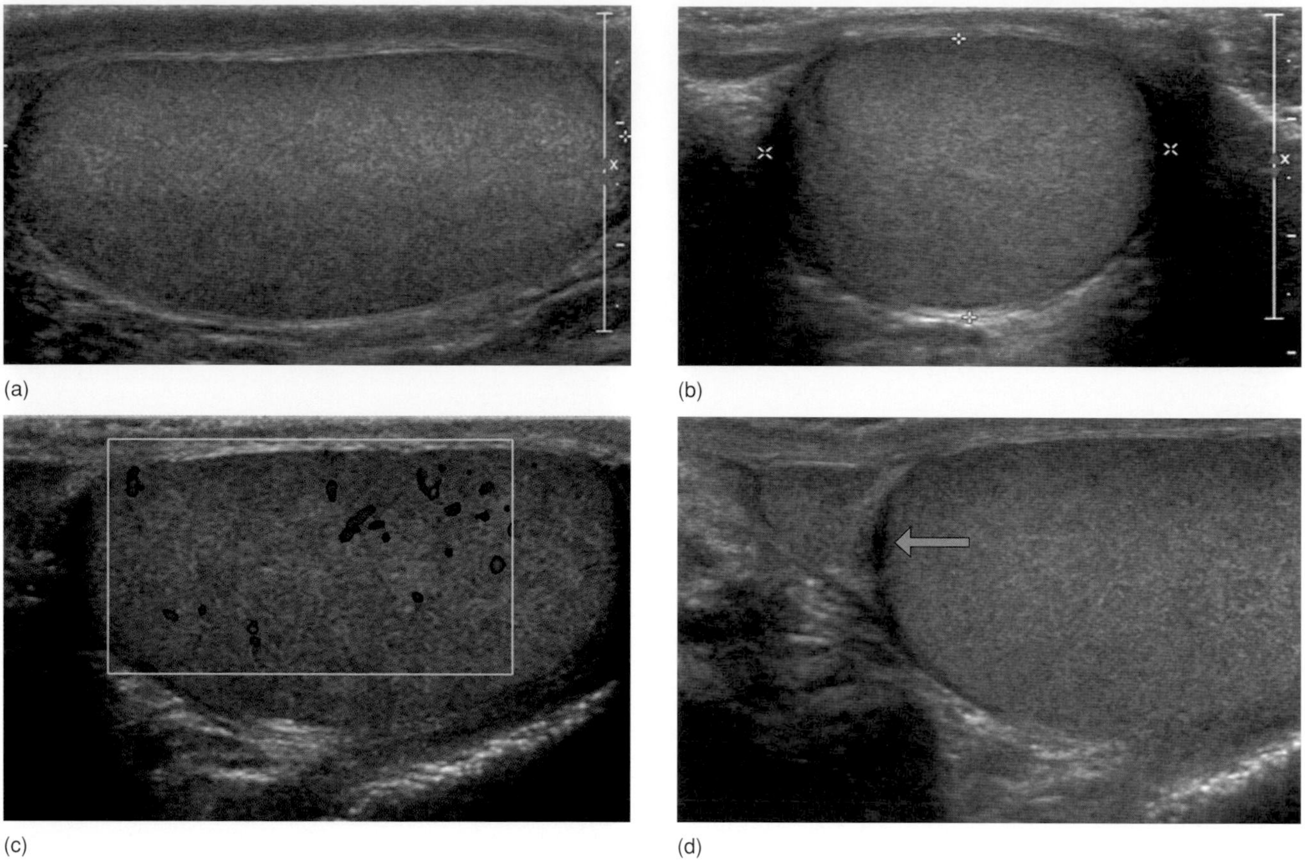

(a)

(b)

(c)

(d)

Figure 6.3 Longitudinal and transverse ultrasound scans of a normal testis (a & b). Normal testicular parenchymal vascularization is also shown (c) and the epididymis (d).

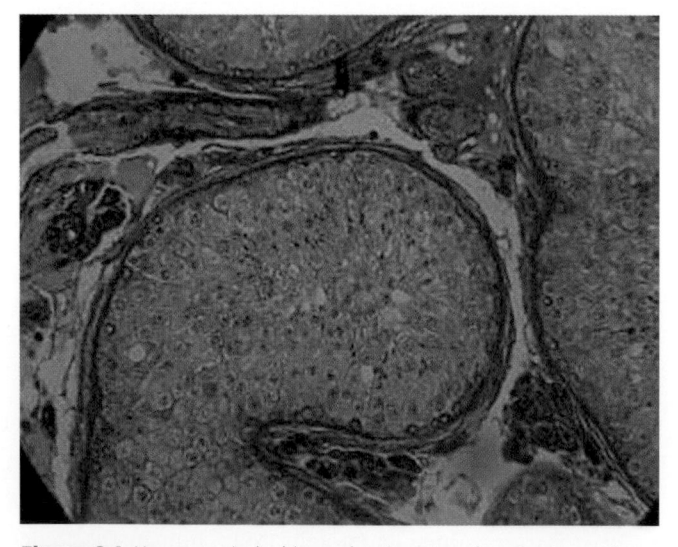

Figure 6.4 Human testicular biopsy showing normal spermatogenesis.

Testicular cancer

Definition and epidemiology

Testicular cancer originates primarily from the germ (95%) and stromal cells (5%) of the testis, and rarely from the epididymis and the rete testis. It accounts for 4–6% of all male urogenital tract cancers and is the most common malignancy in the 15–35 age group.

Germ cell tumors are almost always malignant. Nongerm cell tumors include tumors arising from the stromal cells, primary and secondary tumors from hematopoietic cells, and, rarely, other metastatic tumors.

Etiology

The etiology of testicular cancer is not fully known. The established risk factors include previous testicular cancer, cryptorchidism, positive family history, infertility, and intersex syndromes. Testicular dysgenesis syndrome is also a risk factor. However, some studies reveal a rising number of testicular cancers in patients with normal seminal parameters.

Signs and symptoms

Most testicular cancers are detected by chance by the patient as a lump or painless swelling of the testis (Fig. 6.5). Approximately one-third of patients complain of a sensation of heaviness or fullness in the lower abdomen or scrotum. A dull or heavy pain is reported in 20% of cases, confirming that the presence of pain does not exclude the diagnosis of testicular cancer. In approximately 10% of patients, testicular cancer is associated with acute pain, usually caused by hemorrhage or infarction, mimicking torsion or epididymitis. Frequently, the only symptom reported by the patient is a vague discomfort in the scrotum. Only a minority (< 6%) present with symptoms of metastatic disease.

Hormonally active tumors may present with endocrine abnormalities and related symptoms, most commonly gynecomastia.

Diagnosis

When a testicular tumor is clinically suspected, an ultrasound of the testes must be performed, distinguishing between extratesticular and intratesticular masses, as the vast majority of the latter are malignant.

Magnetic resonance imaging (MRI) can offer additional diagnostic information in differentiating selected cases, while computed tomographic (CT) scans are mainly used for staging purposes. No imaging technique can provide a histological diagnosis. An important adjuvant investigation in a suspicious testicular mass is the measurement of cancer serum markers. Cancer markers also have a well-established role in staging, prognosis, and follow-up.

Testicular tumors are divided into two groups on the basis of their clinical and biological behavior: (i) germ cell tumors (Figs 6.6 & 6.7); and (ii) sex cord and stromal tumors (Fig. 6.8 & Table 6.1).

Table 6.1 World Health Organization's pathological classification of germ cell tumors and sex cord and stromal tumors*

Germ cell tumors
- Intratubular germ cell neoplasia
- Seminoma (including cases with syncytiotrophoblastic cells)
- Spermatocytic seminoma (mention if there is sarcomatous component)
- Embryonal carcinoma
- Yolk sac tumor
- Choriocarcinoma
- Teratoma (mature, immature, with malignant component)
- Tumors with more than one histological type (specify percentage of individual components)

Sex cord/gonadal stromal tumors
- Leydig cell tumor
- Malignant Leydig cell tumor
- Sertoli cell tumor
  - Lipid-rich variant
  - Sclerosing
  - Large cell calcifying
- Malignant Sertoli cell tumor
- Granulosa cell tumor
  - Adult type
  - Juvenile type
- Thecoma/fibroma group of tumors
- Other sex cord/gonadal stromal tumors
  - Incompletely differentiated
  - Mixed
- Tumors containing germ cell and sex cord/gonadal stromal (gonadoblastoma)

Miscellaneous nonspecific stromal tumours
- Ovarian epithelial tumours
- Tumors of the collecting ducts and rete testis
- Tumors (benign and malignant) of nonspecific stroma

*Adapted from Eble JN, Sauter G, Epstein JI, Sesterhenn IA (eds). (2004) WHO histological classification of testis tumours. *Pathology and Genetics of Tumours of the Urinary System and Male Genital Organs*. IARC, Lyon, France.

Imaging tests

The following imaging tests may be performed:
• *Testicular ultrasonography and MRI:* Distinguish between and characterize extratesticular and intratesticular masses.
• *Computed tomography:* Search for distant metastases and perform staging.

Laboratory findings

The following laboratory tests may be needed:
• *Cancer markers*: Alpha fetoprotein (αFP), human chorionic gonadotropin (β-hCG), carcinoembryonic antigen (CEA), and placenta-like alkaline phosphatase (PLAP) are most specific, while lactate dehydrogenase (LDH) and ferritin are less specific.

• *Endocrine investigation*: Endocrine disorders may be detected with various hormonal assays. These include testosterone, follicle-stimulating hormone, luteinizing hormone, prolactin, and estradiol levels.

• *Testicular biopsy*: If a tumor is found, a transinguinal exploration of the testis should be performed, and if a malignant tumor cannot be ruled out an orchiectomy should follow.

• *Semen analysis*: Both testicular cancer per se and its treatment may have negative effects on the patient's potential fertility. Sperm banking should be offered prior to therapy, preferably before any orchiectomy.

Treatment

Surgery

Radical orchiectomy is performed through an inguinal incision, and the entire testicle and spermatic cord are excised at the level of the internal inguinal ring. Further treatment is decided by histological diagnosis, stage, and risk classification (for example nerve-sparing retroperitoneal lymph-node dissection).

Radiation and chemotherapy

Seminomas are extremely sensitive to both radiation therapy and chemotherapy. Nonseminomas are less sensitive to radiation therapy and treatment options are monitoring or adjuvant chemotherapy. The primary treatment is always cisplatin-based chemotherapy: bleomycin, etoposide, and cisplatin (BEP) for nonseminomas and, usually, etoposide and cisplatin (EP) for seminomas.

Illustrations (Figs 6.5–6.8)

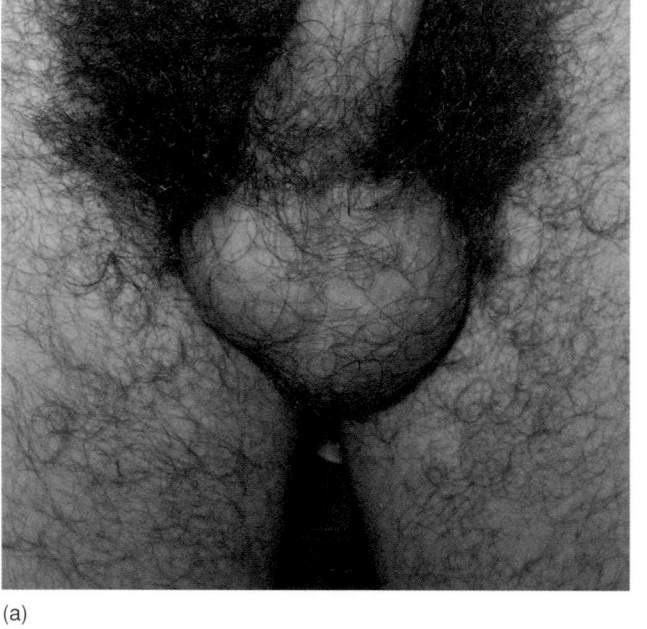

(a)

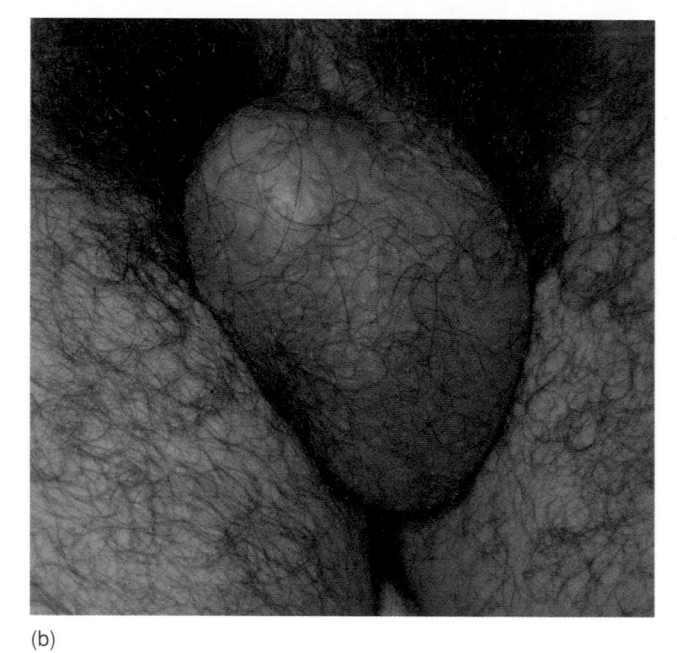

(b)

Figure 6.5 Physical examination showing patient with a painless swelling of the left hemiscrotum (a & b).

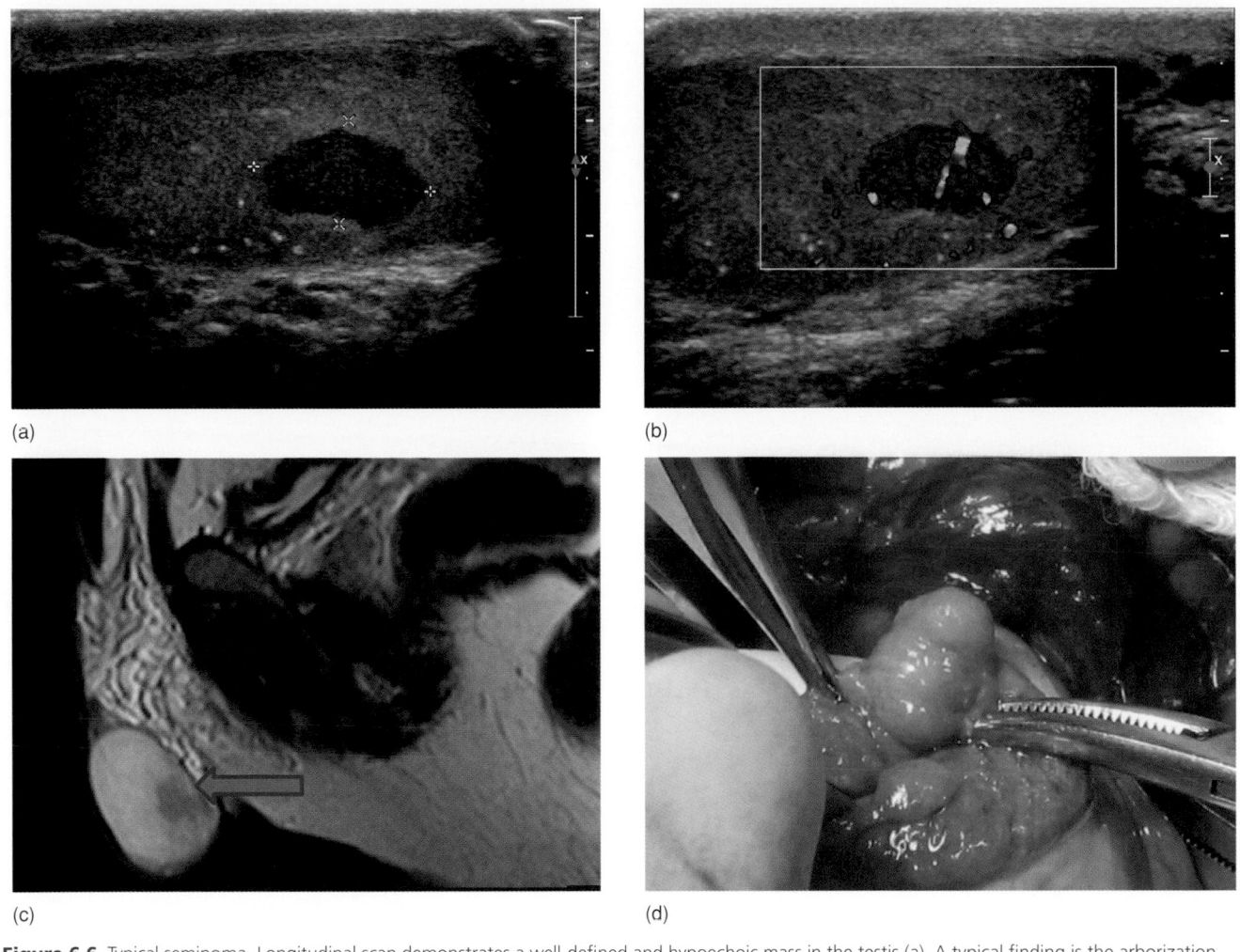

(a)

(b)

(c)

(d)

Figure 6.6 Typical seminoma. Longitudinal scan demonstrates a well-defined and hypoechoic mass in the testis (a). A typical finding is the arborization (b) of high-flow, low-resistance vascular branches within the lesion. The same lesion on magnetic resonance (MR) T-2 weighted turbo spin echo (TSE) high resolution image acquired on sagittal plane (c). Surgery confirmed the presence of seminoma (d).

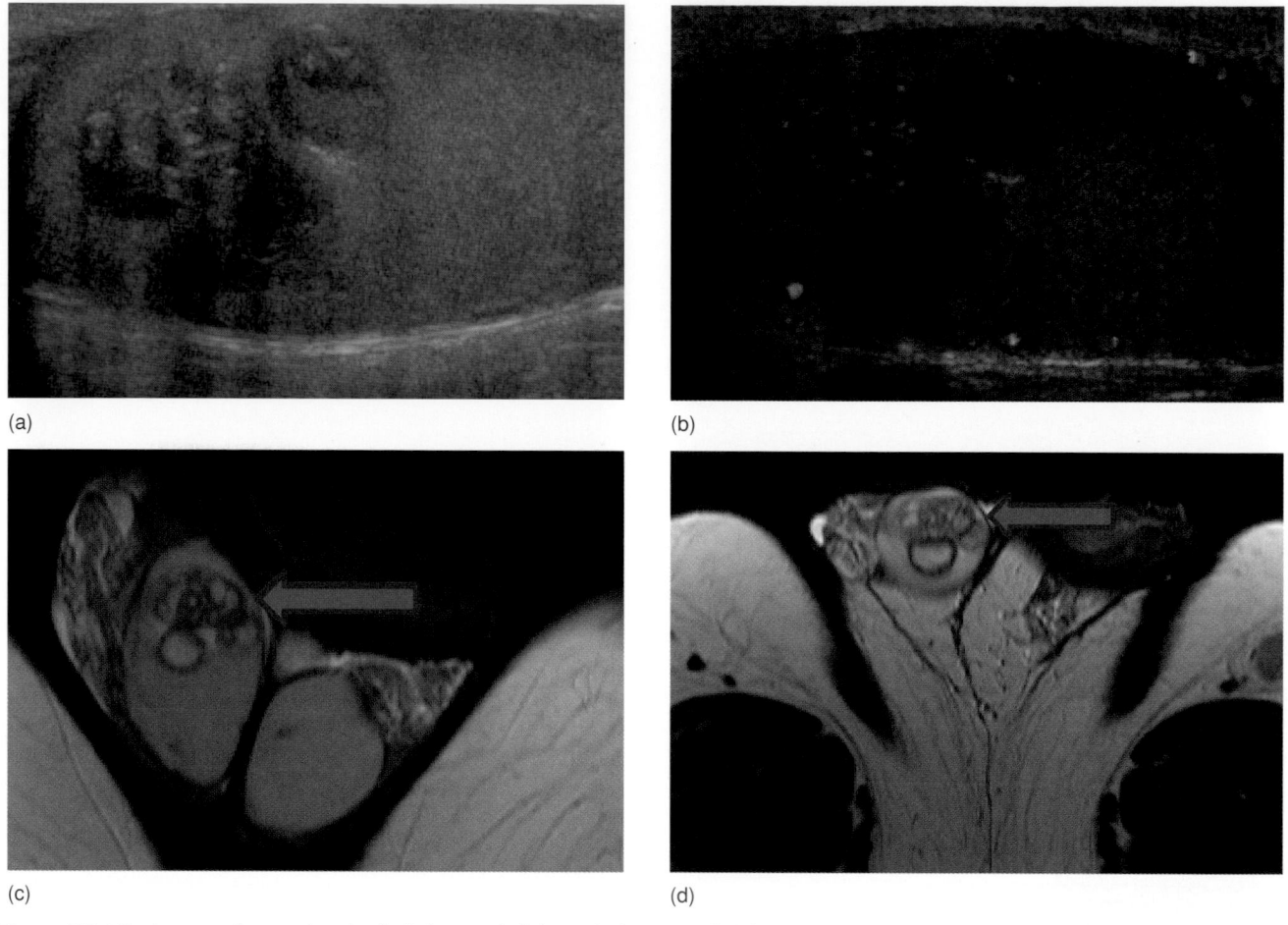

(a)

(b)

(c)

(d)

Figure 6.7 Mixed germ cell tumor. Longitudinal ultrasound of the testis shows a well-defined heterogeneous complex mass with cystic areas (due to tumour necrosis) and hyperechogenic foci (due to calcifications). The mass was hard on palpation (a). Color Doppler interrogation of the mass shows peripheral vascularity (b). The complex mass (arrow) seen on magnetic resonance (MR) T-2 weighted turbo spin echo (TSE) high resolution images, respectively acquired on coronal and axial plane (c & d).

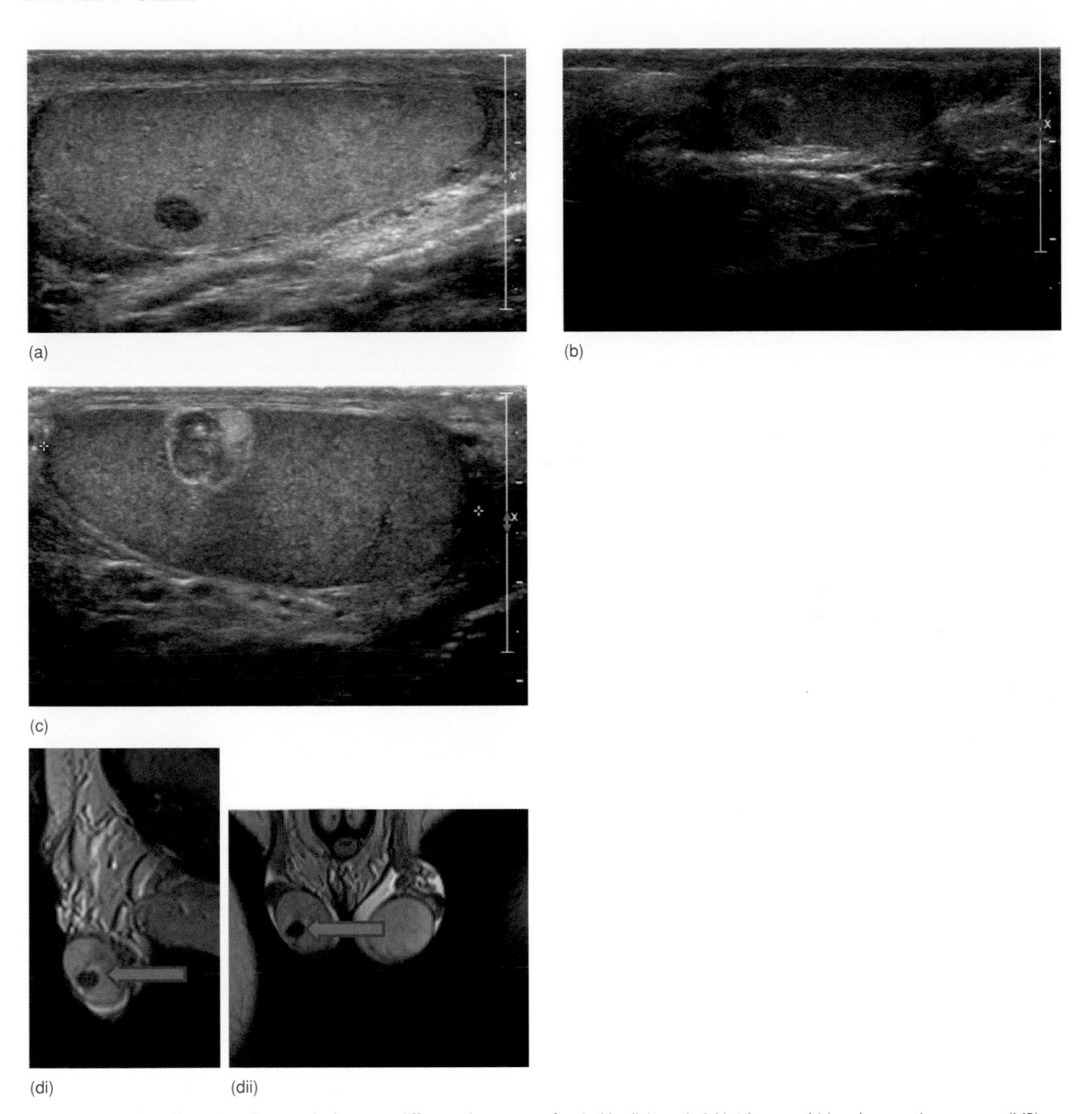

Figure 6.8 Leydig cell tumors. Ultrasounds show two different phenotypes of typical leydigioma (a & b). Ultrasound (c) and magnetic resonance (MR) images (di & dii) show an atypical leydigioma. In the MR T-2 weighted turbo spin echo (TSE) images (di & dii), the lesion is hypointense (arrow) compared to the normal testis tissue on the sagittal and coronal planes.

Cryptorchidism

Definition

Cryptorchidism is the absence of one or both testicles in the scrotum due to an arrest of the process of testicular migration along the normal anatomic path. It is a relatively common finding in pediatric practice, and in some cases may be associated with other disorders of the genital–urinary tract. The incidence varies from 21% in preterm to 1.8–4.0% in full-term boys.

There is progressive histological testicular damage. Importantly, cryptorchid boys have a significantly increased risk of infertility and testicular cancer.

Etiology

There are multiple causes of cryptorchidism and the precise etiologic factors are still largely unknown; however, abnormalities in both functional anatomic and hormonal factors during embryogenesis and testicular descent are involved. Due to a similar increase over the last century in other male reproductive diseases, such as hypospadias, testicular cancer, and a drop in sperm count, environmental factors have recently been suspected.

Signs and symptoms

Cryptorchidism is usually unilateral (bilateral in 25–30% of cases). The only clinical sign is the absence of one or both testicles in the scrotum, which appears reduced in volume. The testis, when palpable, is often decreased in volume and softer than the contralateral testis. Other genital malformations may be present.

Diagnosis

Diagnosis may be made through an andrological check-up, including a thorough physical examination to assess the location and morphology of the testis, if palpable. There is screening at birth and at 3 months to discriminate between permanent and transient undescended testis, of which the latter is most frequent.

The cryptorchid testis may be located at any point along the descent route. Description of the location of the affected testis should be noted: intra-abdominal, inguinal, or prescrotal.

Imaging tests

When the testis is not palpable, it must be determined whether there is a testis or not, and if so where it is located. Standard abdominal and inguinal imaging with ultrasound (Fig. 6.9), computed tomography (CT), and magnetic resonance imaging (MRI) (Fig. 6.10) are useful, and laparoscopic assessment is generally recommended to confirm the existence and location of the testis.

Ultrasound is useful only for identifying testes in the inguinal canal or in the prescrotal region and should be the initial imaging procedure. However, the undescended testis is generally smaller and hypoechoic due in part to greater ultrasound attenuation by the overlying tissues. It is often elongated and softer (easily compressed by the probe). Care must be taken not to confuse an inguinal lymph node with a cryptorchid testis.

Ultrasound is also useful for both therapeutic monitoring of testicular descent in patients undergoing hormone treatment and monitoring patients after orchidopexy and in followup for early detection and staging of possible malignant degeneration.

Laboratory findings

Laboratory tests are as follows:

• *Genetic screening*: Karyotype, especially where there are associated hypospadias or multiple malformations.
• *Endocrine investigations*: Depending on clinical presentation, hormone tests are performed at birth, during the first year, in the peripubertal period, or after puberty, especially when men are assessed for infertility.
• *Other tests*: Include testing for testosterone, follicle-stimulating hormone, luteinizing hormone, prolactin, and estradiol levels.
• *Extent*: The extent of work-up, e.g. tumor markers, depends on the phenotype and results depend on the age at testing.

Treatment

Important complications include infertility and testicular malignancy (most commonly seminomatous tumors or embryonal cell carcinoma).

The cryptorchid testis may descend spontaneously within a year of birth, but otherwise medical treatment (hormonal human chorionic gonadotropin or gonadotropin-releasing hormone) and/or surgery (orchiectomy or orchidopexy, if possible) is necessary to reduce the risk of infertility and cancer.

A recent trend is to propose orchidopexy before 1 year of age if possible, in the hope of preserving fertility.

Illustrations (Figs 6.9 & 6.10)

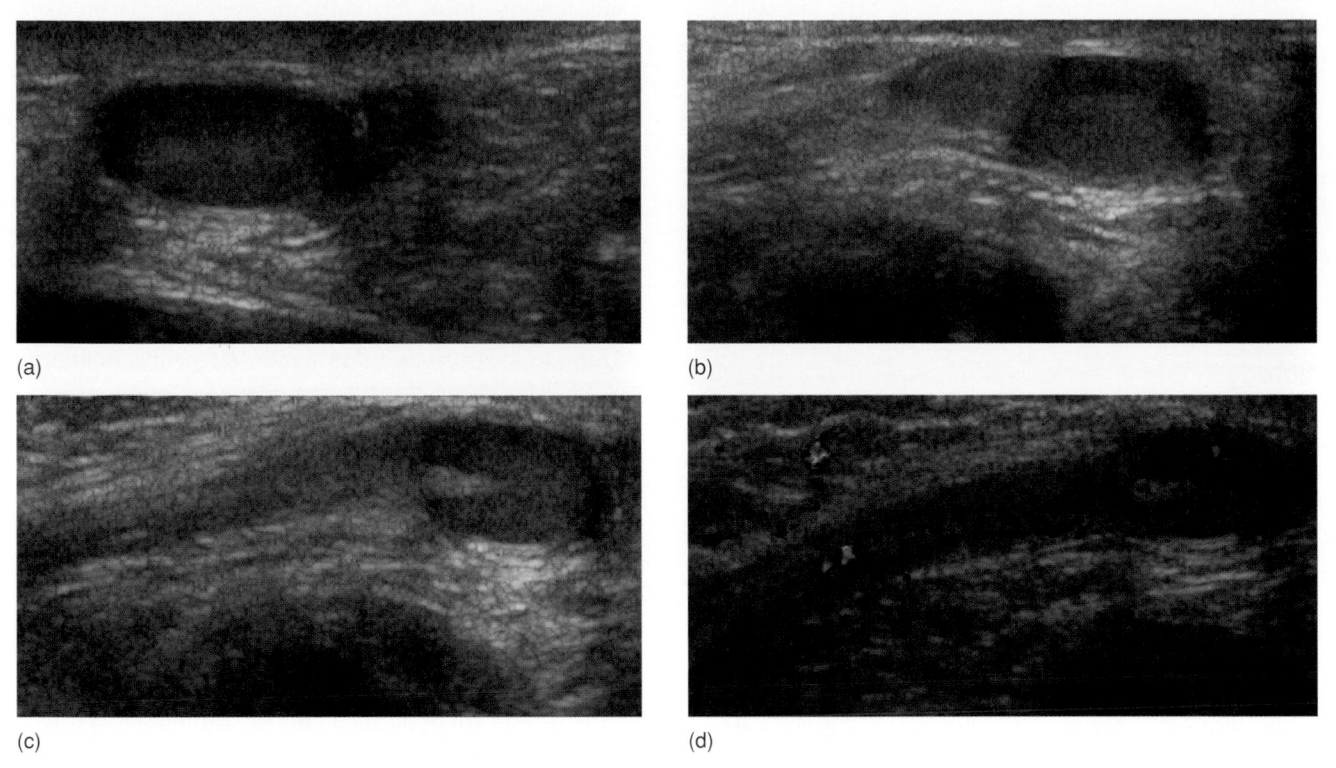

(a)

(b)

(c)

(d)

Figure 6.9 Longitudinal ultrasound scan showing two small and hypoechoic undescended testes situated in the inguinal canal (a & b). Note the hilum in (c), which helps in the identification of the testis. Vascularization of the cryptorchidism testis is shown in (d).

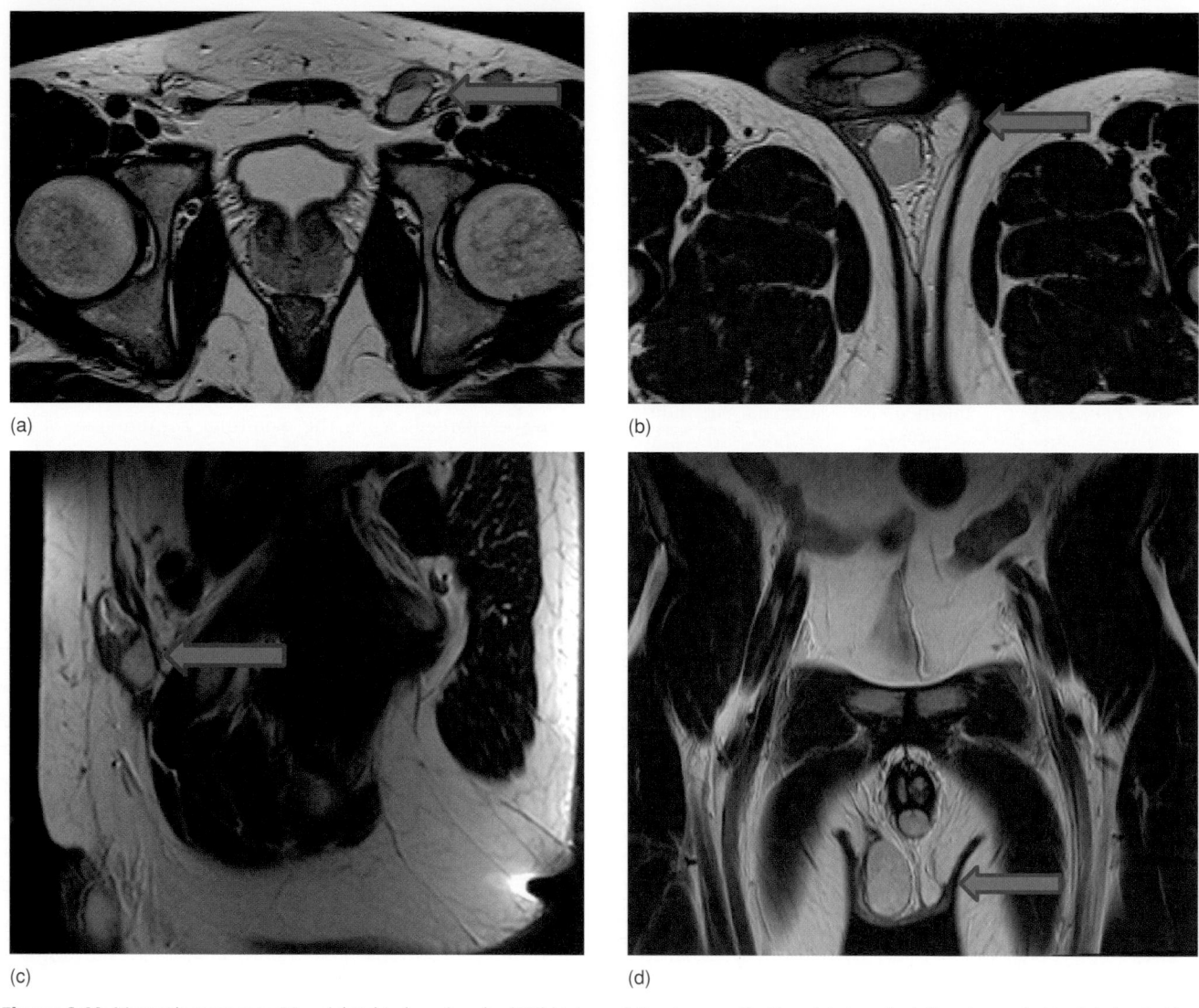

(a)

(b)

(c)

(d)

Figure 6.10 Magnetic resonance T-2 weighted turbo spin echo (TSE) high resolution images. On the axial plane the left undescended testis is located in the inguinal canal (a). The axial and coronal planes show an empty hemiscrotum on the left side (arrow) (b & d). The sagittal scan shows the undescended testis and the right emiscrotal containing the normal testis (arrow) (c).

Gynecomastia

Definition

Male gynecomastia is the enlargement of glandular tissue in the male breast. Physiological gynecomastia is found in newborn infants, pubertal boys, and elderly men. There is a high frequency of gynecomastia in the general population.

Etiology

Pathologic gynecomastia may be caused by a decrease in the production and/or action of testosterone, by an increase in the production and/or action of estrogen, or by drug use. However, gynecomastia may also be idiopathic. Increased sensitivity to estrogens may be the cause of unexplained gynecomastia, including gynecomastia in the aging male. Another rare cause of gynecomastia is hyperprolactinemia. The development of gynecomastia seems to depend on individual sensitivity.

Causes of gynecomastia

Estrogen excess

Estrogen excess may be caused by exogenous or endogenous estrogens. Exogenous estrogens include therapeutic or unintentional exposure, including exposure to aromatizable androgens (e.g. athletes). Endogenous estrogens include:
• Increased secretion from testis (Leydig cell or Sertoli cell tumors, stimulation of normal Leydig cells by luteinizing hormone or human chorionic gonadotropin [hCG]).
• Increased secretion from adrenals (feminizing adrenocortical tumors).
• Increased aromatization of androgens to estrogens (aging, obesity, alcoholic cirrhosis, hyperthyroidism, drugs, hCG-secreting tumors, aromatase excess syndrome).

Androgen deficiency

Androgen deficiency may be caused by primary or secondary hypogonadism due to disease, trauma, radiation, or drugs.

Altered serum androgen/estrogen ratio

Altered serum androgen/estrogen ratio may be caused by puberty, aging, refeeding gynecomastia, hepatic cirrhosis, renal failure and dialysis, hyperthyroidism, and drugs.

Decreased androgen action

Decreased androgen action may be caused by:
• Androgen receptor antagonists (spironolactone, cimetidine, bicalutamide, flutamide)
• Absent or defective androgen receptors
• Expansion of CAG repeats in the androgen receptor gene (Kennedy's disease)

Diagnosis

A detailed clinical history and thorough physical examination are often all that are required.

The physical examination should include anthropomorphic measurements, including height, weight, body mass index, and upper and lower body segment measurements. Signs of virilization should be assessed.

A careful genitourinary examination is also of particular importance. Attention should be paid to Tanner staging, testicular volume, and masses or irregularities along the testes. However, laboratory or radiologic investigations may be necessary to investigate a suspicion of gynecomastia.

True gynecomastia must be distinguished from pseudogynecomastia (Fig. 6.11). In the latter process, only adipose tissue is enlarged, while the glandular components of the breast are normal.

Examination

With the patient in the supine position and hands placed behind the head, the examiner should grasp the breast between the thumb and forefinger and gradually move the digits toward the nipple. In true gynecomastia, a rubbery or firm, mobile, disk-like mound of tissue will arise concentrically beneath the nipple–areolar complex; in pseudogynecomastia, no such disk is palpated. Eccentric breast masses, especially those fixed to underlying tissues, are uncommon in pubertal boys. Their presence raises concern for other masses listed on the differential diagnosis. Worrisome signs that may indicate more serious disease include hard or firm breast tissue, unilateral growth, location outside the nipple–areolar complex, and overlying skin changes, such as dimpling or nipple retraction.

Although gynecomastia is usually bilateral, it may also be unilateral.

Imaging tests

The following imaging tests may be needed:
• B-mode ultrasonography allows assessment of the gland size and structure (Fig. 6.12).
• The investigation of male breast enlargement by mammography appears to be a useful and reliable method (Fig. 6.13).

Laboratory findings

Laboratory testing includes:
• *Endocrine evaluation*: The initial laboratory evaluation usually consists of thyroid function tests, testosterone, follicle-stimulating hormone, luteinizing hormone, prolactin, estradiol, and hCG.
• *Fine needle biopsy*: Cytology of fine needle aspirates is a very reliable method for the diagnosis of breast lesions.

Treatment

Treatments for male gynecomastia include reassurance, pharmacotherapy, and surgical correction.

Pharmacologic

Although several hormonal therapies have been investigated for the treatment of gynecomastia, none are currently approved for use in adolescents by the US Food and Drug Administration. Despite this, treatments used include androgens, danazol, antiestrogens, and aromatase inhibitors. Testosterone therapy has shown no beneficial effect, and carries the risk of further stimulating breast development if aromatized to estradiol. A nonaromatizable androgen, dihydrotestosterone (DHT), has also been used.

Surgery

The treatment of choice for gynecomastia is surgery of the enlarged tissue. There are a great variety of procedures:

- Semicircular, intra-areolar incision, and resection of tissue
- Nipple transposition on a single derma flap
- Free nipple graft after excision of redundant skin and breast tissue
- Transaxillary approach
- Suction-assisted lipectomy

Radiotherapy

Radiation therapy is sometimes used to prevent gynecomastia in patients with prostate cancer prior to estrogen therapy.

Illustrations (Figs 6.11–6.13)

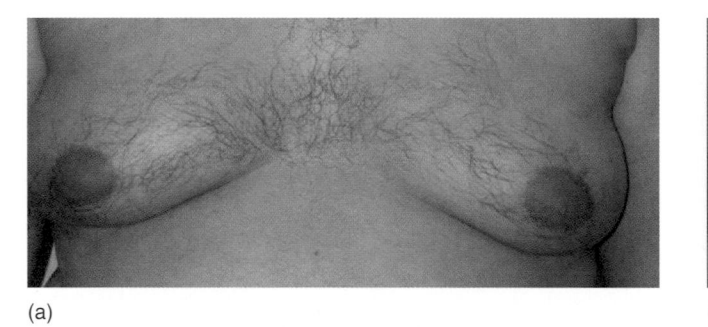

(a)

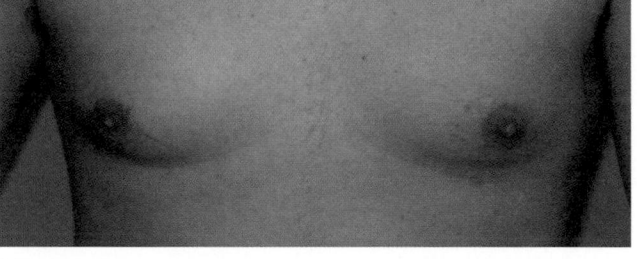

(b)

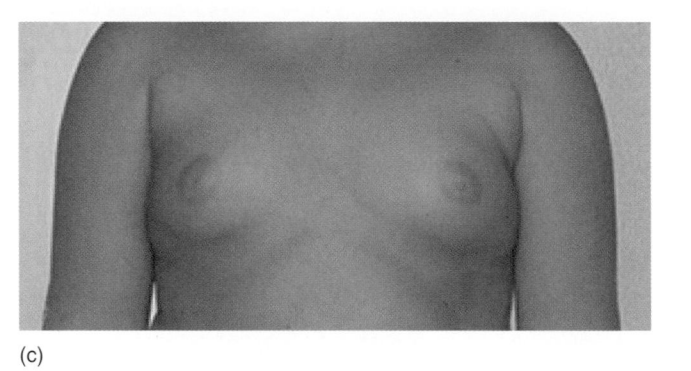

(c)

Figure 6.11 Physical examination showing true gynecomastia (a & b) and pseudogynecomastia (c).

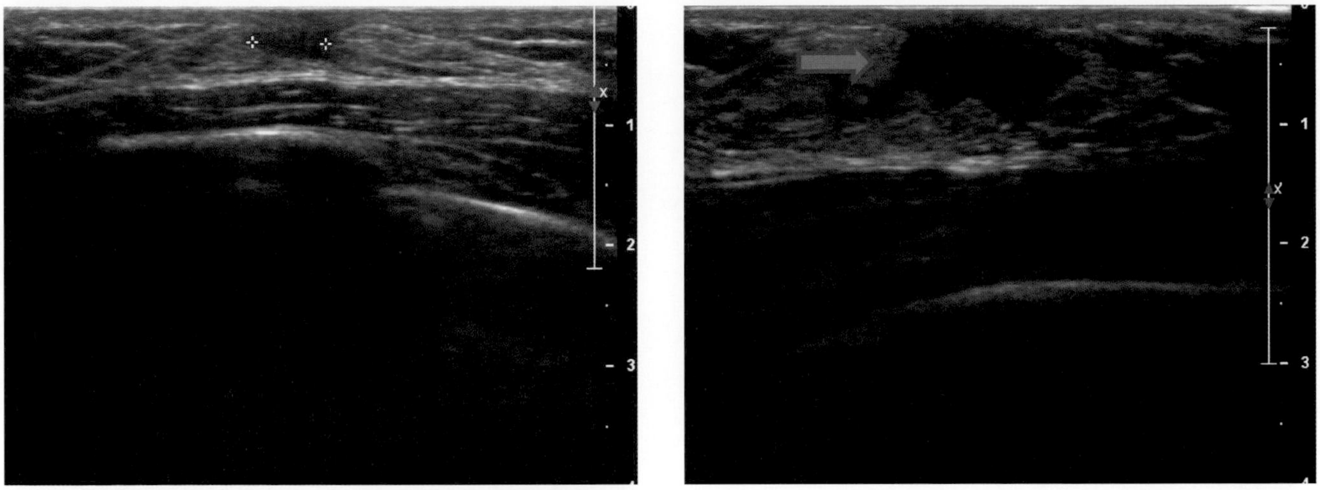

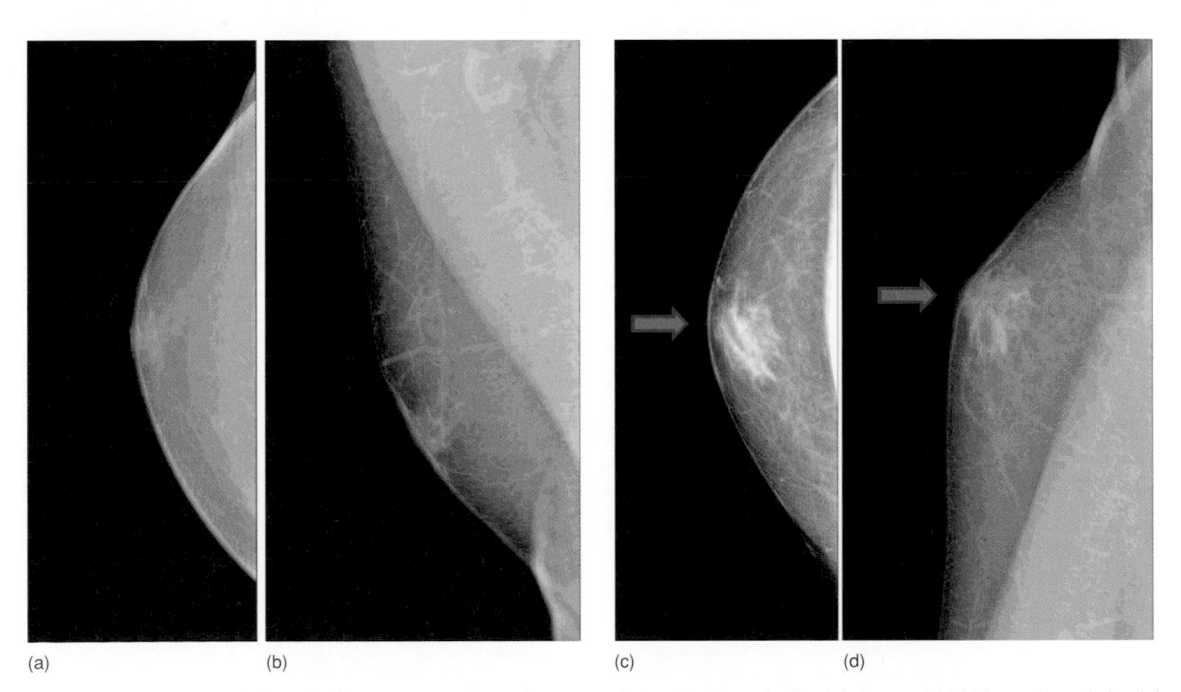

(a)

(b)

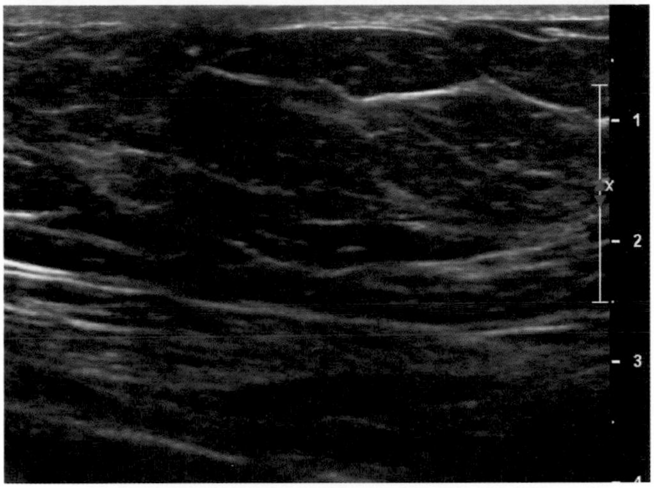

(c)

Figure 6.12 Transverse ultrasound images show a normal male breast (a); a case of gynecomastia with an enlargement of glandular tissue (b); and a case of pseudogynecomastia with only enlarged adipose tissue (c).

(a) (b) (c) (d)

Figure 6.13 Craniocaudal and mediolateral oblique mammograms show normal glandular tissue in the right breast (a & b) but enlarged glandular tissue in the left breast arrows (c & d).

Klinefelter syndrome

Definition

Klinefelter syndrome (KS) – first described by Harry Klinefelter in 1942 – is an endocrine disorder characterized by gynecomastia, small, firm testes, hypogonadism, and a high level of follicle-stimulating hormone. It is the most common chromosomal disorder, affecting 1 in 500 men, and is a frequent cause of hypogonadism and infertility.

Etiology

Klinefelter syndrome is caused by extra X chromosomes, usually acquired through nondisjunction during maternal or paternal gametogenesis. The most common karyotype is 47,XXY (80%). The remaining 20% have higher grade chromosome aneuploidies (48,XXXY; 48,XXYY; 49,XXXXY), 46,XY/47,XXY mosaicism, or structurally abnormal X chromosomes.

Signs and symptoms

The KS phenotype is typically characterized by tall stature, narrow shoulders, broad hips, sparse body hair, gynecomastia, and small, firm testes (Fig. 6.14). However, its high variability and the fact that symptoms rarely present simultaneously can make diagnosis more difficult.

The clinical picture of patients varies according to age:
• Before puberty only discrete physical anomalies may be noticed, e.g. slightly lower than normal testicular volume or long-legged.
• A history of maldescended testes is often recorded.
• At puberty, characteristic skeletal proportions begin to develop. These patients are generally of average height or taller.
• During puberty, painless bilateral gynecomastia of varying degrees is often recorded.
• In adolescence and after puberty, small, firm testes and varying symptoms of androgen deficiency are often recorded.
Patients with chromosome mosaics generally show very few clinical symptoms and the testes may be normal in size.

Diagnosis

Klinefelter syndrome is often not diagnosed until adulthood, due to the extreme variability of its clinical presentation.

A suspected diagnosis is based on a combination of typical clinical findings. The most important of these are very low testicular volume and firm consistency of the testes.

In early adulthood the most frequent problems leading to diagnosis may be infertility and/or azoospermia. Later life signs of hormonal testicular failure, such as sexual dysfunction and comorbidities, such as endocrine, metabolic, and cardiovascular diseases, or osteoporosis and autoimmune diseases, may also lead to diagnosis.

Chromosome analysis in lymphocytes confirms the diagnosis of KS. Physical examination and serum hormone quantification help confirm the diagnosis of hypergonadotropic hypogonadism.

Laboratory findings

Endocrine investigations
• Serum testosterone concentrations, which increase during early adolescence (in some patients), decrease by 15 years of age, and are lower than normal in about 80% of adult patients with the 47,XXY karyotype.
• Estradiol, sex hormone-binding globulin, luteinizing hormone, and follicle-stimulating hormone serum concentrations, which are higher than normal in men with KS.
• Follicle-stimulating hormone testing offers the best discrimination, with little overlap with normal individuals, due to the significant seminiferous tubule damage.
• Inhibin B concentrations, which are in the normal range in prepubertal boys with KS but decrease significantly during late puberty, because virtually all germ cells and the majority of Sertoli cells disappear.

Semen analysis
Practically all ejaculates from patients with 47,XXY karyotype show azoospermia. Sperm are observed only rarely. Exceptional cases of spontaneous paternity have been reported.

Testicular biopsy
Histology of the testes generally shows fibrosis of the seminiferous tubules, absence of spermatogenesis, and relative hyperplasia of the Leydig cells (Fig. 6.15). However, the presence of tubules with residual foci of spermatogenesis has also been reported, with meiotic arrest at primary spermatocyte or spermatid stages and foci of normal spermatogenesis.

Imaging tests
The following imaging tests may be needed:
• *Testicular ultrasonography*: Echotexture is generally hypoechoic and nonhomogeneous, with multiple scattered hypoechoic foci (Fig. 6.16).
• *Breast ultrasound*: For gynecomastia.

Treatment

When testosterone serum concentrations are low, lifelong replacement therapy is indicated. If the patient wishes, surgical intervention for gynecomastia may be sought. Testicular sperm extraction, associated with intracytoplasmic sperm injection, offers KS patients the possibility of fatherhood.

Illustrations (Figs 6.14–6.16)

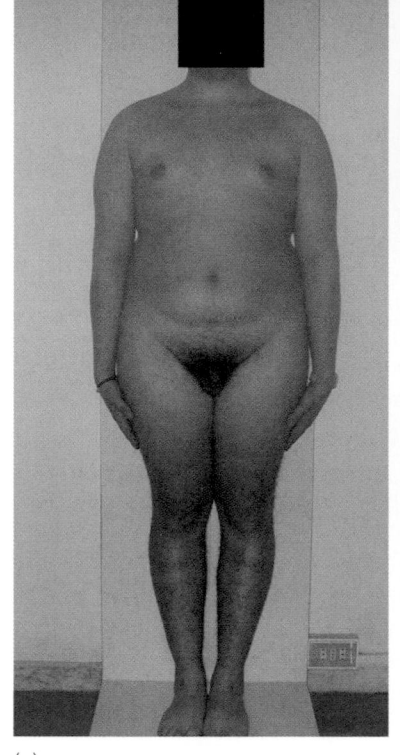
(a)

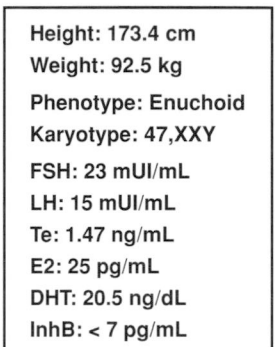
(b)

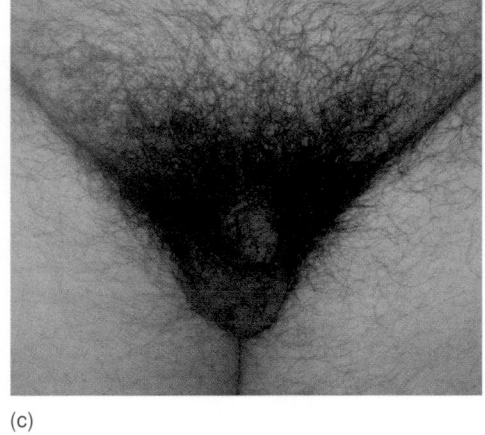
(c)

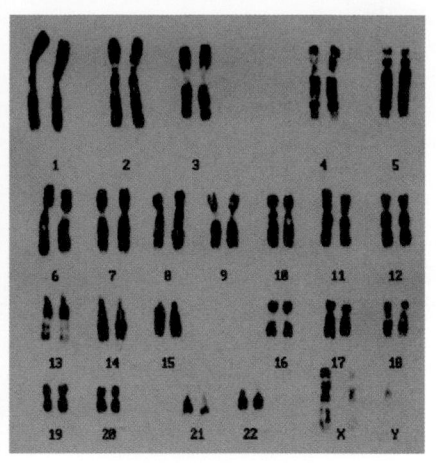
(d)

Height: 173.4 cm

Weight: 92.5 kg

Phenotype: Enuchoid

Karyotype: 47,XXY

FSH: 23 mUI/mL

LH: 15 mUI/mL

Te: 1.47 ng/mL

E2: 25 pg/mL

DHT: 20.5 ng/dL

InhB: < 7 pg/mL

(e)

Figure 6.14 A sixteen-year-old boy with Klinefelter syndrome. Clinical photographs of patient show gynecomastia, small, firm testes, and hypogonadism (a–c). Patient's karyotype and laboratory findings are also shown (d & e).

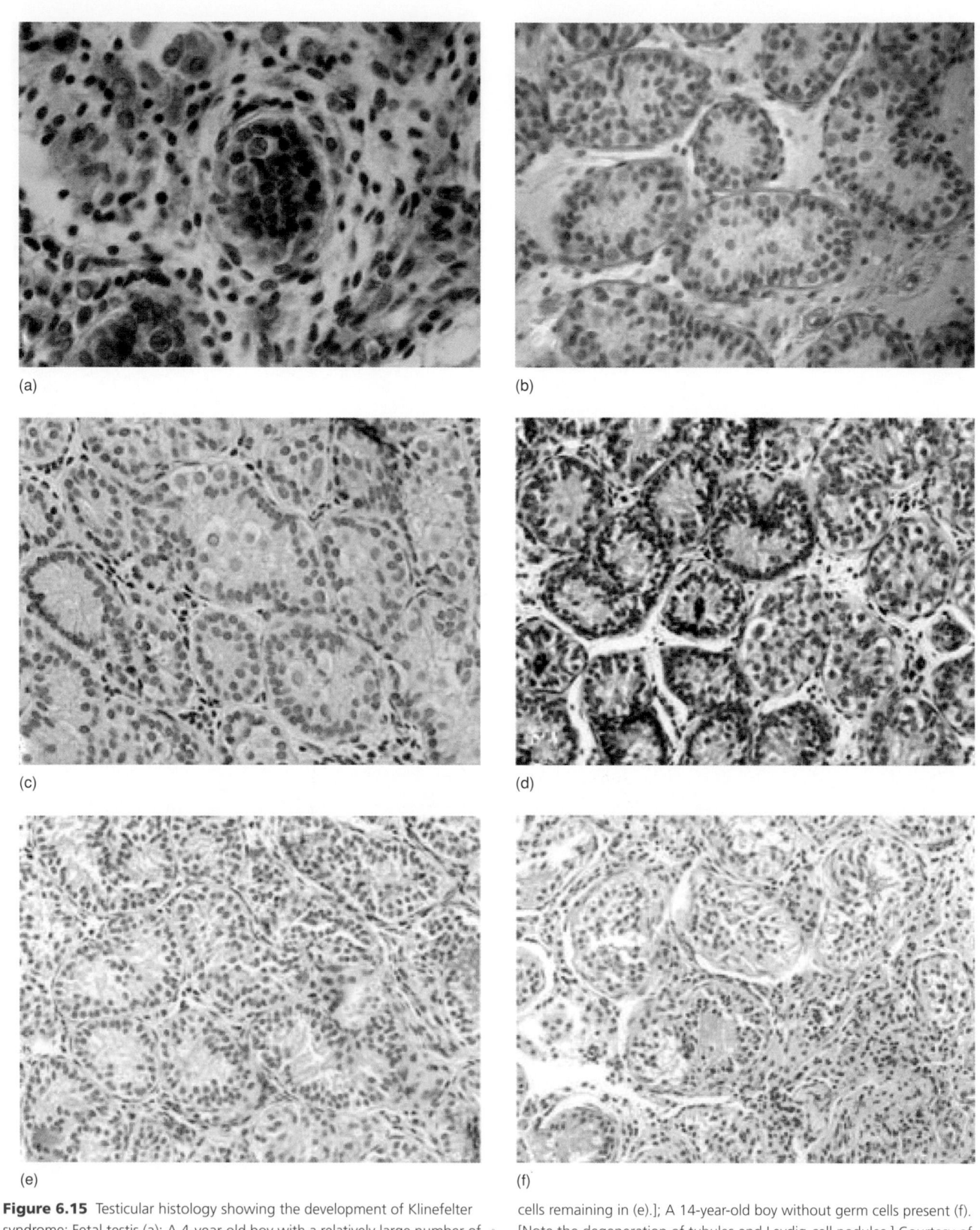

Figure 6.15 Testicular histology showing the development of Klinefelter syndrome: Fetal testis (a); A 4-year-old boy with a relatively large number of germ cells (b); Three prepubertal 10- to 12-year-old boys with variable numbers of remaining germ cells (c–e). [Note a few focally grouped tubules with germ cells visible on the right side of the figure in (d) and no germ cells remaining in (e).]; A 14-year-old boy without germ cells present (f). [Note the degeneration of tubules and Leydig-cell nodules.] Courtesy of Aksglaede L, Wikström AM, Rajpert-De Meyts E, et al. (2006) Natural history of seminiferous tubule degeneration in Klinefelter syndrome. *Human Reproduction Update* **12**(1):39–48.

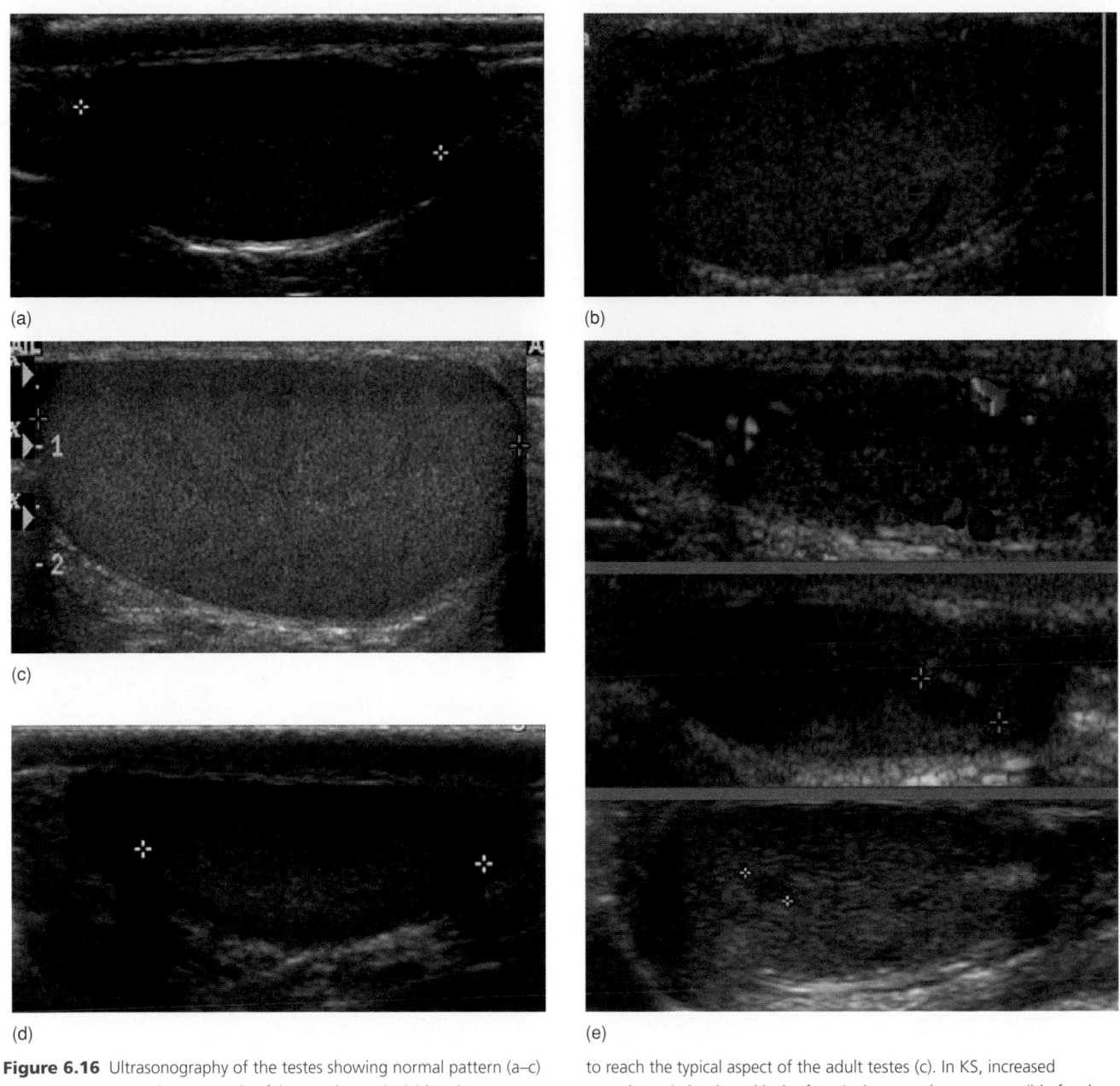

(a)

(b)

(c)

(d)

(e)

Figure 6.16 Ultrasonography of the testes showing normal pattern (a–c) and pattern commonly seen in Klinefelter syndrome (KS) (d & e). Prepubertal testes in KS (d) are undistinguishable from normal prepubertal testes (a). In normal puberty (b), vascular activation occurs, testicular volumes increase and brightness of the echotexture increases progressively to reach the typical aspect of the adult testes (c). In KS, increased gonadotropin levels and lack of testicular growth are responsible for the increased vascularization density (e, top) and acquisition of a nonhomogeneous echotexture. The testes of KS adults often develop multiple scattered hypoechoic foci (e, bottom).

Male infertility

Definition

Infertility is defined by the World Health Organization as the inability of a couple to achieve conception or bring a pregnancy to term after 1 year or more of regular, unprotected sexual intercourse. It is a major health problem, affecting 15% of couples in the reproductive age group.

Male infertility is the cause in approximately 30% of such couples, while detectable abnormalities can be found in both partners in another 30%.

Infertility is classified as primary when there has never been a pregnancy. Secondary infertility applies when the man has at some time impregnated a woman, regardless of whether or not she is his current partner and regardless of the outcome of the pregnancy.

Etiology

Several conditions can interfere with the complex mechanisms underlying spermatogenesis and cause a reduction in sperm quality and production.

The various causes of male infertility include varicocele; endocrine diseases; chromosomal abnormality; cryptorchidism; anabolic steroid abuse; gonadotoxin exposure; primary testicular failure; congenital bilateral absence of the vas deferens; ejaculatory duct obstruction; prostate diseases; infectious and immunological diseases; and some systemic diseases.

The most common cause of correctable male infertility is a varicocele. In about 30–40% of cases, no obvious cause or altered hormone concentration can be found. This is known as idiopathic infertility.

Diagnosis

For all infertile men, a detailed clinical history and physical examination is recommended to identify potentially correctable causes.

Clinical history should include questions about frequency and timing of sexual intercourse; duration of infertility and any previous fertility; childhood illnesses and developmental problems; systemic medical illnesses and previous surgery; and sexual history, including sexually transmitted infections and exposure to gonadal toxins.

At the physical examination, the physician should carefully examine the body habitus, any gynecomastia, olfactory sensations, and secondary sexual characteristics, and perform a complete genitourinary examination.

If sexual and ejaculatory function are normal and intercourse occurs with adequate frequency and at the right time, semen analysis is essential. This is one of the basic objective parameters used to evaluate male fertility. Double readings are necessary to ensure a representative sample.

If spermatozoa are present in the ejaculate, the diagnostic classification of semen parameters will be oligozoospermia (reduced number), asthenozoospermia (change in motility), teratozoospermia (change in morphology), or any combination of these (Figs 6.17 & 6.18). The term cryptozoospermia is used when no sperm are seen in the fresh preparation but some are found in the sediment after centrifugation.

Men in whom no sperm at all are detected in either the fresh preparation or after centrifugation are classified as azoospermic. Investigations are needed to differentiate between obstructive and primary testicular azoospermia.

Laboratory findings

Laboratory tests may include:
- *Semen analysis*: Macroscopic examination and microscopic investigation (Table 6.2).
- *Antisperm antibodies*: The mixed antiglobulin reaction and the immunobead test are commonly used to assess the presence of antisperm antibodies.
- *Postejaculate urine analysis*: For men with persistently low-volume ejaculate.
- *Endocrine investigation*: Endocrine disorders can be detected with various hormone assays. These include testosterone, follicle-stimulating hormone, luteinizing hormone, prolactin, and estradiol levels. Inhibin B could be useful to assess spermatogenic function.
- *Genetic screening*: For men with azoospermia or severe oligozoospermia, genetic testing consists of karyotype and Y-microdeletion testing. In cases of suspected obstructive azoospermia, cystic fibrosis screening is recommended.

Table 6.2 Human semen examination*

Macroscopic investigation
Appearance of the ejaculate
Liquefaction
Viscosity
Volume $\geq$ 1.5 mL
PH $\geq$ 7.2

Microscopic investigation
Counting of spermatozoa
- $\geq$ 39 $\times$ 10^6 per ejaculate
- $\geq$ 15 $\times$ 10^6 per mL

Motility
- Total motility: progressive motility (PR) + nonprogressive motility (NP) $\geq$ 40%
- Progressive PR $\geq$ 32%

Morphology
- Normal forms $\geq$ 4%

Nonsperm cells
- Peroxidase-positive cells concentration < 1.0 $\times$ 10^6 per mL

*Adapted from *WHO Laboratory Manual for the Examination and Processing of Human Semen*, 5th edn, 2010.

• *Testicular biopsy*: In cases of azoospermia, testicular biopsy is used to examine the testicular parenchyma for spermatogenesis (Fig. 6.19).

Imaging tests

Ultrasound and magnetic resonance imaging (MRI) are the techniques commonly performed:

• *Scrotal ultrasound*: This is useful in the evaluation of the testicles and extratesticular scrotal structure.

• *Transrectal ultrasound and MRI*: These tests may yield pertinent information about the distal ductal system and prostate gland. An MRI is also used to evaluate the brain and sella turcica in cases in which an abnormality of these areas is suspected on the basis of hormonal assays.

Treatment

The therapeutic strategies for absent, deficient, or disturbed spermatogenesis may be classified as etiological or empirical whether or not a possible cause of the altered sperm parameters is found.

If neither surgery nor medical therapy are appropriate, assisted reproduction can be initiated. From a male infertility viewpoint, the choice of technique (intrauterine insemination, in-vitro fertilization, or intracytoplasmic sperm injection) depends mainly on the degree of impairment of total motile sperm concentration.

Illustrations (Figs 6.17–6.19)

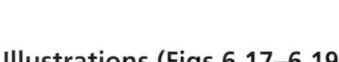

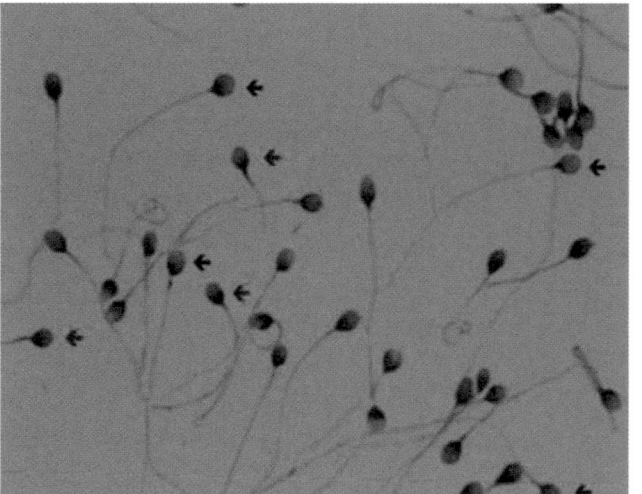

(a)

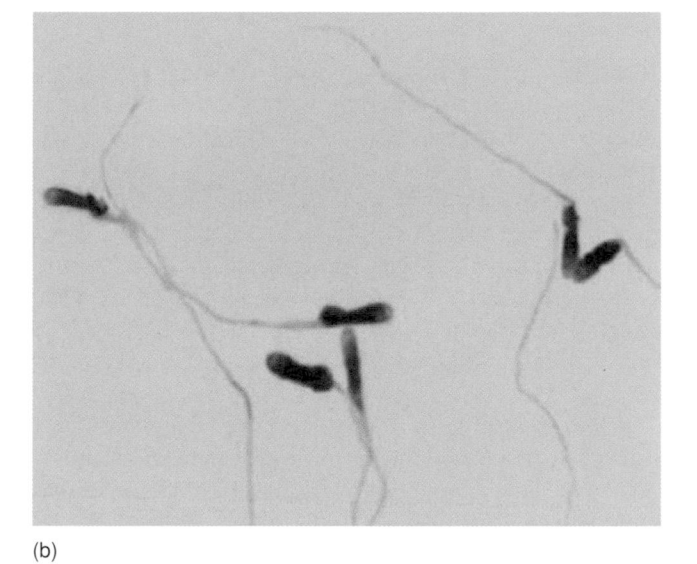

(b)

Figure 6.17 Semen analysis: Blue arrow shows a normal head; red arrow shows a small head (a); Tapered heads (b). Sperm stained with May–Grünwald–Giemsa 1000 × . Courtesy of Gandini L, Lombardo F, Dondero F, & Lenzi A. (2004) *Atlante di Seminologia*. Carocci Editore, Rome, Italy.

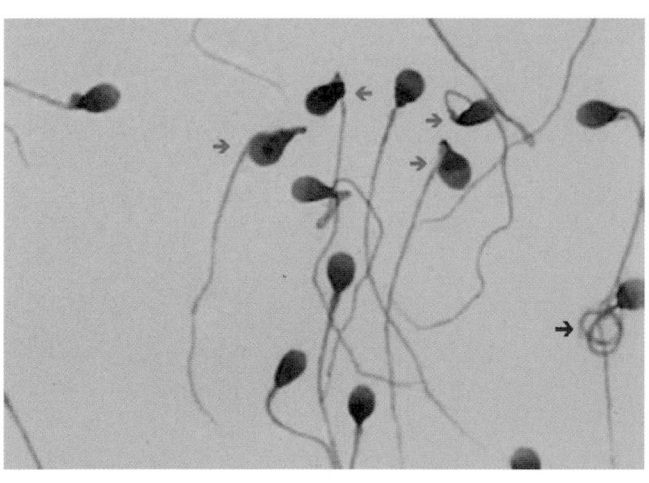

Figure 6.18 Semen analysis. Green arrow shows bent neck; red arrow shows a coiled tail. Sperm stained with May–Grünwald–Giemsa 1000 × . Courtesy of Gandini L, Lombardo F, Dondero F, & Lenzi A. (2004) *Atlante di Seminologia*. Carocci Editore, Rome, Italy.

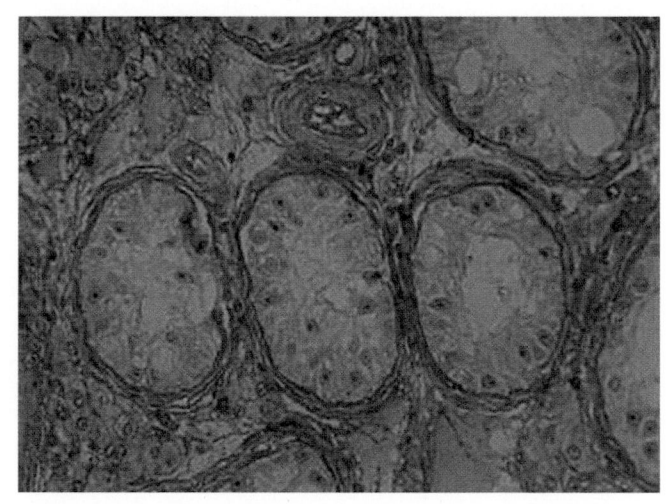

Figure 6.19 Human testicular biopsy showing Sertoli cell syndrome.

Varicocele

Definition

Varicocele is an enlargement of the pampiniform venous plexus associated with a variable degree of blood reflux in the internal spermatic veins. It can cause testicular and epididymal malfunction.

Etiology

The etiology is unclear and probably multifactorial. Most varicoceles are due to incompetent valves in the testicular veins whilst a minority are caused by vein obstruction. They may be primary (idiopathic) or secondary:

• *Primary varicoceles* are due to incompetent or absent valves in the spermatic veins. They are more common on the left, where the left spermatic vein enters perpendicular to the left renal vein.

• *Secondary varicoceles* are due to pressure from a mass on the spermatic vein in the retroperitoneum or marked hydronephrosis of the kidney. They can also occur with thrombosis of the inferior cava vein.

Varicocele is found in about 10–20% of the general male population and up to 40% in infertile men. A higher incidence is also found in athletes (about 30%). Varicoceles are 10 times more common on the left than on the right.

Signs and symptoms

The clinical presentation is variable. There may be a visible or palpable mass of tortuous veins, sometimes tender, which may feel like a "bag of worms." Patients with varicocele generally report few or no symptoms. They may sometimes feel a sensation of weight in the scrotum, particularly during physical exertion. Generally the testis volume is reduced on the effected side and the echotexture is less homogeneous.

Diagnosis

Clinical varicocele is a readily palpable dilatation of the veins in the scrotum at rest or during Valsalva maneuver. Subclinical varicocele cannot be manually detected but is seen on ultrasonography.

Clinical stages

Dubin and Amelar devised a useful clinical grading system for palpable varicoceles:

• *Grade 1*: Palpable only during Valsalva maneuver.
• *Grade 2*: Palpable without Valsalva maneuver.
• *Grade 3*: Visible and palpable without Valsalva maneuver (Fig. 6.20).

If there is any clinical doubt about the diagnosis or its cause, a more accurate classification is required. Color Duplex, Color Doppler ultrasonography is recommended.

Imaging tests

Ultrasounds (Figs 6.21 & 6.22) should be performed with the patient in both a supine and standing position. The ultrasound appearance of varicocele consists of multiple, hypoechoic, serpiginous, tubular structures 2.5 mm in diameter and above, creating a tortuous multicystic collection that is usually best seen adjacent or proximal to the upper pole of the testis and epididymis or lateral to the testis. Large varicoceles can extend posteriorly and inferiorly to the testis. Varicoceles > 3–4 mm in diameter are usually clinically apparent. The sensitivity and specificity of varicocele detection approaches 100% with Color Doppler ultrasound. If an obstructive varicocele is suspected, ultrasound examination of the kidneys and retroperitoneal organs is performed.

Laboratory findings

The following laboratory tests may be needed:

• *Semen analysis*: Semen analysis usually reveals oligozoospermia with reduced sperm motility (asthenozoospermia) and a lower percentage of sperm cells with normal morphology (teratozoospermia).

• *Endocrine investigation*: Blood tests may reveal a marginal reduction in testosterone and higher gonadotropin (follicle-stimulating and luteinizing hormone) concentrations.

Treatment

Therapy is aimed at arresting the reflux of blood in the spermatic and collateral veins.

Surgical treatment (preferably with an above-inguinal approach) can be performed by laparoscopy or through microsurgical techniques. The surgery should not injure the testicular artery and may be complicated by hydrocele, which would require a second operation.

More recently, radiological embolization with the Seldinger approach has gained momentum. Retrograde venography from the renal veins shows the anatomy and location of the veins and refluxes into the spermatic veins on both sides; embolization is then performed by super-selective catheterization (Fig. 6.23).

Illustrations (Figs 6.20–6.23)

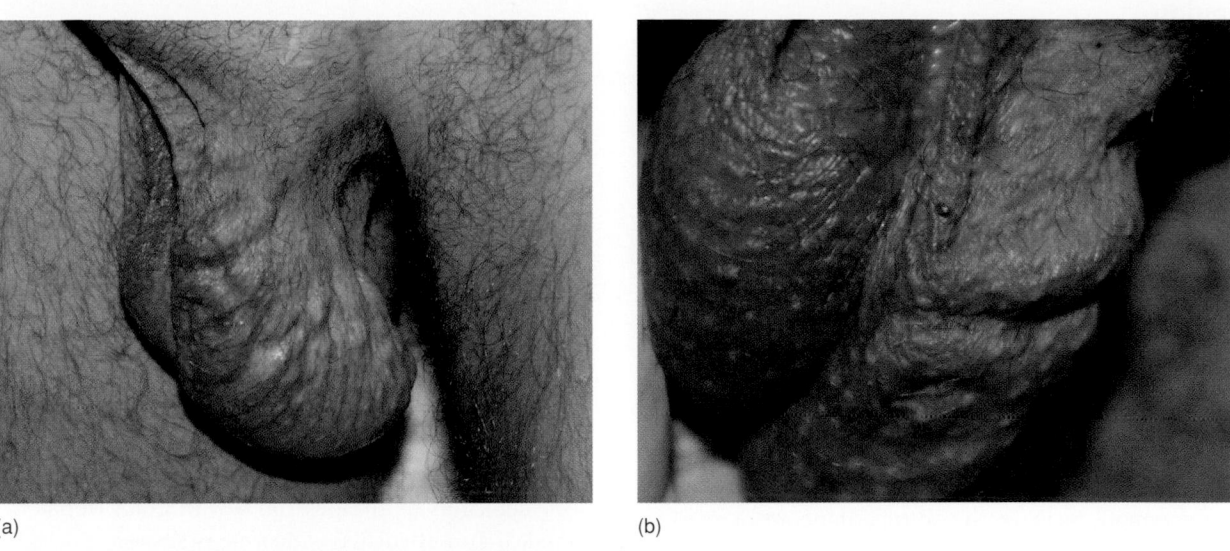

(a)

(b)

Figure 6.20 Physical examination showing varicocele, clinical grade 3 (a & b).

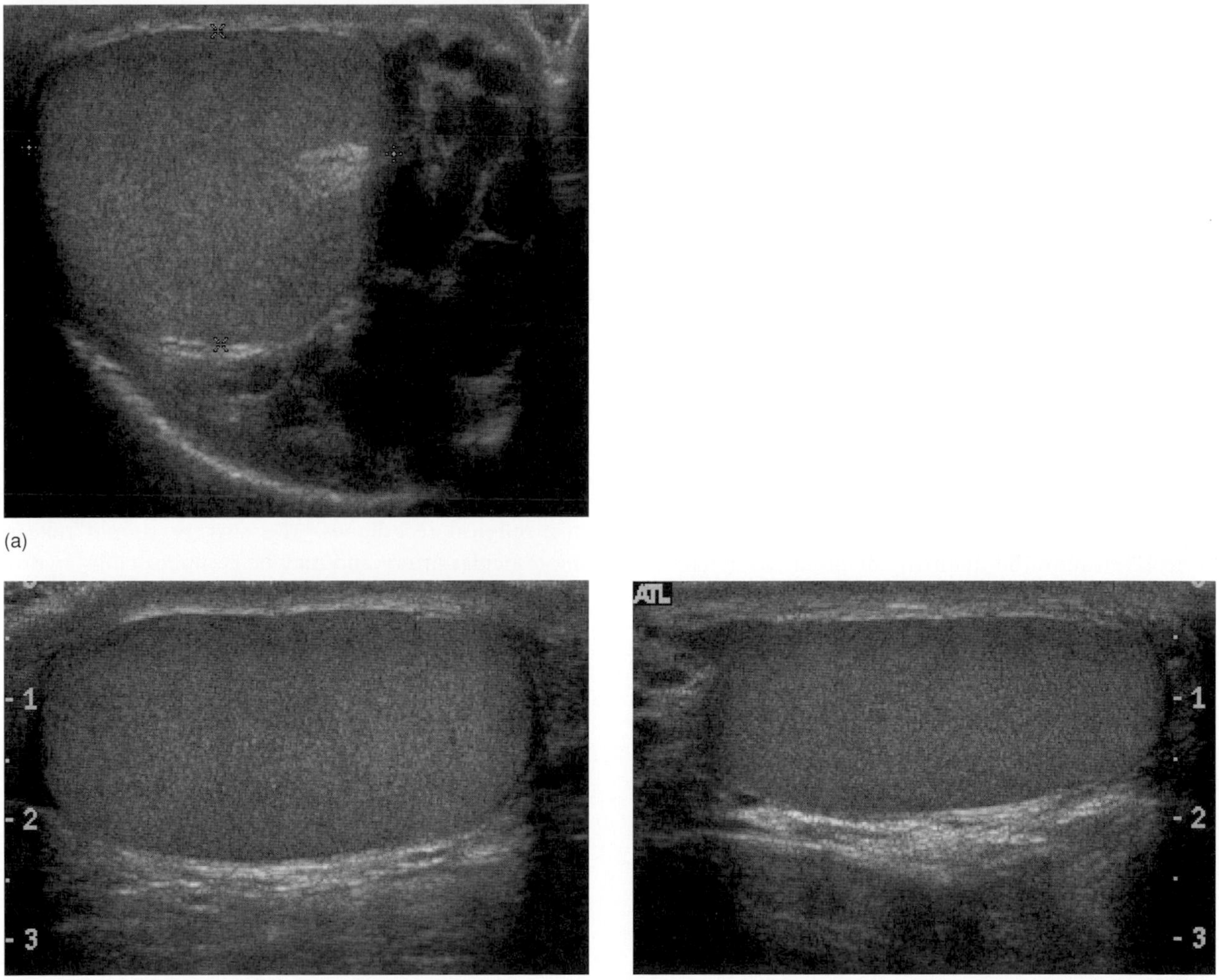

(a)

(b)

(c)

Figure 6.21 Ultrasounds showing multiple, serpiginous, tubular structures > 2.5 mm in diameter (a) and left testicular dysmetria (b & c).

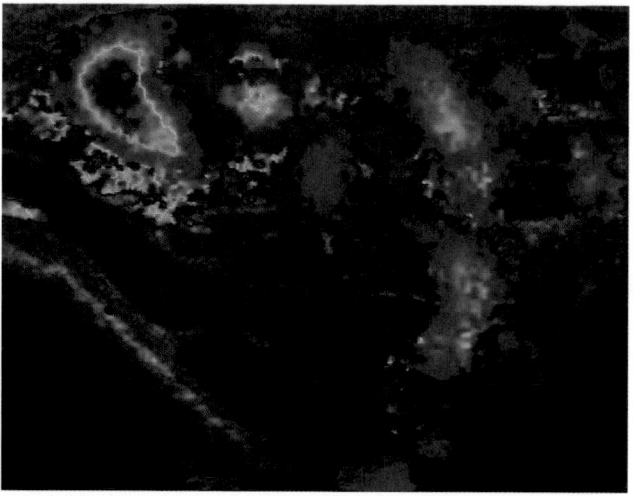

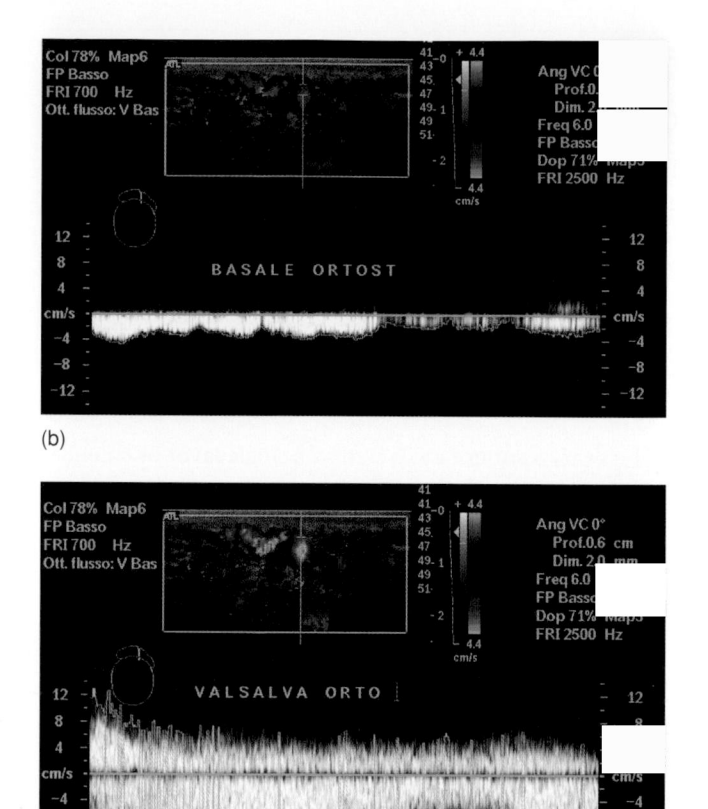

(a)

(b)

(c)

Figure 6.22 Color Doppler study showing color flow signal in multiple, hypoechoic, serpiginous, tubular structures (a), retrograde flow at rest (b), and/or during Valsalva maneuver (c).

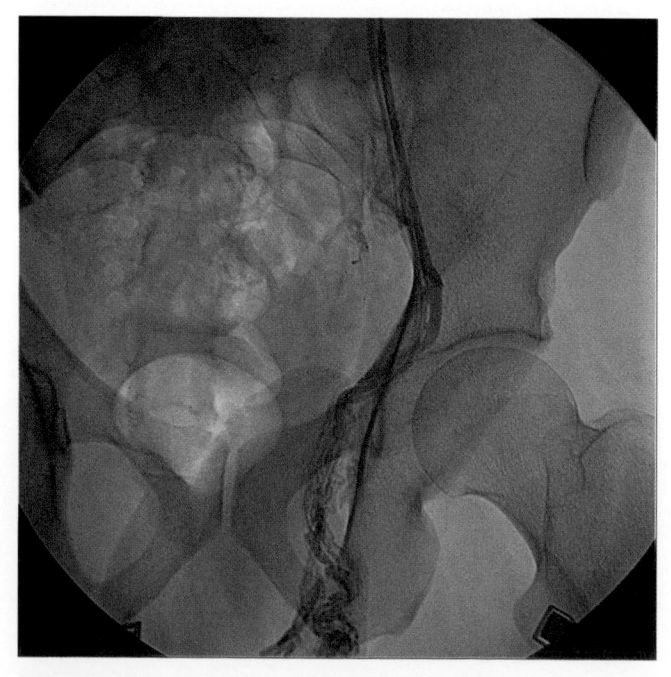

Figure 6.23 Venography showing location of the reflux.

Female gonads

Ovary

Definition

The ovary is an ovum-producing reproductive organ, often found in pairs as part of the vertebrate female reproductive system (Figs 6.24 & 6.25). Ovaries in females are homologous to testes in males, in that they are both gonads and endocrine glands.

In normal adult women the ovaries are oval-shaped bodies each 2.5–5.0 cm in length and 1.5–3.0 cm in width (Table 6.3).

The ovary's surface is covered by a single layer of cuboidal epithelium, also called *germinal epithelium*. Fibrous connective tissue forms a thin capsule, the *tunica albuginea*, immediately beneath the epithelium (Fig. 6.25).

The ovary is divided into an *outer cortex* (very cellular connective tissue stroma in which the ovarian follicles are embedded) and an *inner medulla* (composed of loose connective tissue, blood vessels, and nerves).

Function

The functions of the ovary are:
1 To regularly produce a single Graafian follicle that secretes estradiol (E_2) and ovulates a mature oocyte at about midpoint in the menstrual cycle.
2 To produce an endocrine structure, the corpus luteum, which secretes large amounts of E_2 and progesterone (P) that act on the uterus to prepare it for implantation of the embryo.
The ovary's cyclic nature is regulated by the anterior pituitary gonadotropins follicle-stimulating hormone (FSH) and luteinizing hormone (LH).

Folliculogenesis

Preantral period – gonadotropin-independent phase

The preantral follicle develops through three major events: (i) The recruitment of a *primordial follicle* into the pool of growing follicles; (ii) the growth and differentiation of the oocyte; (iii) the acquisition of FSH and LH receptors in the granulose and theca cells – *the secondary follicle*.

Antral period – gonadotropin-dependent phase

The secondary follicle fills up with clear fluid and reaches 400 µm in diameter – *the tertiary* or *graafian follicle*.

Table 6.3 Ovarian volume by age

Age	Ovarian volume
< 2 years	< 0.7 cm³
Childhood	0.75–0.86 cm³
6–11 years	1.19–2.52 cm³
After puberty	1.8–8.7 cm³

The process of *cavitation* begins to remodel granulosa cells to develop theca interna and externa, producing an oocyte.

Ovulation

On or about the 15th day of an ideal 28-day cycle, the preovulatory follicle secretes the egg-cumulus complex. The process requires the combined action of FSH, LH, and P, which induce meiotic maturation of the oocytes or resumption of meiosis.

Luteogenesis

After ovulation the follicle transforms into an endocrine organ, the *corpus luteum*, which produces P and E_2 during the luteal phase of the cycle. *Luteinization* then occurs – the lutein cells differentiate. If the egg is not fertilized, the corpus luteum undergoes apoptosis – *luteolysis* – and is expelled via menstruation.

Hormone synthesis

The estrogen-secreting granulose cells and the androgen-producing theca cells respond respectively to pituitary FSH and LH.

The human ovary produces three main classes of steroid hormone: C-18 estrogens, C-19 androgens, and C-21 progestins from cholesterol and enzymes involved in steroid biosynthesis and metabolism under the control of gonadotropins (Figure 6.24).

A high concentration of estrogens leads to the ovulatory surge of LH, which in turn stimulates luteogenesis.

Follicular growth culminating in the corpus luteum requires both FSH and LH.

Follicle-stimulating hormone promotes proliferation of granulose cells and induces the gene expression involved in E_2 biosynthesis.

Estradiol and P synergize with gonadotropins to maintain a regular menstrual cycle and promote ovarian growth (granulose cells of the dominant follicle highly express P receptors at the time of LH surge).

Progesterone maintains the secretory endometrium.

Physiological androgen secretion by the ovary has paracrine and autocrine functions.

Androgens have complex actions on granulose cells, amplifying the effect of FSH during intermediate stages of follicular development on aromatase expression and P production.

Imaging tests

Imaging testing includes:
• *Pelvic ultrasonography (abdominally, transvaginally)*: Ovaries appear lateral to the uterus and vary in their relative position within the pelvis (Fig. 6.25).
• *Ultrasonographic follicular monitoring*: Ovarian follicles recruited grow to 8–12 mm in diameter. The dominant follicle selected reaches about 22–30 mm.

Laboratory findings

The following laboratory assessments are needed:
- Assessment of physiologic hormone secretion:
  - FSH, LH, and E_2 at 7-day cycle
  - FSH, LH, and E_2, P at 14 and 21-day cycle
- Assessment of anterior pituitary hormone secretion
- Evaluation of ovarian and adrenal androgen secretion
- Evaluation of fertility by measuring inhibin A, anti-müllerian hormone (AMH) levels

Treatment

Treatment of ovary diseases is discussed in the separate entries.

Illustrations (Figs 6.24 & 6.25)

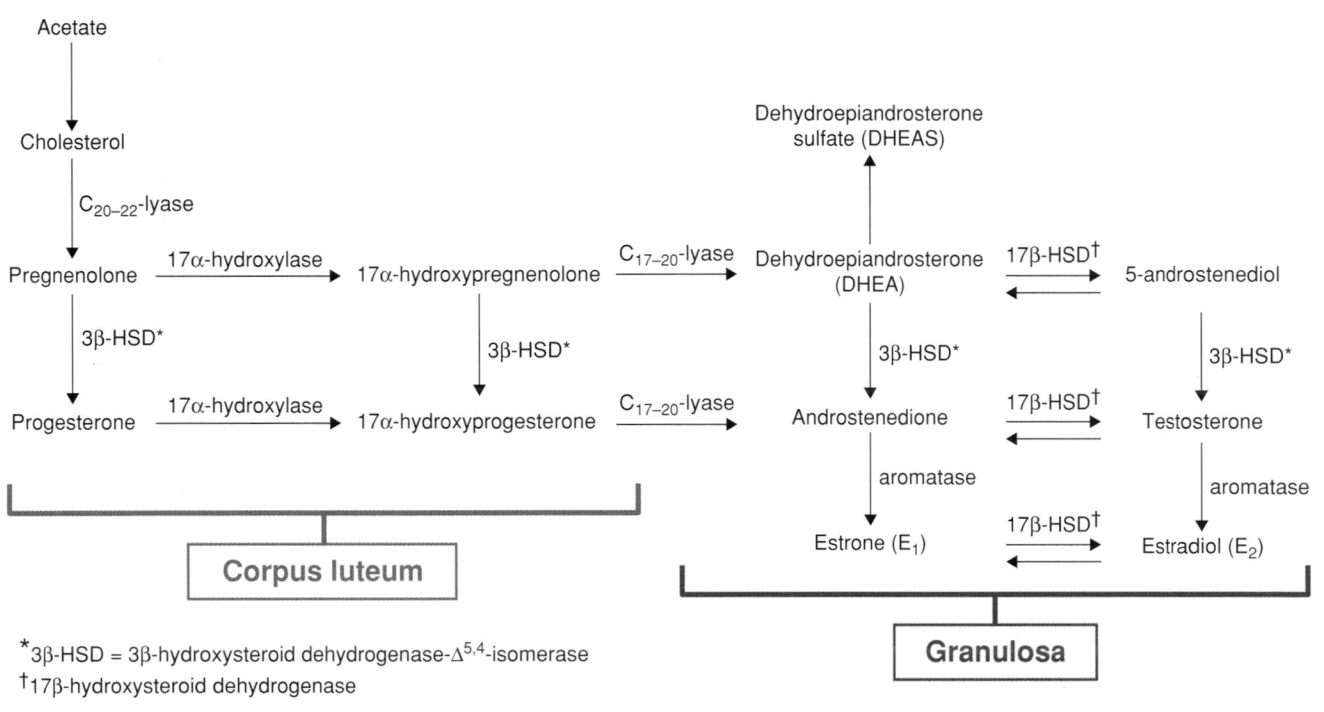

*3β-HSD = 3β-hydroxysteroid dehydrogenase-$\Delta^{5,4}$-isomerase
†17β-hydroxysteroid dehydrogenase

Figure 6.24 Flowchart showing ovarian steroid biosynthesis.

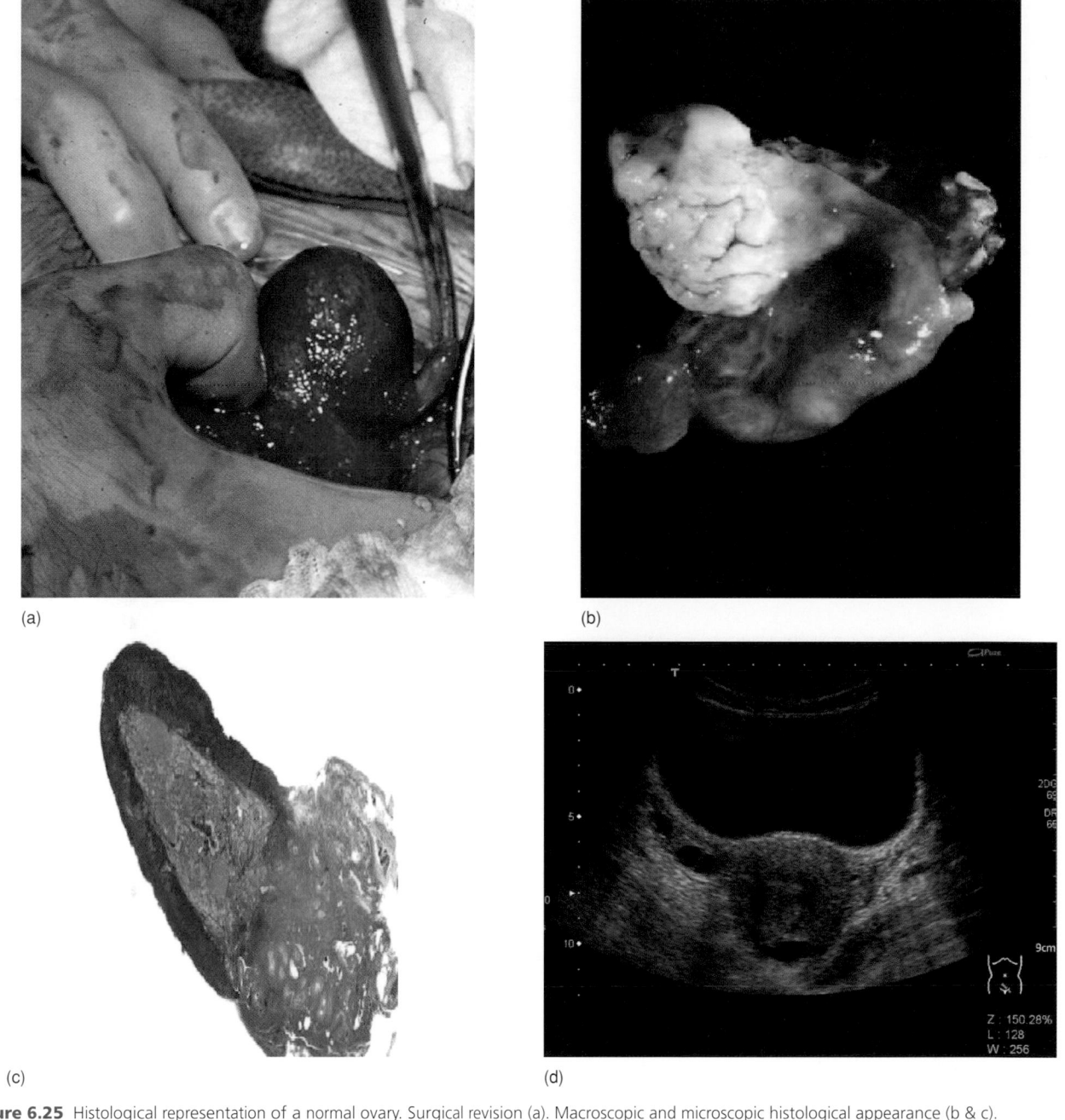

(a)

(b)

(c)

(d)

Figure 6.25 Histological representation of a normal ovary. Surgical revision (a). Macroscopic and microscopic histological appearance (b & c). Ultrasonographic representation of normal ovary (d).

Ovarian cancer

Definition and epidemiology

Ovarian cancer is characterized by tumors that originate from the surface of the ovary "epithelial" (> 90%), or from the egg cells "germ cell tumor," or supporting cells "sex cord/stromal." Ovarian cancer may produce steroid hormones directly or produce a steroid nucleus, which can be converted to a functioning compound. Each year 200 000 new cases are diagnosed worldwide.

Etiology

Lifestyle and genetic factors include:
- *Age*: The risk of ovarian cancer increases with age.
- *Pregnancy*: The risk of ovarian cancer decreases with pregnancy.
- *Alcohol*: Alcohol intake over 40 g per day increases the risk for ovarian cancer.
- *Genetics*:
  - Mutations of the *BRCA1* or the *BRCA2* gene account for 5–13% of ovarian cancers.
  - Ashkenazi Jewish women have a higher risk of both breast and ovarian cancer (at an earlier age than the general population).
  - A family history of hereditary nonpolyposis colorectal cancer (HNPCC EN also known as Lynch II syndrome – uterine cancer, colon cancer, or other gastrointestinal cancers) is associated with a higher risk of developing ovarian cancer.

Signs and symptoms

The following are signs and symptoms of ovarian cancer (Fig. 6.26):
- *Menstrual disturbance*: Anovulation, amenorrhea, oligomenorrhea.
- *Clinical hyperandrogenism*: Hirsutism, acne, seborrhea, androgenic alopecia.
- *Virilization*: Clitoral enlargement and deepening of the voice.
- *In children:* Isosexual pseudoprecocity.
- *Symptoms related to pelvic mass:*
  - Bloating, pelvic, or abdominal pain
  - Pain in the back or legs
  - Diarrhea, gas, nausea, constipation, indigestion, difficulty eating
  - Urinary symptoms (urgency or frequency)
  - Pain during sex
  - Abnormal vaginal bleeding
  - Trouble breathing
- Clinical features of *Peutz–Jeghers syndrome* in *sex cord stromal tumor with annular tubules (SCTAT)*:
  - Melanocytic macules (pigmented spots) around the mouth, eyes, hands, feet, and genital areas
  - Gastrointestinal polyps
  - Small intestine intussusception
- Rapid breast enlargement, and occasionally colostrum secretion in adults (choriocarcinoma)
- Meigs syndrome (Fig. 6.27)
- *Paraneoplastic events:*
  - Hypercalcemia
  - Zollinger–Ellison syndrome
  - Hypertension due to hyper-reninism
  - Cushing syndrome
  - Carcinoid syndrome

Diagnosis

Specific markers

Specific markers include:
- *Hormonal assessment* in secreting tumors
- *Histology* – see Table 6.4
- *Electron microscopy* demonstrates in SCTAT (composed of simple and complex ring-like solid tubular structures) that some cells lining the tubules contain Charcot–Böttcher bundles of filaments

Imaging tests

Imaging tests may include pelvic ultrasonography and magnetic resonance imaging (MRI) (Figs 6.26–6.30). Computed tomography (CT) may also help in the detection of distant metastases.

Laboratory findings

Endocrine investigations
Endocrine findings include:
- Increased total urinary estrogens
- Overproduction of estrogens, androgens, hCG, and, rarely, progesterone, corticosteroids, and ACTH
- A baseline plasma total testosterone (TT) level in the male range (> 350 ng/dL; 12 nM) usually indicates an iridizing tumor, which should in any case be suspected with a level > 200 ng/dL; 7 nM
- Lack of androgen suppression on prolonged (96 h) dexamethasone test: TT outside normal range
- Inhibin and progesterone are elevated in SCTAT
- Teratomas with specialized tissue (thyroid or pituitary cells) produce specific secretory products.

Specific markers
Specific markers include:
- Serum alpha-fetoprotein (AFP) and lactate dehydrogenase (LDH) increased in young girls and adolescents with ovarian tumors
- Increased markers for CEA, GICA, CA125, CA19-9
- Elevated placental lactogen (choriocarcinoma)

Table 6.4 Classification and histology of cancers and tumors of the ovary.

	Classification	Histology
Ovarian epithelial carcinoma	Serous tumor	It contains clear fluid and has a smooth lining composed of columnar epithelial cells with cilia
	Endometrioid tumor	In association with endometriosis and concurrent primary endometrial carcinoma
	Mucinous cystadenocarcinoma	Contains complex multiloculated cyst but with exuberant solid areas in places. It usually presents with omental metastases which cause ascites
Sex cord-stromal cell tumors	Granulosa cell tumors	Pattern with Call–Exner bodies
	Thecomas	Ill-defined masses of rounded vacuolated cells, abundant lipid
	Luteinized thecomas	Lutein cells, singly or in nests
	Sertoli–stromal cell tumors (androblastomas)	Sertoli cells, Leydig cells, indifferent stromal cells, or all three. Five degrees of differentiation: well-differentiated, intermediate differentiated, poorly differentiated (sarcomatoid), tumors with heterologous elements, and retiform type
Steroid cell tumors	Steroid cell tumors, not otherwise specified (lipid cell tumor)	Polygonal cell, from medium to large size, with slightly granular to eosinophilic cytoplasm
	Stromal luteoma	Rounded nodule of lutein-type cells growing in nests and cords
	Leydig (Hilar) cell tumors	Reinke's crystals in the cytoplasm (light or electron microscopic examination)
Gonadoblastoma		Discrete cellular aggregates composed of an intimate admixture of germ cells, sex cord, and, sometimes, stromal cells
Germ cell tumor	Choriocarcioma	Cytotrophoblasts and syncytiotrophoblasts without the presence of chorionic villi
	Teratomas	*Struma ovarii*: normal thyroid tissue. *Carcinoid*: discrete cellular masses and rests separated by fibromatous stroma. The peripheral cells of the islands often contain reddish-brown argentaffin granules visible on routine staining. The trabecular carcinoid has long wavy parallel 1–2-cell-thick ribbons of cells. The eosinophilic cytoplasm contains argyrophilic granules. *Struma carcinoid* presented both struma and carcinoid typically intimately admixed. *Teratoma containing pituitary adenoma*

Treatment

Surgery

Surgical treatment options are:
• *For stage I granulosa cell tumors in postmenopausal woman*: Total hysterectomy and bilateral salpingo-oophorectomy.
• *For younger woman*: Unilateral salpingo-oophorectomy (if the disease has not spread beyond the ovary) (Fig. 6.30).

Chemotherapy

Chemotherapy options are:
• Intraperitoneal chemotherapy for patients with stage IIIC epithelial ovarian adenocarcinomas

• Surgery and combination chemotherapy with methotrexate, dactinomycin, and chlorambucil in choriocarcinoma
Note that tearatoma is not sensitive to chemotherapy.

Radiation

Radiation therapy is not effective for advanced stages.

Illustrations (Figs 6.26–6.30)

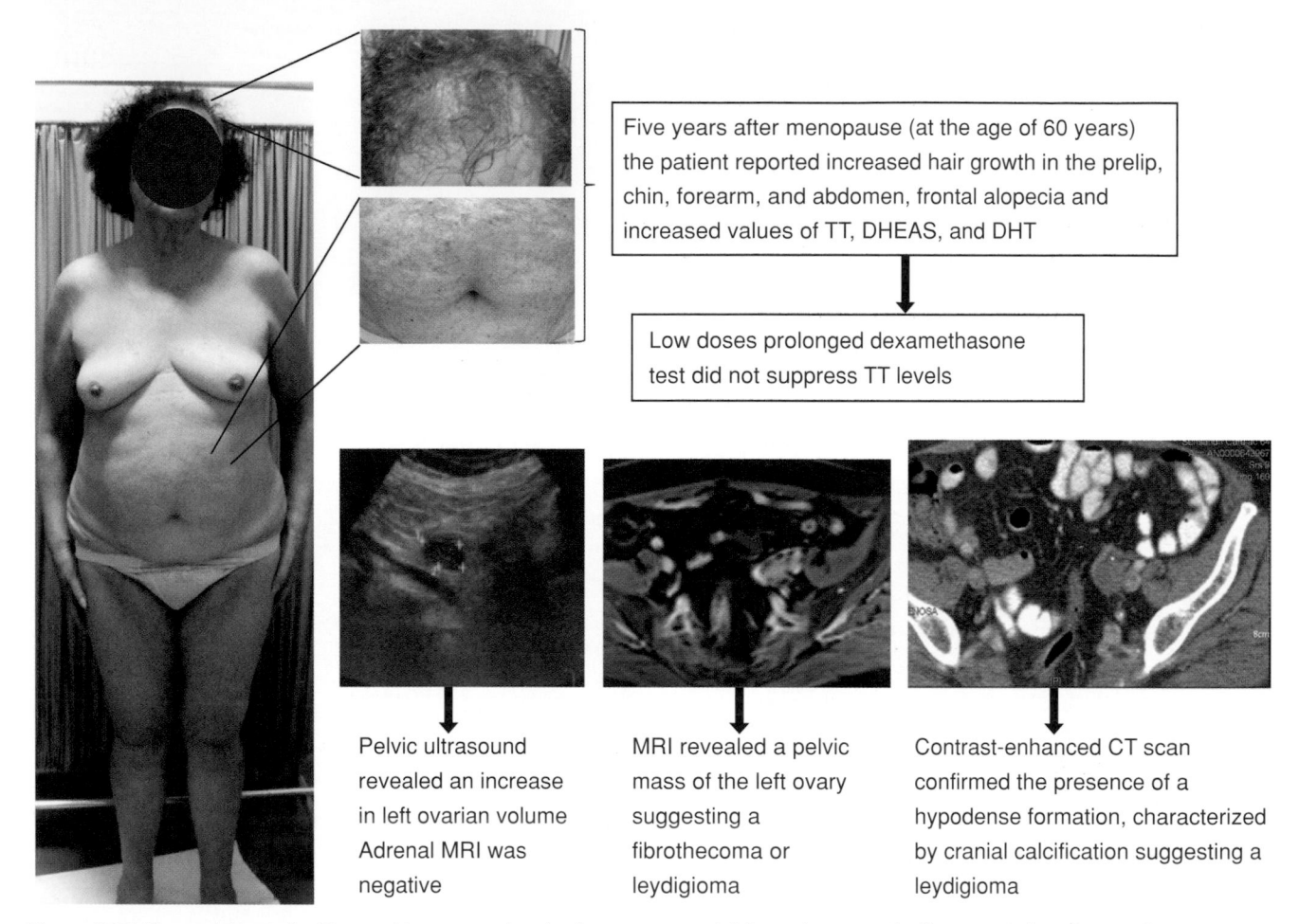

Five years after menopause (at the age of 60 years) the patient reported increased hair growth in the prelip, chin, forearm, and abdomen, frontal alopecia and increased values of TT, DHEAS, and DHT

Low doses prolonged dexamethasone test did not suppress TT levels

Pelvic ultrasound revealed an increase in left ovarian volume Adrenal MRI was negative

MRI revealed a pelvic mass of the left ovary suggesting a fibrothecoma or leydigioma

Contrast-enhanced CT scan confirmed the presence of a hypodense formation, characterized by cranial calcification suggesting a leydigioma

Figure 6.26 The special case of a 70-year-old woman undergoing hysterectomy and right oophorectomy for fibromatosis since the age of 42. CT, computed tomography; DHEAS, dehydroepiandrosterone sulfate; DHT, dihyrotestosterone; MRI, magnetic resonance imaging; TT, total testosterone.

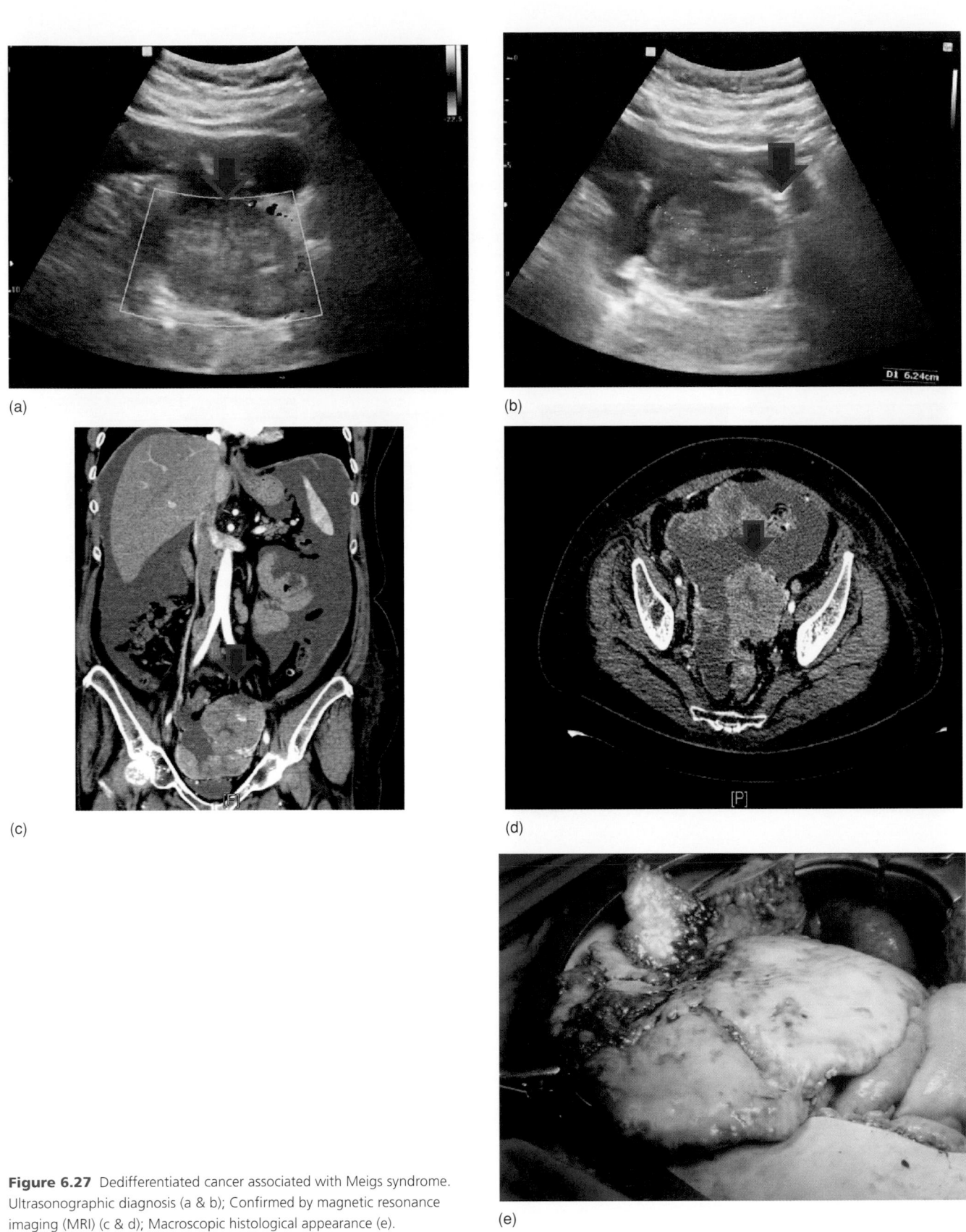

Figure 6.27 Dedifferentiated cancer associated with Meigs syndrome. Ultrasonographic diagnosis (a & b); Confirmed by magnetic resonance imaging (MRI) (c & d); Macroscopic histological appearance (e).

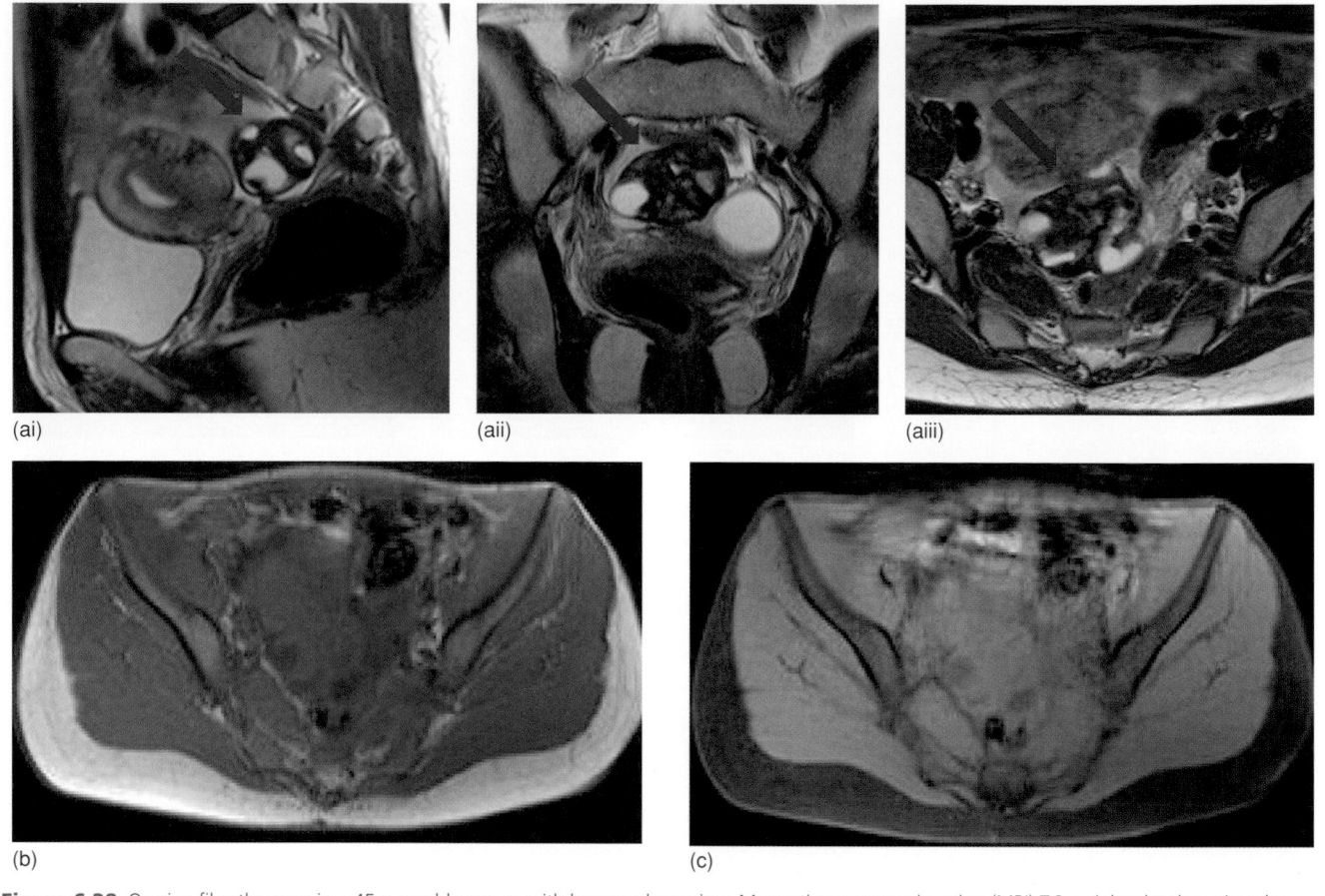

(ai)　　　　　　　　　(aii)　　　　　　　　　(aiii)

(b)　　　　　　　　　(c)

Figure 6.28 Ovarian fibrothecoma in a 45-year-old woman with hyperandrogenism. Magnetic resonance imaging (MRI) T-2 weighted turbo spin echo (TSE) sequence, acquired on sagittal (ai), coronal (aii), and axial (aiii) planes show an intensive mixed-signal probable ovarian mass. MRI T-1 weighted axial plane, with (b) and without (c) fat-saturation (FATSAT), did not show blood or fat component.

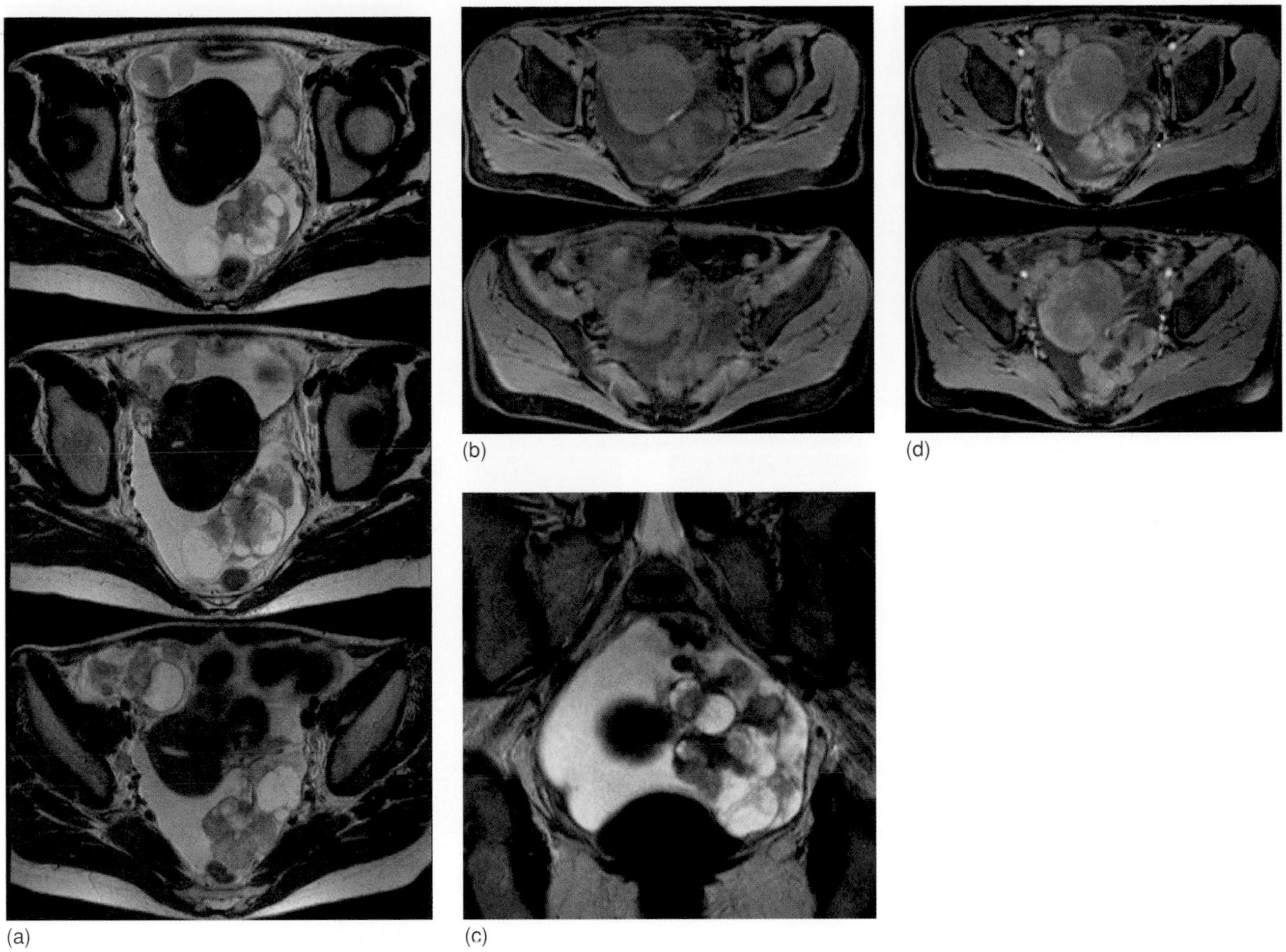

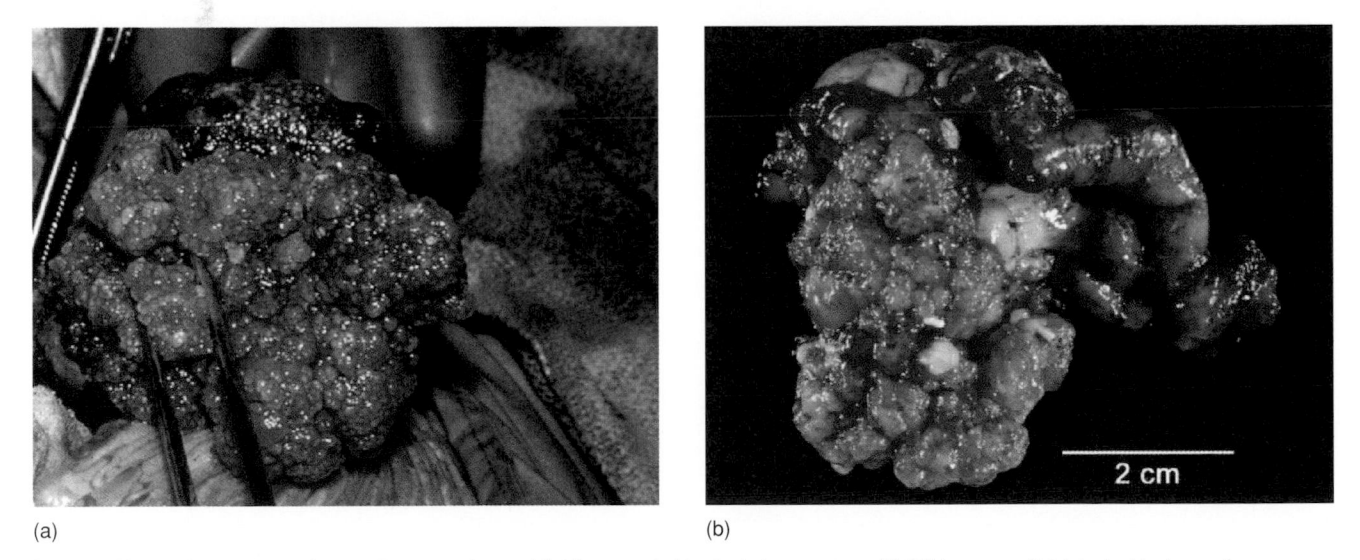

(a)

(b)

(c)

(d)

Figure 6.29 Bilateral cystadenocarcinoma. Both ovaries are filled with expansive complex lesion with cystic and solid components, clearly visible on T-2 weighted images (a–c). T-1-weighted images indicate the absence of fat or blood component (d). There is concurrent massive pelvic effusion.

(a)

(b)

Figure 6.30 Ovarian serous carcinoma: Serous carcinoma (a); Macroscopic histological appearance (b); Wide range of histological features of serous boderline ovarian tumors (c); Hierarchical proliferation of serious borderline ovarian tumors (d); Nonhierarchical proliferation of serous borderline ovarian tumors – trimmed tree or Medusa-like (e). Courtesy of Piero Luigi Alò, Section of Pathology, Department of Experimental Medicine, Sapienza Università di Roma, Italy.

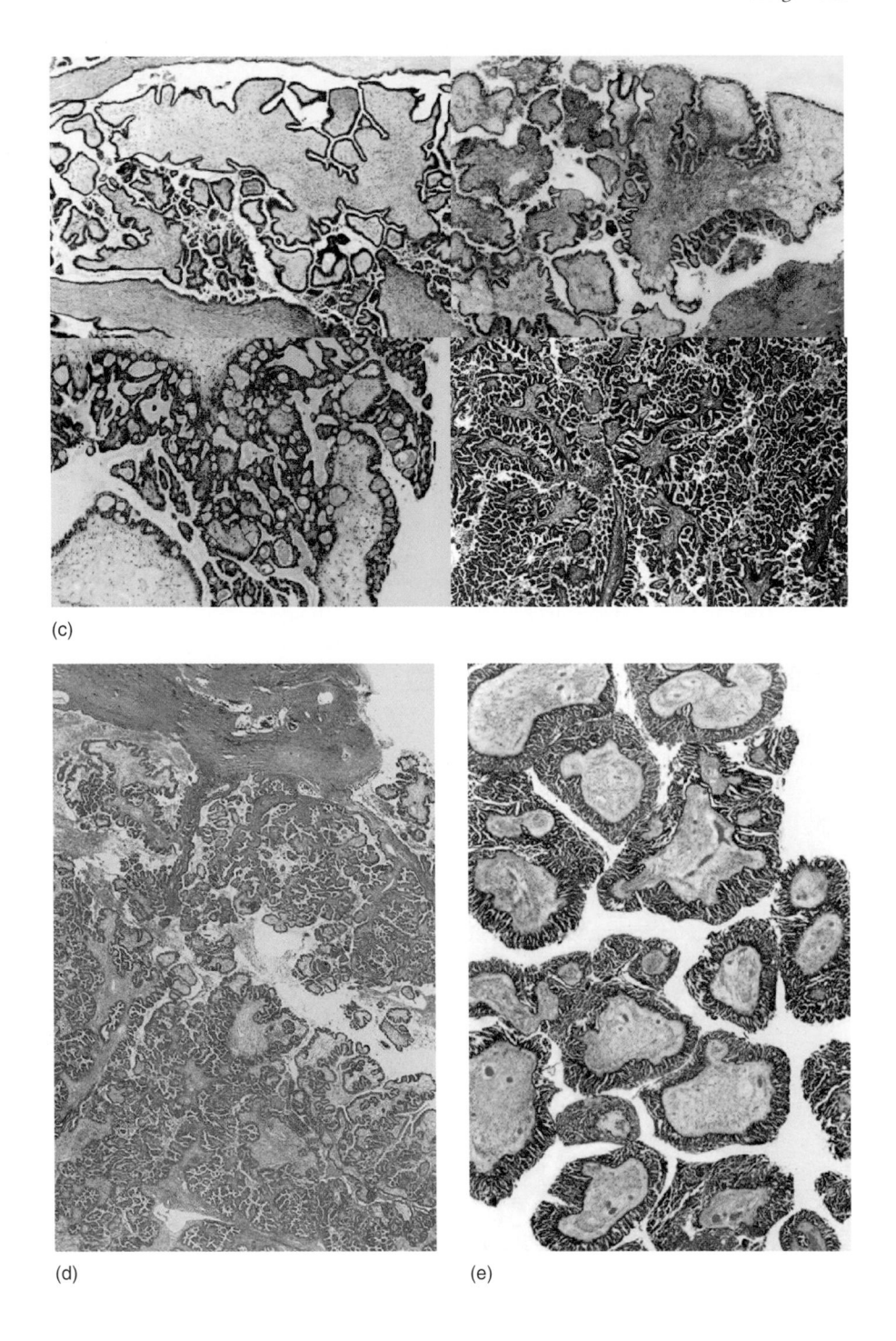

(c)

(d)   (e)

Figure 6.30 (*Continued*)

Ovarian cysts

Definition

An ovarian cyst is a collection of fluid within an ovary surrounded by a very thin wall of about 2 cm diameter or more (Fig. 6.31).

Etiology

Follicular cysts

Follicular cysts result from continuous gonadotropin stimulation of the developing follicle without the mid-cycle surge of luteinizing hormone (LH) (Fig. 6.32). Autonomous follicular cysts may be a component of McCune–Albright syndrome.

Corpus luteum cysts

Corpus luteum cysts (less common than follicular cysts) develop after the ovary releases its egg and the formed follicular cyst changes into a small hormone-producing "yellow body," also known as the corpus luteum. If the yellow body reaches > 3 cm, it is referred to as a cyst. Smokers have a twofold increased risk of these cysts.

Ovarian cysts

Ovarian cysts are frequently detected in Carney's complex.

Endometriomas

Endometriomas/"chocolate" cysts (endometriosis of the ovaries) develop when implants of cells that line the uterine cavity become transplanted and form small cysts on the outside of the ovary (Figs 6.33 & 6.34). They respond to hormone stimulation during the menstrual cycle and produce many small cysts, which may then occupy and even replace normal ovarian tissue.

Dermoid cyst

A dermoid cyst is a cystic teratoma that contains developmentally mature skin complete with hair follicles, sweat glands, sometimes clumps of long hair, often pockets of sebum, blood, fat, bone, nails, teeth, eyes, cartilage, and thyroid tissue (Fig. 6.35).

Signs and symptoms

Ovarian cysts are typically asymptomatic but the following may be signs and symptoms:
• Pelvic pain (for 24–48 h if cyst breaks or cyst > 10 cm)
• In endometriomas, pain may be worse at different points of the menstrual cycle
• Menstrual irregularities
• Infertility with endometriomas adhering to the pelvic side wall (and hence interfering with the ovulatory mechanism)
• Transiently follicular ovarian cysts may be functional in prepubertal girls and induce the acute onset of breast development due to ovarian estradiol secretion, and sexual precocity that reverses following spontaneous resolution of cysts

Ovarian cyst associations

Ovarian cysts may be associated with:
• Autonomous follicular cysts may be a component of McCune–Albright syndrome: polyostotic fibrous dysplasia, café-au-lait spots (see "Café-au-lait macules" in Chapter 7), gonadotropin-releasing hormone-independent precocious pseudopuberty, cardiovascular disorders, hyperthyroidism, intramuscular myxomas, Cushing syndrome
• Ovarian cysts are also frequently detected in Carney's complex:
  ○ Endocrine lesions – primary pigmented nodular adrenal dysplasia, testicular tumors (large cell calcifying Sertoli cell tumor, Leydig cell tumor, pigmented nodular adrenal rest tumors), pituitary (growth hormone and prolactin-secreting micro- and macro-adenomas), thyroid (hyperplasia, carcinoma, Hürtle cell tumor), and ovarian (ovarian cysts, endometrioid, or mucinous adenocarcinoma) lesions
  ○ Neuroendocrine lesions – cardiac, skin/mucosal (oropharynx, eyelids, ears, trunk, axilla, genital tract) and breast myxomas
  ○ Spotty pigmentation (lentigines, ephelides, blue nevi, café-au-lait macules [see "Café-au-lait macules" in Chapter 7]) and junctional, atypical, or compound nevi
  ○ Psammomatous melanotic schwannoma
  ○ Osteochondromyxoma

Diagnosis

Diagnosis is made by transvaginal and abdominal ultrasound and pelvic examination.

Imaging tests

Imaging tests include:
• High-resolution ultrasonography (Fig. 6.32):
  ○ Ovarian cysts ≤ 4 cm in diameter
  ○ Solitary cysts occurring outside pregnancy are typically ≤ 8 cm in diameter (cysts are lined by granulosa cells, theca cells, or a combination of both)
• Exclusion of developing ovarian cysts in uterus (rare during childhood)
• Differential diagnosis with polycystic ovary (see "Polycystic ovary syndrome" section of this chapter)
• A computed tomography (CT) scan and/or magnetic resonance imaging (MRI) are indicated to exclude ovarian cancer (Figs 6.32–6.35).

Laboratory findings

Specific markers include elevated levels of CA125 for diagnosis of endometriomas.

Treatment

Treatment depends on the type of cyst:

• *Follicular cysts*: These cysts usually involute spontaneously in 3–6 weeks (they may occasionally rupture and bleed). Oral contraceptives markedly reduce the risk of their formation.

• *Corpus luteum cysts (often rupture on the right)*: Steroid contraceptives may cause more rapid cyst involution and markedly reduce the risk of formation.

• *Endometriomas/"chocolate" cysts (can rupture and bleed)*: Treatment is by surgical excision.

• *Dermoid cysts*: Dermoid cysts are almost always benign. Malignant dermoid cysts usually develop into squamous cell carcinoma in adults and endodermal sinus tumor in babies and children. Treatment may be by surgical excision.

• *Cysts > 5 cm in diameter*: Any cysts of this size that fail to involute may require surgery to exclude a neoplastic cause.

Illustrations (Figs 6.31–6.35)

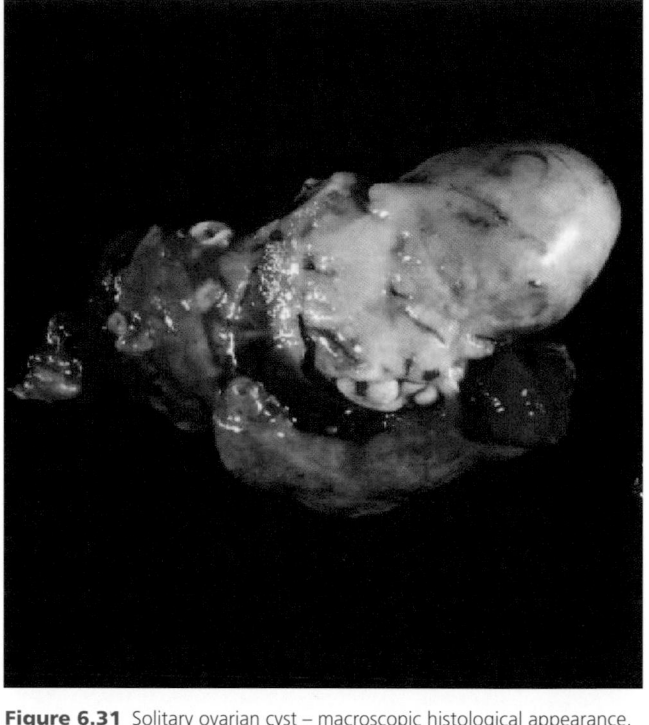

Figure 6.31 Solitary ovarian cyst – macroscopic histological appearance.

CHAPTER 6 Gonads

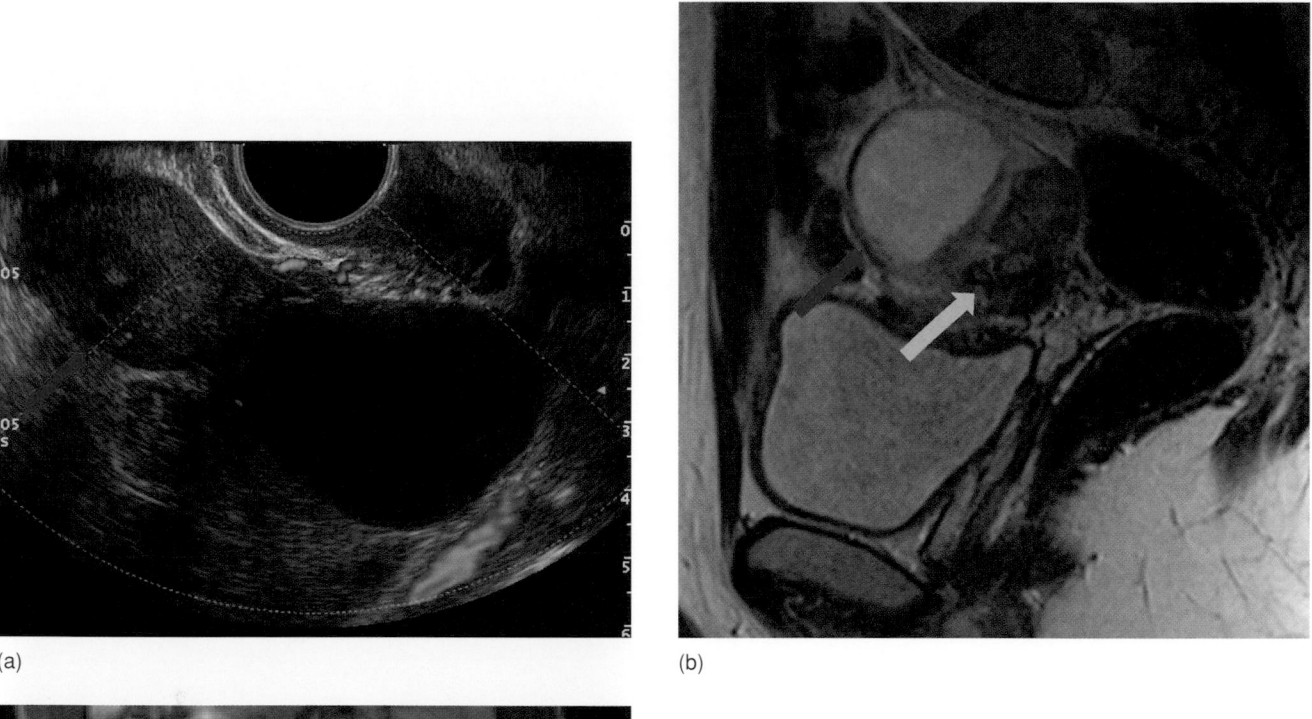

(a)

(b)

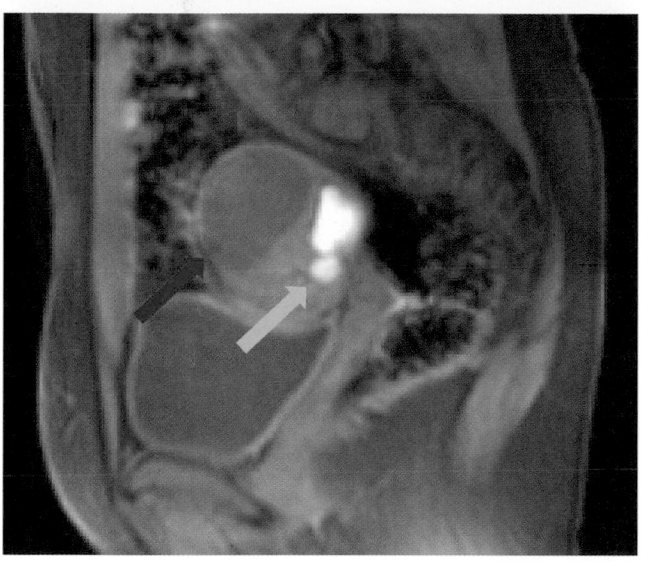

(c)

Figure 6.32 Ultrasonographic diagnosis of follicular cyst of 6 cm in diameter in a 28-year-old women with pelvic pain (a). Magnetic resonance imaging (MRI) in T-2 weighted turbo spin echo (TSE) sagittal confirms the formation of heterogeneously hypointense fluid collections at the front (red arrow) and back (yellow arrow) (b). The MRI T-1 FLASH 2D–fat saturation (FAT-SAT) image shows a probable simple functional cyst (front, red arrow) and an endometrioma (back, yellow arrow) (c).

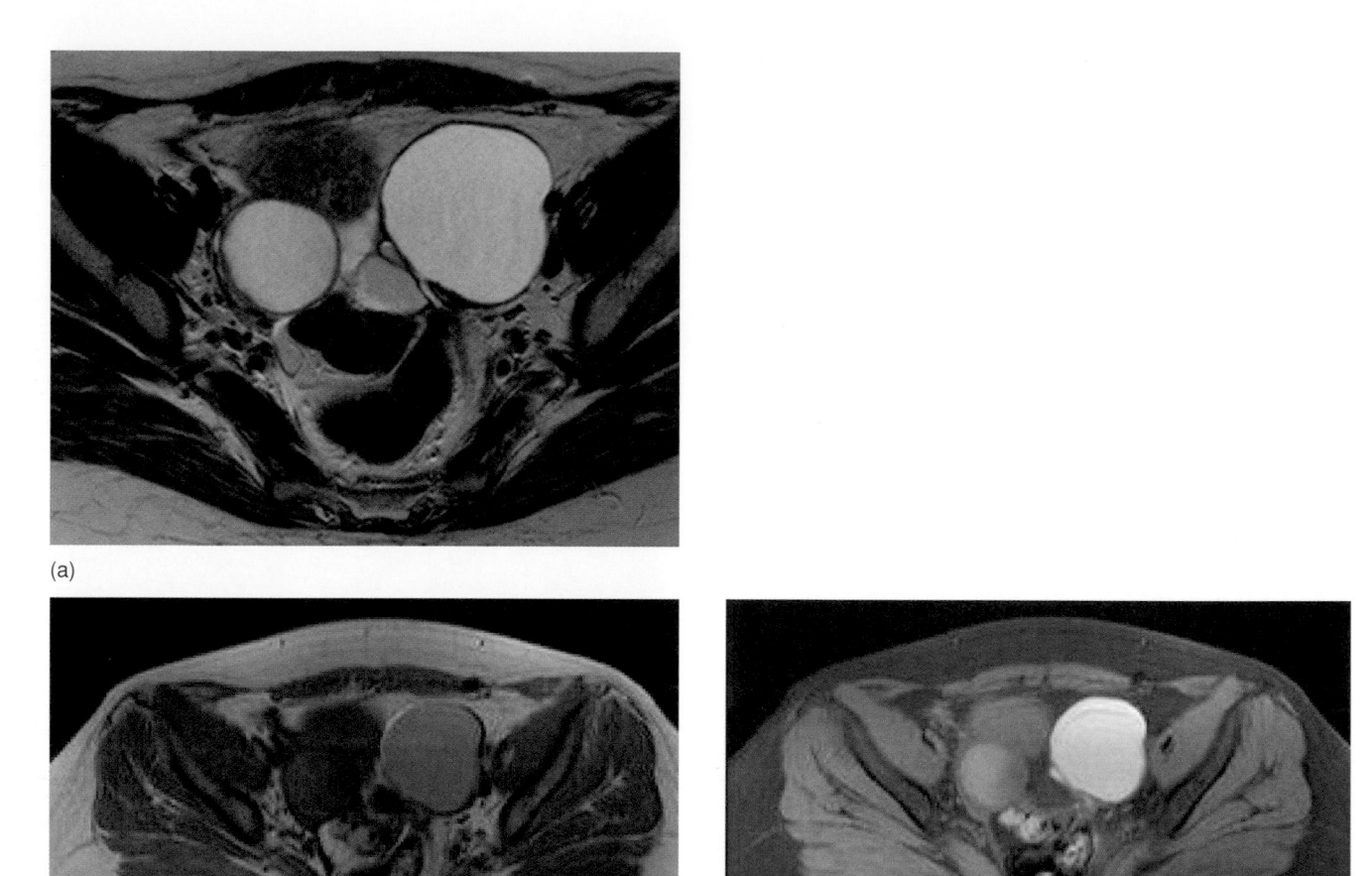

(a)

(b)

(c)

Figure 6.33 Imaging of endometriomas and functional ovarian cysts. Magnetic resonance imaging (MRI) T-2 weighted turbo spin echo (TSE) axial plane shows some ovarian formations with fluid content (two on the left, one on the right) (a). The MRI T-1 sequences without (b) and with (c) fat saturation (FAT-SAT) show an endometriosis ovarian cyst on the left. High signal intensity in FAT-SAT shows the typical breakdown products of hemoglobin. The other two formations are simple cysts.

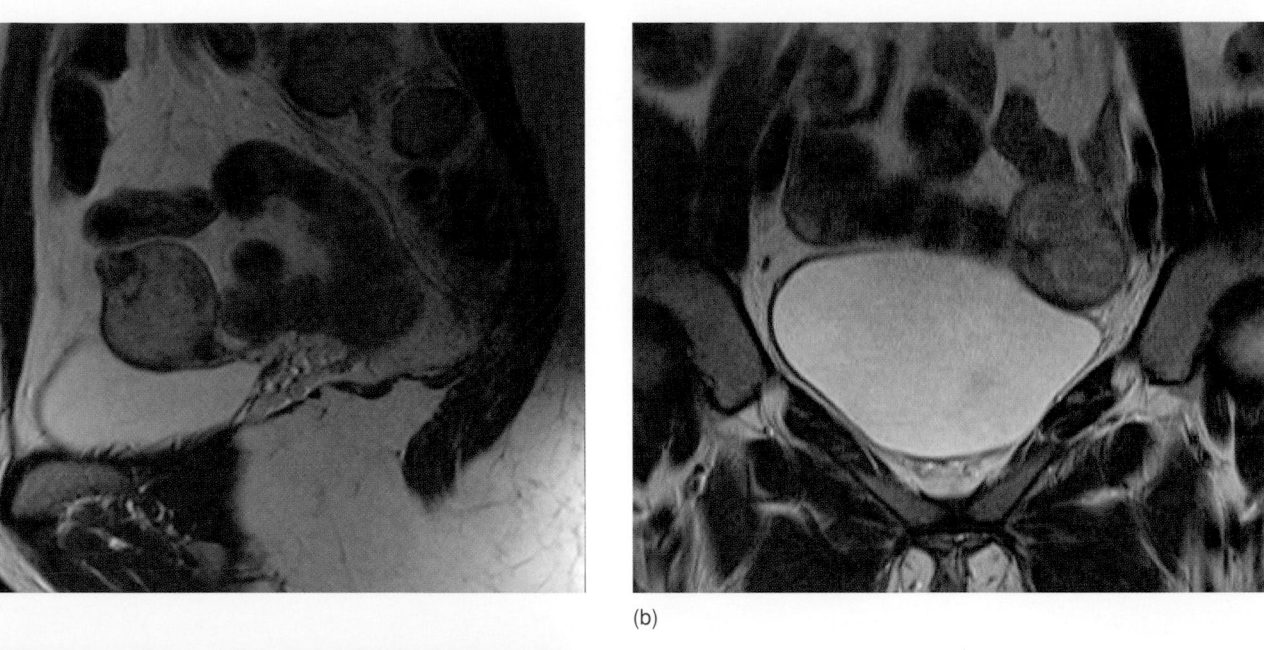

(a)

(b)

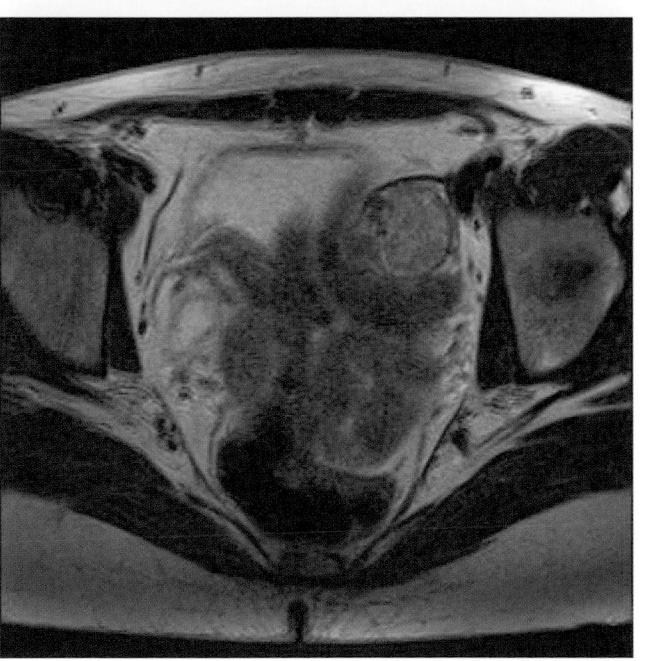

(c)

Figure 6.34 Imaging showing endometrioma developing into endometrial cancer. Magnetic resonance T-2 weighted high resolution imaging obtained in sagittal (a), coronal (b), and axial (c) planes show a heterogeneous formation. This proved to be left ovarian endometrial cancer in a patient suffering from endometrioma who had previously undergone hysterectomy for uterine fibromas and endometriosis.

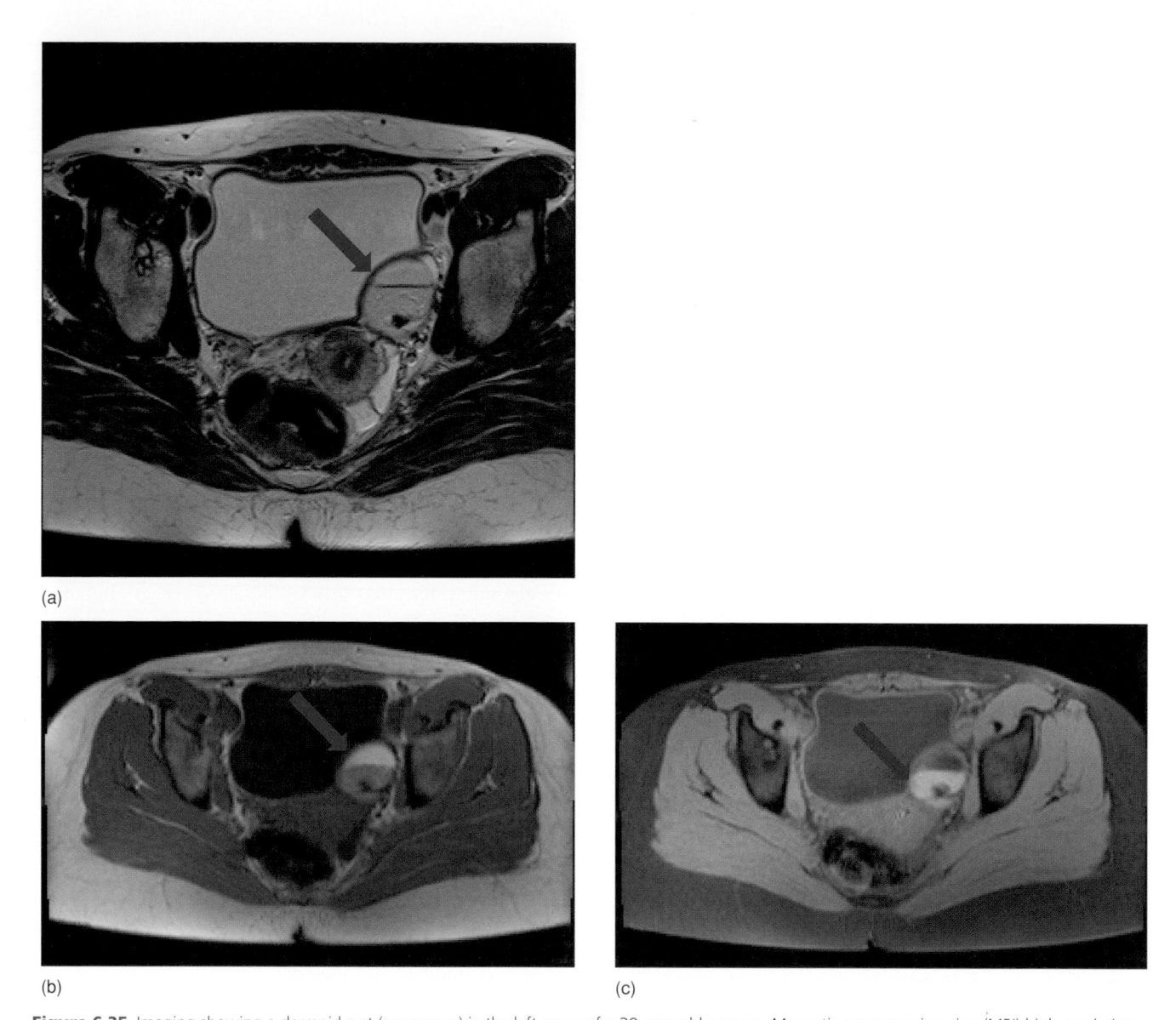

(a)

(b)

(c)

Figure 6.35 Imaging showing a dermoid cyst (see arrows) in the left ovary of a 39-year-old woman. Magnetic resonance imaging (MRI) high-resolution turbo spin echo (TSE) T-2 axial plane (a): An oval image with mixed signal intensity. MRI T-1 FLASH 2D without (b) and with (c) deletion of adipose tissue signal with a fat component mixture, striking in fat saturation (FAT-SAT) image. There is also a Rokitansky nodule (hypointense).

Amenorrhea

Definition

Amenorrhea is defined as either the absence of periods at age 16 (primary amenorrhea) or the absence of periods for more than 6 months (secondary amenorrhea).

Etiology

Primary amenorrhea (Fig. 6.36)

The etiology of primary amenorrhea is as follows:
• *Genital tract disorders*: Transverse membrane; imperforate hymen or incompletely canalized vagina; complete failure of the Müllerian duct system (Mayer–Rokitansky–Küster–Hauser syndrome – absence of a uterus, vaginal agenesis, normal karyotype, and external genitalia (Fig. 6.37); association of abnormalities of the urinary tract with absence of the uterus and/or vagina; endometrial abnormalities (iatrogenic, Asherman syndrome).
• *Disorders of sexual differentiation*: Congenital androgen synthesis disorders (normal XY karyotype); complete androgen insensitivity syndrome (Morris syndrome); partial androgen insensitivity syndrome.

Secondary amenorrhea (Fig. 6.38)

The etiology of secondary amenorrhea is as follows:
• *Physiologic causes*: Pregnancy; lactation.
• *Hypothalamus–pituitary disorders*: Hyperprolactinemia (prolactin-secreting tumor; centrally acting medications, including dopamine antagonists); pituitary disease (nonprolactin secreting pituitary infarction, e.g. Sheehan syndrome; generalized hypopituitarism including after pituitary surgery).
• *Hypothalamic amenorrhea*: Nutrition/exercise disorders; idiopathic hypogonadotropic hypogonadism (IHH).

Primary ovarian failure

Primary ovarian failure may be caused by the following:
• *Iatrogenic*: Surgery; chemotherapy; radiotherapy.
• *Environmental*: Smoking; viral infections.
• *Autoimmune*: Premature ovarian failure (POF) (an association with other autoimmune diseases).
• *Abnormal karyotype*: 46,XY gonadal dysgenesis (Swyer syndrome with streak gonads; uterus and fallopian tubes are normal); 45,X0.
• *Genetic disorders with a normal karyotype*: Fragile X permutations; galactosemia; carbohydrate-deficient glycoprotein syndrome type 1 (CDG1); inhibin-B gene mutations; follicle stimulating hormone (FSH) receptor gene mutations.
• *Resistant ovary syndrome*.

Extraovarian endocrine diseases

Extraovarian endocrine diseases that may cause amenorrhea are:
• Hypothyroidism (due to prolactin)
• Hyperthyroidism (due to sex hormone-binding globulin)
• Cushing syndrome
• Adrenal carcinoma
• Congenital adrenal hyperplasia (CAH)
• Hyperandrogenism

Signs and symptoms

Signs and symptoms of amenorrhea are:
• Galactorrhea (in pathologic hyperprolactinemia)
• Dyspareunia, vaginal dryness (associated with estrogen deficiency)
• Critical body weight = 15% below ideal body weight (anorexia nervosa and bulimia)
• Anosmia (Kallmann syndrome)
• Specific physical findings of Turner syndrome (see "Turner syndrome" section of this chapter) and other genetic disorders
• Pelvic swelling and a bulging septum at the introitus in genital tract disorders

Diagnosis

An algorithm for diagnosis of amenorrhea is shown in Fig. 6.39.

Imaging tests

The following imaging tests (Figs 6.36–6.38) may be needed:
• Magnetic resonance imaging (MRI) of the sella turcica
• Pelvic and abdomen ultrasonography
• Computed tomography (CT) or MRI to study adrenal glands' and ovaries' morphology and/or masses (Fig. 6.37)
• Intravenous pyelography and/or ultrasonography may reveal duplex ureters or the absence of one kidney and collecting duct system

Laboratory findings

Laboratory findings may include:
• *In pregnancy*: Elevated human chorionic gonadotropin (hCG) levels in blood or urine.
• *In hypothalamic–pituitary disorders:* Reduction in pulsatile secretion of Luteinizing hormone (LH); LH and FSH ≤ normal range for follicular phase; estradiol (E_2) < 50 pg/mL; gestodene test negative.
• *In hyperprolactinemia*: Prolactin (PRL) > 20 ng/mL (Friesen Standard); reduced or elevated levels of thyroid-stimulating hormone (TSH) and low levels of free thyroxine (FT_4) and free triiodothyronine (FT_3); gestodene test negative.
• *Hypopituitarism*: Decreased secretion of pituitary hormones.
• *In primary ovarian diseases:* Elevated gonadotropin concentrations, with FSH > LH and negative gestodene test.
• *In POF*: Autoantibodies to ovarian tissue (and to steroid secreting cells in general) and elevated FSH concentrations.
• *In Morris syndrome*: Male levels of testosterone in plasma.
• *In polycystic ovary syndrome (PCOS)*: Assessment of biochemical markers of PCOS (see "Polycystic ovary syndrome"

section of this chapter) accompanied by a positive gestodene test.

Treatment

A problem-oriented approach to the treatment includes:

• *In PRL-secreting pituitary adenoma:* Treatment with the dopamine agonist cabergoline. Treatment should be stopped immediately if pregnancy is diagnosed.

• *In hypopituitarism:* Specific multiple therapy.

• *In hypothalamic disorders:* Induction of ovulation with pulsatile gonadotropin-releasing hormone (GnRH) and/or gonadotropin treatment.

• *In POF:* Long-term low-dose estrogen replacement therapy and oocyte donation for fertility.

• *In genital tract disorders:* Surgical correction.

• *In endometrial abnormalities:* Short-term treatment with estrogen (iatrogenic) or surgery.

• *In Morris syndrome:* Surgical removal of intra-abdominal testes as soon as growth and breast development are complete.

Illustrations (Figs 6.36–6.39)

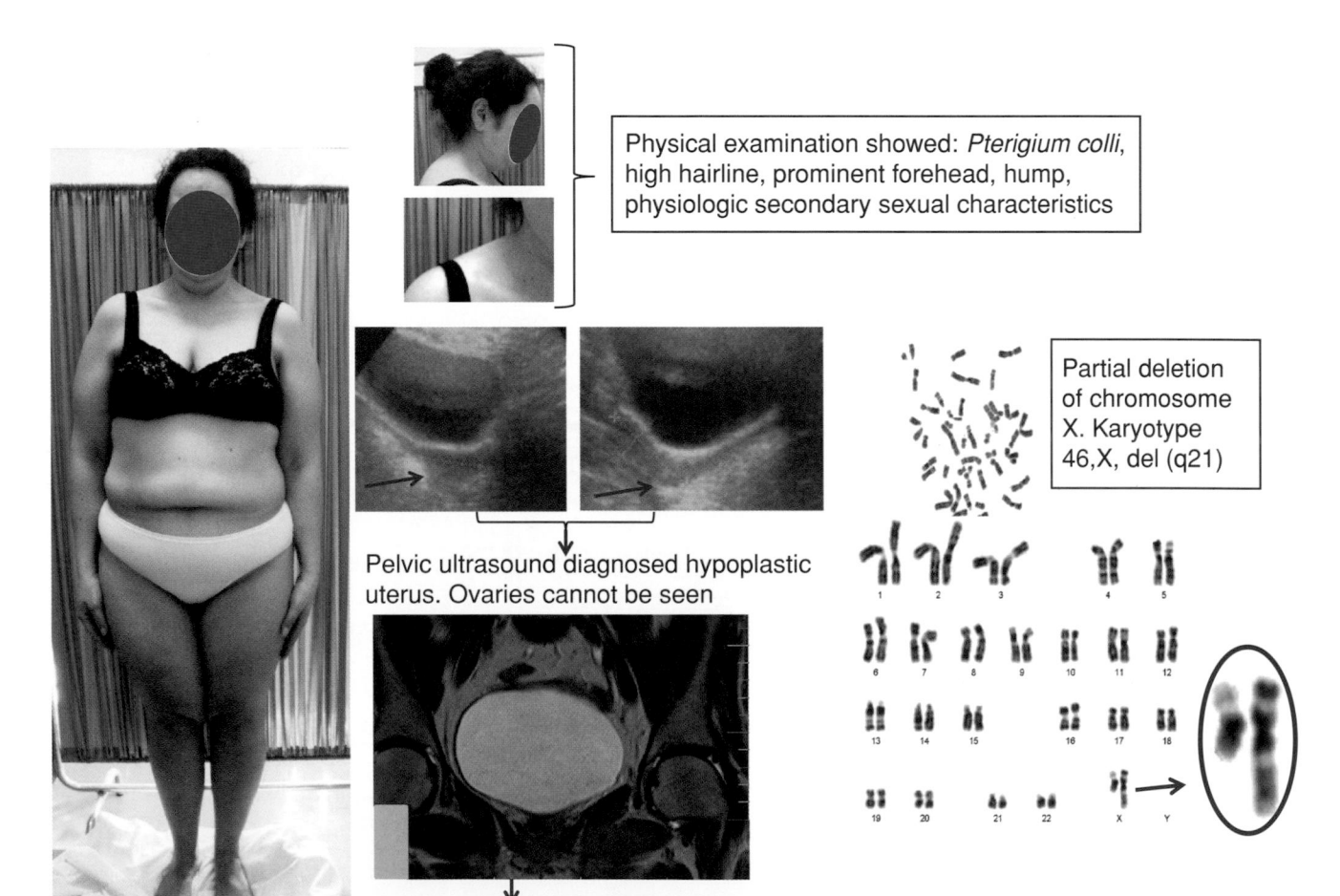

Physical examination showed: *Pterigium colli*, high hairline, prominent forehead, hump, physiologic secondary sexual characteristics

Partial deletion of chromosome X. Karyotype 46,X, del (q21)

Pelvic ultrasound diagnosed hypoplastic uterus. Ovaries cannot be seen

MRI confirmed gonadal dysgenesis

Figure 6.36 A 32-year-old woman with primary amenorrhea.

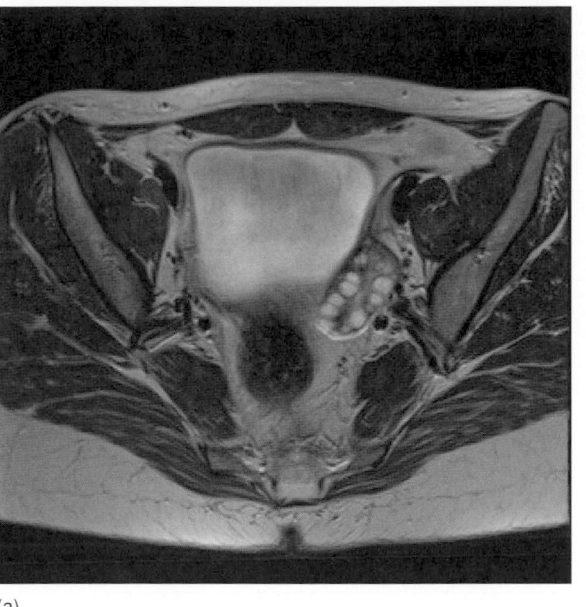

(a)

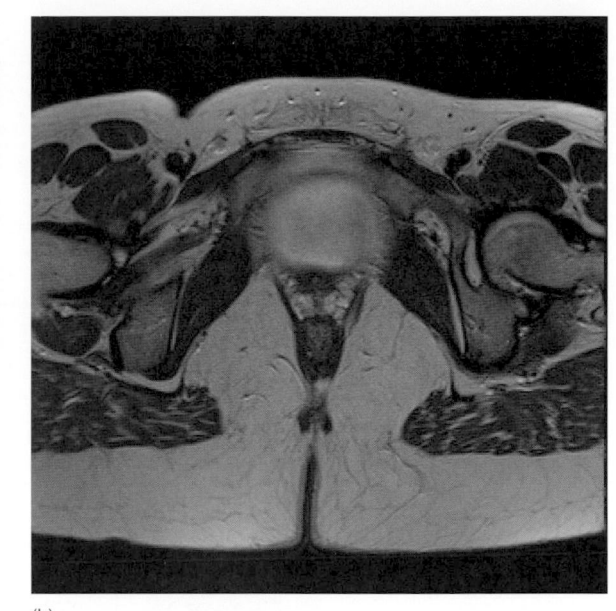

(b)

Figure 6.37 A 19-year-old woman with primary amenorrhea. Magnetic resonance imaging (MRI): T-2 weighted sequence in the axial plane shows a micropolycystic left ovary (a). MRI: T-2 weighted sequence in the axial plane shows that the patient has no uterus or vagina due to Rokitansky syndrome (b).

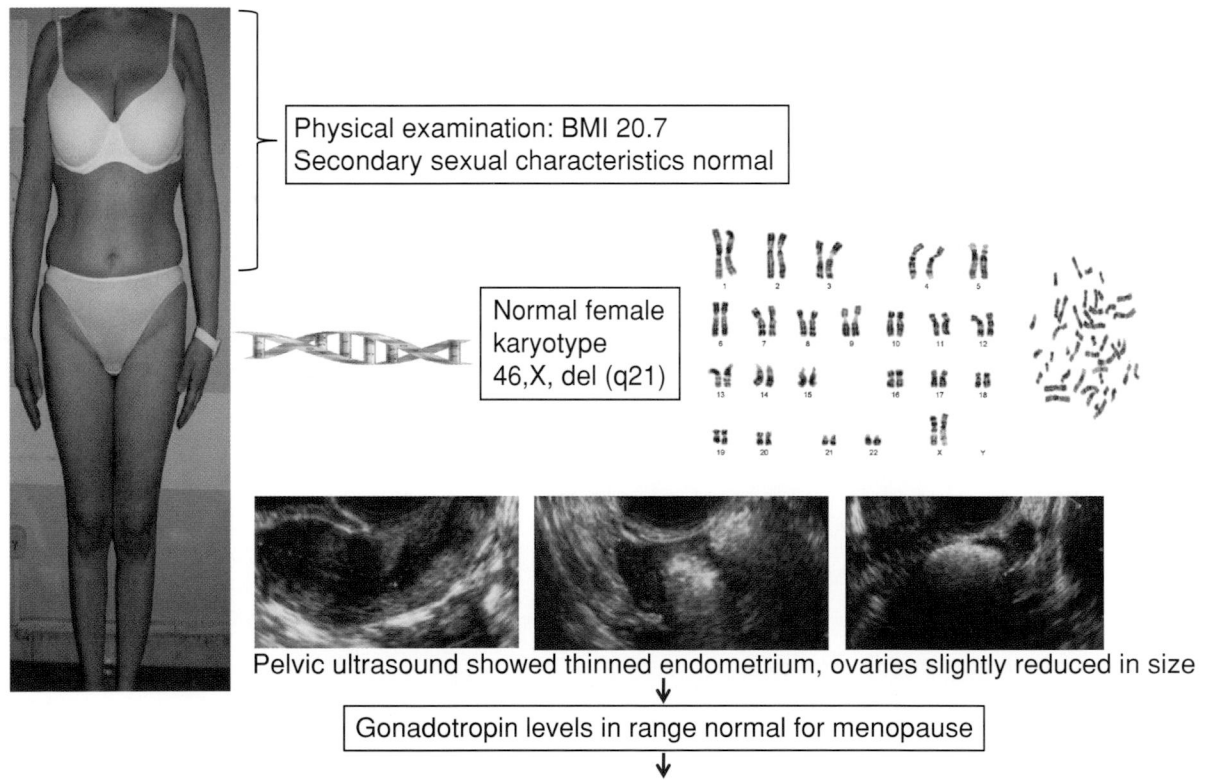

Physical examination: BMI 20.7
Secondary sexual characteristics normal

Normal female karyotype
46,X, del (q21)

Pelvic ultrasound showed thinned endometrium, ovaries slightly reduced in size

Gonadotropin levels in range normal for menopause

The patient received a diagnosis of POF and and is now taking estrogen–progestin

Figure 6.38 A 26-year-old woman with secondary amenorrhea showing vasomotor symptoms.

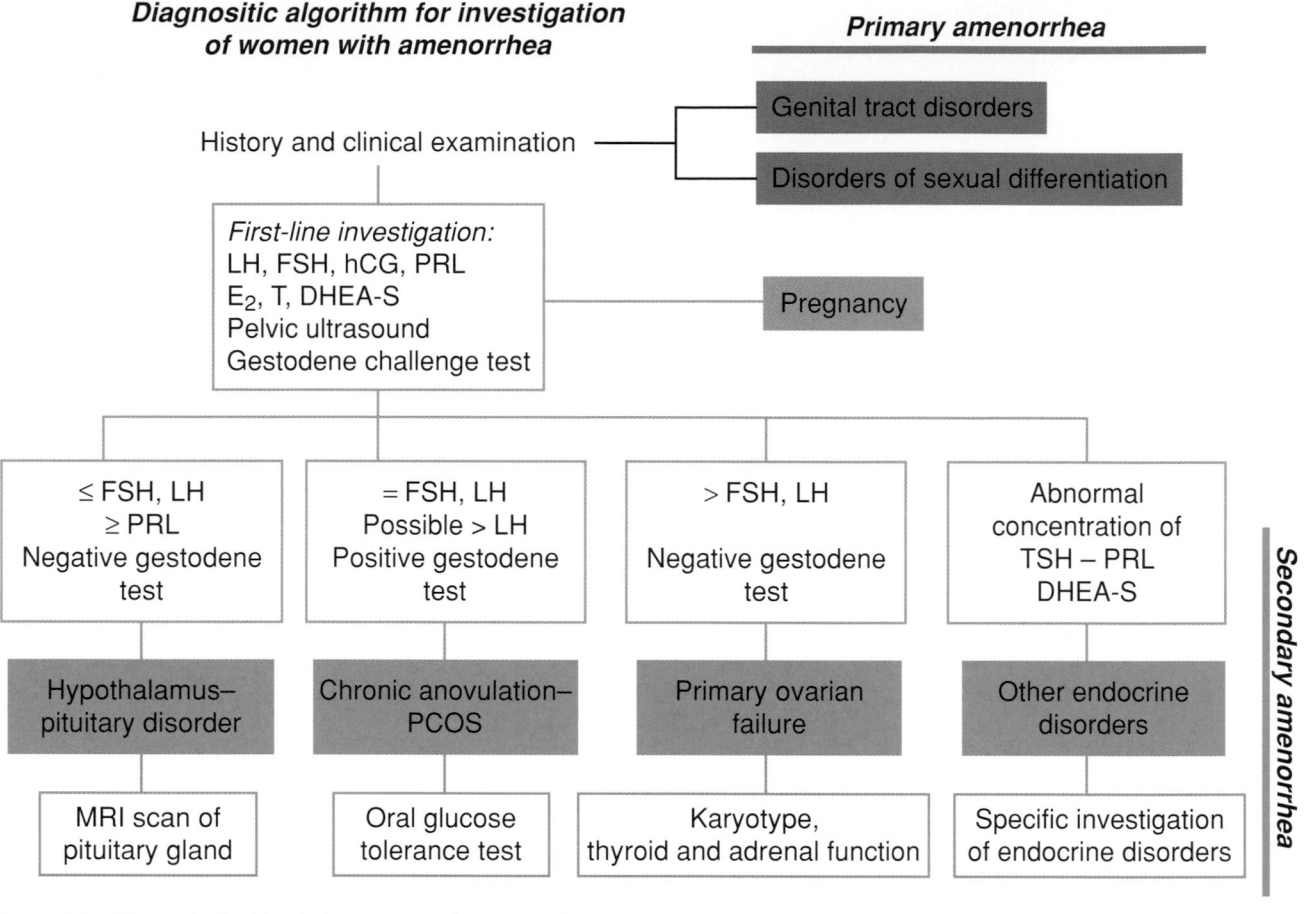

Figure 6.39 Diagnostic algorithm for investigation of women with amenorrhea. DHEA-S, dehydroepiandrosterone sulfate; E$_2$, estradiol; FSH, follicle-stimulating hormone; hCG, human chorionic gonadotropin; LH, lutenizing hormone; MRI, magnetic resonance imaging; PCOS, polycystic ovary syndrome; PRL, prolactin; T, testosterone.

Hyperandrogenism in women

Definition and etiology

Hyperandrogenism in women is a disorder of factors physiologically controlling the biosynthesis, secretion, and action of androgens (Figs 6.40–6.42). There are several clinical presentations:

• *Adrenal hyperandrogenism*: Premature adrenarche; functional adrenal hyperandrogenism (FAH); congenital adrenal hyperplasia (CAH); Cushing syndrome; hyperprolactinemia; acromegaly; abnormal cortisol action/metabolism; adrenal neoplasms.

• *Gonadal hyperandrogenism*: Ovarian hyperandrogenism (functional ovarian hyperandrogenism/polycystic ovary syndrome [PCOS]; adrenal virilizing disorders; ovarian steroidogenic blocks; syndrome of extreme insulin resistance; ovarian neoplasms); true hermaphroditism; pregnancy-related hyperandrogenism.

• *Peripheral androgen overproduction*: Obesity; idiopathic.

Functional abnormalities are much more common (found in 50% of cases of hyperandrogenism and PCOS) than tumors (found in < 1%).

Signs and symptoms

Cutaneous manifestations of excessive androgen are variable and include (Figs 6.41 & 6.42):

• Male pattern baldness
• Hirsutism – excessive male pattern hair growth in women, defined by a total score ≥ 8 on a modified Ferriman–Gallwey scale
• Acne
• In rare cases, muscle and clitoral hypertrophy

Diagnosis

Diagnosis is made by:

• Assessment of the pattern and degree of hair growth
• Screening for hyperandrogenemia by measuring blood levels of total (TT) and free (FT) testosterone, sex hormone-binding globulin (SHBG), cortisol, androstenedione, dehydroepiandrosterone sulfate (DHEAS), and 17-hydroxyprogesterone (17-OH-P) in the follicular phase
• Low dose prolonged dexamethasone androgen-suppression test to establish the pattern of androgen response, administering 2.0 mg in divided doses by mouth for 4 days
• Corticotropin (ACTH) (Synachten) test when CAH is suspected
• Glucose and insulin metabolism assessment

Imaging tests

Ultrasound, computed tomography (CT), or magnetic resonance imaging (MRI) will usually reveal any adrenal or ovary masses, or cysts.

Laboratory findings

Regarding laboratory findings (Fig. 6.40):

• A normal plasma TT does not exclude an important hyperandrogenic disorder (virilizing CAH, PCOS).
• A baseline plasma TT level in the male range (> 350 ng/dL; 12 nM) usually indicates a virilizing tumor, which should in any case be suspected with a level > 200 ng/dL; 7 nM. A baseline DHEAS level > 800 μg/dL (18.5 μM) suggests an adrenal tumor.
• Normal suppression of androgens by dexamethasone is most specifically indicated by normalization of plasma TT and FT.
• Normal adrenal suppression is indicated by a reduction of serum cortisol < 50 nmol/L at 48 hours and a 50% reduction in androstenedione and DHEAS.
• Inadequate cortisol suppression indicates Cushing syndrome, glucocorticoid resistance, or noncompliance.
• Subnormal suppression of TT with normal adrenal suppression is usually due to PCOS. Cortisol suppression indicates virilizing tumor, true hermaphroditism, or, in pregnancy, human chorionic gonadotropin (hCG) -related disorders.
• Baseline levels of 17-OH-P in the normal range for follicular phase and/or a high response after 30–60 min of intravenous bolus of 250 μg ACTH distinguishes between noncarriers, carriers, untypical cases, and heterozygotes of 21-hydroxylase deficiency.
• A normal response to the ACTH test suggests excessive growth hormone (GH), hyperprolactinemia, or idiopathic hyperandrogenism.
• Hyperinsulinemia is found in PCOS and insulin resistance syndrome.

Treatment

Treatment for female hyperandrogenism depends on the etiology. A problem-oriented approach to the treatment includes:

• Combination estrogen–progestin (relatively effective)
• Antiandrogens (substantial efficacy)
• Gonadotropin-releasing hormone (GnRH) agonists (in short-term use < 6 months)
• Glucocorticoids (effective in lowering the adrenal component of androgen excess)
• 5-Alfa-reductase inhibitors (not specific)
• Ornithine decarboxylase inhibitors (minimal efficacy topically)
• Clomiphene citrate (moderately effective)
• Biguanides and thiazolidinediones (modest effects on hirsutism)

Illustrations (Figs 6.40–6.42)

Dexamethasone test

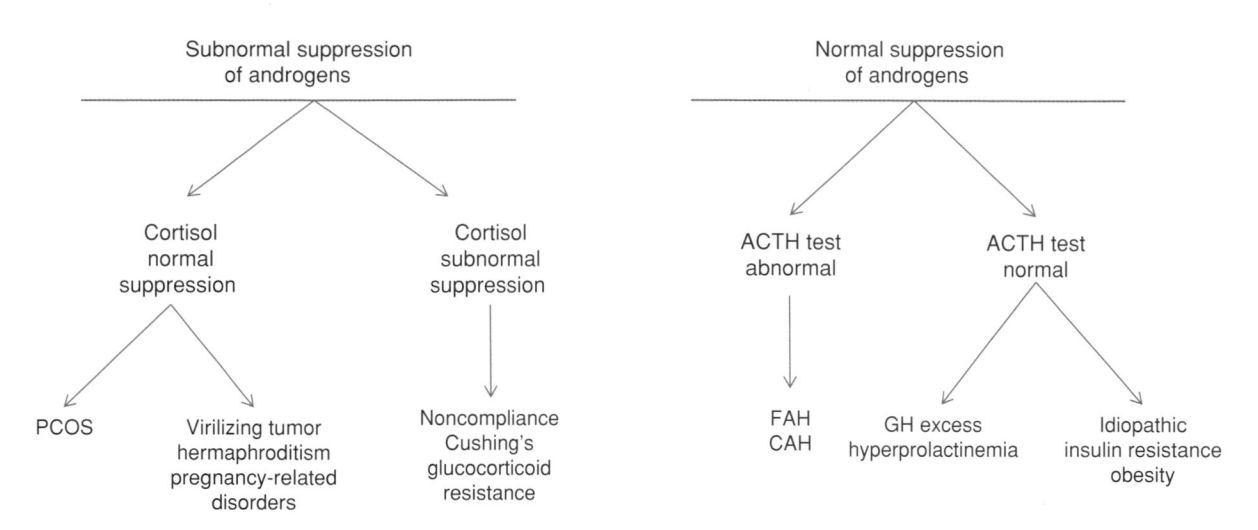

Figure 6.40 Algorithm for the differential diagnosis of hyperandrogenism. ACTH, corticotropin; CAH, congenital adrenal hyperplasia; FAH, functional adrenal hyperandrogenism; GH, growth hormone; PCOS, polycystic ovary syndrome.

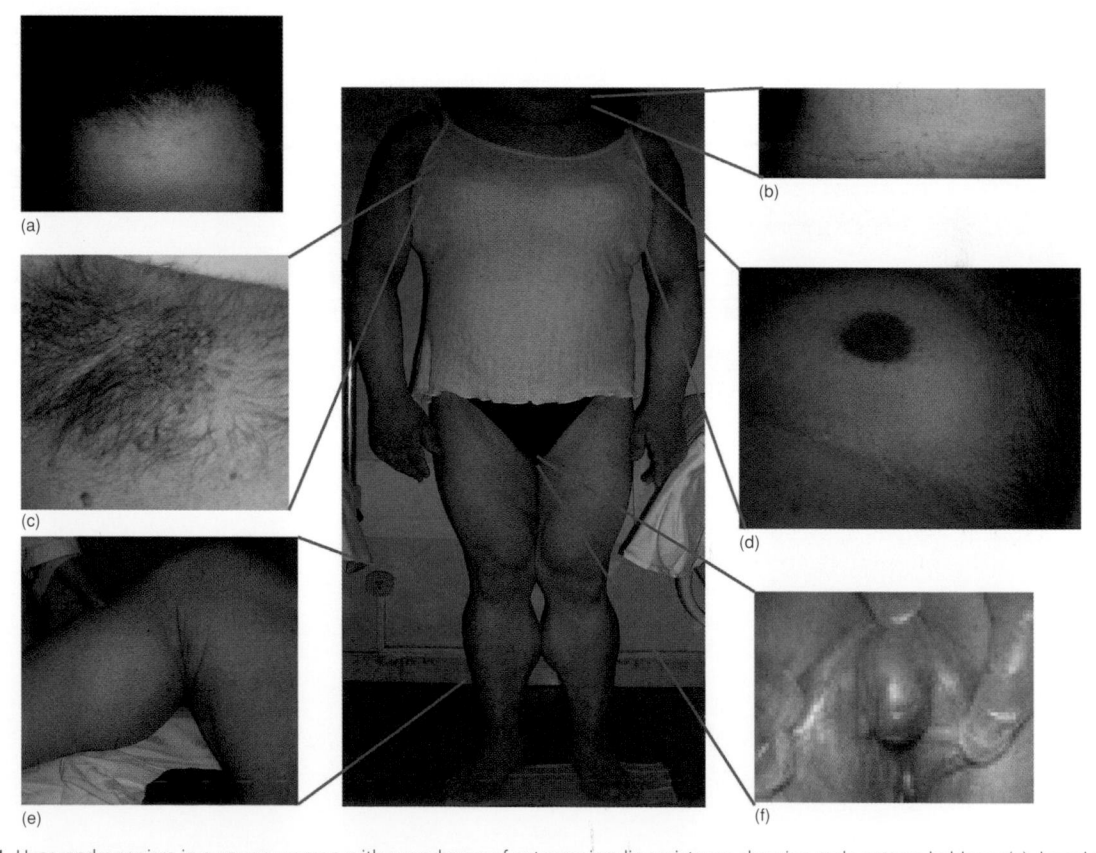

Figure 6.41 Hyperandrogenism in a young woman with a syndrome of extreme insulin resistance showing male pattern baldness (a), beard (b), axillary hair (c), male pattern chest hair (d), hypertrophic muscle mass (e), clitoromegaly (f). See also Fig. 6.42.

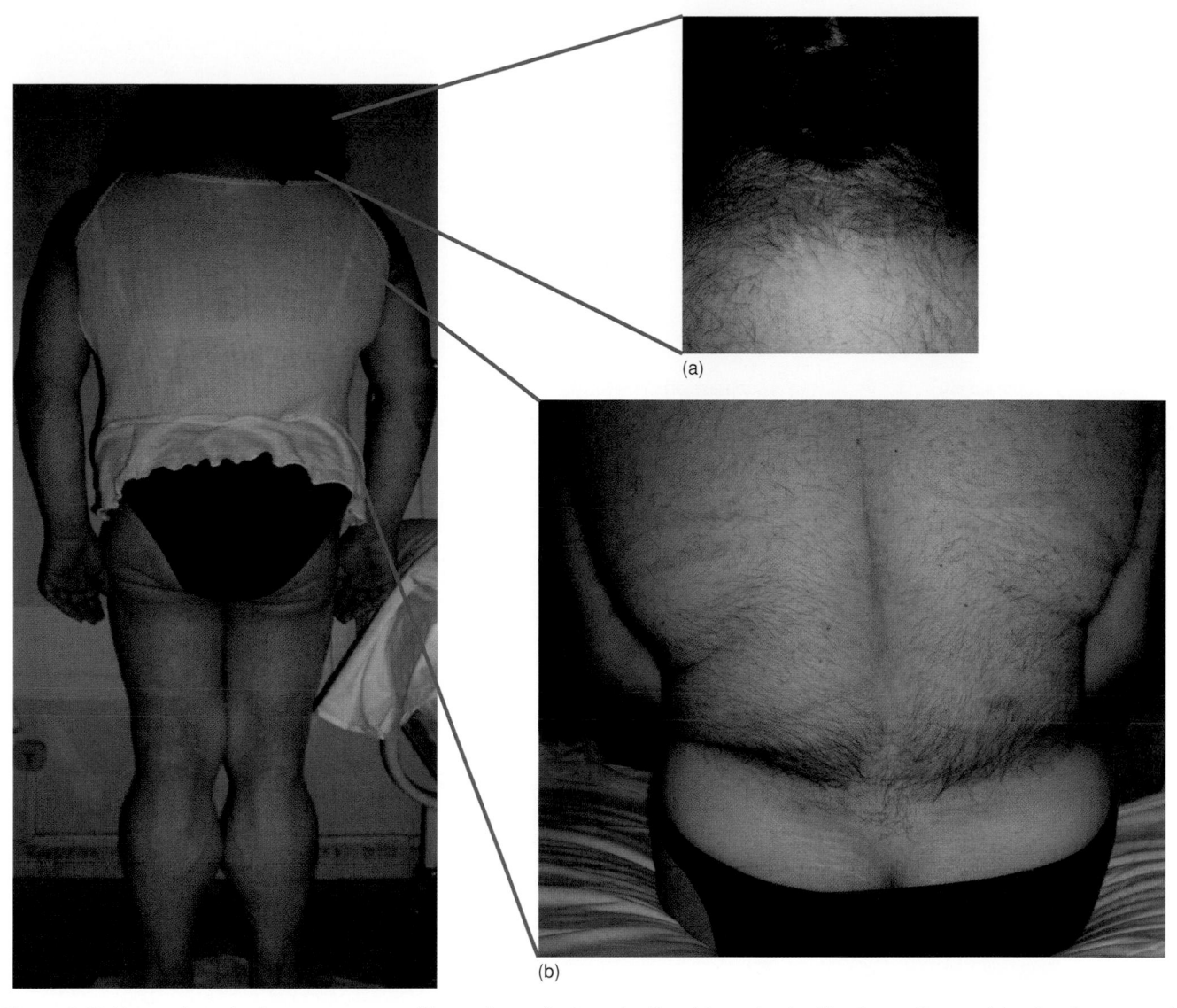

(a)

(b)

Figure 6.42 Hyperandrogenism in a young woman with a syndrome of extreme insulin resistance showing hirsutism on the nape (a) and on the upper and lower back (b). See also Fig. 6.41.

Polycystic ovary syndrome

Definition

Polycystic ovary syndrome (PCOS) is a common endocrine condition in women of reproductive age. It is associated with numerous reproductive disorders (hyperandrogenism, hirsutism, menstrual dysfunction, infertility, pregnancy complications), metabolic disorders (insulin resistance, impaired glucose tolerance, type 2 diabetes mellitus, adverse cardiovascular risk profiles), and psychological conditions (increased anxiety, depression and worsened quality of life). The syndrome was first described by Stein and Leventhal in 1935.

Etiology

Both the reproductive and metabolic features of PCOS are correlated with insulin resistance (IR).

The mechanisms of the impaired glucose utilization in PCOS remain largely unknown, but seem to involve a combination of an abnormal defective insulin response of insulin-sensitive tissues and inappropriate B-cell response to the increased demand.

Insulin resistance is a key factor in the etiology of PCOS, with excess insulin stimulating ovarian androgen production (potentiating luteinizing hormone [LH] effect on ovarian theca cells) and decreasing hepatic sex hormone-binding globulin (SHBG) production, thus possibly increasing the delivery of free androgens to target tissue. The excess in local ovarian androgen production may also cause premature follicular atresia and possibly contribute to anovulation.

Genetic, environmental, and other factors may be involved, including obesity, ovarian dysfunction, and hypothalamic pituitary abnormalities (rapid frequency of gonadotropin-releasing hormone [GnRH] pulses and an increase in the frequency and amplitude of LH pulses).

Insulin resistance is the only common finding in women with PCOS, independent of obesity.

Lean women with PCOS show PCOS-specific IR or intrinsic IR.

Signs and symptoms

The following are signs and symptoms of PCOS (Figs 6.43 & 6.44):

• *Menstrual disturbance*: Anovulation, amenorrhea, and oligomenorrhea.
• *Clinical hyperandrogenism*: Acne; seborrhea; androgenic alopecia; hirsutism (male-pattern excessive growth of terminal hair in women). The degree of hirsutism should be scored, e.g. with Ferriman–Gallwey score (see "Hyperandrogenism in women" section of this chapter).
• *Signs of IR*: Obesity or abdominal obesity; acanthosis nigricans (see "Acanthosis nigricans" section of Chapter 7).

Diagnosis

The European Society for Human Reproduction and Embryology/American Society for Reproductive Medicine Consensus Statement (*Fertil Steril* 2004;81:19 2004a, b) defines PCOS as two out of three of the following: oligo- and/or anovulation, or clinical and/or biochemical signs of hyperandrogenism, or polycystic ovaries (PCO) (Fig. 6.45) and the exclusion of other etiologies. The Androgen Excess Society position statement (*Clin Endocrinol Metab* 2006;91:4237) defines PCOS as hyperandrogenism (hirsutism and/or hyperandrogenemia) and ovarian dysfunction (oligo-anovulation and/or polycystic ovaries) and the exclusion of other androgen-excess related disorders. Other etiologies or related disorders refer to: congenital adrenal hyperplasia; androgen-secreting tumors; Cushing syndrome; 21-hydroxylase-deficient nonclassic adrenal hyperplasia; androgenic/anabolic drug use or abuse; syndromes of severe insulin resistance; thyroid dysfunction; or hyperprolactinemia.

Imaging tests

The main imaging tests are pelvic ultrasounds for ovarian morphology (Figs 6.43 & 6.44). Polycystic ovaries are defined as the presence of 12 or more follicles measuring 2–9 mm in each ovary and/or increased ovarian volume (> 10 mL or cm^3). Ultrasound criteria are nonspecific for diagnosis.

Laboratory findings

The endocrine and metabolic investigations for PCOS are:

• *Assessment of biochemical hyperandrogenism*: Total testosterone (free and bound to SHBG), free testosterone (measured by equilibrium dialysis), or calculated (free androgen index) and SHBG concentration.
• *Assessment of IR*: Abnormal hyperinsulinemic response to oral glucose tolerance test (OGTT) is specific in lean and obese women with PCOS.
• *Assessment of dyslipidemia*: Higher triglycerides and lower high density lipoprotein cholesterol (common in PCOS, independent of body mass index).
• *Assessment of pituitary–gonadal axis*: Some 75% of patients with PCOS have elevated mean serum LH levels.

Treatment

The treatment options for PCOS are:

• *Lifestyle changes*:
  ◦ Weight loss: Specific diet (high protein, low carbohydrate, and low glycemic index)
  ◦ Exercise
• *Pharmacological therapy*:
  ◦ Metformin (improves ovulation, menstrual cyclicity, and, potentially, hirsutism and IR).
  ◦ Combination therapy – if ≥ 6 months of Metformin is ineffective add oral contraceptive pill (OCP) $\pm$ antiandrogen or cyclic progestins.

∘ Metformin and the OCP are not approved specifically for PCOS by most regulatory authorities but are recommended by international and national endocrine societies and are evidence based.

• *Hirsutism treatment:*
  ∘ Cosmetic/laser therapy
  ∘ Eflornithine cream may induce a more rapid response
• *Infertility therapy*:
  ∘ Clomiphene, gonadotropins, and in-vitro fertilization

Illustrations (Figs 6.43–6.45)

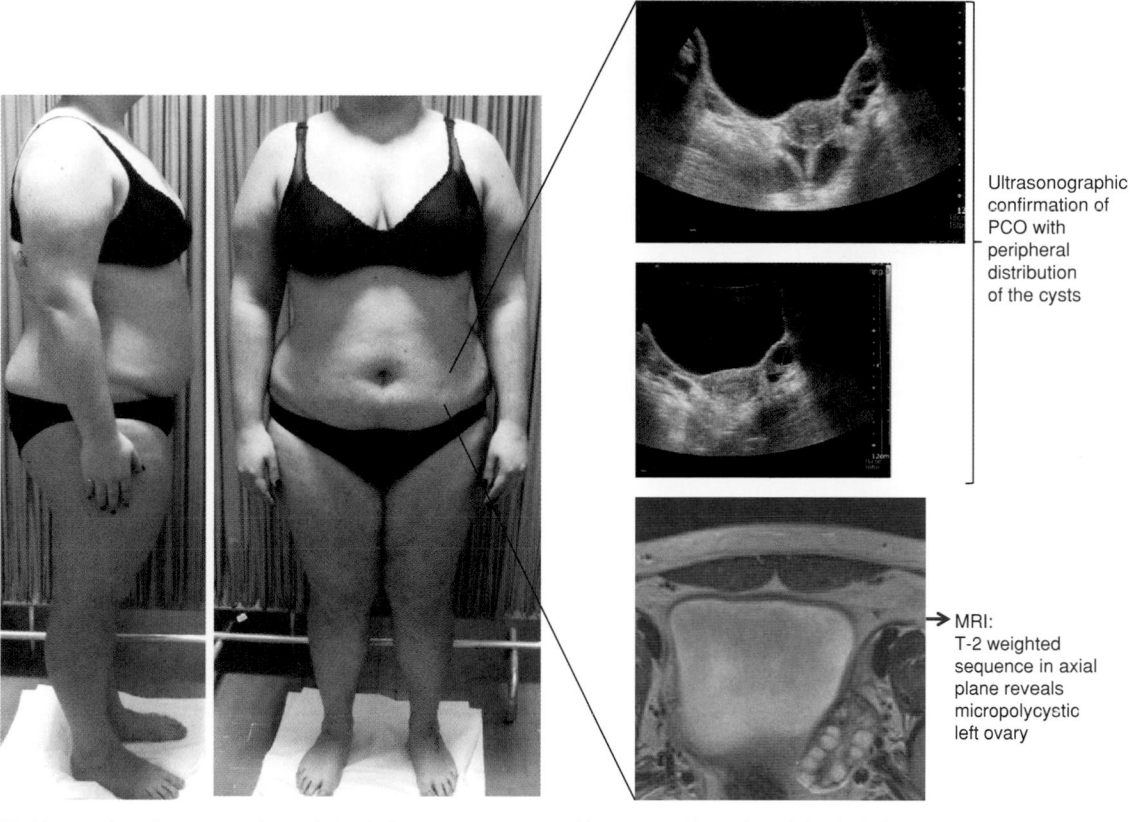

Ultrasonographic confirmation of PCO with peripheral distribution of the cysts

MRI: T-2 weighted sequence in axial plane reveals micropolycystic left ovary

Figure 6.43 Obese polycystic ovary syndrome (PCOS) phenotype. A 22-year-old woman with grade II abdominal obesity (body mass index = 36; waist circumference = 106 cm), insulin resistance, secondary amenorrhea, hyperandrogenism (Ferriman–Gallwey score = 19).

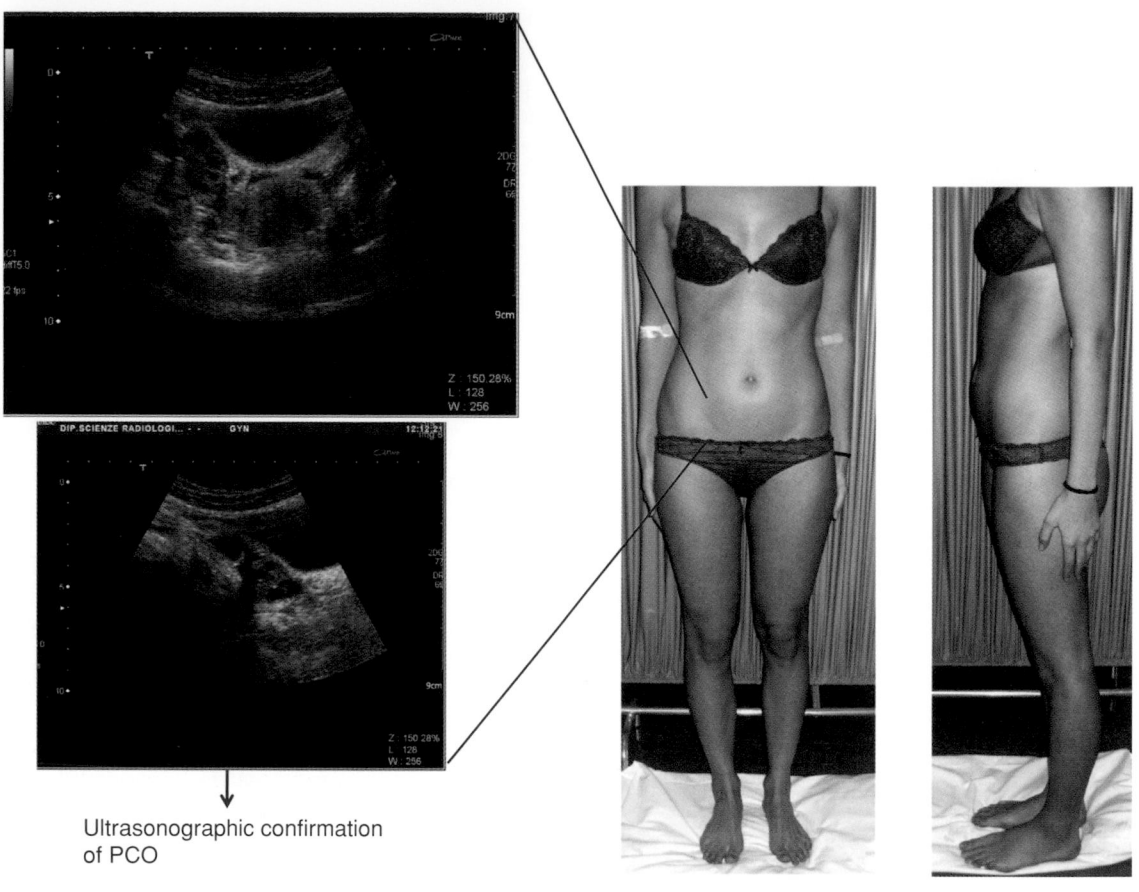

Ultrasonographic confirmation
of PCO

Figure 6.44 Lean polycystic ovary syndrome (PCOS) phenotype. A lean 23-year-old woman (body mass index = 21; waist circumference = 65 cm), with insulin resistance, secondary amenorrhea, acne, and without hyperandrogenism (Ferriman–Gallwey score = 6).

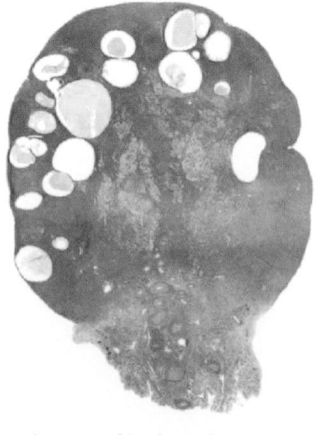

Figure 6.45 Polycystic ovary – histological appearance.

Turner syndrome

Definition

Turner syndrome is a condition causing sexual infantilism, webbed neck, and cubitus valgus that occurs in female patients with gonadal dysgenesis due to an X chromosomal abnormality. It was first described by Ullrich in 1930, featured by Turner in 1938, and recognized by Ullrich in 1945.

Etiology

The cause of Turner syndrome is the total or partial absence of one of the two X chromosomes in some or all of the body cells. The loss of an entire chromosome is observed in about 60% of the patients.

Turner syndrome is the result of a nondisjunction that occurs either before zygotic formation or in the first or second postzygotic division. If an X chromosome is lost by faulty distribution during later cell division, this results in 45,X/46,XX mosaicism. Partial X chromosome losses may also occur from either transverse division.

Signs and symptoms

The main characteristics are abnormal physical features, short stature, and gonadal dysgenesis. The prevalence for mental retardation is no greater than in the general population.

Abnormal physical features

Physical findings indicating Turner syndrome include:
• Short, thick, webbed neck
• Dysmorphic face (fishlike mouth, hypertelorism, epicanthus, ptosis of the eyelids, prominent ears, high-arched palate, micrognathia)
• Low posterior hairline
• Congenital lymphedema (puffy hands and feet at birth)
• Broad childlike chest
• Hypoplastic or inverted nipples
• Cubitus valgu
• Short fourth metacarpals
• Multiple pigmented nevi
• Abnormal fingernails
• Cardiovascular (aortic coarctation) and kidney abnormalities (horseshoe kidney)
• Delayed bone age and osteoporosis
• Auricular malformation, recurrent otitis media, loss of hearing function
• Intestinal telangiectasia, celiac disease, inflammatory bowel disease
• A tendency to keloid formation
• Increased frequency of chronic lymphocytic thyroiditis, diabetes mellitus, and rheumatoid arthritis

Short stature

Short stature is an almost constant finding with reduced length and weight at birth. Postnatal growth lies in the normal range for the first 2–3 years and then decreases. The reduced final height is mainly due to a lack of pubertal growth spurt. The ultimate mean height is below the third percentile (139–147 cm), but also depends on the parents' height. Body proportions are also altered (increased upper-to-lower segment ratio).

Gondal dysgenesis

Gondal dysgenesis leads to:
• Delayed puberty
• Primary amenorrhea
• Premature ovarian failure (in mosaic forms)
Spontaneous pregnancy is an exceptional event.

Variants

A variant is 45,X/46,XY mosaicism. This causes masculinization at birth (from clitoromegaly alone to ambiguous genitalia without palpable gonads).

Diagnosis

Gonadal dysgenesis should be suspected in all short girls with unexpected primary or secondary amenorrhea, and girls with lymphedema. Diagnosis is made by genetic confirmation of 46,X,r(X) or 45,X karyotype or 45,X/46,XX mosaicism (Fig. 6.46). The only disorder that has a similar overall picture is Noonan syndrome.

Imaging tests

Heart and kidney ultrasound tests are needed.

Laboratory findings

Laboratory testing involves:
• *Gonadotropin levels*: Plasma and urinary gonadotropins, particularly follicle-stimulating hormone (FSH), are unambiguously elevated during infancy, childhood, and > 10 years of age.
• *Growth hormone levels*: Growth hormone levels measured over 24 hours or during sleep are below normal from age 8.
• *Adrenal steroids*: Adrenal steroids are normal.
• *Thyroid hormones*: Thyroid hormones are usually normal, although subclinical thyroid dysfunction may be present.
• *IgA-antiendomysial antibodies (EMA)*: These are a good immunologic marker for use in screening for celiac disease.

Treatment

Treatment involves:
• *Growth*: Recombinant human growth hormone (rhGH, 0.60–1.82 IU/kg per week) in six or seven subcutaneous injections. Growth hormone therapy increases final height by a mean of about 5 cm and is indicated in shorter girls. Therapy should be initiated before 10 years of age.

- *Pubertal development*: Estrogen replacement for development of secondary sexual characteristics and menstruation.
- *Fertility*: The rare patients who are able to conceive should undergo prenatal diagnostic techniques. In sterile patients, artificial fertilization techniques may be used.

- *Osteoporosis*: Specific therapy is required. Long-term estrogen therapy does not prevent bone loss.
- *Heart or vascular anomalies*: Specific surgery may be required.
- *Pterygium colli*: Plastic reconstruction may be needed.
- *Pigmented nevi*: Sun exposure should be moderated.

Illustrations (Fig. 6.46)

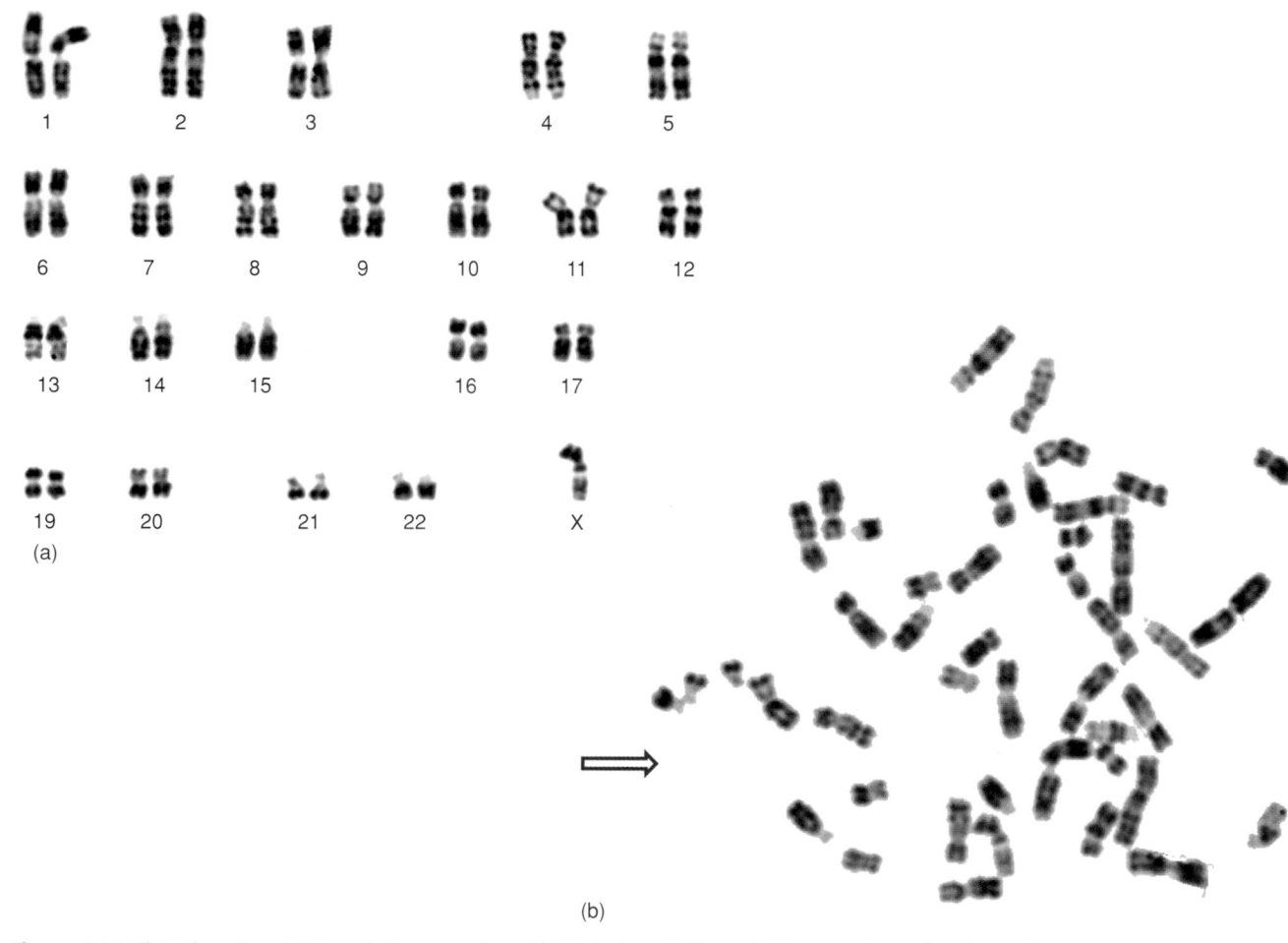

Figure 6.46 Classic karyotype 45,X seen in Turner syndrome (a). Metaphase 45,X seen in Turner syndrome (b, red arrow).

7 Mucocutaneous Manifestations of Endocrine Disorders

Acanthosis nigricans

Definition
Acanthosis nigricans is a hyperpigmented, hyperkeratotic skin lesion.

Etiology
Acanthosis nigricans is caused by factors that stimulate epidermal keratinocyte and dermal fibroblast proliferation.

Benign form
In the benign form the factors involved are marked hyperinsulinemia; defects in the genes involved in insulin signaling; activation of insulin-like growth factor 1 (IGF-1) factors due to high circulating levels of insulin; and stimulating glucose take-up by muscle tissue and epidermal cell propagation. Other suggested mediators include other tyrosine kinase receptors (epidermal growth factor receptor [EGFR] and fibroblast growth factor receptor [FGFR]).

Familial and syndromic forms
Signs generally include obesity, hyperinsulinemia, hyperandrogenism, and craniosynostosis. These forms have been further divided into insulin-resistance syndromes and fibroblast growth factor defects.

Insulin-resistance syndromes
Insulin-resistance syndromes are associated with mutations in the insulin receptor (leprechaunism, Rabson–Mendenhall syndrome); peroxisome proliferator-activated receptor gamma (type 1 diabetes with acanthosis nigricans and hypertension); 1-acylglycerol-3-phosphate O-acyltransferase-2 or seipin (Berardinelli–Seip syndrome); lamin A/C (Dunnigan syndrome); and the Alström syndrome gene.

Fibroblast growth factor defects
Fibroblast growth factor defects include activating mutations in *FGFR2* (Beare–Stevenson syndrome) and in *FGFR3* (Crouzon syndrome with acanthosis nigricans, thanatophoric dysplasia, severe achondroplasia with developmental delay, and acanthosis nigricans [SADDAN]).

In women with hyperandrogenism, most of whom have polycystic ovary syndrome (PCOS), acanthosis is found clinically in 5–30%, and may be much more common when assessed by skin biopsy.

Malignant acanthosis nigricans
In malignant acanthosis nigricans, stimulating factors secreted by or in response to the tumor are responsible for the condition. Transforming growth factor (TGF)-α has a similar structure to epidermal growth factor (EGF) and may well be involved. Both TGF-α and EGF have both been found in gastric adenocarcinoma cells, and EGFR expression has been found in skin cells within acanthosis nigricans lesions.

The malignant form is far less common, with only 2 in 12 000 cancer patients showing signs of acanthosis nigricans. It is most frequently associated with gastrointestinal adenocarcinomas (70–90%). About 18% of cases predate the diagnosis of malignancy.

Signs and symptoms
Acanthosis nigricans presents as symmetrical, hyperpigmented, hyperkeratotic velvety plaques (Fig. 7.1). These may be papillomatous in the most severe cases (Fig. 7.2). Acrochordona (skin tags) are common in the affected areas.

Lesions are most commonly found on the intertriginous areas of the axilla, groin, back of the neck, and over the elbow, but they may cover almost the entire skin surface. The palms, soles, and oral mucosa are not affected. Lesions begin as hyperpigmented macules and patches and progress to palpable plaques.

Imaging in Endocrinology, First Edition. Paolo Pozzilli, Andrea Lenzi, Bart L Clarke and William F Young Jr.
© 2014 John Wiley & Sons, Ltd. Published 2014 by John Wiley & Sons, Ltd.

Pruritus is occasionally reported and may be associated with a higher rate of malignant acanthosis nigricans. This form is clinically indistinguishable from benign acanthosis nigricans, although its onset has been described as abrupt and exuberant.

Diagnosis

Diagnosis may be made by:
• Clinical inspection
• Laboratory assessment of glucose/insulin metabolism via an androgen panel.
• Biopsy. The histologic signs comprise of hyperkeratosis, epidermal papillomatosis, and increased numbers of melanocytes.
The malignant form must be excluded.

Imaging tests

No imaging tests are needed except for ultrasound confirmation of PCOS in selected cases.

Laboratory findings

The following may be found:
• *In type B insulin resistance syndrome*: Low-normal or normal fasting glycemia associated with inappropriately elevated insulin levels (due to insulin receptor antibodies) with suppressed C-peptide and proinsulin.
• *In PCOS and insulin resistance syndrome*: Hyperinsulinemia.
• *In type A insulin resistance syndrome*: Glucose intolerance or overt diabetes and extreme resistance to endogenous and exogenous insulin associated with hyperandrogenism.

Treatment

Management of hyperglycemia and hyperinsulinemia is as follows:
• *In type B insulin resistance syndrome*: Metformin, immunosuppressant, and leptin.
• *In type A insulin resistance syndrome*: IGF-1.
• *In hyperinsulinemia with PCOS*: Low-fat diet, regular exercise, and metformin.
• *In lipodystrophic patients:* Thiazolidinediones.

Illustrations (Figs 7.1 & 7.2)

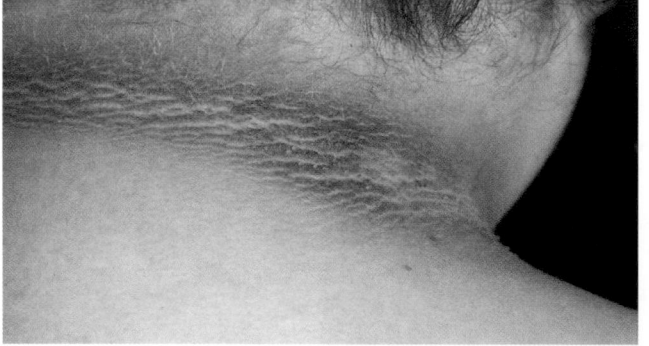

(a)

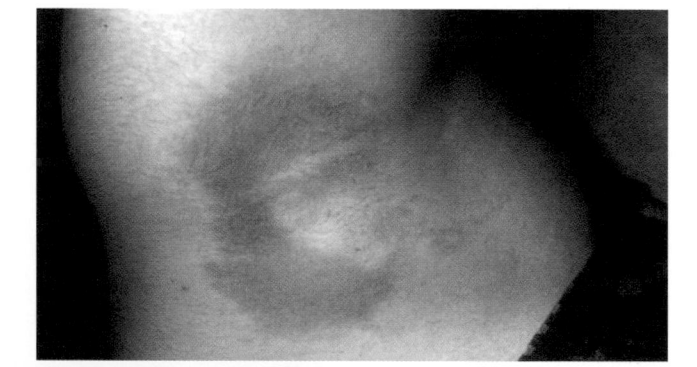

(b)

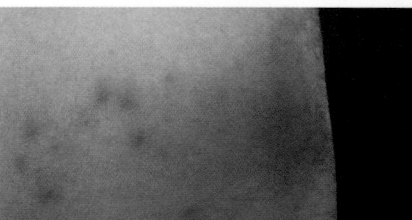

(c)

Figure 7.1 Acanthosis nigricans lesions on back of neck (a), axilla (b), and groin (c).

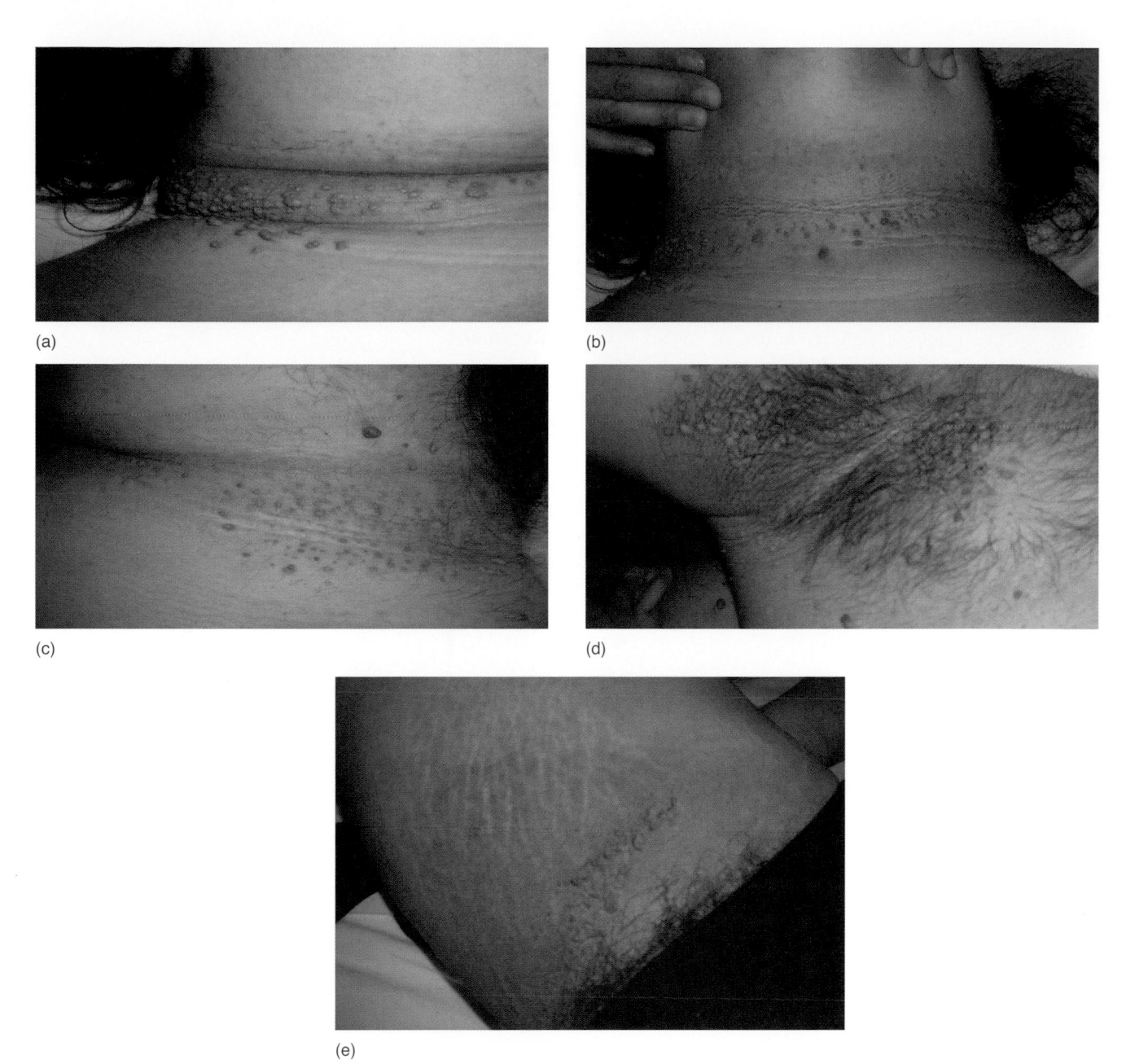

Figure 7.2 Papillomatous variant of acanthosis nigricans (a–e).

Acne

Definition

Acne is a skin disease affecting pilosebaceous units (PSUs) in which a changed keratinization pattern in the hair follicle leads to blockage of sebum secretion.

Etiology

Acne is a multifactorial disease. Genetic factors, stress, androgens, and excess sweating all affect its progression and severity.

Acne eruptions may be induced by:
- *Drugs*: Corticosteroids, oral contraceptives, iodides, bromides, lithium.
- *Chemicals:* Dioxins
- *Endocrine disorders:* Cushing syndrome, polycystic ovary syndrome (PCOS), congenital adrenal hyperplasia (CAH) (see Fig. 7.4), hyperandrogenism.

Hyperresponsiveness to androgen stimulation of sebocytes and follicular keratinocytes leads to the sebaceous gland hyperplasia and seborrhea typical of acne. *Propionibacterium acnes* colonizes the follicular duct and proliferates, contributing to the development of inflammation. Acne is worse in smokers. Cystic acne is more likely to be androgenic, while in idiopathic acne PSUs seem hypersensitive to normal free androgen levels in the blood.

Signs and symptoms

Acne presents as exposed pustules, papules, nodules, and cysts. Lesional polymorphism is the main feature (face, back, and chest). Distended PSUs may take the form of open (blackheads) or closed (whiteheads) comedones. In severe cases, inflammatory papules and nodules merge to form draining sinuses, leading to long-term scarring and, in rare cases, malignant changes.

Postinflammatory lesions may present as macular pigmentation and scars (hypertrophic, keloid scars, ice pick scars, depressed fibrotic, and atrophic macules, perifollicular elastolysis). Postinflammatory hyperpigmentation and seborrhea are common in pigmented skin.

Diagnosis

The severity of acne can be determined in various ways, but the Leeds Revised Acne Grading System (a numerical pictorial grading system) is the fastest, most accurate, and most reproducible.

The psychological impact should be assessed with tools such as the Assessment of the Psychological and Social Effects of Acne (APSEA) questionnaire or the Cardiff Acne Disability Index.

Imaging tests

No imaging tests are needed except in selected cases:
- *In PCOS*: Ultrasound confirmation.
- *In Cushing syndrome or CAH*: Adrenal computed tomography (CT) for diagnostic management.

Laboratory findings

Laboratory findings are as follows:
- *Assessment of pituitary–adrenal axis diseases*: Corticotropin (ACTH), cortisol, urinary free cortisol, and dexamethasone suppression test for adrenal secretion (Cushing syndrome). Baseline levels of 17-OH-P and its response to Synacthen test (CAH).
- *Assessment of biochemical hyperandrogenism*: Total (TT) and free testosterone (FT), dehydroepiandrosterone sulfate (DHEAS), androstenedione, dihydrotestosterone (DHT), and evaluation of androgen suppression in prolonged dexamethasone test (96 h). An increase in FT concentration is seen in half of the cases of persistent mild acne in adolescents.
- *Assessment of insulin resistance*: Abnormal hyperinsulinemic response to oral glucose tolerance test (OGTT) in PCOS.

Treatment

Treatment depends on the etiology and the degree of acne.

Etiology

- *In PCOS:* Combination estrogen–progestin (+ cosmetic and dermatologic management); drospirenone (a spironolactone analog) + ethinyl estradiol, to reduce androgen levels.
- *In CAH:* Glucocorticoids (prednisone 5–10 mg or dexamethasone 0.5 mg at bedtime) are more effective to treat excessive adrenal androgen.
- *In Cushing syndrome:* Ketoconazole (a synthetic imidazole antifungal agent) has a moderate beneficial effect on acne.
- *In hyperandrogenism:* Binding of androgens to the receptors is inhibited by cyproterone acetate in "reverse sequential" manner (50–100 mg daily from 5th to 15th day of the cycle + ethinyl estradiol 35–50 μg daily from 5th to 26th day of the cycle; spironolactone 100–200 mg daily + estrogen–progestin).

Degree (Figs 7.3 & 7.4)

Mild
- *Topical agents*: Benzoyl peroxide, azelaic acid, retinoids, tretinoin, adapalene.
- *Topical antibiotics*: Clindamycin, tetracycline, erythromycin.
- Or *combined therapies*.

Moderate

• *Oral antibiotics*: Oxytetracycline, erythromycin, minocycline, doxycycline, lymecycline; trimethoprim.
• *Hormone therapy*

Severe

• *Isotretinoin:* A retinoid related to retinol (vitamin A): can lead to permanent remission.

• *Atrophic scarring:* Laser resurfacing, dermal collagen injection, antilogous fat implants.
• *Hypertrophic scarring*: Chemical peels, microdermabrasion, topical corticosteroid cream, intralesional triamcinolone injection, excision, cryotherapy, application of silicone gels.

Illustrations (Figs 7.3 & 7.4)

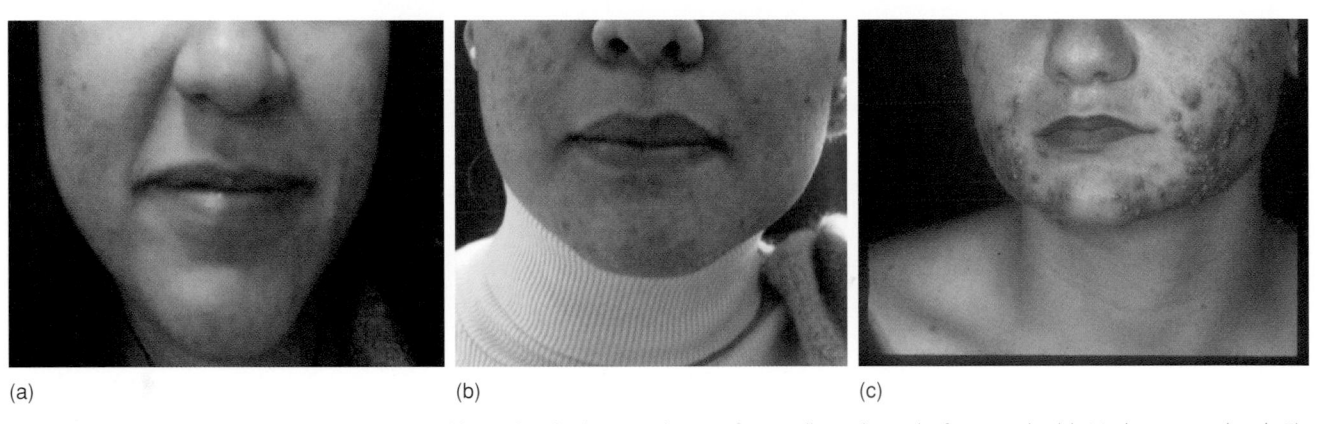

(a)   (b)   (c)

Figure 7.3 Leeds Revised Acne Grading System. Mild acne (grade 2) – comedones, a few small papules and a few pustoles (a). Moderate acne (grade 7) – numerous comedones, small inflammatory papules, numerous pustoles (b). Severe acne (grade 12) – numerous comedones, deeper papules and pustoles, deep and large lesions, cysts, and abscesses (c). Adapted from the Grading System of Lenzi, Isidori, & Giannetta.

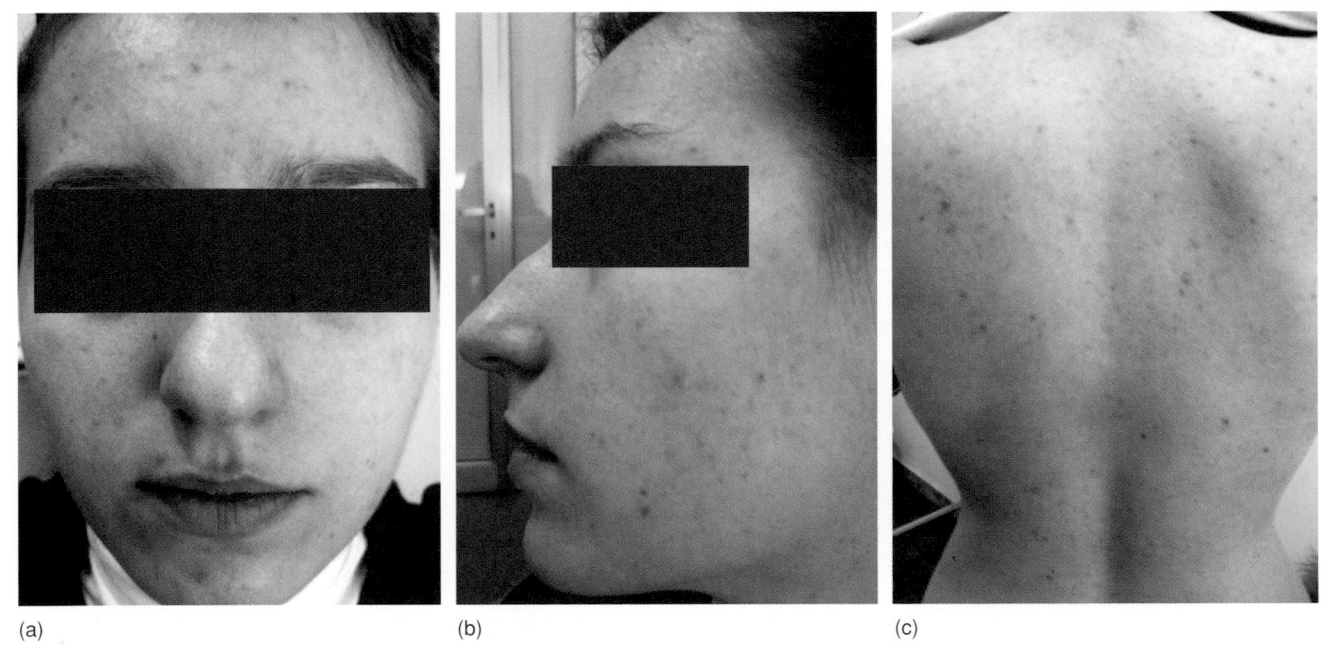

(a)   (b)   (c)

Figure 7.4 A 22-year-old woman with congenital adrenal hyperplasia (CAH) who had mild acne as a unique sign on face (a & b) and on back (c).

Alopecia

Definition

Androgenic alopecia

In men, androgenic alopecia is the gradual replacement of long, pigmented, terminal hairs on the scalp by short, pale, vellus hairs. In women, it is the progressive diffuse loss of hair from the crown with retention of frontal hair line.

Alopecia areata

Alopecia areata is a disease of the hair follicles in the anagen (active growth) phase, characterized by patchy or more generalized hair loss, up to complete loss of scalp hair (*alopecia totalis*).

Etiology

Androgenic alopecia (Fig. 7.5)

In androgenic alopecia, androgens gradually inhibit hair growth on the scalp in genetically predisposed individuals, boosting the intrinsic response of individual follicles.

There is often a family history of androgenic alopecia. Genetic involvement includes a shorter CAG triplet repeat length, mutations of one allele of the steroid metabolism gene *CYP17*, and the X-linked gene for adrenoleukodystrophy. Stress and anxiety are also involved as they increase adrenaline levels and peripheral vasoconstriction, reducing oxygen and nutrients supplied to hair follicles.

In women, androgenic alopecia is also associated with polycystic ovary syndrome (PCOS), hirsutism, and hyperandrogenism.

Alopecia areata (Table 7.1)

The etiology of alopecia areata involves an autoimmune origin plus genetic involvement in autoimmune polyglandular syndromes (APS). In children, alopecia totalis is associated with hereditary vitamin D-resistant rickets (HVDRR).

Signs and symptoms

Androgenic alopecia (Fig. 7.5a–c)

In men, progressive regression of the hair is seen, spreading backwards to join the thinning region on the vertex, resulting in a bald crown.

In women, the front hairline is normally retained; instead, general thinning on the vertex progresses gradually until the vertex becomes bald. Women may also have hirsutism, with or without menstrual abnormalities.

Alopecia areata (Fig. 7.5d)

Table 7.1 lists the signs and symptoms associated with alopecia areata. In addition, HVDRR is associated with total scalp and body alopecia; bone pain; muscle weakness; hypotonia; occasional convulsions; retarded growth; and hypoplasia of the teeth.

Diagnosis

Androgenic alopecia

In men, diagnosis of androgenic alopecia is made based on Hamilton's Grading Scale (modified by Norwood) (Fig. 7.6a). In women, diagnosis is made based on Ludwig pattern stages (Fig. 7.6b).

Alopecia areata

Diagnosis of alopecia areata is made by clinical features, a serologic test for autoantibodies, a function test for the secretion of organ-specific hormones, and genetic tests for mutations in *AIRE* and *HLA-D* genes.

Imaging tests

Imaging tests are needed in selected cases:
• Computed tomography (CT) scan or magnetic resonance imaging (MRI) to provide confirmation of an androgen-secreting tumor.

Table 7.1 Diseases, disorders, and syndromes associated with alopecia areata

APS 1	APS 2-a	APS 2-b	%
Hypoparathyroidism	Adrenocortical insufficiency	Thyroiditis, type 1 diabetes mellitus, pernicious anemia, vitiligo (NSV)	> 40
Malabsorption, *alopecia totalis*, pernicious anemia (juvenile onset), thyroditis chronic, active hepatitis, mucocutaneous candidiasis, adrenocortical insufficiency, ungual dystrophy, enamel hypoplasia, hypogonadism	Thyroiditis Type 1 diabetes mellitus		10–40
Vitiligo Sjögren's syndrome Anterior hypophysitis Type 1 diabetes mellitus	Hypogonadism vitiligo (NSV), alopecia, pernicious anemia (adult onset), myasthenia gravis, celiac disease, rheumatoid arthritis, Sjögren syndrome	Hypogonadism, alopecia (adult onset), myasthenia gravis, celiac disease, rheumatoid arthritis, Sjögren syndrome	< 10

APS, autoimmune polyglandular syndrome.

- Ultrasonography to provide confirmation of PCOS.
- Specific imaging tests for organ-specific disease in APS.
- Tests, if needed, for radiologic features of rickets.

Laboratory findings

Androgenic alopecia
In men:
- Testing would find normal male testosterone (TT) and raised free testosterone (FT), but elevated urinary dehydroepiandrosterone sulfate (DHEAS).
- Normal male androgen levels are sufficient to produce androgenic alopecia in relation to the intrinsic response of the follicles.

In women:
- Assessment of biochemical hyperandrogenism: TT, FT, DHEAS, androstenedione, DHT, and suppression of androgens on prolonged dexamethasone test (96 h).
- Assessment of PCOS.

Alopecia areata
- Assessment of humoral autoimmunity. Autoantibodies against steroidal cell autoantibodies (SCAb); parathyroid; pancreatic beta-cell autoantibodies (AbGAD, AbIA2, AbICA); thyroid (AbTPO, AbTg); transglutaminase, and gliadin; gastric parietal cell; melanocytes; tyrosinase; acetylcholine receptors.

- Assessment of electrolyte levels.
- Assessment of pituitary–adrenal, pituitary–thyroid, pituitary–gonadal axis, and parathyroid function. In HVDRR: normal 25(OH)D, low 24,25(OH)2D, and elevated 1,25(OH)2D serum values.

Treatment

Androgenic alopecia
For androgenic alopecia, the treatment options are:
- *Surgery*: Follicle transplant.
- *Antiandrogens in postmenopausal women:* (a) Cyproterone acetate 50–100 mg/day + estrogen; spironolactone; or (b) 5α-reductase inhibitors.
- *Antiandrogens in premenopausal women:* Finasteride 1 mg/day orally + oral contraceptives to avoid hypospadias in a male fetus.
- *Antiandrogens in men:* Finasteride 1 mg/day orally.
- *Nonhormonal therapy:* Minoxidil (vasodilator) applied topically.

Alopecia areata
For alopecia areata, the treatment option is exogenous glucocorticoid supplements. Given for Addison's disease, these may ameliorate alopecia. Note that alopecia persists in HVDRR despite the treatment of rickets.

Illustrations (Figs 7.5 & 7.6)

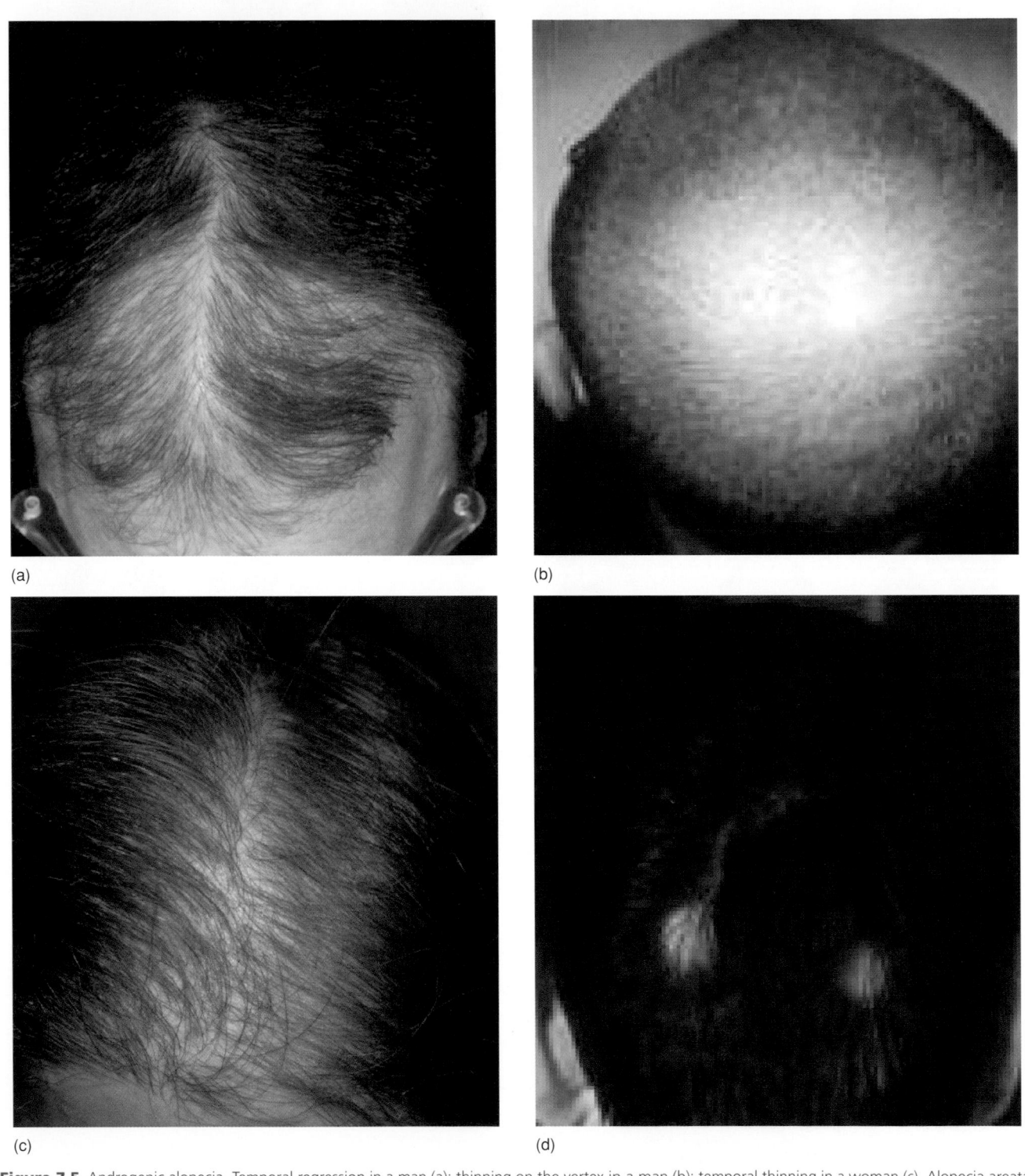

(a)

(b)

(c)

(d)

Figure 7.5 Androgenic alopecia. Temporal regression in a man (a); thinning on the vertex in a man (b); temporal thinning in a woman (c). Alopecia areata in a young man with APS2-b (d).

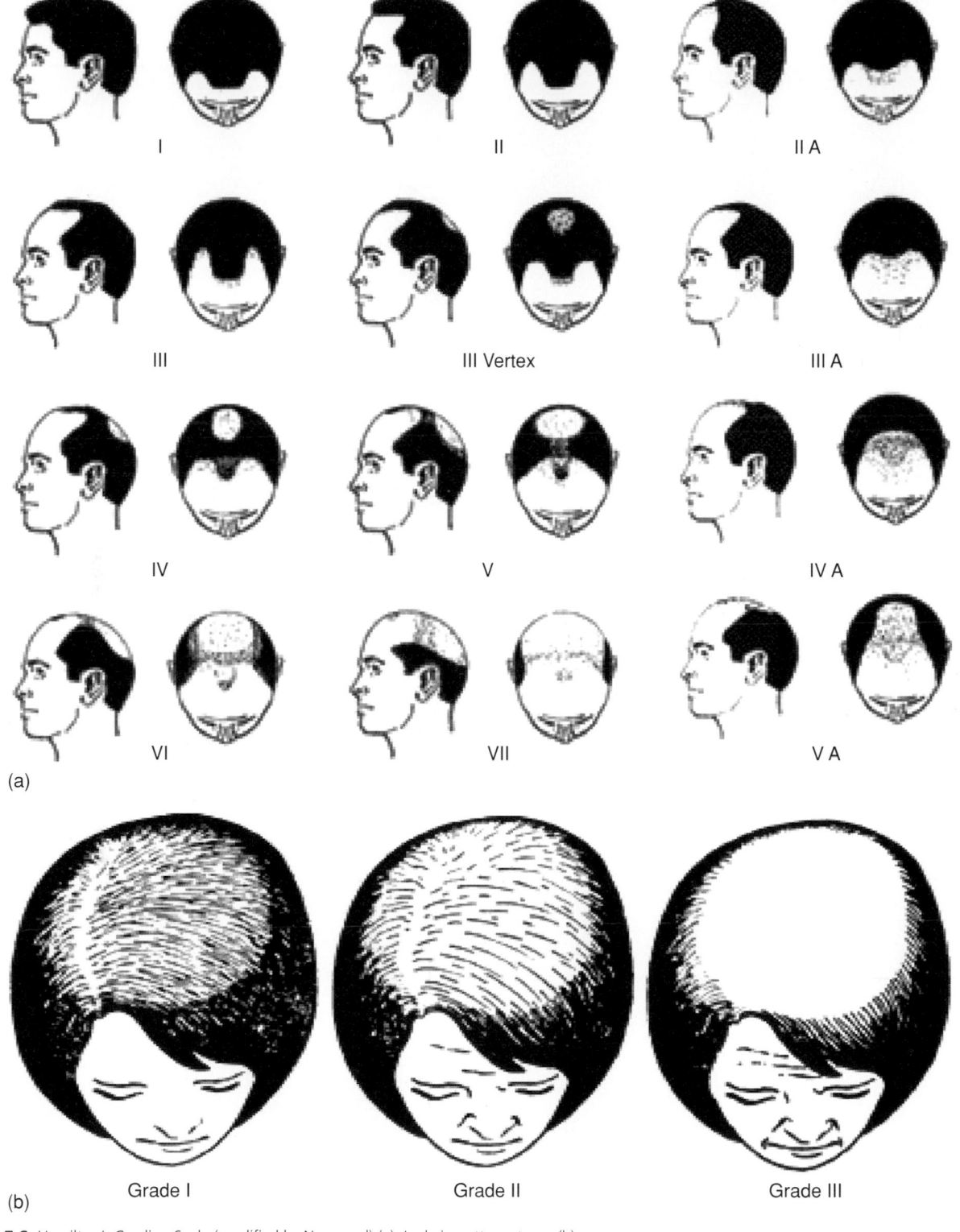

(a)

(b)

Figure 7.6 Hamilton's Grading Scale (modified by Norwood) (a). Ludwig pattern stages (b).

Café-au-lait macules

Definition

Café-au-lait macules (CALMS) are flat, uniformly hyperpigmented, oval macules with a regular or irregular border. They appear during the first year after birth and usually increase in number during childhood.

Etiology

Twenty-five percent of the normal population have 1–3 CALMS. Café-au-lait macules are found in many multimalformation syndromes:

• *Neurofibromatosis type 1* (NF-1 or von Recklinghausen's disease). This is an autosomal dominant genetic disorder with the genotype 17q11.2.

• *Neurofibromatosis type 2* (NF-2). This is an autosomal dominant disorder predisposing to multiple neoplastic lesions with the genotype 22q12.2.

• *McCune–Albright syndrome (MAS)*. This is a sporadic disease due to somatic activating mutations in the gene (*GNAS1*) encoding a subunit of the trimeric guanosine triphosphate-binding protein (Gsa) that stimulates adenylyl cyclase.

• *Biallelic mutations in all mismatch repair genes*. These mutations are due to a biparental inheritance of *PMS2* mutations.

• *Multiple endocrine neoplasia type 1* (MEN-1). This is an autosomal dominant syndrome due to heterozygous mutations on 11q13.

• *Carney complex*. This is an autosomal dominant inheritance syndrome with incomplete penetrance in those with *PRKAR1A* mutations.

Signs and symptoms

Distribution of CALMS (Fig. 7.7a)

Café-au-lait macules may appear on the forehead, neck area, trunk and buttocks, and along the lines of Blaschko. Spotty pigmentation may also occur around the mouth.

Neurofibromatosis CALMS: presentation and appearance (Fig. 7.7b)

In neurofibromatosis, CALMS present as pale brown macules 0.5–20.0 cm in size, found on any cutaneous surface (especially on the trunk). Borders are smooth and regular (i.e. "coast of California"). Macules appear in childhood.

McCune–Albright syndrome CALMS: presentation and appearance (Fig. 7.7c)

In McCune–Albright syndrome, CALMS have a more irregular border (i.e. "coast of Maine") than in neurofibromatosis. Macules may not be conspicuous in childhood. They usually do not cross the midline, are usually on the same side as the main bone lesions, and have a segmental distribution.

Associations

Neurofibromatosis associations
Associations with NF-1:

• *Tumors*: Optic gliomas; meningiomas; astrocytomas.

• *Skin lesions*: CALMS; neurofibromas; freckling in axilla or groin.

• *Risk of developing*: Rhabdomyosarcoma; pheochromocytoma; duodenal carcinoid; neurofibrosarcoma and glioma; Lisch nodules on eyes; pseudoarthrosis tibia; macrocephaly.

Associations with NF-2:

• *Tumors*: Vestibular schwannoma; acoustic neuroma.

   ◦ *Skin lesions*: Occasional CALMS; neurofibromas; pigmented plaques; subcutaneous peripheral nerve swellings; cutaneous schwannomas.

   ◦ *Risk of developing*: Glioma; meningioma; juvenile cataracts; juvenile subcapsular lenticular opacities.

Associations with NF-6:

• No neurofibromas, only CALMS, occurring in two generations.

Other associations

• *McCune–Albright syndrome*: CALMS; polyostotic fibrous dysplasia; sexual precocity; hyperfunction of multiple endocrine glands.

• *Biallelic mutations in all mismatch repair genes*: Colon, hematologic, and central nervous system tumors, and/or neurofibromatosis-like signs.

• *Multiple endocrine neoplasia type 1*: Pituitary gland, pancreas, and parathyroid gland tumors; peptic ulcer disease; facial angiofibromas; collagenomas; CALMS; subcutaneous lipoma.

• *Carney complex*: Primary pigmented nodular adrenal dysplasia; testicular tumors, pituitary and ovarian lesions; neuroendocrine lesions; spotty pigmentation (liver spots, freckles, blue nevi, CALMS and junctional, atypical, or compound nevi); psammomatous melanotic schwannoma; osteochondromyxoma.

Diagnosis

Neurofibromatosis type 1

For diagnosis of NF-1 at least two of the following clinical features are required (NIH Consensus Statement. *Arch Neurol Chicago* 1988;45:575):

• Six or more CALMS > 5 mm in prepubertal and > 15 mm in postpubertal individuals.

• Two or more neurofibromas or any type 1 plexiform neurofibroma.

• Freckling in the axillary or inguinal regions.

• Optic glioma.

• Two or more Lisch nodules (iris hamartomas).

• A distinctive bony lesion such as sphenoid dysplasia or thinning of the long bone cortex with or without pseudoarthrosis.
• A first-degree relative (parent, sibling, or offspring) with NF-1 based upon the above criteria.

Multimalformation syndromes

Genetic testing is needed to diagnose multimalformation syndromes. Skin biopsy may also be required to diagnose epidermal hypermelanosis with rare macromelanosomes.

Imaging tests

Imaging tests may be needed for associated organ-specific diseases.

Laboratory findings

• *McCune–Albright syndrome:* Elevated serum estradiol and prepubertal luteinizing hormone (LH) response to LH-releasing hormone (LHRH), consistent with LHRH–independent puberty. Free triiodothyronine (FT$_3$) and free thyroxine (FT$_4$) and cortisol may also be raised.
• *Multiple endocrine neoplasia type 1:* Hyperparathyroidism; elevated levels of gastrin, insulin, glucagon, vasoactive intestinal peptide (VIP), pancreatic polypeptide (PP), and somatostatin; hyperprolactinemia or elevated levels of growth hormone (GH), corticotropin (ACTH); hypopituitarism; hypercortisolemia; hyperaldosteronism.

Treatment

Treatment consists of laser therapy in selected cases.

Illustration (Fig. 7.7)

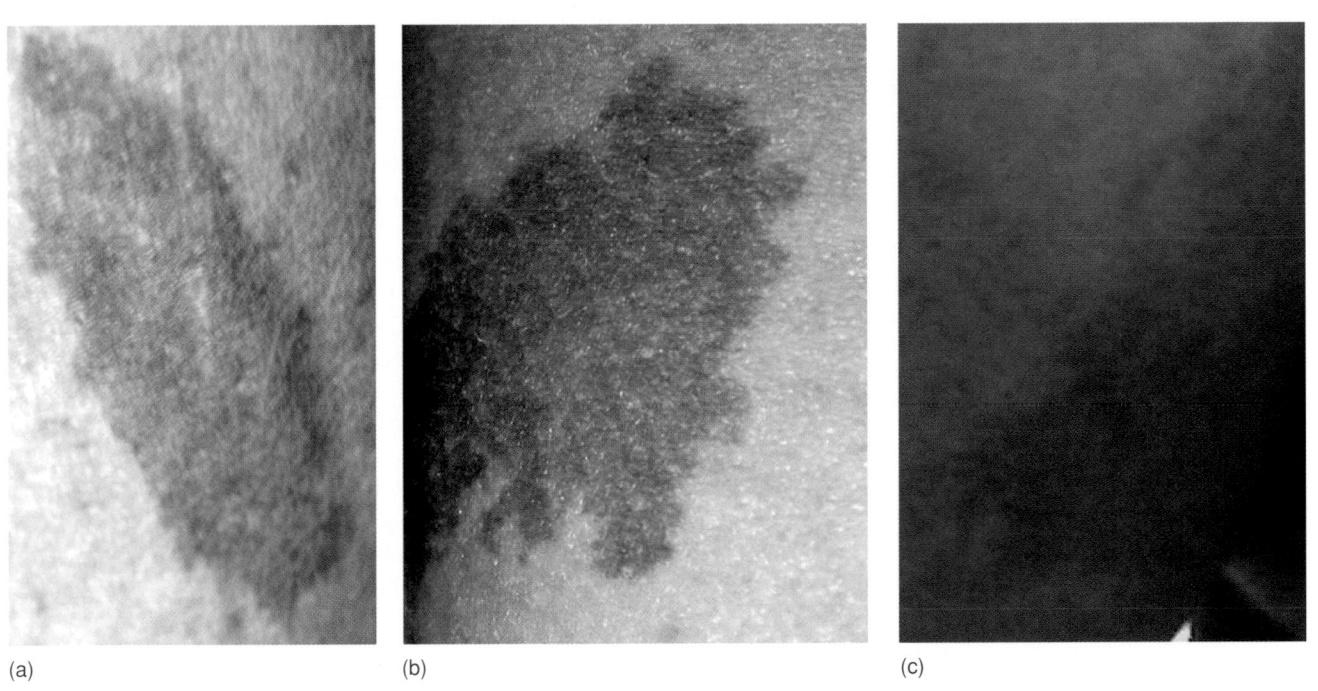

(a)   (b)   (c)

Figure 7.7 Café-au-lait spots. A café-au-lait macule present since birth on a healthy young woman – regular borders, no changes in size or number (a). A café-au-lait macule in neurofibromatosis with smooth regular borders ("coast of California") (b). A café-au-lait macule in McCune–Albright syndrome with irregular border ("coast of Maine") (c).

Mucocutaneous neuromas

Definition
Mucocutaneous neuromas are benign nerve sheath tumors, including mucosal neuromas (localized on the tongue, lips, inside of cheeks, palate, and gums – but also the conjunctiva, cornea, and pharyngolarynx) and cutaneous neuromas (on the face and, less often, on the trunk).

Etiology
Usually considered typical of multiple endocrine neoplasia type 2B (MEN-2B; Wagenmann–Froboese syndrome), mucocutaneous neuromas are a rare autosomal dominant neurocristopathy. In most cases, genetic analysis has shown a germline mutation at codon 918 in exons 15 and 16 of the RET proto-oncogene (10q11.2).

Signs and symptoms
Mucosal and cutaneous neuromas are usually nonpigmented dome-shaped or pedunculated papules measuring from a few millimeters to 1 cm in diameter.

Multiple mucosal neuromas involve all mucosal surfaces and are considered to be a pathognomonic feature observed in almost 100% of patients with MEN-2B. They are present at birth or appear during early childhood and are usually painless and associated with pruritis from infancy. They are also present throughout the gastrointestinal tract. Isolated mucosal neuromas may also occur in MEN-2B.

Cutaneous neuromas are covered by normal skin. Cutaneous lesions are characterized first by pain, like an electric shock, sometimes triggered by rubbing of clothes, before involvement of the skin. A few months later, a red brown papule of 2 ± 5 mm in diameter may appear at the painful site (Figs 7.8 & 7.9).

Both mucosal and cutaneous neuromas are associated with characteristic phenotypic features, including a marfanoid body habitus, coarse facial features, developmental delay, connective tissue abnormalities, muscle wasting, and alimentary tract ganglioneuromatosis. Flushing attacks occur as a result of the pheochromocytoma.

Cutaneous lichen amyloidosis precedes medullary thyroid cancer, which is very aggressive with early metastases.

The most frequent distribution is on the eyelids and/or cornea.

Diagnosis
Clinical features
Clinical features of mucocutaneous neuromas are:
- Characteristics of MEN-2B – medullary thyroid cancer and pheochromocytoma.
- Genetic tests showing *RET* gene mutations (10q11.2).
- Skin biopsies showing well-demarcated, fasciculated lobular dermal nodules without fibrosis and an inflammatory cellular infiltrate, with an increasing number and size of well-circumscribed clusters of small dermal nerves without surrounding inflammation, corresponding to a typical neuroma. No stroma abnormality.
- Immunohistochemical staining confirming both a positive diagnosis for S100 protein and neurofilament and a negative diagnosis for smooth muscle actin.

Imaging tests
Imaging tests for organ-specific diseases may be needed:
- Neck and abdominal ultrasound
- Chest X-ray
- Adrenal computed tomography (CT) scan or magnetic resonance imaging (MRI)
- ^{123}I metaiodobenzylguanidine (MIBG) scintigraphy and Octreoscan study

Laboratory findings
Routine laboratory data are normal but the following evaluations help diagnose mucocutaneous neuromas:
- *Electrolytes and endocrine evaluations:* Serum calcium may be low-normal/normal. Serum phosphate, thyroid function tests, may be normal.
- *Marker evaluations:* Serum calcitonin (before and after pentagastrin challenge) may be indicative of medullary thyroid carcinoma and negative in early stage of the disease. Carcinoembryonic antigen may be increased. Serum and urinary markers for pheochromocytoma may be positive or negative in early stage of the disease.

Treatment
Treatment is by surgical excision of main lesions.

Illustrations (Figs 7.8 & 7.9)

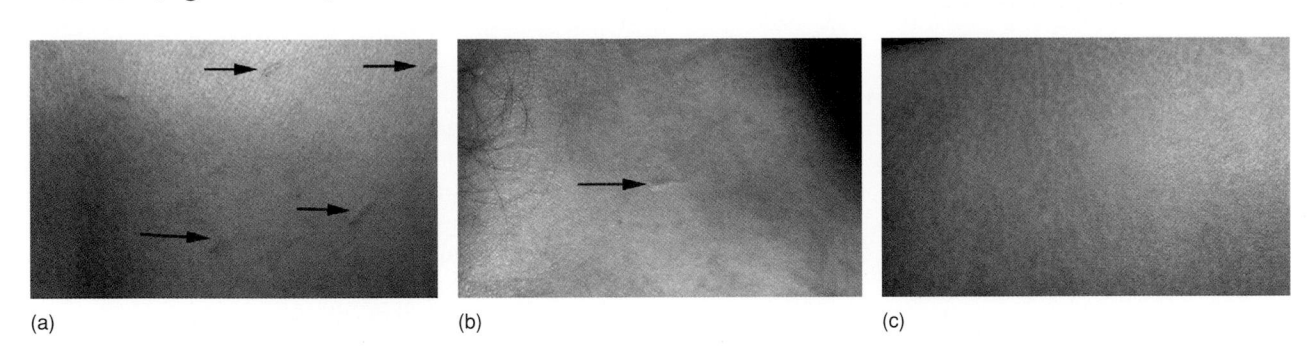

(a)   (b)   (c)

Figure 7.8 Cutaneous neuromas distributed throughout trunk (a, arrows). Note linear configuration of cutaneous neuromas on arms and neck (b, arrow). Pigmented lesions of rippled pattern on interscapular region (c).

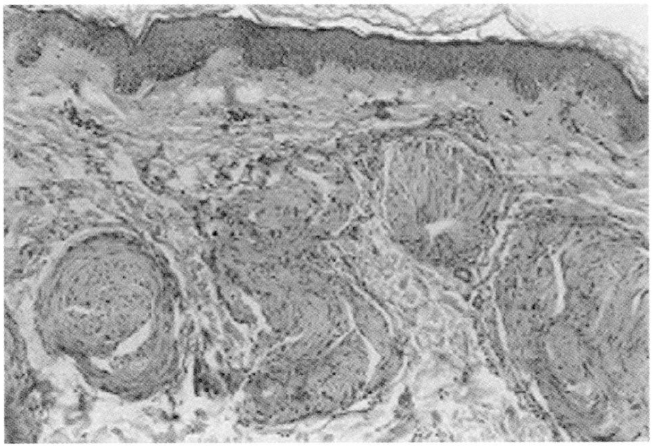

(a)

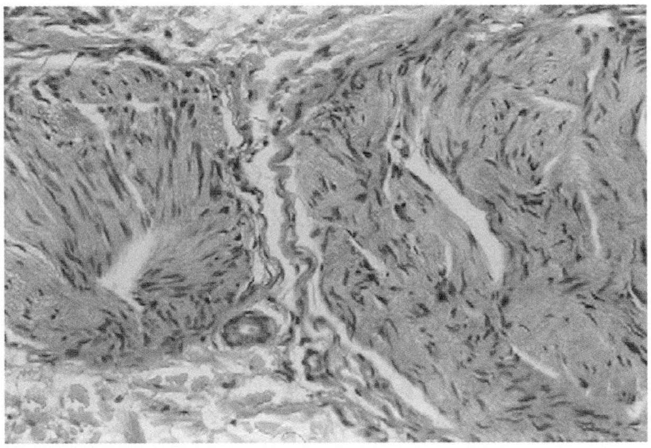

(b)

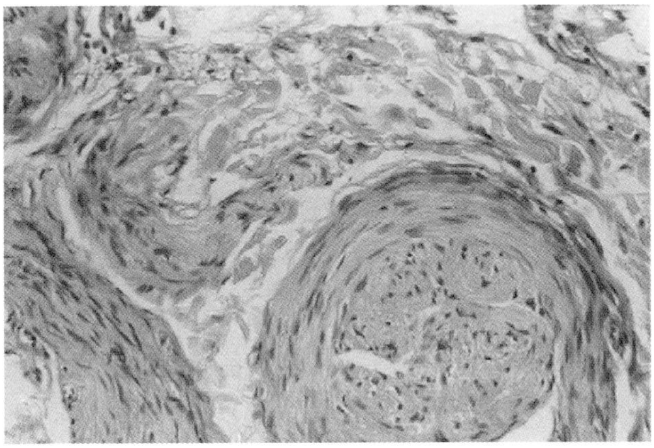

(c)

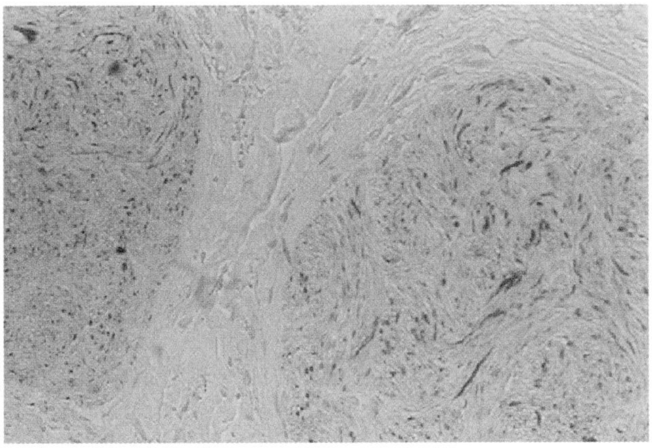

(d)

Figure 7.9 Cutanous neuromas. Panoramic view of thick, tortuous nerve bundles in papillary and mid dermis (a). Longitudinally sectioned thick bundles initiate tiny nodules when cross-sectioned (b). Fascicles composed of slender spindle cells, on cross-section appear as tiny round clear spaces – a clue to their axonal content (c). Abundant axonal content demonstrated by antineurofilament antibody staining (d). (a–c, hematoxylin stain; a–d, original magnification × 100.) Courtesy of Baykal C, Buyukbabani N, Boztepe H, Barahmani N, Yazganoglu KD. (2007) Multiple cutaneous neuromas and macular amyloidosis associated with medullary thyroid carcinoma. *Journal of American Academy of Dermatology* **56**(2): 533–7. Copyright (2010), with permission from Elsevier.

Necrolytic migratory erythema

Definition
Necrolytic migratory erythema (NME) is a paraneoplastic manifestation of glucagonoma syndrome (GS). It presents as a plaque skin disease and was first described by Becker and colleagues in 1942.

Etiology
The cause of the rash is unknown, but direct action of glucagon on the skin, amino acid deficiency, fatty acid deficiency, and zinc deficiency have all been proposed as possible causes.

Signs and symptoms
The skin eruptions present as erythematous erosive patches, papules, scabs, and pigment deposition. The lesions increase in number and size but undergo spontaneous remissions leaving areas of hyperpigmentation, as well as exacerbations and recurrences at another site, without identifiable precipitating factors. The lesions usually start at the groin and perineum and migrate to the distal extremities (Fig. 7.10). The mucosal membranes may be involved (stomatitis, cheilitis, and/or glossitis).

Symptoms of GS include progressive weight loss, diarrhea, vein thrombosis, pulmonary embolism, nail dystrophy, neuropsychiatric symptoms, and other paraneoplastic syndromes (optic atrophy).

When GS is associated with multiple endocrine neoplasia type 1 (MEN-1), signs and symptoms related to other tumors are involved: parathyroids, pancreatic islets (gastrinoma with Zollinger–Ellison syndrome, insulinoma, VIPoma), anterior pituitary (prolactinoma, somatotrophinoma, corticotrophinoma, nonfunctioning), and associated tumors (adrenal cortical, carcinoid, lipoma, facial angiofibromas and collagenomas, thyroid cancer).

Diagnosis

Clinical features
Clinical features of NME are:
• Characteristic triad of GS – pancreatic tumor secreting glucagon, diabetes mellitus (DM), and NME.
• Genetic tests showing mutations of *MENIN* and *MEN1* genes (ch. 11q13).
Skin biopsies are nondiagnostic. Necrolysis of the upper third of the epidermis with vacuolated keratinocytes, leading to focal or confluent necrosis, is similar to biopsy findings with pellagra, zinc deficiency, and necrolytic acral erythema (Fig. 7.10).

Imaging tests
The following imaging tests are needed:
• Specific imaging tests for organ-specific disease in MEN-1.

• Ultrasonography, computed tomography (CT) scan, and magnetic resonance imaging (MRI) to confirm tumor.
• Somatostatin receptor scintigraphy to diagnose metastatic disease.

Laboratory findings

Endocrine and metabolic tests
• Elevated plasma glucagon levels (10–20 times)
• Impaired glucose tolerance
• Mild diabetes
• Normocytic normochromic anemia

In association with MEN-1
• *Hyperparathyroidism*: Increased parathyroid hormone (PTH) levels, symptomatic hypercalcemia.
• *Pancreatic tumors*: Elevated levels of gastrin, insulin, glucagon, vasoactive intestinal peptide (VIP), pancreatic polypeptide (PP), somatostatin.
• *Pituitary tumors*: Hyperprolactinemia, elevated levels of growth hormone (GH), corticotropin (ACTH), or hypopituitarism.
• *Adrenocortical tumors*: Hypercortisolemia and hyperaldosteronism.

Treatment
Necrolytic migratory erythema responds to somatostatin analog therapy, oral and topical zinc, and surgical excision of localized solitary tumor.

Illustration (Fig. 7.10)

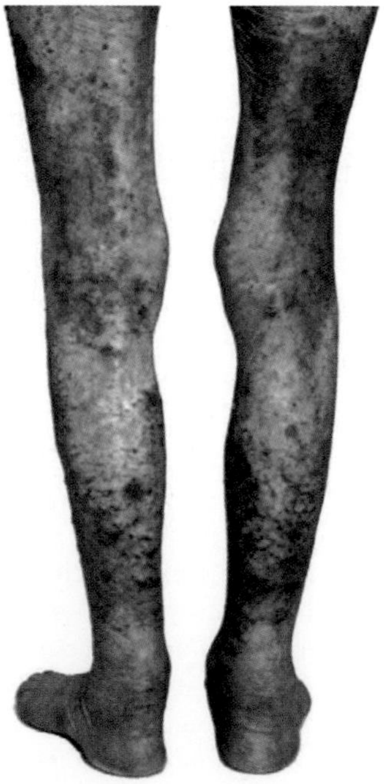

Figure 7.10 Necrolytic migratory erythema with indurated areas, blistering, crusting, and necrosis. Courtesy of Jabbour SA, Davidovici BB, Wolf R. (2006) Rare syndromes. *Clinics in Dermatology* **24**(4):299–316. Copyright (2010), with permission from Elsevier.

Neurofibromas

Definition
Neurofibromas are benign tumors composed of a mixture of Schwann cells, fibroblasts, and mast cells. There are four types:
- *Cutaneous*: The most common type.
- *Subcutaneous*: These present as firm, tender nodules along the course of peripheral nerves. They are described on palpation as feeling like a bag of worms.
- *Nodular plexiform*: These are complex clusters appearing along proximal nerve roots and major nerves. They are similar to subcutaneous neurofibromas. They can cause vertebral erosion with compression of the spinal cord.
- *Diffuse plexiform*: These usually involve multiple nerve fascicles, with serpiginous growth and significant vascularity, rendering complete surgical resection extremely difficult. Plexiform neurofibromas can also undergo malignant transformation to malignant peripheral nerve sheath tumors – neurofibrosarcomas or schwannomas.

Etiology
Neurofibromatosis type 1 (NF-1 or von Recklinghausen's disease) is a autosomal dominant genetic disorder: Genotype 17q11.2.

Neurofibromatosis type 2 (NF-2) is a autosomal dominant disorder predisposing to multiple neoplastic lesions: Genotype 22q12.2.

Neurofibromatosis types 3 and 4 have more numerous cutaneous neurofibromas.

Signs and symptoms

Cutaneous neurofibromas (Figs 7.11 & 7.12)
Cutaneous neurofibromas are soft, fleshy, benign tumors arising from cells in the peripheral nerve sheath. They can invaginate into the underlying dermal defect with light digital pressure (buttonholing). They begin to appear just before or during adolescence, tending to increase in size and number with age. They vary in number from just a few to several hundred, with the highest density over the trunk. Pruritis associated with accelerated growth of neurofibromas may be a prominent and distressing symptom.

Neurofibromatosis type 1 associations (Fig. 7.13)
Associated with NF-1 are:
- Peripheral nerve neurofibromas – associated with optic gliomas, meningiomas, and astrocytomas.
- Skin lesions – café-au-lait spots (see "Café-au-lait macules" section of this chapter), freckling in axilla or groin.
- Risk of developing rhabdomyosarcoma, pheochromocytoma, duodenal carcinoid, neurofibrosarcoma, and glioma.
- Lisch nodules on eyes; pseudoarthrosis tibia; macrocephaly.

Neurofibromatosis type 2 associations
Associated with NF-2 are:
- Central neurofibromas – associated with vestibular schwannoma, acoustic neuroma.
- Skin lesions – occasional café-au-lait spots (see "Café-au-lait macules" section of this chapter), pigmented plaques, subcutaneous peripheral nerve swellings, cutaneous schwannomas.
- Risk of developing glioma, meningioma, juvenile cataracts, and juvenile subcapsular lenticular opacities.

Neurofibromatosis types 3 and 4
Types 3 and 4 have more numerous cutaneous neurofibromas.

Diagnosis
Clinical features
Diagnosis of NF-1 requires at least two of the following clinical features (NIH Consensus Statement. *Arch Neurol Chicago* 1988;45:575):
- Six or more café-au-lait macules (CALMS) > 5 mm in prepubertal and > 15 mm in postpubertal individuals
- Two or more neurofibromas of any type or 1 plexiform neurofibroma.
- Freckling in the axillary or inguinal regions.
- Optic glioma.
- Two or more Lisch nodules (iris hamartomas).
- A distinctive bony lesion such as sphenoid dysplasia or thinning of the long bone cortex with or without pseudoarthrosis.
- A first-degree relative (parent, sibling, or offspring) with NF-1 based upon the above criteria.

Diagnosis may also require genetic tests for NF and skin biopsies.

Imaging tests
Imaging tests for organ-specific diseases may be needed:
- Computed tomography (CT) scan
- Magnetic resonance imaging (MRI)
- ^{123}I metaiodobenzylguanidine (MIBG) scintigraphy
- Octreoscan
- Fluorescein angiography

Laboratory findings
Endocrine investigations are needed for assessment of pheochromocytoma. Findings would include:
- Increased urinary metanephrine levels.
- Urinary or plasma catecholamines that may be elevated or may be normal.
- Clonidine-suppression test would find no suppression of metanephrine.

Treatment
Treatment would be surgical excision in selected cases.

Illustrations (Figs 7.11–7.13)

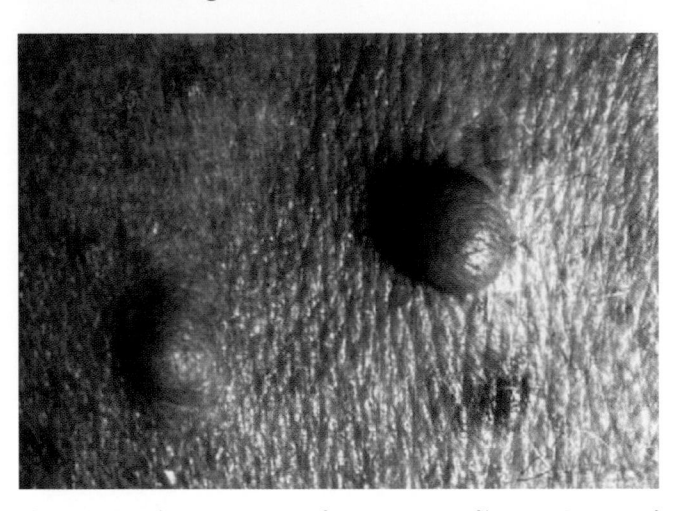

Figure 7.11 Classic appearance of cutaneous neurofibromas. Courtesy of Jabbour SA, Davidovici BB, Wolf R. (2006) Rare syndromes. *Clinics in Dermatology* **24**(4):299–316. Copyright (2010), with permission from Elsevier.

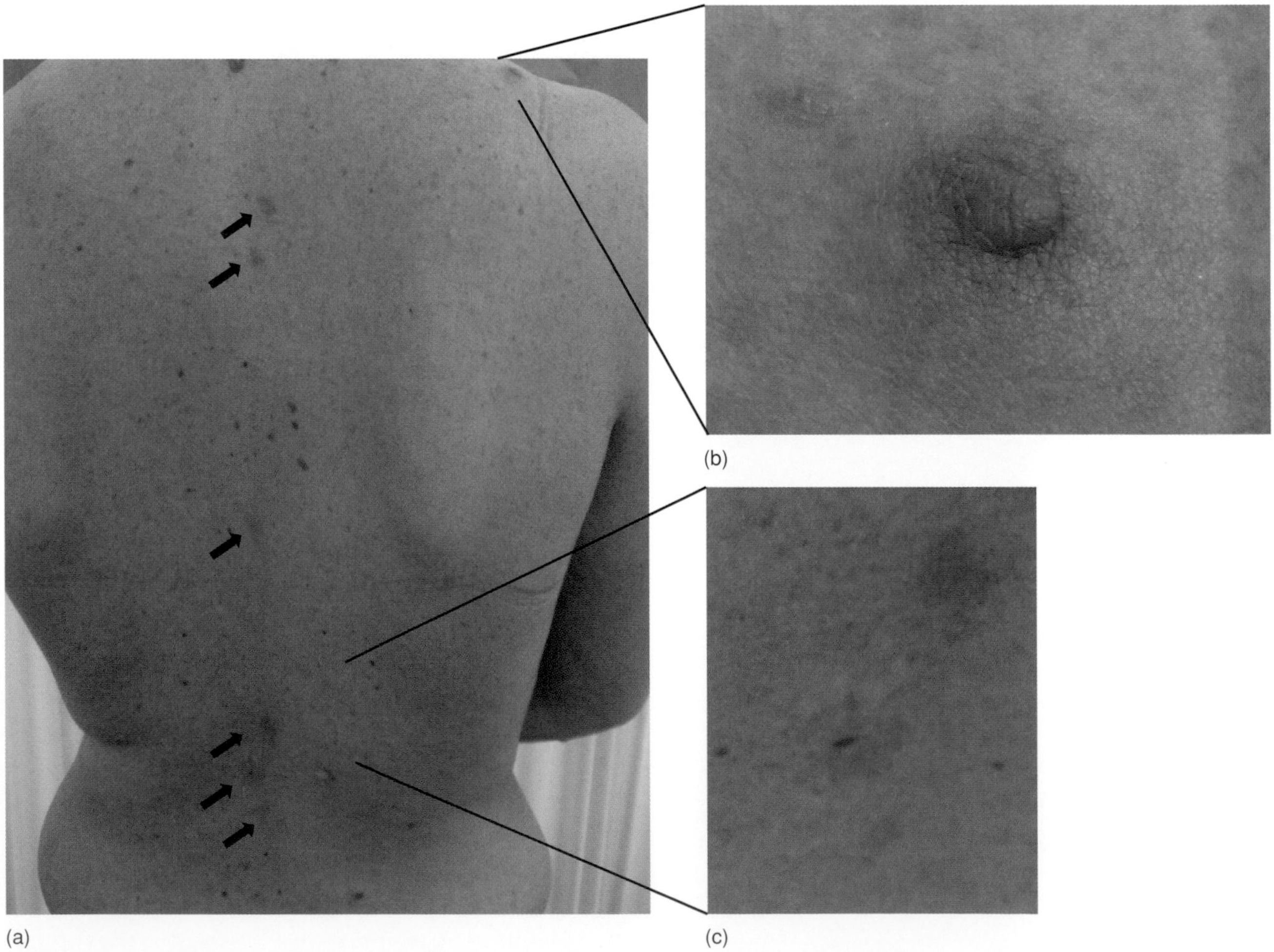

(a)

(b)

(c)

Figure 7.12 Cutaneous neurofibromas. A woman's back with cutaneous neurofibromas shown by arrows (a). Close-up of one of the cutaneous neurofibromas (b). Close up of three of six café-au-lait macules on the woman's back (c). There are 10 macules in all on the woman's body.

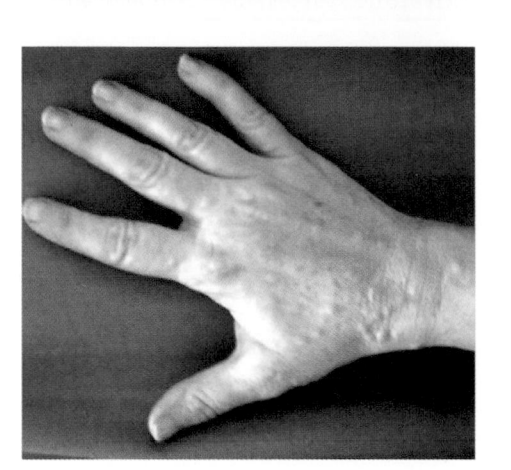

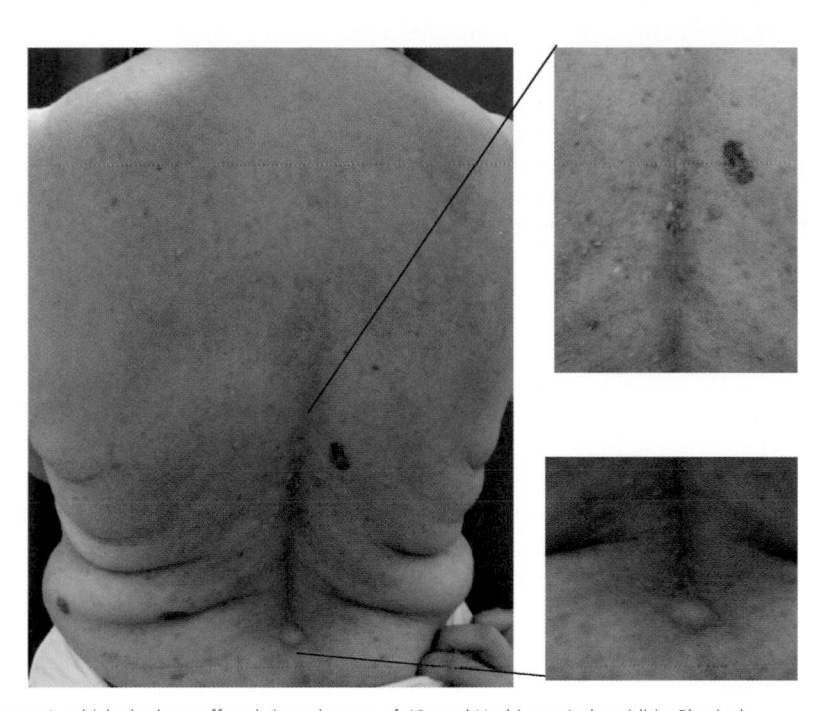

Figure 7.13 A 61-year-old woman with neurofibromatosis type 1, which she has suffered since the age of 40, and Hashimoto's thyroiditis. Physical examination shows skin lesions all over her body. There is no spinal involvement.

Vitiligo

Definition

Vitiligo is a multifactorial, noncontagious disorder causing patches of skin depigmentation that can spread over the entire body.

Etiology

The cause of vitiligo is unknown.

Depigmentation arises from the loss of functioning melanocytes. Impaired antioxidative defenses lead to the accumulation of reactive oxygen species (ROS), to which melanocytes are sensitive. Mitochondrial membrane lipid peroxidation may participate in ROS overproduction.

Oxidative stress and autoimmunity are involved in the pathogenesis, and genetic predisposition makes vitiligo melanocytes more susceptible to triggering factors.

Keratinocytes and melanocytes are affected and apoptosis, aging, or melanocytorrhagy are the ultimate effects of the complex deregulation.

Nonsegmental vitiligo (NSV) – the most common form – may run in families. It is usually progressive and may be associated with autoimmunity (autoimmune polyglandular syndrome [APS]).

Segmental vitiligo (SV) frequently stabilizes a few years after its onset. It may be associated with changes in the blood flow and nerve fibers of the affected skin.

Signs and symptoms

The patches are generally distributed over the body, often in a symmetrical manner. The first areas affected are usually around the eyes, anus, penis, genitals, and nails and, more generally, the face, neck, hands (Fig. 7.14), forearms, and groin. They appear as white patches with well-defined, possibly hyperpigmented margins; the skin is undamaged.

In areas covered by hair, there may be loss of hair and beard (Fig. 7.15).

Vitiligo patches are susceptible to sunburn and scalds.

Associations

See Table 7.1 (page 211) for diseases, disorders, and syndromes associated with vitiligo.

In addition, in primary autoimmune adrenal insufficiency vitiligo is associated with weakness, fatigue, orthostatic hypotension, anorexia, nausea, vomiting and diarrhea, loss of appetite and weight loss, hyperpigmentation, and adrenal calcification (Fig. 7.16).

Diagnosis

Diagnosis is made through clinical features, serologic testing for autoantibodies, function testing for the secretion of organ-specific hormones, and genetic testing for mutations in *AIRE* and *HLA-D* genes.

Imaging tests

Specific imaging tests are needed for organ-specific diseases in APS. In addition, in primary autoimmune adrenal insufficiency computed tomography (CT) scans or magnetic resonance imaging (MRI) are needed for confirmation of adrenal calcification.

Laboratory findings

Endocrine and autoimmune evaluations

For assessment of *humoral autoimmunity* the following tests are needed:
• *Autoantibodies against*: Steroidal cell autoantibodies (SCAb); parathyroid; pancreatic β-cell autoantibodies (AbGAD, AbIA2, AbICA); thyroid (AbTPO, AbTg); transglutaminase and gliadin, gastric parietal cell, melanocytes, tyrosinase, acetylcholine receptors.
• *Electrolyte abnormalities*: Hyponatremia, hyperkalemia, hypercalcemia.
• *Assessment of*: Pituitary–adrenal, pituitary–thyroid, and pituitary–gonadal axes, and parathyroid function.

For diagnosis of *adrenal insufficiency*, Synacthen and insulin tolerance testing with cortisol values < 18 μg/dL (500 nmol/L) are needed.

Treatment

Treatment consists of:
• Protection against the sun with clothing and/or sun cream (high SPF > 40, narrow-band UVB 311–12 nm).
• Immunomodulatory and photosensitizing drugs.
• The combined action of psoralen and UVA light (PUVA), surgical techniques, vitamin D analogs, and pseudocatalase leads to gradual repigmentation.

Illustrations (Figs 7.14–7.16)

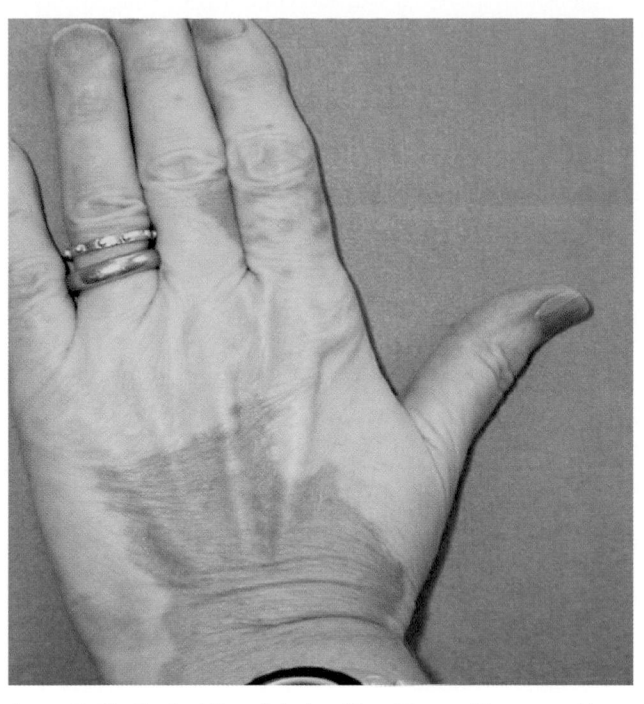

Figure 7.14 Classic vitiligo of the hand in a 63-year-old woman with pernicious anemia (adult onset), thyroditis, and Sjögren syndrome.

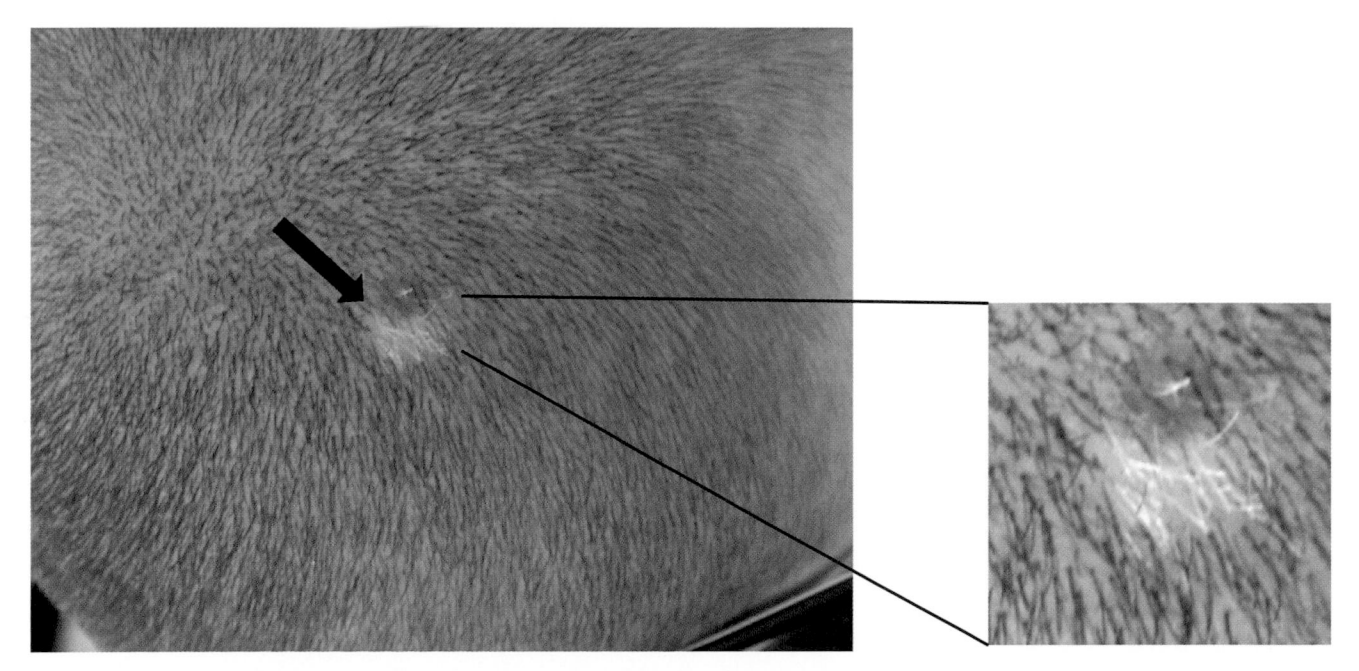

Figure 7.15 A rare case of piebaldism – vitiligo of the scalp associated with hair depigmentation.

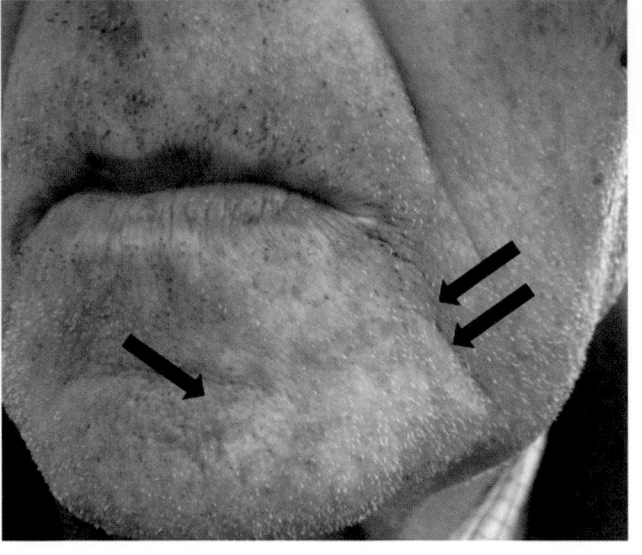
(a)

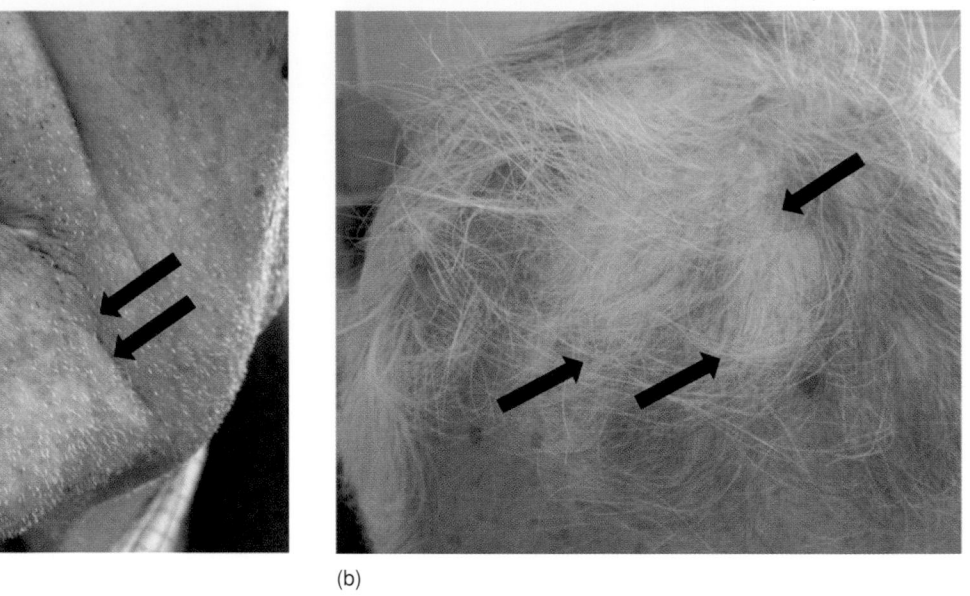
(b)

Figure 7.16 A 76-year-old man with primary late-onset autoimmune adrenal insufficiency and vitiligo of the chin and mouth (a) and scalp (b).

Index

Note: page numbers in *italics* refer to figures, those in **bold** refer to tables.

Imaging in Endocrinology, First Edition. Paolo Pozzilli, Andrea Lenzi, Bart L Clarke and William F Young Jr.
© 2014 John Wiley & Sons, Ltd. Published 2014 by John Wiley & Sons, Ltd.

Index

bone density
  familial high bone mass phenotype due to Lrp5
      mutation 138
  osteogenesis imperfecta 147
  skeletal fluorosis 141
bone disorders
  Charcot osteoarthropathy 81, *83*
  fibrous dysplasia 125–6, *127–8*
  hungry bones syndrome 104
  hyperparathyroid bone disease 122, *123, 124*
  metabolic 121, 129
  osteitis fibrosa cystica 103, *105,* 122, *123*
  osteogenesis imperfecta 145–8, *148–9*
  osteogenic sarcoma *116*
  osteolysis 152
  osteomyelitis *84*
  osteonecrosis of jaw 101, *102*
  osteopetrosis 129–31, *131*
  osteopoikilosis 134
  osteoporosis–pseudoglioma syndrome 150,
      150–1
  primary hyperparathyroidism 103
  progressive diaphyseal dysplasia 135, *136*
  sclerosing 129–42
  skeletal fluorosis 141, *142*
  see also osteomalacia; osteoporosis; osteosclerosis
bone formation
  chronic kidney disease 121
  osteomalacia 117
  Paget's disease 113, 114
  progressive diaphyseal dysplasia 135
  sclerosing bone disorders 129
bone pain
  Erdheim–Chester disease 139
  fibrous dysplasia 125–6
  osteomalacia 118
  Paget's disease 113
bone resorption
  Paget's disease 113
  sclerosing bone disorders 129
BRCA1 and *BRCA2* genes 181
breast cancer, adrenal gland metastases from 74,
  75
brittle bone disease *see* osteogenesis imperfecta
bromocriptine 27, 35
brown tumors, primary hyperparathyroidism 103,
  106

cabergoline 35
café-au-lait spots (macules) 215–16, 220, *221*
  distribution 215, *216*
  fibrous dysplasia 125, *127*
  pheochromocytoma 65, *66*
calcinosis, tumoral 143–4, *144–5*
calcitonin 114
calcitriol 109, 110
  chronic kidney disease 122–3
  pseudohypoparathyroidism 112
calcium
  deficiency in osteomalacia 117
  intake 104
  see also hypercalcemia; hypocalcemia
calcium gluconate 110

calcium supplementation
  chronic kidney disease 123
  hypoparathyroidism 109, 110
  osteomalacia 119
  pseudohypoparathyroidism 112
Camurati–Engelmann disease *see* progressive
      diaphyseal dysplasia
carbergoline 27
carcinoid tumor, metastatic *46*
cardiovascular disease
  chronic kidney disease 121
  diabetes mellitus 76–7, *77–9*
Carney complex 52, *53*
  café-au-lait macules 215
  ovarian cysts 188
carotid body tumor 68, *70*
catecholamine-secreting paraganglioma 65, 68,
  69–71
cathepsin K gene mutations 132
cerebrovascular disease 77
Charcot osteoarthropathy 81, *83*
children
  craniopharyngioma 22
  gigantism 25
  hypophosphatasia 153
  infantile osteopetrosis 129, 130
  melorheostosis 134
  progressive diaphyseal dysplasia 135
  pycnodysostosis 132
cholesterol 76, 77
chondrocalcinosis 153
chronic autoimmune thyroiditis *see* Hashimoto's
      thyroiditis
chronic kidney disease (CKD) 121–3, *123–4*
  fractures 122, *123*
  hyperparathyroid bone disease 122, *123,
      124*
  osteoporosis 123
  rugger-jersey spine *123*
  stages 121
  tumoral calcinosis 143
  vascular calcification 122
chronic kidney disease–metabolic bone disease
      (CKD–MBD) 122
Chvostek's sign 109
cinacalcet 104, 123
codfish vertebrae 118, *119*
collagen disorders
  diabetes mellitus 80, *81*
  mutations in osteogenesis imperfecta 147
congenital adrenal hyperplasia (CAH) 55–6,
      57
  acne 209, *210*
  11β-hydroxylase deficiency 55, 56
  17α-hydroxylase deficiency 55, 56
  21-hydroxylase deficiency 55, 56, *57*
  3β-hydroxysteroid dehydrogenase deficiency
      55, 56
  lipoid 55, *56*
connective tissue defect, osteogenesis imperfecta
      145, 146
coronary artery stenosis *79*
coronary heart disease 77, *78, 79*

corpus luteum cysts 188, 189
corticotroph adenoma of pituitary 31, *32*
corticotropin (ACTH)
  Cushing syndrome 29, 52
  Nelson syndrome 31
  pituitary carcinoma 35, *36*
corticotropin-secreting pituitary tumor 29, *30*
cortisol
  adrenal venous sampling 61
  Cushing syndrome 29, 52
cosyntropin 61, **62**, 63
cranial sutures, pycnodysostosis 132
craniofacial bones, fibrous dysplasia 126, *128*
craniopharyngioma 22, *23*
  cystic fluid 22, *23*
  magnetic resonance imaging 22, *23*
  suprasellar 22, *23*
craniosynostosis, acanthosis nigricans 206
Crouzon syndrome 206
cryptorchidism 156, 163, *164–5*
  definition 163
  infertility 173
Cushing syndrome 29, 30, *36*
  acne 209
  adrenal-dependent 52, *52–4*
  adrenocortical carcinoma 50, *51*
  imaging 29, *30*
  pituitary-dependent 31
  signs/symptoms 52
  subclinical 47–8
  treatment 31, 52
cutaneous lichen amyloidosis 217
cutaneous neuromas 217, *218*
CYP17A1 gene mutations 55

de Quervain's thyroiditis *see* subacute thyroiditis
denosumab 101
dermoid cysts 188, 189, *193*
dexamethasone suppression test 198, *199*
diabetes insipidus 33
  pituitary metastases 45
diabetes mellitus 76–94
  cardiovascular disease 76–7, *77–9*
  collagen disorders 80, *81*
  skin diseases 80, *80–1*
  type 1 in primary adrenal failure 63
diabetic dermopathy 80
diabetic foot 81–2, *82–5*
  angiography 82, *85*
  angioplasty 82, *86*
  blood vessel damage 81
  bone reabsorption 81, *83*
  Charcot osteoarthropathy 81, *83*
  clinical stages 82
  deformation 81
  femoral artery stenosis *85*
  gangrene 82, *84, 86*
  nervous system damage 81
  neuropathic foot 81, *82–3*
  osteomyelitis *84*
  popliteal artery stenosis 82, *84*
  ulcers 81, 82, *83, 84, 86*
  vascular foot 81